IS THIS YOUR CHILD'S WORLD?

ALSO BY DORIS J. RAPP, M.D.

Is This Your Child?

IS THIS YOUR CHILD'S WORLD?

*How You Can Fix the Schools and
Homes That Are Making Your
Children Sick*

Doris J. Rapp

M.D., FAEM, FAAP, FAAA
Clinical Assistant Professor of Pediatrics at the State
University of New York at Buffalo
Board Certified in Environmental Medicine, Pediatrics,
and Pediatric Allergy

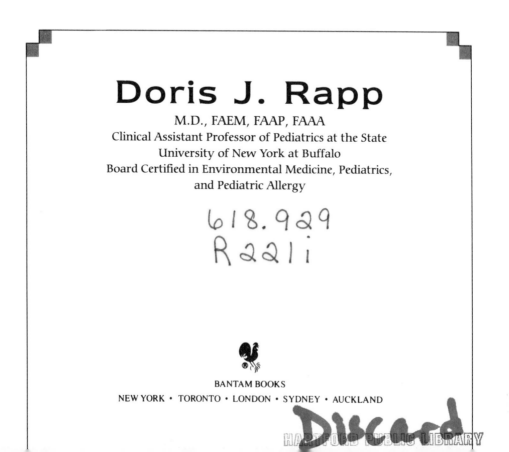

BANTAM BOOKS
NEW YORK · TORONTO · LONDON · SYDNEY · AUCKLAND

IS THIS YOUR CHILD'S WORLD?

A Bantam Book / October 1996

Cover art copyright © 1996 by Tom Tafuri Graphic Design
Book design by Stanley S. Drate / Folio Graphics Co. Inc.

Library of Congress Cataloging-in-Publication Data

Rapp, Doris J.
    Is this your child's world? : how you can fix the schools and homes
that are making your children sick / Doris J. Rapp,
        p.   cm.
    Includes bibliographical references and index.
    ISBN 0-553-10513-2
    1. Environmentally induced diseases in children—United States.
    2. Environmentally induced diseases—United States.   3. Sick
building syndrome—United States.   4. School buildings—
Environmental aspects—United States.   5. School buildings—Health
aspects—United States.   6. School children—Health and hygiene—
United States.   I. Title.
RJ383.R37   1996
618.92'98—dc20   96-9398
                                                                    CIP

Published simultaneously in the United States and Canada

Bantam Books are published by Bantam Books, a division of
Bantam Doubleday Dell Publishing Group, Inc. Its trademark,
consisting of the words "Bantam Books" and the portrayal of a
rooster, is Registered in U.S. Patent and Trademark Office and in
other countries. Marca Registrada. Bantam Books, 1540 Broadway,
New York, New York 10036.

PRINTED IN THE UNITED STATES OF AMERICA

FFG   10   9   8   7   6   5   4   3   2   1

To the many students and teachers who have not only so generously shared their personal health problems but also allowed me to videotape their reactions during allergy testing. A better understanding of their illnesses will help others who have had similar experiences so they too can recognize that they are truly ill and can be helped. It is hoped that their experiences will encourage others to recognize the urgent need for more effective, better, easier, less expensive, and practical ways to cope with environmental illness.

To Lou, Teddy, and Katie, who were all neglected, much too often and too long, so this book could be written.

CONTENTS

PART I

EVALUATING THE PROBLEM AND FINDING THE CAUSE

PART II

WHAT YOU CAN DO ABOUT A SICK SCHOOL

PART **VI**

SOME FINAL CONSIDERATIONS

■

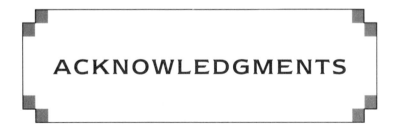

ACKNOWLEDGMENTS

Wendy McCurdy and **Richard Trubo,** for their advice and guidance in the final rush editing and extensive revisions so this book would not have to wait another year before being born.

Linda Hankins, my superlative personal secretary. This book truly could not have been written without her most exceptional ability and knowledge. If fate had not intervened, the book would have been completed much earlier. She and her dedicated team, Sally Ann Czermerys, Nancy Drost, and Martha Baines all helped to patiently check and recheck this manuscript.

Pat Schlifke, my office manager, who so ably and consistently was there to help finalize this book. She worked above and beyond in every way to help accomplish what needed to be done.

Christine Hartnett, P.A., Karen Kochinski, P.A., and **Joann Brown, R.N.,** who so generously helped to reread the manuscript and recheck the resources.

Cindy Rose and **Ralph Melillo** who rechecked resource information, repeatedly.

Joseph Miller, M.D., Mobile, AL, the magnificent and exceedingly wise teacher and caring physician who so generously shared his knowledge about environmental medicine.

George Shambaugh, M.D., Chicago, IL, a most generous ENT authority who suggested that Phil Donahue ask me, rather than him, to be on his talk show—a turning point in my life and career.

William Rea, M.D., Dallas, TX, who is the world's authority on chemical sensitivities. No one has given so much of himself, in so many ways, to help people with these problems. His books about chemical sensitivities are a must for all up-to-date physicians.

Rosalind Anderson, Ph.D., West Hartford, VT, whose exceptional bioassay techniques with mice have helped to document the many dangers in everyday household products.

Kalpana Patel, M.D., Buffalo, NY, a caring colleague and friend whose knowledge of environmental medicine is exceptional.

John Laseter, Ph.D., Richardson, TX, who so generously shared his extensive biochemical expertise in measuring and documenting chemical pollution all over the world.

Theodore Simon, M.D., Dallas, TX, and **Thomas J. Callender, M.D.,** Lafayette, LA, whose advanced radiographic imaging techniques have helped to demonstrate and objectively document brain changes caused by small exposures of chemicals.

Mary Lamielle, Voorhees, NJ, and **Irene R. Wilkenfeld,** Granger, IN, whose special educational programs and information have informed so many about the significance of the school environment for health and learning.

Mark Jackson and **Russell Olinsky,** engineers, who helped provide and review the technical material on ventilation and indoor air quality.

To the videographers, especially **David Collins,** who so diligently helped to videotape, edit, and catalog the reactions of many children and teachers to allergy testing.

To all the students and teachers described in this book who generously allowed me not only to share their private histories but to visually demonstrate their personal responses during challenge testing in videotapes produced by the Practical Allergy Research Foundation (PARF). We owe them a tremendous amount of gratitude for helping the many others who might have been similarly affected by detrimental exposures within a school or home.

To **John Pangborn, Ph.D., Billie Sahley, Ph.D., Philip Broughton, M.D., Susan Busse, M.D., Alexander Bralley, Ph.D., Nancy Didriksen, Ph.D., John Boyles, M.D., Jonathan Wright, M.D., Douglas Seba, Ph.D., James Neubrander, M.D., Albert Donnet, Ph.D., Natalie Golos, John Milder, Irene Wilkenfeld,** and others for their generous help and specialized advice on various aspects of this book.

PREFACE

Is Your School Environmentally Sick?

Every single day students and teachers are exposed to environmentally unsafe schools and homes that can compromise their overall health and mental capabilities. Throughout the United States the problem has become so serious—sometimes even devastating—that our abundance of sophisticated modern drugs can no longer relieve their symptoms. Special-education teachers are unable to effectively cope with the soaring number of children diagnosed with hyperactivity or other behavior and learning difficulties in school.

As you read this book, you'll find much of the problem lies in America's school buildings. Many schools built in the 1970s were designed to last only twenty to thirty years. No wonder a February 1995 U.S. government report admitted that approximately 25,000 or one-third of all schools (which educate about 14 million children) now need extensive repair and/or replacement. These figures reflect only the significant problems related to lead, asbestos, radon, underground storage tanks, plumbing, sewage, termites, ventilation, and structural inadequacies. They do not even consider the additional, and at times, more significant role of dust, molds, chemicals, foods, and germs.

▪ THE DILEMMA OF CHILDREN AND TEACHERS

More and more children and teachers feel unwell day after day at school and do not understand why. Nor do they understand why they feel better within a few hours of arriving home. The children are confused and upset; the teachers are bewildered because children learn very well and behave appropriately one day but not the next. Is this due to an emotional problem or could it be related to how they teach?

Parents are equally perplexed because their children seem unable to remember things as well as they once did, or to learn at a level comparable to their natural ability. At certain times or in specific rooms, these youngsters cannot think clearly or recall things they know. Sometimes these changes are apparent only at home and not at school.

In addition, there are the inexplicable mood and behavior changes that students (and teachers) may experience. Why do they suddenly become upset or angry, or cry more easily than usual, but only when they are either at school or at home? Why do their actions become progressively more inappropriate from Monday to Friday afternoon but improve by Sunday night? When this happens to adults, they're embarrassed and worry that someone might notice; they repeatedly ask themselves, what could possibly be wrong?

■ HOW DO OTHERS REACT?

When children and adults experience perplexing illnesses due to allergies or toxic reactions, they suffer not only from the environmental contact but also from psychological stress. Too often, they are not believed when they tell others how they feel, and they do not know where to turn for help. Too often, responsible, loving parents wonder what they have done wrong, while their equally perplexed children are often frightened and justifiably discouraged because they believe they are "bad." To make matters worse, no one seems able to explain what is going on. When parents finally find treatment that sets their child's health and life back on course, all too often the family's insurance company refuses to pay for it.

Sometimes a medical evaluation can end by instilling a feeling of personal inadequacy or failure in a child, or even worse, with an accusation of malingering. Some children or adults are told simply that "it is all in your head" or that they must "learn to live with it."

However, as you'll learn in this book, our environment can trigger serious physical, neurological, and psychological problems. Environmental illness can be every bit as real as that caused by germs. The symptoms of allergic and chemically induced sicknesses extend far beyond those typical of asthma, hay fever, intestinal, and skin problems. Increased fatigue, moodiness, depression, irritability, hyperactivity, aggression, and an inability to focus and remember can all be part of the big, perplexing picture.

The frustrating and often debilitating diseases caused by exposures to chemicals and natural allergens—such as dust, molds, and pollen—are not confined to schools. Our other surroundings, including homes, workplaces, and even the outdoors, can be equally problematic. No place, however, is more critically important to the continued vitality of our society than our schools, which are largely responsible for the competence and welfare of coming generations.

■ THE CHALLENGE

Environmental illnesses are taking a toll upon our children day by day. Whether slowly or quickly, they can progressively harm any part of the human body—doing damage that can last for years or even a lifetime. Our youngsters are expected to learn not only in very old school buildings but newer well-insulated, heat-efficient, highly chemicalized buildings with windows that allow the entrance of light but not air.

So our current challenge is much more than increased dust and molds; these factors can be important, but they have been around for a long time. The major new kid on the block is the seventy thousand chemicals that presently permeate what we eat, breathe, touch, and smell. We can no longer wait for our government to protect us. *We have to make the connection between cause and effect so we can create a personal pocket of protection for our children, families, and friends, to help ensure America's future.*

■ THE ANSWER

As parents, educators, and physicians, we can tip the scales in favor of our children's health. How? We can help them by avoiding unnecessary exposures to chemicals, dust, molds, pollen, and known problem or pesticide-containing foods. No, we don't have to live in a glass house atop a windy mountain—but we should clean with safer products and improve our personal environment as much as possible. This book provides the insight you will need to cope with schools that are not up to par environmentally. The same recommendations are also applicable in the home (an environment that is infinitely easier to control). For the vast majority of children, teachers, and families, such changes do not need to be extensive or expensive.

In terms of diagnosing environmental illness, newer specific provocation/neutralization techniques can not only pinpoint the causes but provide fast and effective relief of the symptoms. Still other faster and better ways to deal with these problems are promised, but they need much more critical evaluation before they can be seriously discussed. For now, the ultimate key to better health is *prevention*. To accomplish it, everyone needs to develop an increased awareness of what can cause ill health, inappropriate behavior, and an inability to learn.

■ WHAT THIS BOOK CAN DO

I hope that this book will sound a wake-up call, leading to a serious attempt to curtail the spread of this new, critical, universal problem. Environmental illnesses, especially those due to the many unsuspected chemicals present in our modern world, are capable of causing an immense variety of health problems. They are impairing the health, well-being, and potential of many children and adults. *We urgently need to address these issues by recognizing the causes and removing them, and by more quickly and effectively treating the individuals who have already lost their health and learning ability.* We must do this immediately, for the sake of present and future generations. We must stem the present focus on drug-oriented medicine. A desire for ever-increasing economic reward has engulfed nearly every vestige of old-fashioned common sense, foresight, and compassion. We need to return to the sensible priorities of yesterday.

I am hopeful that the information in this book will motivate the movers in society to take substantive action that will produce tangible results. The more we learn and the more effectively we apply what we know, the more secure everyone's future will be.

Some, of course, will vigorously disagree with information in these pages. Frankly, that is fine. Let them try to prove their point of view. Through dialogue we can eventually confirm or negate what this book discusses. No progress can be made if everything is done exactly as it has always been done, but if we work together, we can find more meaningful answers for tomorrow.

■ HOW I BECAME AN ENVIRONMENTAL MEDICAL PHYSICIAN

Strange as it may be, although my parents had no college education, I was positive at the age of four that I was destined to become a physician. After earning both a bachelor's degree, magna cum laude, and a master's degree at the University of Buffalo, I entered medical college at New York University in 1951, then returned to Buffalo to study pediatrics for three years, followed by training and research in allergy and immunology for another two years.

I certainly wasn't always a believer in environmental medicine, but after twenty years of traditional pediatric allergy practice, I attended a food allergy conference in 1975. It not only changed my practice of medicine; it changed my life. I realized that for two decades I had missed the diagnosis of food allergy repeatedly. At this conference I learned how diets could be conducted in such a way that they would detect and treat food sensitivities, and for the first time I became aware of the immense scope of symptoms that foods can cause. I was introduced to a more precise and better way to test for food and other allergies. This technique is called provocation/neutralization. It involves testing different concentrations of each possible allergenic item separately, then watching to see its effect. Initially, I felt an immense skepticism about this entire approach. It was inconceivable to me that I had not been taught these concepts in my previous medical training if they were truly valid. Afterward, in an attempt to disprove what I had heard, I tried what I had learned at the conference. When I found that these new ideas were indeed incredibly helpful, I felt like a mouse in a cheese factory. Never before had I believed that medicine could be so rewarding and exciting for both my patients and myself!

In time I found that many well-qualified doctors remained highly skeptical, and would not listen or even look at the clinical histories of success, my presentations at medical conferences, and my published research. That was when I decided that the best and fastest way to help desperate parents was to write books and

---

WHAT YOU'LL LEARN IN THIS BOOK

This book will increase your awareness by explaining:

- *How to anticipate which children and adults may be most prone to develop an environmental illness.*

- *How to recognize that someone may be ill by noticing changes in how they look, act, behave, write, draw, and learn.*

- *How to recognize whether an illness is related to inside or outside environmental factors, and how to determine which complaints may be partially or entirely due to some other health or behavioral problem.*

- *How to pinpoint the most likely school- or home-related causes of learning, behavior, or health problems.*

- *How to decide who should take the initiative to find appropriate solutions.*

- *How to prioritize your options, so you know what should be done first, and when and why.*

- *How to find physicians who have special expertise in environmental illness.*

- *How to find qualified scientific investigational teams to evaluate potentially unsafe buildings.*

- *How to locate information and resources to resolve the problems of sick buildings.*

- *How to encourage school administrators, legislators, and builders to become more aware of environmental illness and to implement practical, cost-effective changes.*

- *How to use these same guidelines to improve your home and work environment.*

- *How to find lawyers who have the interest and experience to help those with environmental illnesses.*

---

even to speak on television about these newer methods. The videos that we made at our center vividly and accurately demonstrated and documented what happened to our patients who took this knowledge and sharing many steps further. The skeptics insisted that the videotaped children were accomplished actors. They sincerely believed if a young child seemed hyperactive from eating food or from an allergy skin test, he or she was just acting out or needed a nap. To help convince them, I conducted and published clinical scientific studies and presented evidence at conferences that showed changes in the blood and the brains of some of the children who were reacting. We continued to videotape as many of the children's responses as possible so that others could see that our magnificent human bodies can respond in a highly individualized manner, in minutes, to a drop of an allergy extract or a whiff of a chemical. It is most disappointing that twenty years later, many academic and clinical medical colleagues continue to refuse to look at the evidence, read the literature, observe, learn, and then try P/N allergy testing. Those who do this, very frequently incorporate Environmental Medicine (EI) into their practice.

The negativity of some physicians does not alter what is happening. There is no doubt that dietary adjustments, P/N or SET allergy extract treatment, changes made in homes, chemical avoidance, and improved nutrition can be immensely helpful for many children. These methods, however, are time-consuming, expensive, and lifestyle-altering, particularly when continued medical supervision and repeated allergy testing and treatment are necessary. For that reason I have currently stopped my usual practice of environmental medicine and am investigating other methods that may prove to be more helpful and much less expensive. It is my sincere desire to start a large education and treatment center where we can apply the methods that have already been so helpful. In addition there is a need to more fully investigate other methods that have been poorly documented in spite of repeated anecdotal reports of success. Many parents who have shared their genuine despair with me in my practice and their multitude of letters and phone calls indicate an urgent and desperate need of immediate help. If this book is successful and the center becomes a reality, it should be possible to help not only children and their parents, but also openminded educators, physicians, psychologists, and dieticians.

■ GETTING STARTED

This book contains absolutely everything I can think of that might help you to recognize what is interfering with your child's or your own well-being and then eliminate it. I have tried to anticipate your needs and questions and provide exact references and resources, including addresses and phone numbers. Several sections will provide more details than you want or need but which others might find essential. Read only the parts that are pertinent to your child's (or your own) well-being.

I have not written this book to stir up still more anger and frustration in a world that is already overburdened with both. Rather, I want it to provide meaningful, practical answers for the questions most commonly asked, and provide sensible directions for those who are affected and concerned. Whenever possible, the general therapeutic approach I have followed throughout is:

■ What solutions are fast, safe, easy, and inexpensive?
■ What solutions are better but more expensive?
■ What solutions are best but expensive?

The trajectory of our fast-paced, modern society calls for some immediate critical midcourse corrections. As an Indian chief once said, "Where man walks, the earth hurts." Now the children also hurt. We can no longer tolerate what is happening. The youngsters of today are America's future.

Doris J. Rapp, M.D.

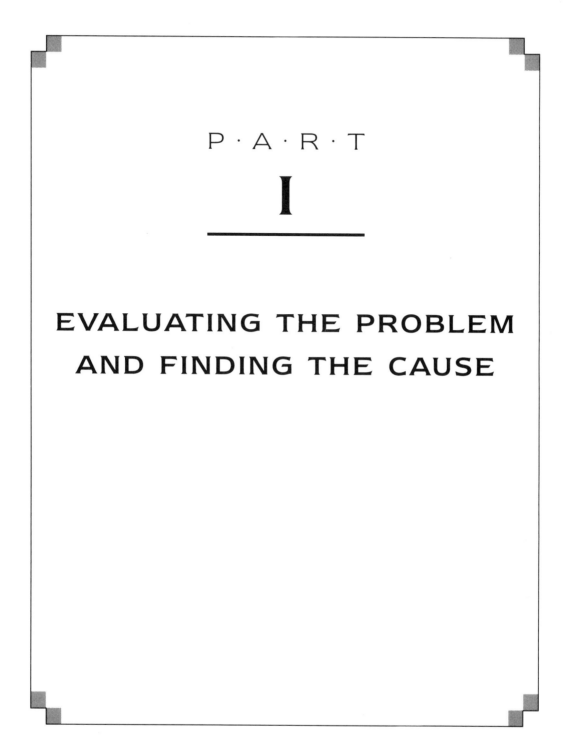

P·A·R·T

I

EVALUATING THE PROBLEM AND FINDING THE CAUSE

INTRODUCTION
FOR PART I

In the next five chapters, we'll evaluate how to find solutions to your child's problem. Millions of children enter their classrooms in all parts of our country each morning, and although many are being exposed to all kinds of substances, only a few become sick. The children who have these environmental illnesses tend to be poorly understood by educators, physicians, and parents. Their complaints are often not recognized or misdiagnosed, frequently leading to years of physical or emotional illnesses and learning problems.

Chapters 1 through 5 are designed to guide you toward helping your child—specifically, by determining whether he or she actually has an EI and what may be causing it. You'll be shown clearly how to do your own detective work. Thousands of concerned parents have used these techniques and discovered the basis of their child's—or their own—illness. In this process, they have become experts in recognizing environmental illness and ultimately informed, effective advocates for their children. Some children have suffered from unrecognized EI for years, until this kind of parental intervention occurred.

A PLAN OF ACTION

Here's a quick overview of what you'll find detailed in the next few chapters:

- In Chapters 1 and 2, you'll get a sense of the most common symptoms experienced by children and teachers in "sick schools." These complaints typically include some combination of nasal congestion, fatigue, aching muscles, blurred vision, burning skin, and abdominal discomfort, as well as a variety of learning or behavior difficulties. If the source of these problems is not properly identified and eliminated, the symptoms can progress to such an incapacitating level that a few youngsters will have to stay away from school and rely on home teaching for their education. You need to become familiar with how to recognize these school-related symptoms, and how they can change in time if no one suspects what's really wrong.

■ Chapter 3 is one of the key chapters in this entire book. It introduces and explains the concept of the "Big Five"—a systematic way to pinpoint the specific causes of an EI. It will explain exactly how you can evaluate the following five key variables. These include a simple check of your child's:

1. Symptoms, behavior, and memory
2. Appearance
3. Writing and drawing
4. Breathing
5. Pulse

I'll explain how you can analyze these characteristics, evaluating each of them in your child both before and after eating, exposure to chemicals, and activity inside and outside both your home and your youngster's school. The "Big Five" can help you pinpoint the exact location or contact that is causing your youngster to be ill or to have learning difficulties. You'll be aided in this process by a system of organized record-keeping that can help you easily recognize cause-and-effect relationships. I'll also introduce you to some dietary adjustments you can make, which often provide answers in three to seven days. With this fast, simple approach, you can often resolve problems that may have disrupted the life of your child—and sometimes your entire family—for years.

■ In Chapters 4 and 5, your own investigative skills will become more sharply honed. You'll look for and identify specific changes in your child's appearance and speech that indicate an EI. Many environmentally ill youngsters, for example, have a characteristic look, a rapid way of speaking, or even unusual sounds such as clucking or barking. They can exhibit sleepiness, hyperactivity, aggression, or vulgarity.

Your child may also demonstrate sudden and characteristic handwriting and drawing changes. You'll find plenty of examples of how chemicals and other exposures can keep youngsters from writing properly. This in turn can certainly interfere with their ability to learn and progress normally in school.

The well-being of your child is too important to delay or ignore the opportunity to find out why he or she doesn't feel or act right. The answers are readily available if someone will take the time to learn what to do and exactly how to do it. Read and follow the guidelines in these next few chapters carefully, and you will have taken a giant step toward helping your youngster regain and maintain a better quality of health and a higher level of learning.

1 ⟨ Which Students and Teachers Are Affected?

Our present environment is causing a growing number of children to routinely feel unwell. If you are a teacher, there may be many children in your own school who, too, are hyperactive or fatigued, or who misbehave. In addition, an expanding number do not feel well enough to attend school. Some claim they have trouble thinking clearly at school; others appear to have similar complaints predominantly at home.

These children may be suffering from an environmental illness caused by something in their school or home surroundings. Too often, parents and teachers suspect other medical or emotional factors underlie their child's illness, leaving the real cause undiagnosed and the illness improperly managed.

Every parent owes it to his or her child to ask: Is my youngster the problem, or is it something in the environment?

■ WHAT IS ENVIRONMENTAL ILLNESS?

Environmental illness (EI) is a name for an assortment of medical problems that can affect almost any area of the body (see Table 1.1). In addition to typical allergy symptoms such as asthma, hay fever, and itchy skin, those who have EI tend to intermittently or constantly have some combination of the following health problems: headaches, inordinate fatigue, hyperactivity, pain in muscles, legs, or joints, persistent bowel problems, embarrassing bad breath, constant congestion, irritating twitches, and/or a wide range of behavioral and emotional problems ranging from leg-wiggling to depression.

One of the most distressing problems caused by EI is what is called "brain allergies" or "brain fog." People with this problem sometimes or frequently cannot think clearly, remember or learn at a level comparable with their innate ability.

Many of the subtle, less obvious forms of environmental allergic illness

TABLE 1.1

Symptoms of Environmental Illness

Nose	Year-round or seasonal stuffiness, watery nose, sneezing, nose-rubbing
Ears	Repeated fluid formation behind eardrums, ringing in ears, dizziness
Face	Pallor, dark eye circles, puffiness below eyes
Glands	Tender, swollen lymph nodes in neck
Chest	Congestion or asthma
Aches	"Growing pains" or aches in the head, back, neck, muscles or joints that is unrelated to exercise
Intestines	Bellyaches, nausea, vomiting, bloating, bad breath, gas, belching, diarrhea, constipation, or excessive appetite
Bladder	Accidents in the daytime or at night, need to rush to urinate, burning or pain with urination, excessive thirst
Skin	Itchy rashes, hives, excessive perspiration, night sweats, cold hands and feet

are not recognized or even suspected by parents, educators, and health providers.

■ WHAT CAUSES EI?

Many factors in schools and homes contribute to EI. The ones we usually hear about are asbestos, lead, and radon. But environmental illnesses typically also involve some form of poor air quality, particularly due to excessive dust or molds, or to chemical pollution in or around a building. Other frequently unsuspected factors are foods and beverages and seasonal pollen. Any of these factors, whether alone or in combination, can unquestionably trigger serious health, behavior, and academic problems.

It is ironic that although we send our children to school to learn, environmental factors in some schools obstruct their ability to do exactly that. We must recognize and eliminate the causes of EI, so we can prevent these health and learning problems.

■ HOW CRITICAL IS THE PROBLEM?

In our environmentally conscious society, damage caused by chemicals has become a major concern. Chemicals and other environmental factors are causing enormous havoc and distress, in the lives of some children. The long-term consequences can be catastrophic. The American Lung Association estimates that 3.7 million American children presently have asthma; this figure represents an increase of 200 percent in the past twenty years. This is related, in part, to environmental factors.[1] This is alarming, but the situation is threatening to jump off the scale, according to a report from a special legislative committee of the Commonwealth of Massachusetts. This report estimates that fully 50 percent of current health problems are caused by a deteriorated indoor air quality. The cost is thought to be more than $100 billion a year.[2] We must all ask how large a role the environment plays in the everyday health problems of our children and ourselves. Is it worth it to correct this type of problem?

■ WHAT ARE ITS EFFECTS?

Let's look at another serious problem and the role that EI may play in it. In 1993, more than two million schoolchildren were receiving activity-modifying drugs, such as Ritalin, so they could sit still long enough to learn.[3] In 1995, the figure doubled to approximately four million. By the year 2000, the projected number can soar as high as eight million. We need to be seriously concerned about the rapidly expanding number of children who are being treated for hyperactivity with Class 2 narcotics, especially if faster, easier, safer treatments are available.

But an even more important consideration is *why* such drugs are thought to be needed in the first place. What are we doing wrong? Any veteran teacher will tell you that the increase in Ritalin is not solely due to an increased awareness of hyperactivity. Think back to when you were in school. Do you recall that hyperactivity was rampant among your classmates?

In one survey of Arizona undergraduates, 66 percent said they became ill after they were exposed to pesticides, automobile exhaust, paint, new carpets, or perfume. Fifteen percent claimed they became ill from four of these five common substances listed in the survey.[4]

Many children and adults suffer daily consequences from routine exposure to dust, molds, foods, and chemicals. It is really not difficult for parents to eliminate the problem substances from their homes, but we must strongly urge our school systems to make similar corrections. As you will see, it is often easy to pinpoint the problem, but remediation can be costly. Yet the costs of not correcting these problems may be far higher, and related to much more than money.

Our schools, in fact, should take the lead in identifying, treating, and preventing environmental illness. We can do the most good in the shortest period of time by making schools our top priority, and in this book, you'll learn what needs to be done and how to do it. By increasing their own awareness and knowledge, parents and teachers can do much to eliminate environmental factors that potentially may harm the health of everyone. About 14 million students are trying to learn in approximately 25,000 schools that are in dire need of extensive repair or replacement.[5] Improving these learning environments deserves our prompt attention.

■ WHO IS MOST LIKELY TO BE AFFECTED?

An estimated 20 percent of all Americans spends time in a school building every day, and many of them are particularly at risk because they are prone to allergies.[6] At least 15 to 20 percent of the population has typical allergies and allergic relatives. In my personal experience, these individuals are often the first to be adversely affected by their environment because they already have typical hay fever, asthma, eczema, or hives. Some are also prone to repeat infections because their immune systems are not up to par. Many have:

■ a history of these health problems, sometimes dating back to infancy
■ a characteristic facial appearance
■ characteristic activity and behavior patterns
■ sudden, inexplicable changes in how they feel, look, act, write, or draw
■ an erratic inability to learn or remember

Each of these problems will be discussed in detail later in this book. The following chapters in Part I will enable you to recognize some of the characteristics typical of environmental illnesses. This information can aid parents to help their family members, and it can enable teachers to relieve their own symptoms and assist their students so they feel better and academically perform well in school.

A TYPICAL CHILD'S HISTORY

Ryan

The story of four-year-old Ryan illustrates many typical aspects of childhood environmental illness. His history exemplifies many of the issues I'll discuss in this book.

Ryan also shows how extremely simple and easy it can sometimes be for parents to find specific solutions to their child's serious health and learning problems. The knowledge Ryan's parents acquired not only helped them to understand many of the perplexing health problems related to his previous exposures, it ultimately prevented future health and learning difficulties.

One major clue strongly suggested that Ryan had a school-related environmental illness: He felt fine before he went to school—but he was always ill by the time he came home.

Ryan was initially brought to our medical center because his mother noticed that after he attended school two afternoons a week, he became so fatigued he could barely stand up and he clung to her. His teachers complained that he was sometimes very antsy. His face twitched frequently. He could not tolerate the school gymnasium; it caused him to become so weak that he had to be carried out bodily after only a few minutes.

Ryan genuinely enjoyed school, so it was unlikely that an emotional problem was the cause of his difficulties. But because his symptoms were much worse at school, his mother went to his classroom to look around. She observed that the tabletops in his room and in the nap area were sprayed with a popular aerosol disinfectant several times each afternoon. To see whether this disinfectant played any role in his problems, we decided to deliberately expose him to a little bit of it. We sprayed a four-inch spot of the disinfectant onto a paper towel and placed it a few feet away from him. In thirty minutes, Ryan was obviously different. He could no longer hold a pencil. He clung excessively to his mother, whined, and appeared exhausted. They were the same types of complaints that his mother noted after school. Ryan's symptoms were relieved in only a few minutes with oxygen. Figures 1.1a to d and 1.2a to c show the changes in his handwriting and drawing during the test.

Writing
before exposure

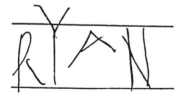

Normally alert

Writing
during exposure

Whining, crying, tired

Writing
at peak of reaction

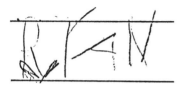

Unable to write

Writing after
oxygen treatment

Normally alert

FIGURE 1.1

Effects of a Disinfectant Aerosol on Ryan's Handwriting

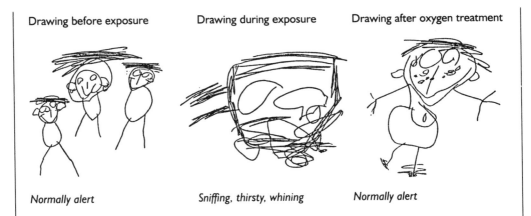

Drawing before exposure   Drawing during exposure   Drawing after oxygen treatment

Normally alert   *Sniffing, thirsty, whining*   *Normally alert*

FIGURE 1.2
Effects of Disinfectant Aerosol on Ryan's Drawing

Identifying the Cause

Phenol is a major offending ingredient in many common disinfectants. When Ryan was tested for a sensitivity to this chemical using the provocation/neutralization method (see Chapter 13), he could barely stand, walk, hold up his head, or even grasp a pencil after ten minutes. This reaction was similar to his reactions at the end of each school day and also after his exposure to the disinfectant. When he was treated with a phenol allergy extract, he walked normally again in ten minutes and could write as before.

With permission from Ryan's school, three simple, inexpensive, yet important changes were made:

- The disinfectant was replaced with one that did not adversely affect him.[7]
- His parents placed an air-purifying machine in his classroom (see PARF under Resources for sources of these machines).
- Safer floor-maintenance cleaning products and waxes were used on the gym floor (see Resources).

Within four weeks after these changes were made and the allergy treatment began, Ryan had improved 75 percent. His parents made some changes in their home environment, started the Rotation Diet (see Chapter 3), improved his overall nutrition, eliminated or reduced his exposure to household and other chemicals, and gave him allergy extract therapy. In another two months the boy no longer had facial twitches. His extreme fatigue, inexplicable clinging, and "clump on the floor" episodes were no longer evident. His headaches, muscle aches, and antsy periods had disappeared.

Five years later, Ryan continues to do extremely well. His mother knows, however, that exposure to certain chemicals continues to cause specific symptoms to flare up, usually when he enters a store or mall, or their church. His mother remains cautious because when gasoline is put into the family car, he routinely becomes tired, and the chemicals on new clothing, for example, make him antsy.

One can only wonder how Ryan would be today if the correct diagnosis had not been made. How fortunate that his school agreed to diminish his exposure to the offending chemicals. Making these changes helped not only Ryan but all the children in his class. In fact, once an air purifier was installed and environmentally safer cleaning agents were used routinely in Ryan's classroom,[8] his teacher commented that the other students "seemed to have less illness." Allergic children, in particular, have fewer symptoms in classrooms that are environmentally cleaner.

If your own children have an environmental illness, their problems are far from insurmountable. Sometimes significant improvement can occur, at any age, in a matter of hours or days after

- a few simple changes are made in a school, home, or work area
- obvious adverse chemical exposures are avoided
- an easy allergy diet is followed
- provocation/neutralization allergy extract therapy is begun
- improved nutrition therapy
- any yeast overgrowth is treated

■ WHAT CAN RYAN TEACH US?

Ryan's problems are typical of so many children who have environmental illnesses. Looking in more detail at his experiences can help you begin to determine whether environmental illness is present in your own child—or in yourself. If you see any similarities between Ryan's symptoms and that of your own child, an environmental exposure may be the cause. If the same medical complaints are present in your child, you may be able to help your child if you follow the example set by Ryan's mother.

MALES PREDOMINATE IN EARLY CHILDHOOD

It has long been apparent that during early childhood, boys are more likely to have allergies and/or environmental illness than girls. The ratio of boys to girls with this problem is about 4:1. After puberty, however, girls and women definitely become more affected. This is particularly true with chemical sensitivities. One possible explanation is that postpubertal males appear to be able to excrete chemicals from their bodies one to five times more rapidly than females.[9]

In general, regardless of their sex, children tend to bounce back to normal more quickly after environmental exposures are reduced than do chemically sensitized allergic adults. One reason is because the immune systems of children are more apt to be more resilient than those of adults. Youngsters tend to respond faster and better to appropriate therapy.

RYAN'S FAMILY HISTORY OF ALLERGIES IS TYPICAL

Both of Ryan's parents had allergies. In fact, most children with environmental illnesses have allergic parents and/or relatives. It is actually unusual to find a child with significant EI who does not have close relatives with asthma, hay fever, and/or skin allergies. In a school setting allergic students and teachers appear to be the first to manifest some form of EI. They are the "canaries in the coal mine" who warn the others that something has gone awry.

RYAN'S HISTORY BEFORE BIRTH AND DURING THE FIRST TWO YEARS

In many environmentally ill individuals, some form of allergy dates all the way back to infancy. Long before Ryan began school, he had both subtle and obvious evidence of allergies. Yet in spite of numerous clues, it can be very easy to miss the correct diagnosis for years. With earlier recognition and treatment, many of Ryan's health problems might have been prevented.

Surprisingly, Ryan may even have had evidence of allergies *before* birth. He kicked so hard in the womb and hiccupped so constantly that his mother's abdomen hurt. All babies, of course, move in the uterus, but some unborn infants who become environmentally ill children tend to be so active in the uterus that their mothers complain that they were bruised from the inside.

As a toddler, Ryan already suffered from hay fever and became excessively wiggly during the pollen season. His parents saw that food dyes made him hostile and aggressive. By the age of two, he had diarrhea and other intestinal symptoms during the summer months. No one knew why. Although there are many causes for these problems, allergies and environmental illness are usually not given enough serious consideration.

ALLERGY TREATMENT

By the age of three, Ryan had been seen by an allergist and treated with a routine allergy extract. Within an hour after each shot, however, he would suddenly feel ill. At first his arm would swell and become very hot. He would wet his bed that night. The next day he would act as if he had the flu. He would become extremely tired, develop a slight fever, and complain about a headache and nausea. This reaction to the treatment always lasted for two full days. Then he would feel and act fine—that is, until the following week, when he would receive his next injection. At that time the identical symptoms would recur. Because of her son's repeated adverse reactions, Ryan's mother eventually stopped his allergy treatments, even though she had been reassured that his symptoms could not possibly be related to his injections. Immediately after the extract therapy was discontinued, his weekly episodes stopped. Although Ryan's type of response to allergy injections is rare, some individuals, especially adults, do feel worse in some manner after every allergy treatment.[10] The cause is often a sensitivity to the phenol preservative routinely used in most allergy extract treatments.

HEADACHES AND MUSCLE ACHES

By the age of three, Ryan also had developed headaches and muscle aches that recurred from April to October. Even though these months corresponded to the time of seasonal allergies, no one suspected that allergies were the cause. Headaches and muscle aches, both very common health problems, can remain undiagnosed for years because pollen and molds are not commonly recognized as a possible cause of these types of symptoms. These problems, however, can be due to pollen when it is warm, molds when it is rainy, and dust, dust mites, and molds when it is cold. Foods and chemicals also can adversely affect these body areas at any time of the year.

Because the main emphasis in today's medicine is temporary drug relief rather than the detection and elimination of causative factors, some children (and adults) needlessly experience head and muscle aches for years. As a parent, however, if you become more observant, you can often figure out the cause and help your doctor to provide more effective treatment for your child.

THE ALLERGIC TENSION FATIGUE SYNDROME

By the age of four, Ryan had the characteristic symptoms of Allergic Tension Fatigue Syndrome. These symptoms include tension, fatigue, nervousness, withdrawal, hyperactivity, and/or moodiness. (See Table 1.2; notice how easily these symptoms could be confused with those of Attention Deficit Hyperactivity Disorder.) Affected allergic children usually have one or more of them.

Sometimes Ryan was too tired to lift his head, and at other times he cried, seemed too sad, or would suddenly and inexplicably become wiggly and unable to sit quietly. These problems, for example, stopped after the floor wax and cleaning materials used for the gym-floor maintenance were

TABLE 1.2

Symptoms of Allergic Tension Fatigue Syndrome

- Hyperactivity; wild, unrestrained behavior
- Extreme talkativeness; explosive speech, stuttering, and hoarseness
- Inattentive, disruptive, and impulsive actions
- Short attention span; inability to concentrate, remember details, or carry out instructions
- Mental confusion or sluggishness
- Restless legs; finger-tapping
- Clumsiness and incoordination
- Tremors, tics, or jerking twitchy muscles
- Insomnia; disturbing nightmares
- Nervousness and irritability; a short temper
- High-strung, excitable, agitated behavior
- Fatigue, weakness, drowsiness, weariness, exhaustion, or listlessness; a lack of energy and ambition
- Depression or extreme silliness
- Despondency, sullenness, withdrawal
- Moodiness, crying, extreme sensitivity to criticism
- Extreme sensitivity to odors, light, sound, cold, touch, and pain
- Loss of desire to play
- Difficulty with schoolwork, especially reading and writing

changed, so that he was no longer exposed to those chemicals. However, he could not remain calm whenever he was exposed to perfume in church or to the odor of formaldehyde in polyester clothing in department stores.

CHEMICAL SENSITIVITIES

Typical allergies unquestionably make some people prone to chemical sensitivities. The phenol in Ryan's allergy extract when he was three years old, and the phenol in the disinfectant aerosol when he was four, certainly caused his behavior to change. Over time, other specific odors also caused discrete changes in his behavior, such as the odor of gasoline, which caused extreme fatigue. Exposure to fireplace smoke caused inordinate lethargy and very stiff joints. Few adults would give such exposures a second thought even though they commonly cause illness.

By the time Ryan was four, he had as many as ten temper tantrums a day, especially in the summer. The cause? His family lived in an area where lawn sprays were used frequently, and pesticides were applied every three weeks to control insects. In retrospect, these chemicals probably contributed not only to his summer flare-ups of symptoms but to the chemical sensitivities he developed when he attended school.

Although many school-related health problems are directly caused by common allergenic substances (dust, molds, pollen, pets, foods), the major unrecognized factor is a sensitivity to chemicals. Ryan later was found to be sensitive to many common allergenic substances, including phenol, formaldehyde, and hydrocarbons.

Fortunately, Ryan's condition was never misdiagnosed as psychological, emotional, or academic in nature. This happens to all too many children and adults who have unrecognized environmental illness.

▪ HOW COMMON IS ENVIRONMENTAL ILLNESS?

The symptoms of environmental illness can clearly be much broader than classic hay fever and asthma. If your school or home is not environmentally sound, the range of your own child's physical, behavioral, and learning problems can be varied and perplexing. It appears that any area of a body can be affected—and that the problem in society at large is widespread.

In a recent survey by the American Academy of Pediatrics and the National PTA, 71 percent of teachers stated that they are now seeing more children with health problems than ever before. Up to 20 percent of American children have developed chronic illnesses.[11] Youngsters also now have a variety of perplexing learning and behavior problems that were simply not evident a few decades ago; hence the need for special-education teachers and classes has grown immensely. New social attitudes about childrearing cannot be blamed for all these changes; nor can ADHD. Environmental illness is certainly one major unsuspected factor in this increase in health and learning problems.

Asthma and allergic coughing, for example, are very common complaints, particularly in children who attend dusty and/or moldy schools. As noted earlier, the incidence of asthma has increased enormously in the past twenty years. A person whose chest is affected by allergy has a tendency to cough excessively after exercise, laughter, cold drinks, or exposure to cold air. Initially, the cough progresses to asthma only when an infection is present. **But if the cause is not found and eliminated**, the asthma will eventually occur suddenly at any time and for no apparent reason.

HOW OFTEN ARE TEACHERS AFFECTED?

Teachers may be more ill now than they were in the past. A survey conducted in 1992 found a 17 percent increase in skin irritation among teachers since 1989.[12] In 1993, 47 percent of surveyed New York teachers said they had inexplicable fatigue and drowsiness on a daily or weekly basis.

Breathing problems, such as irritable or reversible airway disease, will tend to become more severe or frequent when the person attends a dusty school, lives in a moldy building or enters any building that has been renovated recently, because of the many chemicals used during construction.

■ HOW WIDESPREAD IS CHEMICAL SENSITIVITY?

We have no real statistics about the incidence of sensitivity to chemicals such as perfume, pesticides, and formaldehyde, because chemical sensitivities are so frequently unsuspected, misdiagnosed, or disbelieved. Physicians who practice environmental medicine estimate conservatively that it affects at least 25 to 50 percent of today's population.

As you'll learn throughout this book, it is really quite easy to tell whether you or your child has a chemical sensitivity. Chemically sensitive individuals smell odors that others don't notice. Many become ill or behave differently after even a slight whiff of an odor or aroma, especially from:

- perfume, tobacco, or gas furnace vapors
- automobile or truck exhaust fumes
- a gasoline smell
- chemical odors in malls, restaurants, or churches
- neighborhood air after lawn sprays are applied

Your child's symptoms may also increase after exposure to:

- fingernail polish or remover, marking pens, or typing correction fluid
- a new magazine or book, or fresh newsprint
- freshly dry-cleaned or fabric-softened clothing
- cleaning preparations, scouring powder, waxes, or polishes
- disinfectants or deodorizers
- lawn sprays, pesticides, or termiticides

■ GENERALIZED SCHOOL PROBLEMS

The presence of environmental illness becomes particularly evident when many youngsters return to school in the fall. Some find they become ill at the same time with similar complaints each year. When a new factor is introduced into the school and suddenly a rash of similar health problems becomes evident, the environment should be a prime suspect. According to a survey conducted by New York State's largest teachers' union, an estimated 10 percent of the schools in the state now have some form of indoor air pollution that is causing a variety of health problems.[13] If schools in which only a part of a building is affected are included, the proportion rises to 50 percent! In a recent report by the Occupational Safety and Health Administration, over 50 percent (15 out of 29) of state university campuses had indoor air-quality problems. Of that group, 73 percent had Sick Building Syndrome, which means that the school buildings were making students and/or teachers ill. Airborne chemicals were an additional problem in 67 percent of this group.[14]

Thus, both old and new nursery, preschool, elementary, middle, high school, and college buildings are causing varying degrees of illness in a rapidly expanding group of students and teachers. No one knows the statistics related to homes. Regardless of whether the source of the problem is at school or at home, many of those who are affected are completely unaware of the reason that they are ill or cannot learn.

■ THE LONG-TERM EFFECTS OF ENVIRONMENTAL ILLNESS

The impact of environmental illness upon individuals and upon society at large is immense and can no longer be ignored. A growing number of children require home teaching and must adopt a sharply limited lifestyle because they simply cannot tolerate the ordinary daily exposures at school or elsewhere. These problems are not always short-term. Even after an environmental illness is recognized, many of those affected (regardless of age) must remain on guard for many years. Transferring to a new chemically laden school or an older dusty and moldy one, moving to a new or recently remodeled home, binging on craved foods or beverages, developing a severe infection, or any significant new emotional stress may precipitate a relapse lasting hours, days, or weeks.

The sooner an EI is diagnosed and appropriate therapy is started, the better. Prompt treatment can help diminish learning problems in children, as well as prolonged periods of ill health with all the associated secondary psychological, social, or emotional difficulties. The lives of environmentally ill children and adults can be turned around, with the help of the newer and different diagnostic and treatment approaches described in this book.

NOTES

1. This information was reported on ABC's *World News Tonight with Peter Jennings*, May 20, 1994. See also *Human Ecologist*, vol. 55 (Fall 1992), p. 6 (see For Further Reading).

2. Commonwealth of Massachusetts, Special Legislative Committee on Indoor Air Pollution, "Indoor Air Pollution in Massachusetts, Final Report" (Boston, 1989).

3. James Swanson et al., "More Frequent Diagnosis of Attention Deficit Hyperactivity Disorder," *New England Journal of Medicine* (Oct. 5, 1995), p. 944.

4. Iris Bell, "Self-Reported Illness from Chemical Odors in Young Adults Without Clinical Syndromes or Occupational Exposures," *Archives of Environmental Health*, vol. 48 (1993), pp. 6–13.

5. General Accounting Office, Report to Congressional Requesters, *School Facilities: Condition of America's Schools* (February 1995).

6. Environmental Protection Agency, *Indoor Air Quality Tools for Schools*. Write to EPA, Indoor Air Division, 66071, 401 M Street S.W., Washington, D.C. 20460.

7. Such disinfectants are described in A. Berthold-Bond, *Clean and Green* (Woodstock, NY: Ceres Press, 1990).

8. Doris Rapp, *Is This Your Child?* (New York: William Morrow, 1991).

9. William J. Rea, *Chemical Sensitivity*, vol. 3 (Chelsea, MI: Lewis Publishers, 1995).

10. D.J. Rapp, *Allergies and Your Family* (Buffalo, NY: Practical Allergy Relief Foundation, 1989), D.J. Rapp, *Allergies and the Hyperactive Child* (Buffalo, NY: PARF, 1989).

11. American Academy of Pediatrics, *School Health: Policy and Practice* (1993). For a copy, write to the AAP at 141 Northwest Point Boulevard, P.O. Box 927, Elk Grove Village, IL 60009-0927.

12. "Is Your Building Sick?" *New York Teacher*, vol. 34, no. 9 (Jan. 25, 1993), p. 13.

13. "Access to Employee Exposure and Medical Records," *Federal Register*, May 23, 1980.

14. American Academy of Pediatrics, *School Health: Policy and Practice*, 1993.

2 ⟨ Typical Symptoms of Environmental Illness

Whether it is a single child or a number of students, a teacher or an adult, everyone affected by an environmental illness shares typical symptoms. Even so, EIs tend not to be properly identified. Individuals are frequently misdiagnosed, and it is not uncommon for them to be told their symptoms are prolonged flu, anxiety, or that their complaints are "all in their heads."

The first step toward proper treatment is to identify a possible EI in your child or yourself. Let's look more closely at these common symptoms.

■ DO THESE SYMPTOMS SOUND FAMILIAR?

Preschool children with environmental illness tend to whine, cling, say the same phrase over and over, repeatedly remove their clothing, or become withdrawn or untouchable. At times they scream when anyone approaches or touches them. Some pull away and say, "Nobody likes me." A few cower in dark corners, behind chairs, and under tables. Surprisingly, some adults behave similarly, especially after eating the wrong foods or being exposed to certain chemicals.

More common and even more challenging to handle are the young children who seem fine most of the time, and then for no obvious reason suddenly switch from a darling adorable Dr. Jekyll to a hostile, aggressive, vulgar, hyperactive Mr. Hyde. At times, children's inappropriate behavior takes the form of being so overly happy or silly that they laugh uncontrollably. In contrast, other children become excessively quiet, irritable, tired, or placid, and in those youngsters the correct diagnosis can be missed for many years. In that sense, the youngsters who misbehave, hit, bite, spit, punch, pinch, kick, destroy, or become vulgar are actually more fortunate because their actions prompt a definitive need for immediate medical attention.

Here are some other typical examples: A child (or an adult) may write and draw without difficulty before lunch, yet be unable to do anything well in the afternoon. A child may think, remember, and learn easily for an hour or even a day, but then, after an exposure to a chemical odor such as a lavatory deodorizer, adamantly refuse to comply with the simplest request or suddenly seem incapable of learning. Children who are sensitive to milk or juice may suddenly wet their pants or need to urinate more frequently or urgently than other students. Those with intestinal complaints may belch, pass gas, or soil their underpants after eating a problem food. Others may have leg aches in the daytime or at night, or have embarrassing face twitches or tics. It is possible for discrete areas of the brain—as well as the nose, lungs, bladder, bowels, or muscles—to be affected by an allergy. As a result, some children have never had a day when they truly felt well.

If the causes of EI are not identified, the children usually become quite embarrassed by their behavior and suffer repeated blows to their self-esteem because of frequent reprimands. They often feel inadequate and depressed because at times they inexplicably act so spacey or appear to be dumb, lazy, bad, or different. Their mothers often wonder how they have failed; what have they done wrong?

And what about teachers and parents who have EI? Adults can develop similar symptoms in response to environmental exposures. They, too, can feel confused, perplexed, bewildered and depressed, when, for no apparent reason, they suddenly become irritable, moody, angry, sad, aggressive, vulgar, or can't think clearly.

■ THE PROBLEM OF MISDIAGNOSIS

Symptoms like these often lead doctors to make a wrong diagnosis. As I pointed out in Chapter 1, many allergic children are mistakenly thought to have Attention Deficit Hyperactivity Disorder (ADHD). Repeated scientific studies have indicated that as many as 66 percent of ADHD-diagnosed children actually have an unrecognized food allergy causing their symptoms.[1] This means that about two-thirds of hyperactive children may not need an activity-modifying Class II narcotic drug such as Ritalin. Rather, they need to have their food sensitivities detected (which is often possible within three to seven days after a simple one-week elimination diet—see Chapter 3).

Others act inappropriately when they are exposed to dust, mold, or chemicals. It is not uncommon for EI learning-disabled children to fall through the cracks because no one is quite sure how to label them. Some have intermittent specific learning problems, emotional disabilities, Tourette's Syndrome or autismlike symptoms. Others have characteristics typical of a cognitive or Pervasive Developmental Disorder (PDD). These labels provide a name for their problem, but no insightful explanation for the cause of the problem. In reality, for a number of these children, the correct partial or total diagnosis is more appropriately what allergists call the Allergic Tension Fatigue Syndrome, as mentioned in Chapter 1. It encompasses many of the symptoms so characteristic of environmental illness (see Tables 1.1, 1.2, and Chapter 15). Parents and teachers can sometimes identify the cause of these overlapping diagnoses, if they start to ask when and why certain changes occur.

■ SYMPTOMS CAN CHANGE WITH TIME

More and more individuals seem to be affected by EI at earlier ages because of the continued widespread chemical contamination and pollution of our food, water, and air, and our homes, schools, and workplaces. As we have seen, environmental illness frequently can be traced all the way back to infancy and sometimes even before. Many EI children were hyperactive or hiccuped excessively in the uterus because of the foods their mothers ate, the beverages they drank, or the odors that they smelled.

The symptoms that occur in an infant can be quite different from those that occur later in childhood. That is, as a child grows, the manifestations of EI may change, fooling both parents and doctors into believing the problem has been "outgrown. In reality, the child merely has different symptoms *in response to the same contact or food.*

As an example, let's look at the range of different illnesses related to a dairy sensitivity. The following shows how symptoms typically change over time:

■ *In fetuses*, the dairy products a mother ingests "to make a healthier infant" can cause excessive hiccupping and vigorous, painful movements.
■ *In infants*, breast or milk formula tends to cause colic or intestinal discomfort, constipation or possibly diarrhea, extreme discontent with screaming and poor sleep, recurrent ear infections, excessive drooling and perspiration. Some walk at nine months or earlier and head-bang, and/or crib-rock so vigorously that the crib is broken.
■ *In toddlers*, milk is most apt to cause congestion, severe leg aches or weak legs, clumsiness, a tendency to whine, and a refusal to wear clothing. Some of these youngsters gag and repeatedly vomit clear or frothy mucus. Many develop the behavior commonly called the "terrible twos" which then persists through the threes and fours. At times, some affected toddlers are hyperactive—others are so excessively fatigued, their parents are distressed because they can be so drowsy they are difficult to arouse.

■ *In children*, milk often causes nose congestion, hay fever, throat-clearing, clucking throat sounds, a chronic cough, wheezing, nose, ear, chest, or sinus infections, bed-wetting beyond five years, erratic schoolwork, constipation, bad breath, irritability, and tantrums.

■ *In adolescents and adults*, the major symptoms are diarrhea or constipation, fatigue, irritability, and temper outbursts. Environmentally ill adults tend to love cheese and may either crave or detest milk. They often have hay fever and/or asthma, also from dairy, but in time, their milk sensitivity can cause them to develop an irritable bowel, colitis, Crohn's disease, tight joints, arthritis, high blood pressure, or heartbeat irregularities.

In each age group the symptoms may either subside or persist. In some people they can increase in number and become progressively more severe with time. At any point, one set of milk-related symptoms can subside, only to recur in a new form that is not readily recognized as being caused by dairy products. In three to seven days after all forms of milk and dairy products are eliminated from the diet, or after milk allergy extract therapy is begun, these types of symptoms often significantly diminish or subside (see Chapter 15).

Of course, many other medical illnesses can cause any of the above complaints, but if you have allergies in your family and could not tolerate milk as an infant, a missed dairy allergy can certainly cause a spectrum of illnesses that can persist for a lifetime.

■ WHAT ABOUT SCHOOL-RELATED SYMPTOMS?

Once a child begins school, new EI symptoms develop that are often directly related to the classroom environment. The typical symptoms that bother environmentally ill students, teachers, and school employees are listed in Table 3.1. Major complaints include extreme fatigue, burning eyes, numb skin, nasal congestion, headaches, muscle aches, and abdominal cramps. Most affected individuals will have several to many of these symptoms. (Table 3.2 provides additional insight to help you identify more symptoms.)

If the environmental cause of an illness is limited to a specific area of a school, then it's possible that only a few students will be affected. If, however, the cause is more generalized and related to more extensive renovations or ventilation problems, it will affect many individuals throughout a school within a few days, sometimes in hours. On any given day, symptoms tend to begin within a few minutes to several hours after school begins. Many become increasingly ill as the day and/or week progresses. Initially, the symptoms subside one to four hours after the affected students or teachers return home. Eventually, however, the recurring symptoms become more severe, and they may not subside until Sunday night or after a long school vacation. The more severe an environmental illness is, the longer it will take the individual to recover.

SYMPTOMS AT HOME

If your child is well at school but routinely becomes ill within a few hours of arriving home, or seems worse on weekends, think about what in your home could be causing a problem. Note if your child feels better or entirely well when visiting relatives, on vacation, or at camp. In some youngsters, a change in location makes no difference because they are exposed to the same dust, molds, and chemicals at school *and* at home. Similarly, if a favorite food is a problem, symptoms will be evident wherever that child goes.

■ HOW SYMPTOMS PROGRESS

Typically, a severely chemically sensitive child will experience a headache within a very few minutes after entering a polluted school, then gradually develop extreme fatigue, muscle aches, a loss of appetite, and nausea as the morning passes. These symptoms are often mistakenly attributed to the flu. Commonly, the child develops a burning or soreness in his eyes and throat, or complains about a metallic or strange taste in his mouth. Classical hay fever symptoms, accompanied by congestion or coughing are commonly noted. The latter can progress to difficulty breathing, and then to asthma or wheezing. Itchy skin, irritability, numbness, tingling, or twitches of the fingers or face can also occur. By the end of the school day, some children even develop blurred or double vision.

Sensitive teachers have a similar spectrum of symptoms. Some become so confused that they can't tell time, remember their students' names, or prepare their lesson plans. Understandably, they are frequently much too embarrassed to mention these problems to anyone. They are perplexed and frightened when they suddenly "lose control" and act in a most unnatural and inappropriate manner.

Unless the cause is found and eliminated, the illness progresses so that the child's or teacher's symptoms tend to become more intense and more frequent, even incapacitating. A simple occasional headache may begin to throb, so it becomes so painful that the person sobs, rocks back and forth in agonizing distress, or has to lie on the floor. Their joints sometimes ache so badly and constantly that it is difficult for them to walk or climb stairs; some children can't climb stairs, run or play. Their face or body muscles can twitch until they hurt. The fatigue can become so extreme that a child cannot hold up his or her head; sometimes a youngster's head will fall forward onto a desk or directly into a book with a loud thump. After school, a previously active teenage boy may enter his home, flop onto the floor, and cry because he is too tired to play ball. The progressive worsening of any medical complaint indicates more serious trouble—not for a more effective pill, but for the urgent need to find and eliminate the cause.

■ WHO IS MOST SUSCEPTIBLE TO ENVIRONMENTAL ILLNESS?

Although allergic students and teachers are usually the first to manifest symptoms of environmental illness in a particular school, nonallergic individuals can also be affected. Your own child's potential to develop an EI will depend on his genetics and immune system, as well as any previous exposures to allergens and chemicals. The type, frequency, intensity, and duration of these exposures are key variables.

As a parent, your challenge is to recognize and help remedy the causes of an environmental problem as quickly as possible. Allergic children and teachers will often provide the first clue that something is not right, thereby alerting the entire staff, because they suddenly don't feel, behave, or remember appropriately when they are in school. As I'll discuss later in this book, harmful exposures must be eliminated as soon as possible.

IS A SCHOOL-RELATED ILLNESS BECOMING WORSE?

In evaluating your child's EI, here are some key questions to ask:

- Do his symptoms continue for more than a few hours after your child leaves the school building?
- Do they last through the weekend until Sunday night?
- Do they persist until there is a long school vacation?
- Are ordinary exposures to chemicals, which never caused symptoms before, no longer tolerated well? If even the most minute exposure to any odor is now causing symptoms, your child is experiencing the typical "spreading phenomenon." This means that a single or prolonged chemical exposure caused a sensitivity which has expanded or spread so that many chemical odors now trigger symptoms.

Ultimately, a highly chemically sensitive child or adult will need to make adjustments in his lifestyle. Avoidance of churches, workplaces, large department stores, new buildings, malls, restaurants, movies, libraries, hospitals, hair salons, and barber shops, as well as gatherings such as weddings and parties might become necessary. Odors that were previously not even noticed can become severely problematic.

ONE CHILD'S HISTORY

Liza

Liza's history clearly illustrates the symptoms of chemical sensitivities and their tendency to remain unidentified for years. Although most children have milder and fewer health problems, Liza's medical history is exceptionally severe, and some youngsters certainly do have a similarly wide array of symptoms. The surprise is how frequently these symptoms fit into a typical pattern that is characteristic in both children and adults who have environmental illness.

The Onset of Liza's Symptoms

Liza's problems began with a natural gas leak in a stove and a malfunctioning furnace in her family's home. (The leaks could just as easily have come from a faulty gas furnace or ventilation system in a school.) No one in the family realized that the leaks were taking place, so her entire family continued to be exposed to the gas over a period of several years. At the time the exposure began, Liza was only one year old. Although she cried and whined constantly, no one knew why. Her repeated episodes of bronchitis perplexed her doctors.

Each family member subsequently manifested a variety of symptoms as a result of the ongoing exposure. At first, they tried to adapt. Then, one by one, they all developed confusing health problems caused by their continued but unrecognized exposure to chemical odors.

In time, it became clear that Liza's ability to learn had been affected. The problem was first evident at age four, when she could not concentrate and remember during her swimming lessons because of what later turned out to be a chlorine sensitivity. Learning problems due specifically to chlorine, however, were not obvious again until she was twelve years old.

Liza's Chemical Sensitivities Continue Unrecognized

Over time, Liza developed many other symptoms. She experienced chronic recurrent infections and headaches, mainly during the cold winter months. Her major symptom, however, was severe leg aches. Usually this problem suggests a dairy allergy, but that was not true for Liza. Ever since she was a toddler, her parents had to spend hours to rub her legs every evening or during the night to ease her leg pain. At times she would cry for as long as sixteen hours at a stretch because of the pain.

By the time she reached age six, her mother recognized that certain foods seemed to cause Liza's headaches and vomiting. Riding the school bus made her so sick that she would vomit, faint, or sometimes even fall asleep for as long as forty-eight hours. There were periods when she was too weak to walk more than a block or two. No one knew why.

Liza also had recurrent nosebleeds, easy bruising, and rectal bleeding. When she was only six and a half, she experienced vaginal bleeding. Her knees were black and blue—not from a fall while running or playing but from unexplained bleeding inside her joints. Repeated medical evaluations did not provide answers or relief. (The effect of chemicals on the blood, as detailed in the first volume of Dr. William Rea's *Chemical Sensitivity,* was not fully appreciated at that time.)[2]

Symptoms in Other Family Members

Meanwhile, Liza's parents and brother were experiencing health problems too. Her mother complained of severe weakness and tingling in her arms and legs. Although she was too tired to work in the winter, she was energetic and could work full time in the summer. Extensive medical evaluations failed to explain her seasonal symptoms and perplexed numerous medical specialists.

Liza's father also seemed to get worse during the winter. He had persistent headaches and took as many as a hundred Tylenol tablets a week to control his pain. He had dark circles under his eyes and tended to be extremely irritable, again mainly during the colder weather. Years later he developed a brain tumor, which may or may not have been related to his chemical exposures.

Liza's brother had headaches, puffy eyes, a runny nose, and depression. Although he learned easily, sometimes he had trouble concentrating and remembering. His symptoms again were more pronounced during the winter, while during the warmer months, he seemed fine. This observation proved to be valuable in detecting the cause of each family member's problem.

Detecting the Cause

One summer, five years after the stove and furnace leaks began, Liza's family finally became aware of the leak in the kitchen. At that time, they had acquired an electric stove to replace the old gas stove. Three days later Liza's legs stopped aching for the first time in years; she no longer cried with leg pain each night. At the same time, her brother's disposition improved remarkably. Apparently, they concluded, the stove's natural gas leak had been one source of their health problems.

During the fall, however, the weather became colder, and the gas furnace was turned on again. Once more, the entire family had flare-ups of their old symptoms. They investigated and found that the furnace leaked due to improper venting of the carbon monoxide and exhaust fumes. For the first time, they realized why their symptoms had recurred each winter. Surprisingly, they had "adapted" to a degree to exposures from the leaky gas stove and the fumes from the furnace. They subsequently bought a new furnace, switched to electric heat, and corrected the ventilation problems. Thereafter, the recurrent seasonal health problems in each family member subsided.

Liza, however, continued to have intermittent illness. Every time they vacationed or visited someone who had a gas stove, she would wheeze, her legs would ache, and she would bleed in various areas of her body. The "spreading phenomenon" had taken effect. It became evident that even a limited exposure to any chemical odor now caused her to have immediate symptoms.

Liza's Learning Problem

When Liza was twelve years old, an observant teacher provided the critical insight needed to help explain her erratic learning ability. The teacher noticed that Liza's writing had changed dramatically during a particular school assignment. She told Liza's mother about it (see Figure 2.1). The mother recalled that at the time this assignment was written, Liza had been exposed to a minute amount of chlorine bleach. An air duct from the basement laundry room led directly to the bedroom in which Liza had been doing her homework. This ventilation system allowed the chlorine odor to drift into her room.

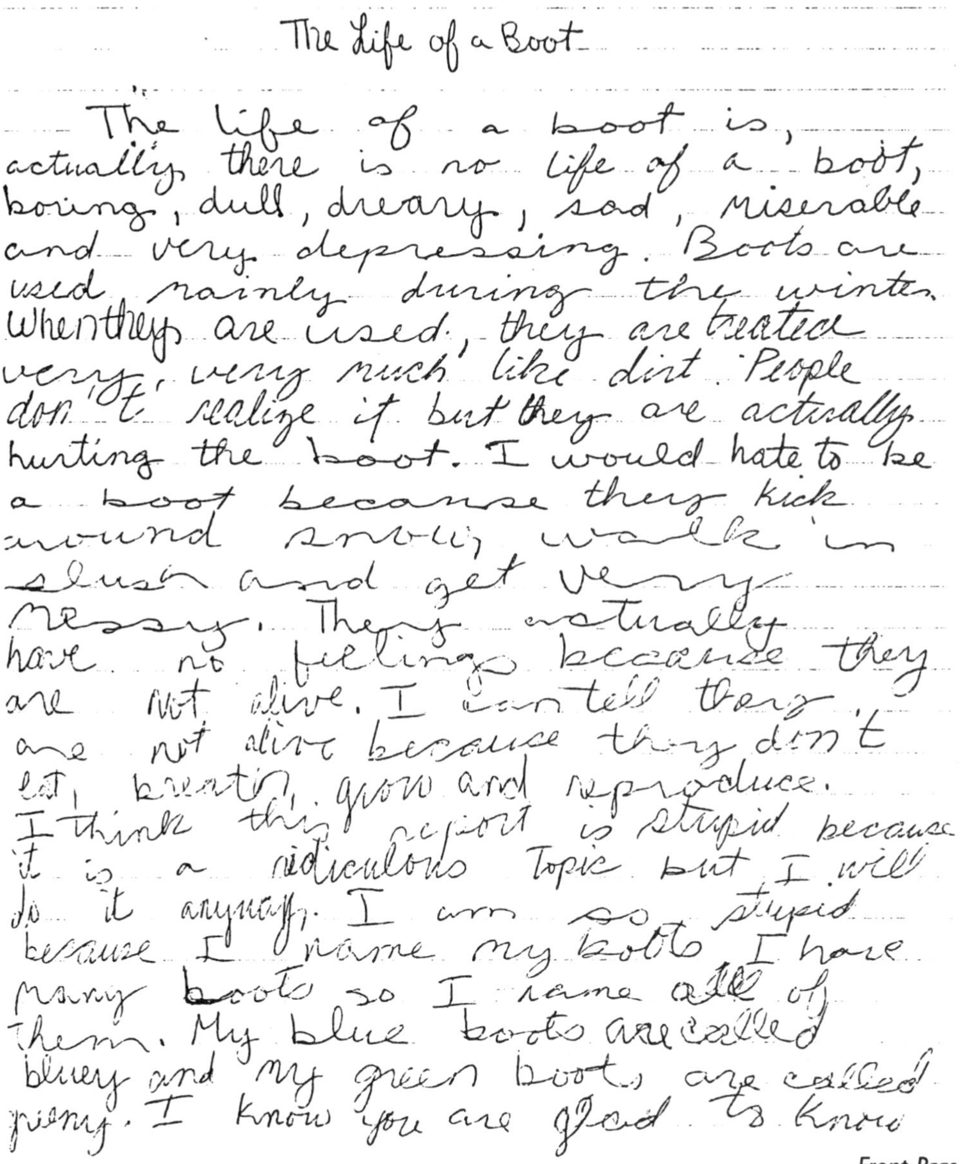

The Life of a Boot

The life of a boot is, actually, there is no life of a boot, boring, dull, dreary, sad, miserable and very depressing. Boots are used mainly during the winter. When they are used, they are treated very, very much like dirt. People don't realize it but they are actually hurting the boot. I would hate to be a boot because they kick around snow, walk in slush and get very messy. They actually have no feelings because they are not alive. I can tell they are not alive because they don't eat, breath, grow and reproduce. I think this report is stupid because it is a ridiculous Topic but I will do it anyway. I am so stupid because I name my boots I have many boots so I name all of them. My blue boots are called bluey and my green boots are called pieny. I know you are glad to know

Front Page

FIGURE 2.1
Note the gradual deterioration of Liza's writing and her ability to express herself.

FIGURE 2.1 (continued)

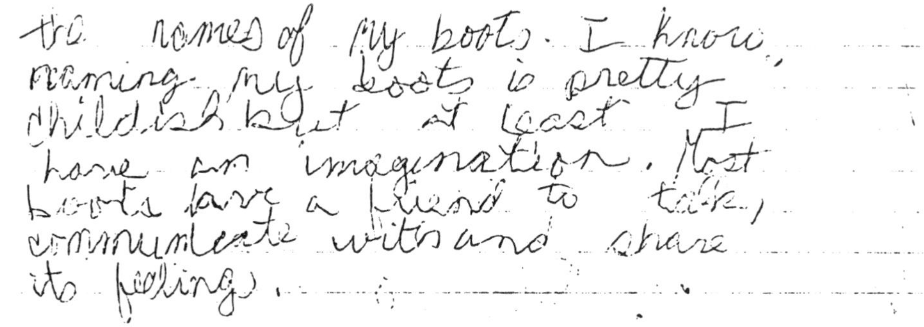

the names of my boots. I know, naming my boots is pretty childish but at least I have an imagination. Most boots have a friend to talk, communicate with and share its feelings.

Back Page

At that time Liza had complained to her mother that the odor caused a headache and intestinal discomfort, and that she felt extremely irritable and tearful. She hadn't been aware, though, that both the content and the penmanship of her composition had markedly deteriorated. When the teacher returned the paper with the note in Figure 2.2, Liza was very embarrassed that she had not recognized the obvious change in her writing or her ability to express herself clearly.

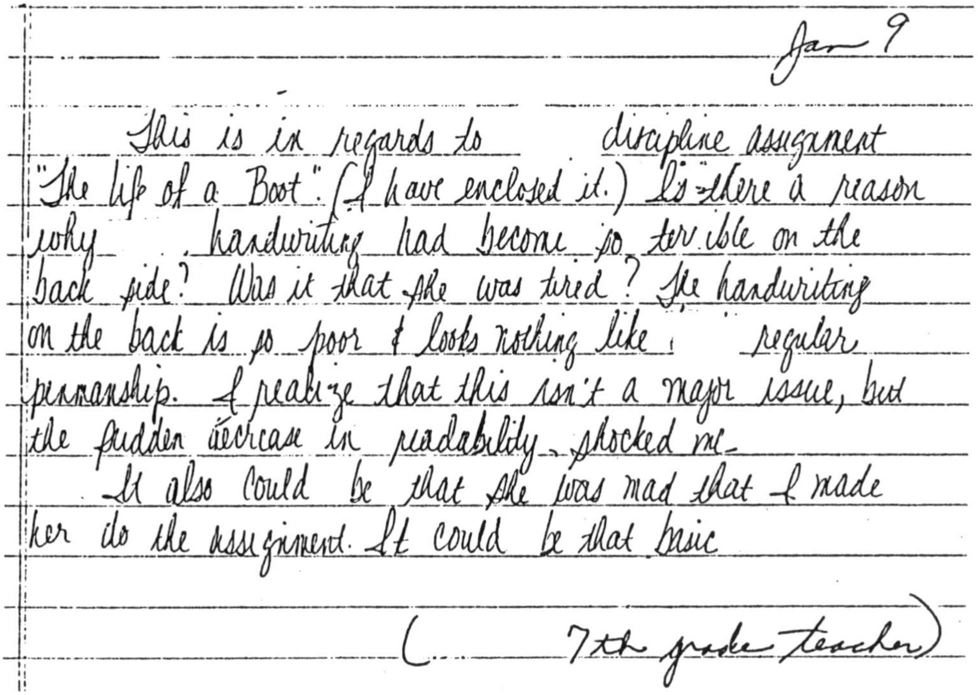

Jan 9

This is in regards to   discipline assignment "The life of a Boot". (I have enclosed it.) Is there a reason why   handwriting had become so terrible on the back side? Was it that she was tired? The handwriting on the back is so poor & looks nothing like   regular penmanship. I realize that this isn't a major issue, but the sudden decrease in readability shocked me.   It also could be that she was mad that I made her do the assignment. It could be that basic

(7th grade teacher)

FIGURE 2.2
The teacher's note.

Solving the Mystery

More pieces of Liza's puzzle gradually began to fit together. Once her parents were made aware of the effect of chlorine on her ability to think, they vividly recalled that a chlorine odor had created similar problems when she was only four years old. After Liza had been swimming in a chlorinated pool, her mother remembered, she would cry more than usual and complained of headaches and leg cramps. While Liza was in the pool, she had seemed unable to follow the simplest swimming instructions. Because of this problem, she ultimately had to discontinue swimming lessons. In retrospect, this reaction was the earliest clue that chlorine interfered with her behavior and her ability to think.

Today, although Liza is living a more normal life, the effects of chemical exposures still linger, sometimes even affecting her ability to learn. Looking back, the sequential pattern of her chemical problems can be summarized as follows:

1. The family had a natural gas leak in their kitchen stove and a furnace leak when Liza was one year old. This initial overexposure to chemicals sensitized her entire family, so they were all ill with different complaints for the next five years and no one knew why.
2. Liza developed a possible unsuspected chlorine sensitivity that affected her thinking when she attempted to take swimming lessons at the age of four. This was the first evidence of the "spreading phenomenon."
3. When Liza was six years old, her family recognized that their gas stove and furnace exhaust system were defective. They finally realized that gas leaks had caused many of their cold weather health problems.
4. When Liza was twelve, her teacher helped her parents recognize that the odor of chlorine had altered her ability to write and think at a level comparable to her ability. As time passed, they recognized the effects that many other chemical odors had on her.

We have no idea how often chlorine or any other chemicals affected Liza before she was twelve. Imagine how much greater her learning problems would have been if her classroom had been located near a swimming pool. Indeed, I have seen some children and teachers experience illness or behavior problems simply because their classroom was adjacent to a pool, a well-sanitized lavatory, or a school print shop.

Once you begin to pay attention to such potential problems, you can sometimes explain your child's present, as well as previous symptoms. It is amazing how often you can actually pinpoint what is making your child or yourself ill.

Meanwhile, use this detailed description of Liza to help increase your own awareness of the possible range and severity of EI symptoms. Most youngsters and their families are not as ill as Liza was. They usually have only one persistent, easily relieved complaint. A few, however, have a multiplicity of perplexing symptoms, and it takes a bit of time and effort to find the cause.

HOW THE BODY ADAPTS TO ODORS

Chemically related EIs often begin when the affected individual becomes increasingly aware of odors. Initially, this awareness helps protect the person. But as this adaptation continues, the odors may no longer be noticed; the child, teacher, or parent may become so accustomed to a smell or exposure that it is not noticed. This period of adaptation varies in length from individual to individual. The duration depends upon the type, degree, and intensity of each stressful exposure, as well as the competency of the person's immune system. Weeks, months, or years later, the body's defenses can falter so much that they no longer protect from offending exposures. During the later stages of chemical sensitivity, some people lose their sense of smell completely. By this time the body defenses are exhausted and can no longer compensate or adequately protect. Elusive intermittent medical complaints such as headaches, irritability, fatigue, muscle aches, weakness, intestinal complaints, unprovoked explosive anger, poor memory, etc., become progressively more evident. School, home, and work exposures and contacts can all cause these types of symptoms.

■ AVOIDING THE LATE STAGES OF CHEMICAL SENSITIVITY

Clearly, it's important to treat a chemical sensitivity early, to prevent severe symptoms and the later stages of illness from developing. Otherwise, regardless of an individual's age, ordinary living can become an overwhelming challenge. Shopping, looking at freshly printed newspaper, studying from certain odorous schoolbooks, visiting a zoo or aquarium, or riding in a school bus, taxi, airplane, or new car may all become off limits. *Once a person is seriously sensitized, any exposure to even minuscule amounts of ordinary and unavoidable chemicals can provoke incapacitating symptoms.*

Chemically sensitized people can be helped, but by the time the correct diagnosis is made, many no longer have the strength, resources, or supportive family and friends to reestablish their health. These consequences can be prevented by the earliest possible recognition and treatment of the environmental illness.[3] Children, in particular, have a limited, well-defined window of time during which they must acquire their education. If they are too ill or if their learning and/or behavior problems are too challenging, their education, career, or their future life may be seriously jeopardized.

<u>NOTES</u>

1. D.J. Rapp, "Does Diet Affect Hyperactivity?" *Journal of Learning Disabilities*, vol. 11 (1978), pp. 56–62; J. O'Shea et al., "Double-Blind Study of Children with Hyperkinetic Syndrome Treated with Multi-Allergen Extract Sublingually," *Journal of Learning Disabilities*, vol. 14 (1981), p. 189; J. Egger et al., "Controlled Trial of Oligoantigenic Treatment in the Hyperkinetic Syndrome," *Lancet 1* (1985), pp. 540–45; Marvin Boris and Francine S. Mandel, "Foods and Additives Are Common Causes of the Attention Deficit Hyperactive Disorder in Children," *Annals of Allergy*, vol. 72 (1994), pp. 462–68; Katherine S. Rowe and Kenneth J. Rowe, "Synthetic Food Coloring and Behavior: A Dose Response Effect in a Double-Blind, Placebo-Controlled, Repeated-Measures Study," *Journal of Pediatrics*, vol. 125, no. 5, part 1 (Nov. 1994), pp. 691–98.

2. William Rea, *Chemical Sensitivity*, 4 vols. (Chelsea, MI: Lewis Publishers, 1991–96).

3. D.J. Rapp, *Is This Your Child?* (New York: William Morrow and Co., 1991).

3 { Fast, Easy, Inexpensive Ways to Find Answers

Each morning, when millions of children enter their classrooms all over the United States, many are being exposed to substances that make them sick. Environmental illnesses, as we have seen, are poorly understood by physicians and parents alike. The problems of these youngsters are often un- or misdiagnosed, frequently leading to years of needless sickness and sometimes to learning problems that can be remedied.

In Chapter 2, I introduced you to key symptoms associated with EI and described how they progress and change over time. Beginning with this chapter, you'll learn how to find out on your own what may be causing your youngster's illness. You'll be challenged to do some detective work. Thousands of concerned parents have used these techniques and discovered the causes of their child's illness. In the process, they have become their youngster's strongest advocate.

■ THE IMPORTANCE OF FINDING THE CAUSES EARLY

A child's entire life can be favorably altered if something that interferes with his or her ability to learn is recognized and treated as early as possible. Drugs can completely relieve a symptom, but the basic illness can march relentlessly onward. For example, a youngster who is hyperactive from molds may sit still after taking an activity-quieting drug, but what happens when the drug is eventually stopped? As a young adult, that individual may experience a recurrence of hyperactivity or some new manifestation of mold-related illness whenever he or she is exposed to a damp environment. This chapter, however, will emphasize the recognition of environmental illness as early as possible, as a first step toward optimal treatment.

If environmental illness is recognized and appropriately treated in the preschool period, for example, it should be possible to prevent or relieve the types of challenges that a person may otherwise face later in life.

THE RISKS OF DOING NOTHING

If EI youngsters are not detected early—and if the cause of their illness is not determined—much more is at stake than poor academic performance. For example, serious secondary psychological and social problems can emerge. It is difficult to feel positive about yourself and your future if you rarely feel well or repeatedly are reprimanded for doing or saying the wrong thing. It is hard to realize your full potential if you feel exhausted, irritable, withdrawn, hyperactive, or aggressive. How can you feel good about yourself if someone is always yelling at you? All children should be given an opportunity to express and expand their natural gifts and innate unique abilities. Those who have EI are definitely discouraged.

If environmentally ill children are treated earlier:

- The number of children requiring special education should decrease.
- The number of students who can't learn at a level commensurate with their ability should diminish.
- They should have a better chance to realize their full potential in both their education and their life.
- Many secondary family, social, and long-term physical and emotional problems may be prevented.

Elimininating the cause of an environmental illness is often more effective and much less expensive than treating the symptoms. The key is prevention, but to stop an illness from developing, you must find and eliminate the cause.

■ STEPS TOWARD EARLY DETECTION

The remainder of this chapter has been divided into three sections:

1. Record-Keeping
This section discusses how to keep written records of your child's symptoms, and the substances to which he or she has been exposed. If done correctly by parents, teachers, and school health personnel, this documentation will organize the information and help provide a wealth of clues to the source of the problem.

2. The "Big Five": How to Pinpoint Why Someone Is Ill
This section explains the "Big Five," a simple, systematic, inexpensive, and fast way to pinpoint exactly what is causing certain individuals to feel unwell, to behave inappropriately, or to be unable to learn at the level consistent with their ability. (Aspects of the "Big Five" will be discussed in even more detail in Chapters 4 and 5—specifically, how a child's appearance, and

handwriting and drawing changes, can reveal how exposures cause health and behavior problems.)

3. Diets That Quickly Detect Food-Related Problems

This section provides easy, inexpensive diets that should give you additional answers in three to seven days.

■ RECORD-KEEPING

When a child or adult does not feel or behave right or can't remember, you should think about the "Big Five" to determine the cause of the symptoms. But first, be prepared to record all pertinent information, preferably in a notebook that has a separate division for each medical or emotional symptom.[1] Detailed records must be kept. List and rate every complaint on a scale similar to this one:

+ = The symptom is slightly or barely evident.
+ + = The symptom is moderately evident.
+ + + = The symptom is severe.

Be sure to date everything and give copies to your physician. For examples of the type of records that can prove most helpful, refer to Tables 3.1 and 3.2. In Table 3.1, you'll find a list of the typical symptoms of environmental illness. There is room on the table for you to write down when a symptom first appeared and if it becomes worse during school hours. This checklist which is helpful in deciding whether environmental illness is a problem for your child. Table 3.2 provides an additional form for record-keeping; it lists questions to ask yourself, to help you figure out what is causing the symptoms. Table 3.3 can help you keep accurate records of the symptoms and when they occur.

TABLE 3.1

Typical Symptoms of Environmental Illness in Schools*

	Date of onset	Is it worse during school hours?
Nose		
Itching, rubbing	_____	_____
Stuffiness	_____	_____
Mucus or congestion	_____	_____
Postnasal drip	_____	_____
Urge to sneeze	_____	_____
Sinus discomfort or facial bone pain	_____	_____
Nosebleeds	_____	_____

	Date of onset	Is it worse during school hours?
Eyes		
Itchiness	_____	_____
Burning	_____	_____
Pain or ache	_____	_____
Tearing	_____	_____
Light sensitivity	_____	_____
Heavy feeling in or around eyes	_____	_____
Dark circles	_____	_____
Bags under eyes	_____	_____
Spacey look; glassy glazed eyes	_____	_____
Frightening or demonic look	_____	_____
Vision		
Blurring, less clarity	_____	_____
Difficulty reading:	_____	_____
Letters mixed up	_____	_____
Words too small or large	_____	_____
Words upside down	_____	_____
Words moving around	_____	_____
Spots, flashes	_____	_____
Too much brightness or darkness	_____	_____
Narrow or tunnel vision	_____	_____
Double vision	_____	_____
Abnormal color vision	_____	_____
Frequent need for new glasses	_____	_____
Throat and Mouth		
Itchiness, soreness, tightness, or swelling in throat	_____	_____
Difficulty swallowing	_____	_____
Throat-clearing	_____	_____
Clucking throat sounds	_____	_____
Weak voice	_____	_____
Hoarseness or choking	_____	_____
Excessive drooling	_____	_____
Bad or metallic taste in mouth	_____	_____
Burning tongue or mouth	_____	_____
Cracked or swollen lips	_____	_____
Ears		
Fullness, blockage	_____	_____
Red earlobes	_____	_____
Ringing in ears	_____	_____
Earches	_____	_____
Hearing loss	_____	_____
Hyperacute hearing	_____	_____

	Date of onset	Is it worse during school hours?
Digestive System		
Bad breath	_____	_____
Nausea	_____	_____
Belching	_____	_____
Bloating	_____	_____
Vomiting	_____	_____
Gagging	_____	_____
Pressure or pain	_____	_____
Cramps	_____	_____
Rumbling, rectal gas	_____	_____
Diarrhea	_____	_____
Constipation	_____	_____
Gallbladder pain (right mid-lower rib cage)	_____	_____
Excessive hunger or thirst	_____	_____
Acid mouth taste	_____	_____
Circulatory System		
Central chest pain	_____	_____
Rapid pulse	_____	_____
Throbbing pulse	_____	_____
Skipped or extra heartbeats	_____	_____
High blood pressure	_____	_____
Spontaneous bruising	_____	_____
Sensitivity to cold	_____	_____
Joints		
Aches, pains	_____	_____
Stiffness	_____	_____
Swelling	_____	_____
Warmth, redness	_____	_____
Muscles		
Tightness, stiffness	_____	_____
Aches, pain, soreness	_____	_____
Nerves		
Tingling in extremities	_____	_____
Numbness of extremities	_____	_____
Fainting	_____	_____
Skin		
Cold hands or feet	_____	_____
Skin rash (local or generalized)	_____	_____
Itchiness	_____	_____
Excessive perspiration	_____	_____

	Date of onset	Is it worse during school hours?
Flushing, hives	_____	_____
Abnormally white or pale face	_____	_____
Red ears, cheeks, tip of nose	_____	_____
Headache		
Migraine (with nausea)	_____	_____
Pressure headache	_____	_____
Stabbing, throbbing, exploding pain	_____	_____
Mood and Behavior		
Depression	_____	_____
Hyperactivity	_____	_____
Irritability	_____	_____
Silliness	_____	_____
Fatigue	_____	_____
Apathy	_____	_____
Dislike of touching or cuddling	_____	_____
Withdrawal	_____	_____
Confusion	_____	_____
Impulsiveness	_____	_____
Lethargy	_____	_____
Insomnia	_____	_____
Excessive sleepiness	_____	_____
Vulgarity	_____	_____
Memory and Learning		
Disorientation	_____	_____
Confusion	_____	_____
Problems remembering or learning:	_____	_____
Names	_____	_____
Past events	_____	_____
New things	_____	_____
Telling time	_____	_____
Poor concentration	_____	_____
Distraction		

*Remember, there are multiple possible causes for all of these symptoms.

TABLE 3.2

If you checked off any symptoms in Table 3.1, ask yourself the following questions:

Have you or any of your family members ever had typical allergies? _____
Hay fever? _____ Asthma or wheezing? _____ Eczema? _____ Hives? _____
Describe it. _____
When did this allergy first occur? _____
How long did it last? _____
Have the symptoms become either **more** or **less** severe? _____
What do you suspect causes the symptoms? _____
Do odors make your child ill? _____
Does your child notice chemical odors **more** or **less readily** than others? _____
When did this first happen? _____
How long do the symptoms last after an exposure to chemicals? _____
Do they last longer now than they did before? _____
Has your child had any major spinal injuries? If so, describe them. _____
_____
Has your child had any surgery or anesthesia? If so, describe it. _____
Is your child taking any medicines? Which ones? At what dose? For how long? _____
Does your child have any drug allergies? _____
   To liquid or tablets? _____
   To which drugs? _____
   What do they do? _____
   When did this first happen? _____
Have there been any recent changes in your child's school or home? What? When? ____
_____
When did your child go to a new or different school or move to a new or different home?
_____
Is anything unusual about the location or building? _____
_____
Do any preexisting medical problems appear to be worse since some school or home
change? _____
What do you think makes your child sick? _____
_____
Does your child have any new health problems? _____
When did they begin? _____
Do any contributing factors make your child feel sick? Is there stress in the family due to
finances, work, relationships, or children? _____
Is there any area or place in the school or home that makes your child feel particularly
well or unwell? _____

In addition, the following table can be very helpful.

TABLE 3.3

Checklist to Detect Possible Environmental Illness or Allergy from Infancy to Old Age

Date _____

Fetal History (in Uterus)
_____Excess hiccups*
_____Excess kicking*
_____Overly active*
_____Overly quiet

Infant History
_____Prolonged screaming/crying*
_____Colic for over 6 months*
_____Excess diarrhea
_____Excess constipation*
_____Excess spitting*
_____Excess vomiting*
_____Nonstop need to be fed
_____Inability to sleep*
_____Extreme head-banging*
_____Excessive crib-rocking*
_____Irritability
_____Excess ear infections by 8
       months*
_____Congestion of nose or chest*
_____Eczema
_____Excessive drooling*
_____Extreme perspiration*
_____Walking before 10 months*
_____Bronchiolitis or wheezy chest
_____Inability to drink milk formulas*
_____Inability to drink soy formulas*

Child History

Nose
_____Symptoms in:
_____ warm months*
_____ cold months*
_____ all year*
_____Stuffy nose*
_____Noisy breathing
_____Watery, runny nose*
_____Sneezes in bouts
_____Upward nose-rubbing*
_____Crease across nose
_____Nose-wiggling*
_____Nose-picking
_____Frequent throat-clearing*
_____Frequent colds*

_____ but not sick*
_____ how often per month?
_____Excessive nosebleeds
_____ how often?
_____Tender nose
_____Number of facial tissues per day

Ears
_____Recurrent ear fluid*
_____On-and-off hearing trouble*
_____Ear-popping
_____Flushed, hot red earlobes
_____Dizziness
_____Ringing in ears

Chest
_____Wheeze (whistle) or asthma with
       infection*
_____ at other times*
_____Cough*
_____ with laughter*
_____ with exercise*
_____ with cold air*
_____ with cold drinks*
_____ at night*
_____ when damp outside*
_____Excessive chest infections*
_____Chronic hoarse voice

Eyes
_____Itchy eyes*
_____Red eyes*
_____Watery eyes*
_____Puffy, baggy eyes*
_____Wrinkles under eyes*
_____Blue/black/red eye circles*
_____Burning eyes
_____Painful eyes
_____Sensitivity to light
_____Frequent squinting/frowning
_____Eye-rubbing*
_____Glassy, glazed, ''spacey'' look*
_____''Demonic'' look*

Skin
_____Pale complexion
_____Eczema or atopic dermatitis*

————Itchy rash on body
————Itchy rash in arm/leg creases*
————Itchy round scaly skin spots*
————Itchy skin—no rash
————Palms extremely wrinkled
————Cracked toes or fingertips*
————Hives or welts*
————Easy bruising
————Tender, sore skin spots
————Swollen face/feet/lips/eyes*
————Puffy fingers or hands
————Sore corners of mouth
————Irritation of mouth corners
————Excess drooling*
————Frequent lip-licking*
————Cracked, dry lips*
————Mottled/bald tongue patches*
————Deep tongue grooves/fissures

Throat
————Excess throat mucus*
————Repeated throat-clearing*
————Itchy roof of mouth
————Ulcers on gums/inside cheeks

Intestines
————Bad breath*
————Frequent bellyaches*
————Frequent nausea*
————Excess rectal gas or belching*
————Bloated abdomen*
————Frequent diarrhea*
————Frequent constipation*
————Itchy rectal area
————Ulcers, gastric or peptic
————Colitis, Crohn's disease

Behavior
————Constant wiggling*
————Irritability*
————Hyperactivity, restlessness
————Moodiness*
————Clumsiness, poor coordination
————Listlessness, tiredness*
————Hostility, aggression*
————Temper tantrums*
————Cries often or easily*
————Unhappiness*
————Excessive nervousness
————Behavior problems*
————Dislike of cuddling*
————Poor balance

————Fainting
————Barking, strange noises*
————Vulgar speech or actions*
————Endless nonsense talking*
————Too much talking*
————Tendency to repeat things
————Poor sleeping*
————Nightmares or night terrors
————Sleepiness in morning*
————Sleepiness after eating*
————Sleepiness after napping
————Unexplained depression*
————Tics or twitching
————Seizures
————Stuttering
————Good vocabulary/inability to
     read
————Poor language development
————Inability to draw, print, or write
————Poor concentration/attention
     span*
————Dislike of loud noises
————Dislike of bright lights
————Dislike of certain odors

Bladder, Kidney, and Urinary Problems
————Wet pants in daytime
————   frequently
————Bed-wetting (after 5 years)*
————   how many times per week?
————Up at night to urinate*
————Recurrent bladder infections
————Other kidney/bladder problems
————Blood in urine
————Urine burns
————Rushing to urinate*
————Difficulty starting urination
————Difficulty stopping urination
————Spraying of bathroom with urine
————Recurring urine problems at
     specific times each year

Miscellaneous
————Headache*
————Neck or shoulder aches
————Backaches
————Leg aches
————Leg cramps*
————Weak legs
————Joint aches
————Tight joints*
————Tingling/numb arms or legs*

_____ Excessive perspiration
_____ Overly sensitive to cold
_____ Excessive infections*
_____ Frequent fever, no infection
_____ Vaginal itching, irritation, or
redness

_____ Irregular heartbeat*
_____ Sudden rapid heartbeat
_____ Unusual body or hair odor
_____ Excessive thirst or appetite*

*Are most frequent symptoms

CONNER'S HYPERACTIVITY SCORE

Your doctor may introduce you to the Conner's hyperactivity score, which is an accepted, simple way to measure your youngster's activity level. Scores between 15 and 30 indicate progressively increasing hyperactivity. Scores below fifteen are considered normal.[2] Scores near 30 indicate problems.

The purpose of the scoring is mainly for comparison. It will enable you to tell if your child's difficulties are staying the same or getting better or worse. If the score is suddenly, consistently too high, ask yourself why. If it suddenly becomes very low, figure out what had this beneficial effect.

TABLE 3.4

Sample Record-Keeping Sheet

Date:

	How does the child feel, behave, or learn*?	How does the child look?	How is the child's writing or drawing?	What is the child's breathing ability (if asthmatic*)?	What is the child's pulse?
Before: Time:	Headache 9 A.M.	ok 10:45 A.M.	ok 10:45 A.M.	350 PFM 10:45 A.M.	80 10:45 A.M.
Exposure: Time:			drank milk 11:00 A.M.		
After: Time:	Headache 11:20 A.M.	ok 11:20 A.M.	ok 11:20 A.M.	250 PFM Wheezing 11:20 A.M.	80 11:20 A.M.

The headache was not caused by the milk because it was evident *before* the milk was ingested and did not become worse *afterward*. However, the breathing became significantly worse, as evidenced by the drop from 350 to 250 in the Peak Flow Meter (PFM) within twenty minutes after drinking milk.

Conclusion: Milk is one possible cause of this child's asthma.

*Other examples of symptoms to record and observe: stuffiness, hives, asthma, cough, bellyache, nausea, irritability, fatigue, anger, hyperactivity, inability to concentrate, or difficulty remembering.

CLUES FROM SCHOOL HEALTH RECORDS

The school health records are another way to document your child's symptoms, and they often help confirm the existence of specific patterned responses. For example, is your child always in the health office on Friday, when the cafeteria serves fish? Some allergic children become ill simply from the odor of cooked fish. If a child is routinely in the principal's office after every school party, this sequence suggests a junk food sensitivity. If a child is a behavior problem or becomes asthmatic each year mainly during the pollen seasons, this indicates a pollen problem. Do you observe any consistent change on rainy damp days, suggesting a mold problem? Does the child develop a headache only after attending art class or when odorous marking pens are used? This suggests a chemical sensitivity. Some children become much worse after exposure to a well-disinfected lavatory, due to the aroma of the chemicals used to clean or "freshen" the room. If a child becomes congested after playing on mats during gym class, think of dust and molds.

Notice if adolescent girls—or female teachers, are in the health office each month at the same time. Just before their menstrual periods, females often crave the very foods or beverages to which they are sensitive. For example, eating chocolate during the menses can totally change how a woman feels and acts. If she doesn't eat or drink favorite foods, she is less likely to change emotionally or physically. The records of the school nurse may reveal a monthly pattern of responses that become evident only after an adverse food or environmental exposure.

Some chemically sensitive females have a significant but unrecognized drop in their white blood count at the time of each menses. The health records of these females can show monthly patterns of infection. Specialists in environmental medicine sometimes can be most helpful in diagnosing and treating this problem (see Resources). They routinely take the time to study records and look for such relationships.

Recurrent monthly cold sores, for example, often respond nicely to treatment with the correct dilution of a flu vaccine; the Premenstrual Syndrome (PMS) also responds well to the correct dilution of progesterone.[3] If a girl or woman has a food craving due to a chocolate sensitivity and cold sores near her menses, a combination of flu vaccine, progesterone, and chocolate allergy extract therapy (after P/N allergy testing) can be immensely helpful.[4]

■ THE "BIG FIVE": HOW TO PINPOINT WHY SOMEONE IS ILL

By using the "Big Five," you can find answers in a surprisingly simple and organized manner. This approach involves comparing the following five variables *before* and then ten to sixty minutes *after* an exposure—that is, before and after eating or drinking, or being in a particular room or area at school or at home. By using it, you can often pinpoint the specific cause of a problem. (Table 3.4 will help you document the information you gather.)

Here are the "Big Five," which you should check whenever applicable:

1. Note how you feel, behave, and think
2. Appearance, how you look
3. Writing and drawing
4. Your breathing
5. Your pulse

The "Big Five" are keys to alert you that something has gone wrong. They should be asked when you or your child suddenly change. Once you know "what" has caused an illness or change in mood or behavior—then ask "when" and "why."

TABLE 3.5

The "Big Five"

Consider each of the following before and after eating or exposures inside each classroom or room at home, outside your school or home, and to all chemicals. Answer these five questions.

Exposure to:

1		2		3		4		5	
How does my child (or do I) feel, behave, and remember?		How does my child (or do I) look?		Is there any handwriting or drawing change?		Is there asthma or a breathing problem present*?		Is there a change in the pulse rate or rhythm?**?	
Before	After	Before	After	Before	After	Before	After	Before	After
____	____	____	____	____	____	____	____	____	____
____	____	____	____	____	____	____	____	____	____
____	____	____	____	____	____	____	____	____	____
____	____	____	____	____	____	____	____	____	____
____	____	____	____	____	____	____	____	____	____
____	____	____	____	____	____	____	____	____	____
____	____	____	____	____	____	____	____	____	____

*Use a Peak Flow Meter if wheezing is a problem. Note a drop of over 10 to 15 percent.
**Check for a pulse increase over 20 beats per minute or a change in pulse rhythm.

1. CHECK HOW YOU FEEL, BEHAVE, AND THINK

It can be difficult to remember when a headache began. Try to recall whether it was before or after eating, entering a room, going outside, or smelling some odor. Learn to observe your child closely when a reaction is taking place. Note everything. Does your child learn well in the morning but poorly in the afternoon? Does this change also occur at home? Does the change occur before or after lunch, a snack, or a party? When does the child have to rush to the lavatory? Do failing grades occur in only one classroom? When does irritability, hyperactivity, fatigue, or an inability to think clearly become evident? If you were not there, you will have to depend on your child's recollection. When is the reaction is over? The answers are often obvious—but only after someone has taken the time to ask. The videotape *Environmentally Sick Schools* vividly documents the many reactions that can occur within minutes after a variety of adverse exposures. (See the list of videos in For Further Reading.)

2. CHECK THE APPEARANCE

Does your child (or do you) look different in some way during school hours or when you are at home or outside? Note obvious changes such as red earlobes, black eye circles, nose-rubbing, puffiness below the eyes, red cheeks, wiggly legs, throat-clearing, or clucking throat sounds. A sudden change in appearance can be an early warning that some form of an environmental illness is about to begin.

In Chapter 4 I'll discuss in detail how you can compare the appearance of your child before, during, and after school, home, or other exposures. Once you identify these changes and determine what was eaten, smelled, or touched just before they occurred, you can easily pinpoint many causes of these types of changes.

3. CHECK WRITING AND DRAWING

Changes in the way your youngster writes or draws, and the content of his writing and illustrations, may indicate an adverse environmental exposure. Have your child write and/or draw before and after each class, snack, or chemical exposure. Do this in every area of your child's school and home. The variety of changes that can become readily apparent is astonishing.

Chapter 5 illustrates many of these characteristic samples of writing and drawing that occur after environmental exposures, eating, or P/N allergy testing. This chapter will provide the details about how you can identify the causes of these variations.

4. CHECK THE BREATHING

If your child (or you) develops asthma, irritable or reactive airway disease, or a cough after exercising, laughing, being exposed to cold air, or drinking cold beverages, the answer is literally only a breath away. (If your child has no breathing problems, skip this step, since it is not necessary.)

Those who have lung problems should learn to use a Peak Flow Meter (PFM) (available from suppliers listed in Resources). Different meters are designed for children and adults. Most children over five years of age can use them accurately. A PFM is merely a hollow plastic tube with a movable gauge. The lips should tightly encircle the mouthpiece. When an individual blows one breath quickly and vigorously into the tube, the air pressure that is generated moves the gauge. The degree of movement is roughly reflected on the graduations on the gauge, so it reflects a person's ability to breathe.

Here are some typical readings. If a child blows 300 before chemistry, biology, gym, or art class, and 200 about fifteen to forty-five minutes later, it means his lungs have gone into spasm. Such a sudden drop must have a cause. A decrease of 15 percent is usually significant (like 100 to 85, or 200 to 170). Keep asking the key question: What did the child eat, touch, or smell? What was different that day in his chemistry, biology, gym, or art class? If the PFM drop occurred at home, look for the same clues. Did it happen after certain cleaning materials or a vacuum cleaner were used? A Peak Flow Meter can be used before and after each meal, in every class, and in every room. Check your child's breathing after any special exposure and in every possible problem area, including the school bus, a cafeteria, gym, lavatory, or pool. Measure how well your child (or you) blows into this instrument when outdoors compared with indoors, or when in a school building compared to your home. Notice if eating, drinking, or chemical exposures cause any significant change.

The downhill course in the learning ability of some environmentally ill children and the careers of many capable adults can be totally reversed by the actions of one caring, knowledgeable individual. Maybe that person can be you.

A PRACTICAL EXAMPLE

One mother knew her son's PFM reading always ranged between 200 and 230. At one time, his breathing level consistently and inexplicably fell to about 150 and he began to wheeze, but this happened only at home, not at school or at our clinic. Detailed discussions revealed nothing new or different about the boy's diet or home environment—except for a possible natural gas leak from the furnace or stove. A furnace leak was finally found. When the leak was eliminated, the PFM again registered above 200, and the asthma disappeared.

Gas leaks can be difficult to detect. If a similar drop in a PFM reading had occurred primarily or only at school, the parents would have tried to find out what in the school building or classroom was causing the problem. There are definite reasons why a child's health becomes either worse or better in a particular place. Learn to find those reasons.

Check your child's PFM readings both before and ten to thirty minutes after the use of any drugs to treat asthma. The propellants that expel the aerosol medications used to treat asthma can contain Freon or chlorofluorocarbons and artificial sweeteners. If these substances cause asthma in your child, his treatment can actually hinder his breathing.[5]

A Basic General Principle: If you can find and eliminate the cause of a health, behavior, or learning problem, it is certainly possible to diminish or eliminate the need for drugs.

---

5. CHECK FOR PULSE CHANGES

Parents, teachers, and older students should all learn to check their pulses. If you are unsure about how to do it, ask any medically trained person, such as a friend who is a nurse, to teach you. It is really very simple. All you need is a watch or clock with a second hand. Put the back of one wrist into the opposite open palm. Curl your fingers around the outer edge of the wrist. Now gently feel that area. One of the first three fingers should feel a pulsating blood vessel. Merely count the beats for a full minute. Normally the pulse ranges from about 65 to 80 beats per minute, but each person has his or her own normal level.

If your child's resting pulse increases by about 20 points over its normal level, you may have found a clue to identifying his problem. Getting to the root of an environmental illness often means learning what causes a pulse to increase significantly when the person is quiet and calm. A resting pulse over 90 to 100 is often indicative of stress within the body. Such a stress could be due to a food or environmental exposure.

Any sudden, unexplained 20-point increase in the resting pulse can be an early warning. Like a silent smoke alarm, the pulse is your own personal and very sensitive warning system. The greater the pulse elevation, the stronger the indication that the body may be at risk. Large pulse increases frequently indicate that an exposure to something has placed the body in the "alert mode."

Keep in mind that a child should be at rest and neither excited nor crying for this change to be significant. A pulse normally goes up if the person exercises, cries, becomes upset, or is stressed. It is a normal response to exertion or an emotionally stressful situation. Moreover, a slight increase of 10 to 15 points is normal after a meal. If, however, there is no obvious reason for a significant increase, you must look for what has caused it. The cause may seem elusive at first, but with a little thought, you can often find it.

Sometimes a pulse change is not an increase but a distinct irregularity. If a pulse is not beating smoothly and regularly, this again provides a clue. In some adults, the pulse can suddenly beat much too quickly, sometimes above 180, or too slowly, in the range of 40 to 50. Notice when this happens. Similarly, some blood pressure elevations are also directly related to offending exposures. *Some cardiac problems, including heart attacks, are en-*

WHAT CAN TEACHERS DO?

Teachers are not hired to be physicians or parents, but with so many single- and working-mother families today, they are sometimes the only people who regularly see youngsters for long enough periods to spot the cause of a problem. They should try to recognize patterns of illness in their students (and also in themselves). They should notice if a child repeatedly has allergic symptoms or feels unwell. Does a particular student seem unable to learn on a particular day of the week, at a specific time, or in a certain place? Does another child's academic performance, behavior, or health seem to differ in some way at certain times of the year, every year? When does a child not look or act right? Does a child have sudden mood swings or act inappropriately?

There is often an obvious explanation when an adorable Dr. Jekyll child switches suddenly to an impossible Mr. Hyde.

Some teachers have become extremely perceptive in this regard because of the many hours and days they spend with children. But for other educators, as well as counselors, psychologists, and physicians, there remains a critical gap of understanding. They can be unaware, uninformed, or disbelieving about the effects of the environment or foods on children's behavior or performance.

Teachers can help raise the awareness of affected students and their parents. In turn, parents can attempt to confirm the teacher's observations by watching their child after school and on weekends. If necessary, teachers should take the time to reflect upon why they *personally* are not feeling right or remembering as well as they should. Do these problems happen at certain times or in specific places within the school?

tirely due to environmental factors, especially to chemical exposures. (Ask if your cardiologist is familiar with the articles and books written by William Rea, M.D.[6] His many research studies provide valid scientific evidence that has turned some lives around.)

HOW ONE FAMILY ILLUSTRATES A GENERAL PRINCIPLE

Findings from the "Big Five" can have implications for more than just the affected youngster. For example, the discovery of one child's sensitivity to chocolate alerted other family members to a food problem common to all of them. An awareness of the effects of chocolate on the little girl's activity and ability to learn eventually enabled her mother and grandmother to recognize that chocolate caused their own symptoms. Whenever the mother ate chocolate, within thirty minutes she would routinely develop spasms or cramps in her heart called PVCs (paroxysmal ventricular contractions). If the grandmother ate chocolate in the evening, she tended to awaken during the night with an alarmingly rapid heartbeat (tachycardia). Her physicians did not recognize the cause of her reaction because the tachycardia did not take place until several hours after eating dinner. In an allergy testing clinic, however, the child's and mother's reactions could be reproduced in ten minutes by replicating an exposure to chocolate. When the grandmother stopped eating chocolate desserts after dinner, her rapid heartbeat at night was no longer evident.

> **I**f a particular food or other item bothers one member of a family, it is not unusual for that same food or item to affect other family members. The symptoms in each individual, however, may be quite different.

WHEN TO DO THE "BIG FIVE"

Not all of the "Big Five" must be checked. For example, there is no need to check your child's breathing if asthma is of no concern. In some individuals, the pulse test repeatedly provides no clues, so skip it. If some other measurable bodily function, such as blood pressure, however, is a problem, check it "before and after," as indicated previously.

The following guidelines describe the situations in which the "Big Five" should generally be checked. Remember, the key question to ask is: What was smelled, eaten, or touched just before some change became evident?

FOODS

Check every food or beverage that your child commonly eats. When time permits, check before and fifteen to sixty minutes after each meal, snack, or party. If a meal causes symptoms, wait five to seven days, preferably until a weekend, for the symptoms to subside. Then deliberately give the child a small portion of each food that was ingested during the problem meal. Check one separate food or beverage item every two hours. Do the "Big Five" before and after each item is ingested, until you find the one that reproduces the changes that were originally noted. In school celebrations, the "life of the party" child is often the one who is sensitive to certain ingredients in junk food.

ROOMS

Check every room inside your child's school and your home. Do the "Big Five" before a student's problem enters each classroom and again after thirty to sixty minutes. Check even the lavatory, auditorium, halls, music room, and basement. Check before and after leaving home and after returning from school. Sometimes it is necessary to check immediately before and after the school bus ride to and from school. Similarly, check each room at home to see if it causes symptoms. Do the "Big Five" at least once for each room, including the cellar, garage, bathroom, family room, and bedroom.

INDOORS AND OUTDOORS

Do the "Big Five" before a child goes outside. After a child has played, does recess or outside play for thirty to sixty minutes cause any significant change? Think about the presence of lawn-cuttings, pesticides, and aerial sprays, as well as asphalt, tar, and paint, and/or wind-blown factory pollution if major changes become evident.

CHEMICALS

If your physician approves, do the "Big Five" before and then again two to ten minutes after your child is exposed to a specific chemical. Suppose your youngster complains or feels worse from a particular smell. First check the normal pulse and breathing, as well as how your child looks, feels, behaves, and writes. Then spray a three-inch spot of the suspect perfume or chemical product on a paper towel. Without telling her what you are doing, tape the paper towel two to three feet away while your child plays a quiet game or reads a story. Look for changes during the next few minutes. Have someone videotape any reactions if you need proof for a skeptical principal, teacher, relative, doctor, psychologist, friend, or insurance company.

Ten to thirty minutes of fresh air or oxygen at four liters per minute will usually stop many reactions to chemical odors rather quickly.

Never purposefully expose yourself or anyone else if you suspect something might cause a severe, life-threatening, or frightening reaction. Always check with your physician first. Do chemical challenges in your doctor's office, unless you have permission to do them at home without supervision.

ALLERGY EXTRACTS

Although most allergic individuals are better after their allergy extract treatments, some definitely become worse. One common reason is that some major allergenic component (dust, molds, and the like) in the extract is in a concentration that an individual does not tolerate well. Others react to the preservative—such as phenol, glycerine, or benzyl alcohol—used in the extract preparation. Once again, do the ''Big Five'' before and again ten to thirty minutes after a dose of extract is administered to your child. Test each bottle of allergy extract separately. If every extract treatment causes symptoms, be very suspicious of the preservative or the substances in which the various components are diluted.

OTHER COMMON ITEMS TO CHECK

Drugs, vitamins, antibiotics, immunization vaccines, and dental anesthetics, among other things, can be checked one at a time, before and after a purposeful exposure.

Do the ''Big Five'' whenever your child starts a new medicine and whenever you are suspicious of a drug or any other form of treatment taken by mouth. *As with chemicals, check with your doctor before you try to test medications. It is best and safest to check out any suspect drugs only at your doctor's office.*

The procedure is simple. You or your doctor places a drop or two of a liquid or a piece of a pill under the tongue for two to three minutes. Then you remove it and see what happens. If one or more of the ''Big Five'' changes significantly in ten minutes, check with your physician before your child takes any more of that prescribed medicine.

Remember, it is possible to be allergic to a new drug or to suddenly become sensitive to a drug *that you've taken repeatedly in the past without difficulty.* Drug sensitivities can arise at any time, sometimes after years of use, so always be alert.

Check the ''Big Five'' for each drug or medicine you routinely use. Although drugs usually relieve illness, at times they cause health problems.

Throughout this entire "Big Five" process, notice whether your child routinely feels worse as the school day or week progresses but seems better a few hours after school or on the weekends. If this happens, it suggests a possible gradual buildup of allergenic substances or other exposures. Find out whether the school is serving wholesome foods in the cafeteria. Serve such foods at home. Check out snacks and vending machines. Is your child swapping lunches? Has the school's water been analyzed for germs, lead, and/or chemicals?

Confusion can arise because some EI children's difficulties are sporadic and seem to appear suddenly for no specific reason. Once you have done the "Big Five," take the time to think about *why* your child is ill in a specific place, at a certain time, or on a particular day. Parents do not have to believe that their children's medical, emotional, and/or learning problems are "all in their head" or that they should "try harder," "learn to live with it," or "discipline better." Psychotherapy is certainly helpful and even necessary for many affected children and parents, but it is often completely ineffective until the environmental aspects of the illness are recognized and appropriately treated.

The key is to keep asking yourself: What did the child eat, touch, or smell in the fifteen minutes to an hour before the problem became apparent? Was it something inside or outside the school or home, perhaps a food or a chemical?

Remember: *Most reactions to offending exposures inside buildings or to foods occur within an hour of the exposure and last for a few minutes or hours. Some delayed food reactions may not occur for eight hours or more. On rare occasions, eating a normal-sized portion of one food will create symptoms that persist for as long as eight days. In contrast, chemicals tend to cause symptoms within seconds or minutes, and they can last for a few seconds or minutes or, at times, for several hours, days, or unfortunately, at times, much longer.*

■ DIETS THAT QUICKLY DETECT FOOD-RELATED PROBLEMS

Special diets are another way to pinpoint the cause of your child's (or your own) symptoms. If you suspect that a food interferes with how your child feels or performs in school or at home, there are two major allergy diets that are quite fast, easy, inexpensive—and can help you evaluate or resolve the problem:

The *Food Elimination Diets* (single and multiple foods) are diagnostic. They confirm if there is a single or multiple food problem.

The *Rotation Diet* is basically a treatment diet.

For the remainder of this chapter, I'll discuss how to use these diets to find the cause of your child's, or possibly your own, difficulties.

> **M**ajor Caution: Do *not* allow anyone to eat any food if you already know causes a severe allergic reaction. Never test any food without your doctor's advice if it has caused serious medical problems in the past. For example: If eggs or peanuts caused immediate throat swelling, or if fish caused severe asthma, it can be unsafe to smell or to eat even a speck of these foods. **Test only those food items that are routinely eaten.** These diets help to determine whether frequently eaten foods are causing problems.

SINGLE FOOD ELIMINATION DIET

If you suspect that a single, frequently eaten food is the cause of your child's problem, try the Single Food Elimination Diet. Merely stop consumption of that suspect food, in *every* form, for seven to twelve days. After twelve days (or sooner, if the symptoms disappear), feed the food again. If there is a true food sensitivity, the symptoms should recur about an hour after a normal-sized portion is eaten on an empty stomach. An empty stomach means nothing has been eaten for at least four hours. (On rare occasions, a child will have to eat the offending food for two or more consecutive days before the symptoms recur.) It is sometimes possible to relieve food-related symptoms within twenty minutes. Try taking Alka Aid (available in health food stores) or Alka-Seltzer Antacid Formula without aspirin in gold foil (available in drugstores), or about 250–500 mg of vitamin C, shortly after symptoms are noted.

Although the symptoms caused by a single food can vary, some food sensitivities commonly occur in several family members. The same food may cause one child to develop headaches, another a stuffy nose, a third hyperactivity, and another to wet the bed. The same food—milk, for example—can be a problem for several generations of a family. You may want to place your entire family on the diet to find out if a variety of symptoms in several family members share one common cause.

THE MULTIPLE FOOD ELIMINATION DIET

PART ONE
The Multiple Food Elimination Diet is a fast, inexpensive method of food allergy detection that can sometimes provide rapid, safe relief from symp-

TABLE 3.6

Multiple Elimination Diet, Part One

Food	Allowed	Forbidden
Cereals	Rice (Rice Puffs only); oats (oatmeal made with honey); barley. Someone who has a gluten sensitivity will react to any grain.	*Foods containing wheat flour (most cakes, cookies, bread, baked goods); corn and popcorn; cereal mixtures (like granola).*
Fruits	All fresh fruits, except citrus; canned fruit, but only if in its own juice and without artificial color, sugar, or preservatives.	*Citrus (orange, lemon, lime, grapefruit). All fruits or juices could cause symptoms, but citrus is the most common.*
Vegetables	All fresh vegetables, except corn and peas; french fries (homemade); potatoes; soy.	*All frozen and canned vegetables; corn, peas, and mixed vegetables.*
Meats	Chicken and turkey (non-basted); Louis Rich ground turkey; veal and beef; pork; lamb; fish, tuna.	*Luncheon meats, wieners, bacon; artificially dyed hamburger meat; ham; dyed salmon and lobster; breaded and stuffed meats.*
Beverages	Water; single herb or plain tea and honey; grape juice, bottled (Welch's); frozen apple juice (Lincoln or pure apple); pure pineapple juice. No corn or dextrose additives.	*Milk; all dairy drinks with casein or whey; fruit beverages except those specified; Kool–Aid, Coffee Rich (yellow dye); 7–Up, Squirt, Teem, cola, Dr Pepper, ginger ale.*
Snacks	Potato chips (no additives); RyKrisp crackers and pure honey; raisins (unsulfured).	*Corn chips (Fritos); chocolate and cocoa; hard candy, ice cream, and sherbet.*
Miscellaneous	Pure honey; homemade oil and vinegar dressing; sea salt; pepper; pure maple syrup; homemade soup.	*Sugar; bread, cakes, and cookies (except special recipes); eggs; dyed (colored) vitamins, pills, mouthwash, toothpaste, medicines, cough syrups, etc.; jelly and jam; Jell-O; margarine and diet spreads (dyes and corn); peanut butter and peanuts; sorbitol (corn); cheese.*

TABLE 3.7

Hidden Sources of Problem Foods

Problem Food	Hidden Sources
Milk and dairy	Yogurt, cheese, ice cream, casein, sodium caseinate, whey
Wheat	Bread, most cereals, cake, cookies, baked goods
Chocolate	Cocoa or cola
Peas	Peanut butter
Citrus	Orange, lemon, lime, grapefruit
Food coloring, food additives, and preservatives	Luncheon meats, sausage, ham, bacon, and packaged baked goods

---

toms which have perplexed everyone for years. It usually helps within a week, and it enables you to pinpoint exactly which food items are causing specific symptoms during the following week or ten days. Use this diet if you suspect that several foods or beverages are bothering your child (or you). A person's favorite foods are usually the major culprits. Sometimes entire families feel dramatically better on this diet in three to seven days. A few people will become asymptomatic as early as the second day or as late as the fourteenth day. (Typical histories of children who responded well and quickly to this diet are discussed in Chapter 8.)

During part one of the diet, your child can eat many foods (as listed in Table 3.6), including *most* fruits, vegetables, and meats, as well as some grains. As the table indicates, however, there are some forbidden foods. Any item that your child craves or eats in excess can be a cause of medical or emotional problems. Be sure to avoid all the hidden sources of common problem foods (see Table 3.7). Read every label of everything your youngster eats or drinks to make sure it is free of the additives he must avoid.

Your child must avoid *all* coffee, tea, alcohol, tobacco, or craved foods, including even mushrooms, sunflower seeds, and the like. Avoid, in particular, any food that is frequently eaten in excess. Note that milk, wheat, chocolate, sugar, and corn are often found in children's favorite foods, such as cookies and cake.

The "allowed" foods can be selected, combined, and eaten in any quantity. If you are a bit suspicious of a particular food, start by giving your child a tiny amount of it and increase it gradually during the day if no symptoms become evident. If you do the "Big Five" just before or 30 to 60 minutes after your child eats only the suspect food, you'll quickly know if that one is a problem. Keep detailed records in a food diary of *exactly* what is eaten and any reaction to it.

For a beverage, you can mix the allowed fruits in a blender with spring water and honey or pure maple syrup. Use this mixture on cereal to replace milk, or combine it with carbonated water to create soda pop.

Improvement noted on day two may greatly increase by day seven, so continue with this part of the diet for seven days. The major object is to see the maximum amount of improvement during the first seven days. If your child feels better in a week or less, begin part two of the diet on the eighth day (see page 57).

A 90 percent improvement means that a major cause of your child's health or learning problem is food. If your child improves 20 percent, foods are probably a smaller part of the illness. Consider dust, pollen, molds, pets, and chemicals as other possible factors.

If your child has *not* improved within a week, recheck the diet records for that week. Were *only* the allowed foods eaten? If your child repeatedly forgot and ate the wrong foods or drank the wrong beverages, the item that was *not* deleted or omitted from the diet may be the culprit. Try part one again, but this time, adhere more strictly to the diet. It is best to do the diet only once, but do it right. School lunches must be brought from home and contain only the allowed foods (see the history of Sidney in Chapter 18. He had an extra year of illness simply because the diet was done poorly the first time).

Some individuals may develop worse symptoms during the first two to three days of part one. Nausea, headaches, congestion, muscle aches, and irritability are common. These are withdrawal symptoms and will usually subside by the fourth day. If your child gets *worse* on the fifth or sixth day, suspect whatever food you substituted for milk or whatever food the child ate in excess while on the diet (such as potatoes). Suppose your child drank apple or grape juice instead of milk. Either may be a cause of the medical complaints. If the symptoms worsen, retry part one, but this time also stop the new food or beverage suspects as well.

If an infection occurs during the diet, stop the diet. It will be too difficult to interpret the results if you continue. If your child always has an infection, he needs the help of an environmental medical specialist. The cause of such a problem can be found by provocation/neutralization allergy testing, without using a diet.

In rare cases, people who were not helped during the first week will dramatically improve when the diet is prolonged. If the first week of the diet did not help, continue with part one for a second week. But if part one of the diet has not helped by the fourteenth day, this particular diet is not going to help you find answers. Your child's health problems may be unrelated to food, or to the foods omitted on this diet. The symptoms may also be due to a frequently eaten item—such as apple juice, grape juice, mushrooms, cinnamon, coffee, tea, tobacco, or alcohol—that was not removed from the diet.

Be sure to do the "Big Five" in the morning and evening of each day during the first week. If the child's writing and drawing change, it suggests that the tested food could be affecting his schoolwork.

PART TWO

During part two of the diet, each food that is normally a part of your child's diet is reintroduced. Add each one at a time, as indicated below.

Day 8 Add milk	Day 13 Add food coloring
Day 9 Add wheat	Day 14 Add corn
Day 10 Add sugar	Day 15 Add preservatives
Day 11 Add egg	Day 16 Add citrus
Day 12 Add cocoa	Day 17 Add peanut butter

The specific details of part two appear on page 59. Now keep in mind that your aim is to have your child eat each food on its specified day to see what effect it has upon how your child feels and conducts himself. (Obtain your physician's advice before you, try even a speck of any food that you know or even suspect is a serious problem or any food that you do not

---

USING AN ALKALI TO HELP RELIEVE FOOD-RELATED SYMPTOMS

Alkali preparations were designed to relieve acid indigestion such as heartburn, but they can also help detect, prevent, and treat many allergic responses to foods. If symptoms develop as you add foods back into your child's diet, Alka-Seltzer Antacid Formula from any drugstore or Alka Aid from a health food store may be used. (People with kidney or heart problems should check with their physician before using either preparation.)

The dose for a child is one-half tablet for a three-year-old, one tablet for a six-year-old, and two tablets for a twelve-year-old or adult (see Table 3.9). Alkali preparations do not help all food reactions, but they do appear to reduce or eliminate roughly two-thirds of such responses in less than twenty minutes.

To be safe, always have your child's usual allergy medications handy so symptoms can be relieved quickly if they occur. If you are concerned, immediately check with your doctor.

If some form of alkali is effective, it suggests that a food allergy is present. Immediately write down everything that your child ate or smelled within the previous few hours. An alkali also can help relieve symptoms from chemical odors.

TABLE 3.8

Common Food Contaminants

Pesticides	Most fruits and vegetables, root vegetables, carrots, beets, potatoes; less, if soil is not contaminated. Most meats, unless raised on organic farms
Hormones	Chicken and turkey, some milk
Fumigants	Nuts, raisins, figs, dates, prunes, dried fruits, grains, dried beans; sometimes chocolate, carob, tapioca, arrowroot
Bleaches	Grains (flour, rice)
Sulfur	Peaches, apricots, nectarines, raisins
Sulfur Dioxide (anti-brown agent)	French fries, fresh fruits, molasses, marmalade
Dyes	Citrus, cherries; sweet or Irish potatoes; butter, oleomargarine; meats such as wieners, bologna, and hamburger; cake decorations; soft drinks
Gas	Apples, pears, bananas with brown streaks (ethylene); roasted coffee (flame exposure); sugar, syrups (bone char filtration)
Wax (paraffin)	Apples, cucumbers, eggplant, peppers, parsnip, turnips, rutabagas, citrus fruits
Chemicals	Saccharine, artificial sweeteners, phenol in food cans, plastic, Styrofoam for packaging, some decaffeinated coffee

Source: Used by permission. Bonnye L. Matthews, *Chemical Sensitivity* (Jefferson, NC: McFarland and Co., 1992).

TABLE 3.9

Alkalai Preparations

	Sodium Bicarbonate	Potassium Bicarbonate	Ratio of Sodium Bicarbonate to Potassium Bicarbonate	Citric Acid
Alka Aid (1 tablet)	360 mg.	180 mg.	2:1	0
Alka-Seltzer Antacid Formula (1 tablet)	958 mg.	312 mg.	3:1	832 mg.*
Baking soda (1 teaspoon)	952 mg.	0	—	0

*Due to this ingredient, it might be a problem for those sensitive to citrus.

routinely eat.) Start with about a quarter of a cup or try a smaller amount, such as half a teaspoon, if there is any reason to be more cautious. Double the amount taken every two to four hours, provided you see no changes in the "Big Five." Gradually increase the amount to a normal-sized portion.

Keep a detailed record of how your child feels at the beginning and the end of each day, and observe him or her carefully for one hour after suspect foods are eaten again. Do any symptoms suddenly reappear? If no symptoms appear during that day, during the night, or the next morning before breakfast, the food is probably all right, and it may be eaten whenever it is desired.

Watch closely to see what happens each day. Do the "Big Five" before and after reintroducing each food. One food may cause a stuffy nose, the next no reaction at all, and the next a bellyache. Some reactions occur immediately; others take several hours. Usually the symptoms caused by a food occur within an hour; however, some food-related symptoms, such as eczema or itchy skin, canker sores, bed-wetting, tight joints, ear fluid, and bowel problems, tend to cause delayed reactions that appear several hours later, so that final decisions can't be made until the next day.

If a test food causes symptoms, your child should stop eating it, in all its forms, until you can secure the advice of your physician. Do not reintroduce another food until the symptoms from the previous one subside.

If Alka-Seltzer in gold foil does not help and the reaction lasts more than twenty-four hours, *do not try* to reintroduce another possible problem food until this reaction has *entirely* subsided.

Not all food reactions are due to foods. They can be due to various additives or chemicals used to grow or preserve them. Washing, cooking, and peeling helps but will not remove all the pesticides or other chemicals (see Table 3.8).

If you are uncertain whether a food causes symptoms, discontinue it until the rest of the foods are reintroduced. Then try that suspect food again at five-day intervals. See if the symptoms recur each time.

Here are some day-by-day guidelines for implementing part two:

Day 8: The day you add milk, give your child lots of it, along with cottage cheese and whipped cream sweetened with pure maple syrup or honey. He should eat no butter, margarine, or yellow cheese, however, unless you are absolutely certain they contain no yellow dyes.

Day 9: The day you add wheat, give your child Triscuits or pure wheat cereal. If these are all right but bread is not, yeast may be the problem. If your child had trouble with milk, be sure not to use any wheat products that contain milk (casein or whey). If you do and your child gets worse, you won't know whether milk or wheat is at fault. Italian bread and kosher bread should not contain milk, but always read the label to be sure. Bake bread if you like, but do not use eggs or sugar. If the milk day caused no problem, milk products can be eaten.

Day 10: The day you add sugar, give your child sugar cubes and add granulated sugar to the allowed foods. If milk or wheat caused trouble, avoid them, or you won't be able to tell whether he tolerates sugar. Many children react within an hour to four to eight sugar cubes eaten by themselves on an empty stomach. Pure water is allowed.

Day 11: The day you add egg, give eggs cooked in the normal way. Custard is allowed, but remember, no milk, wheat, or sugar can be consumed if any of these caused problems. Do not give egg if you already know that egg is a problem. If sugar caused symptoms, use honey or pure maple syrup as a sweetener.

Day 12: The day you add cocoa, give your child dark chocolate with water, cocoa (pure Hershey's cocoa powder), and honey or pure maple syrup. No candy bars are allowed, since most of them contain milk, sugar, and corn. Remember, no milk, wheat, sugar, or egg is allowed if any of these caused symptoms.

Day 13: The day you add food coloring, give Jell-O, jelly, or artificially colored fruit beverages (soda pop, Kool-Aid), Popsicles, or cereal. If you prefer, add food coloring to plain pure gelatin. Try to give him a variety of yellow, purple, and red items because only one of these colors may be causing the reaction. Remember, avoid milk, wheat, sugar, eggs, and cocoa if any of these were a problem.

Day 14: The day you add corn, give corn, cornmeal, and plain popcorn. It is not unusual for only one such form of corn to cause symptoms. (Do not give him cornflakes, which contain sugar, malt, and the preservative BHT.) If milk, wheat, sugar, egg, cocoa, or food coloring caused trouble, do not give any of these. Do not use butter on popcorn if your child has a milk sensitivity.

Day 15: The day you add preservatives, give foods that contain preservatives and food additives. Read every label. In particular, give him luncheon meat, bologna, hot dogs, bread, baked goods, and soups, which commonly contain many preservatives and additives.

Day 16: The day you add citrus, give fresh fruit or lemon, lime, grapefruit, or orange juice. Avoid artificial dyes if food colors were a problem. Fruit "drinks" contain much less fruit than juice.

Day 17: The day you add peanut butter, give your child lots of peanut butter or peanuts. Test for this only if it is a favorite food. Use RyKrisp if no wheat is allowed. Use pure peanut butter without additives from a health food store, or Smucker's. **Don't test peanut or soy products if either caused serious health problems in the past.**

Once you determine which food causes a specific symptom, you must discuss your conclusions with your physician. Some foods cannot be omitted from the diet indefinitely if proper nutrition is to be maintained. Ask your doctor for the help of a dietitian or nutritionist if you have specific diet questions (see Resources).

If your child refuses to go on the diet at all, try offering a reward. Promise a gala party if there is no cheating and if he or she is truly cooperating in every way. The party should take place after both parts of the diet are completed. At that time, allow your child to have the foods that caused the symptoms, providing these were not severe or incapacitating. This will be a double-check, confirming that these foods had that effect. If you prefer not to repeat a reaction, don't give that food again, or try an alkali.

If your child has asthma, add the test food back into the diet with extreme care. It is possible that a problem food could precipitate a sudden, severe asthma attack, even though the child frequently ate it in the past. Have asthma medications on hand during part two of the diet, and use the Peak Flow Meter to help find out exactly what is causing your child to wheeze. If you are concerned, or if his asthma has been severe or frightening in the past, check with your doctor before trying the diet.

If your child is routinely worse (impatient, angry, tired, irritable, headachy, or hyperactive) before meals, consider whether he has hypoglycemia or low blood sugar. If hypoglycemia does turn out to be the problem, provide a small protein snack every hour or two throughout the day. This will reduce his ups and downs. Remember, however, that some children (and adults) have both food allergies *and* hypoglycemia. If they have both problems, they can get worse before and after eating. And the diagnosis is often missed for years.

Once again, do the "Big Five" before and after reintroducing each suspect food in part two.

> The Multiple Elimination Diet should be used only on a short-term basis. It is not nutritionally balanced and should never be used for more than two or three weeks without consulting a physician or a certified nutritionist.

WILL MEDICATIONS AFFECT THE DIET?

Your child can take his usual medications during the food elimination diets. If he improves, you may find that he needs less of some medicines, such as antihistamines, asthma medications, or activity-modifying drugs, by the end of the first week. But check with your doctor before stopping an activity-modifying drug, because if they are tapered too fast, these drugs can cause serious problems in some children. If you can't tell when you miss or are late for a dose, your child may no longer need the drug as often as it is being given.

Try to use only colorless liquid medications or white pills. For small children, crush them and place them in applesauce or mashed potatoes. Pills are best because many liquid medications contain corn, sugar, artificial flavors, and food dyes, all of which may cause symptoms.

Try not to give your child antihistamines or Intal (cromolyn sodium) before a food is reintroduced during part two of the diet. These drugs may prevent a food reaction from taking place. You can purposely use Intal to prevent food reactions at celebrations or parties, however, when it is difficult to control what your child eats. Because Intal prevents food allergies, it can be used to help both the diagnosis and treatment of food sensitivities.

Also, don't try this diet for a week after your child has had a flu, tetanus, or other inoculation. Immediate or delayed vaccine reactions can confuse the interpretation of the diet. Check with your child's physician about any questions you may have regarding any aspect of this plan.

THE ROTATION DIET

The Rotation Diet is a treatment diet. It is often used on a long term basis—for several months or, if necessary, for many years. It may not begin to reduce symptoms for about a month, but in time it often enables a person to eat a wider variety of foods without difficulty, and it quickly indicates if a new food sensitivity develops.

Basically, with the Rotation Diet, no food is eaten any more frequently than every four days. With this diet, the body eliminates ingested foods more fully before they are eaten again. It is thought to help prevent food allergies. It also quickly indicates if a new food sensitivity is present because whenever one begins, the symptoms reappear like clockwork at four-day intervals, when that food is eaten. This approach enables an individual, usually over a period of months, to eat normal amounts of certain foods without difficulty, even though they previously caused mild to moderate symptoms. For detailed examples of the Rotation Diet, see Tables 3.10 and 3.11. This diet cannot be used to treat severe life-threatening food allergies.

TABLE 3.10

A Sample 4-Day Rotation

	Day 1	Day 2	Day 3	Day 4
Meat	beef	turkey	pork or fish	chicken
Vegetable	potato	squash	sweet potato	carrots
Fruit	berries	melon	grape	citrus
Grain	wheat	corn	barley	oats
Sweetening	date sugar	corn syrup	maple syrup	honey
Oil	safflower	corn	olive	soy or peanut
Thickeners	wheat flour	cornstarch	cream of tartar	oat flour
Nuts	filberts	cashews	walnuts/pecans	peanuts

TABLE 3.11

Rotation Diet Sample Food Choices

Day 1	Day 2	Day 3	Day 4	Extras and Substitutes
Meats				
beef, beef liver, lamb, veal, veal liver, goat, moose, venison	turkey, turkey liver, turkey eggs	pork bacon, ham sausage fish: cod, haddock, ocean perch, flounder, halibut, plaice, sole, turbot, monkfish, roughy, tuna, mackerel	chicken, chicken liver, chicken eggs	fish: salmon, trout, herring, sardines, whitefish, yellow perch, clams, scallops, oysters, white perch, yellow bass, crab, lobster, shrimp
Vegetables				
potato, tomato, eggplant, red/green or chili peppers mushroom, yeast	cucumber, zucchini, pumpkin, acorn squash, & seeds of all	turnip, cabbage, radish, kraut, watercress, cauliflower, broccoli	peas, beans, lentils, soybeans, bean sprouts, carob carrots, celery, parsley, fennel, anise, parsnip	beet, swiss chard, spinach[a] lettuce, endive, escarole, romaine, artichoke[b]
bamboo shoot	onion, asparagus, garlic, leek, chives		chestnuts	okra
plantain[a]	corn	sweet potato	olives	yams

	Day 1	Day 2	Day 3	Day 4	Extras and Substitutes
Fruits					
	strawberry, raspberry, blackberry, boysenberry	cantaloupe, honeydew, casaba, watermelon, muskmelon	grape, raisin	citris, orange, lemon, lime, grapefruit, kumquat, tangerine	apricot, cherry, nectarine, peach, plum, prune
	banana		pineapple		
	coconut, dates, palm, cabbage	blueberry, huckleberry, cranberry	rhubarb		guava
	avocado	apple, apple butter	pomegranate	mango	persimmon
	papaya	prickly pear	kiwi	currants, gooseberry	breadfruit, figs
Grains					
	wheat: flour, bread, rolls, graham flour, bran, wheat germ, farina, semolina, gluten flour	corn: starch, meal, grits millet: flour, cereal	barley: flour, pearl barley, barley flakes	oat: flour, oatmeal, oat bread, oat cakes, puffed oats	rye: flour, bread, crackers, noodles quinoa: flour, cereal[a]
	potato: flour, starch, bread	amaranth: flour, cereal, puffed Amaranth	rice: flour, cakes, noodles, snaps, puffed rice, cream of rice cereal	soy flour, pea flour, mung bean noodles flaxseed	artichoke
Sweeteners					
	date sugar	corn syrup, turbinado sugar, molasses, cane sugar	maple syrup, barley syrup	honey	beet sugar, fig syrup
Oils					
	sesame	corn, pumpkin seed, cottonseed	olive, walnut	soybean, peanut, linseed, flaxseed	sunflower, safflower[b]
Thickeners					
	sago starch, potato starch	cornstarch	cream of tartar	oat flour	tapioca starch

Day 1	Day 2	Day 3	Day 4	Extras and Substitutes
Nuts and Seeds				
filberts, hazelnuts, pine nuts	Brazil nuts, cashews, pistachios, pumpkin & poppy seeds	walnuts, pecans, butternuts, hickory	peanuts, caraway seeds, anise seeds	almonds, macadamia nuts, sunflower seeds
sesame seeds, tahini				

ᵃAll items marked ⁽ᵃ⁾ must be used on the same day.
ᵇAll items marked ⁽ᵇ⁾ must be used on the same day.

■ OTHER TESTS

While additional types of tests can also help diagnose your child's problems, those discussed in this chapter can be performed on your own. Others—such as provocation/neutralization (P/N) testing—must be administered by a knowledgeable doctor or nurse. EPD therapy (Chapter 13) also helps food allergies, but this might require several months to a year or two before it helps.

P/N testing involves injecting single drops of progressively weaker dilutions of allergy extract into a child's arm. Any response a youngster may experience to these extracts, such as sudden changes in appearance, behavior, and feelings, are noted and recorded. During the "provocation" phase of testing, a "neutralization" dose of the same extract can be determined by the doctor. This is the dose which stops the reaction caused by a previous symptom-provoking injection. This dose can then be used to help prevent symptoms from occurring in the future, or to treat symptoms that occur within minutes when certain foods are ingested.

Again, although P/N testing can provide information more quickly than the diets in this chapter, it requires the help of medical professionals. For a more detailed description of P/N testing, see Chapter 13.

NOTES

1. See Doris J. Rapp, *Is This Your Child?* (New York, NY, William Morrow & Co., 1991), chap. 9.
2. C.K. Conners et al., "Food Additives and Hyperkinesis: A Controlled Double-Blind Experiment," *Pediatrics*, vol. 58 (1976), p. 154.
3. Joseph G. Miller, *Relief At Last!* (Springfield, IL: Charles C Thomas, 1987).
4. Ibid.
5. Bonnye L. Matthews, *Chemical Sensitivity* (Jefferson, NC: McFarland and Co., 1992).

6. William J. Rea, ''Environmentally Triggered Small Vessel Vasculitis,'' *Annals of Allergy*, vol. 38 (1977), p. 245–51; William J. Rea, ''Recurrent Environmentally Triggered Thrombophlebitis,'' *Annals of Allergy*, vol. 47 (1981), pp. 338–44; William J. Rea and O.D. Brown, ''Mechanisms of Environmentally Vascular Triggering,'' *Clinical Ecology*, vol. 3 (1985), pp. 122–27; William J. Rea and C.W. Suits, ''Cardiovascular Disease Triggered by Foods and Chemicals,'' in *Food Allergy: New Perspectives*, ed. John Gerrard (Springfield, IL: Charles C Thomas, 1980); William J. Rea et al., ''Environmentally Triggered Large-vessel Vasculitis,'' *Annals of Allergy*, vol. 38 (1977), pp. 245–51; Gerald Ross and William J. Rea, ''Environmentally Triggered Hypertension, Part II,'' presented at the eighth annual international symposium on Man and His Environment in Health and Disease, Dallas, TX, Feb. 22–25, 1990; William J. Rea, *Chemical Sensitivity*, 4 vols. (Chelsea, MI: Lewis Publishers, 1991–96).

4 ⟠ Changes in Appearance

Obvious changes sometimes occur in the physical appearance of children and adults who have typical allergies, or food or chemical sensitivities.[1] These changes can be caused by various exposures within their schools, homes, or workplaces. Many of the most common changes are illustrated in Figures 4.1 through 4.25.

Many parents recognize a characteristic "spacey" or at times almost "demonic" look in their child's eyes when he or she suddenly becomes "impossible." Fortunately, only a few see an almost "demonic" appearance which tends to precede a most frightening outburst and total loss of control. These looks are sometimes accompanied by characteristic sounds, such as throat-clearing and clucking. The latter is typical, in particular, of a dairy or milk sensitivity. Some mothers complain that their children develop a "motor mouth" and ramble on about nothing after they eat or are exposed to the wrong thing. Others bark or repeatedly make chicken sounds or other strange noises at home or at school. A few whine and say the same phrase over and over. These typical changes in appearance and speech repeatedly precede or accompany bouts of hyperactivity, aggression, negativity, or vulgarity.

In addition, sometimes adults, in particular, will suddenly develop a hoarse voice along with red ears or cheeks due to food or chemical exposures. Children can also be affected by this, though hoarseness in children is more commonly due to screaming. Other symptoms can include slurred or rapid speech, and a few lose their voice entirely when exposed to certain chemicals.

▪ WHEN DID THE CHANGE OCCUR?

Exactly when these changes occur is usually the key to discovering their cause. Ask yourself **what your child ate, smelled, or touched** immediately before the symptoms became evident. The effects of chemical odors, such as perfume, tend to occur within seconds or a very few minutes. Food reactions are apt to take fifteen to sixty minutes to become apparent. A reaction to dust or molds usually occurs within an hour. You can often pinpoint the cause merely by thinking back over what happened. For example, if red earlobes, a severe headache, or wiggly legs occur half an hour after lunch or a party, it's logical to assume the symptoms are possibly related to something that was eaten. If the problem is eczema, watch the arm and leg creases: these areas commonly become red and itchy *during* meals or immediately after contact with dust, molds, or certain foods. The actual rash, however, will not develop until the next day. Also suspect food sensitivities if your child has any form of intestinal complaints after eating. If dark eye circles and muscle aches routinely occur after gym, art, chemistry, or biology class, or after a shower, suspect a reaction to a chemical exposure. If these changes occur after play on freshly cut grass, suspect grass pollen. If puffy eyes or red ears or cheeks are evident only after exposure to a moldy-smelling basement or mainly on rainy days, suspect molds in that room or in the outdoor air. If a child's nose becomes itchy and drippy, or if asthma and coughing get worse after tumbling on gym mats or play on an old carpet, the cause could be dust, molds, or both. If a youngster becomes wild and uncontrollable and has a peculiar spaced-out look after using a lavatory that smells of scented body preparations, deodorants, or disinfectants, suspect chemicals. (For a videotape showing some of these reactions, see *Environmentally Sick Schools*, listed under "Videos" in For Further Reading.)

Teachers, as well as parents, should learn to watch for dark eye circles, red earlobes, nose-rubbing, skin-scratching, wiggly legs, yawning, and various throaty sounds. Try to correlate these changes in appearance with exposures, or the ingestion of certain foods or beverages. Problems sitting still, learning, walking, and speaking definitely can be associated with any of the above changes in how environmentally sensitive individuals look.

Some characteristic changes in appearance are shown in the following illustrations.

With nose-rubbing, usually the nose is rubbed upward or massaged in a circle because it is itchy.

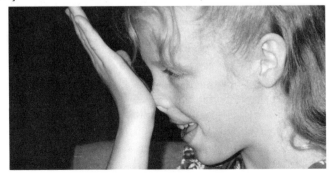

FIGURE 4.1
Typical nose-rubbing.

The allergic nose wrinkle is caused by repeatedly rubbing the nose *upward toward* the ceiling because it itches.

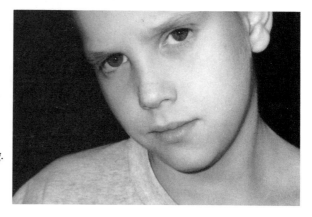

FIGURE 4.2
Nose wrinkle due to upward nose-rubbing.

Puffy eye bags in Figure 4.3 can develop directly below the eyes or somewhat more toward the outer edge of the face. Although these bags can have many causes, in this boy the cause was a dairy sensitivity. (He was evaluated at an allergy clinic and told he had no allergies. Simply stopping milk and all other dairy products helped him significantly.)

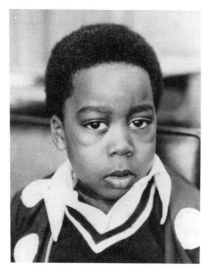

FIGURE 4.3
Puffiness under the eyes.

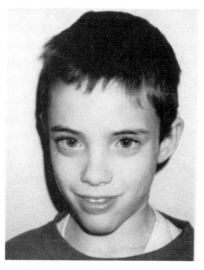

FIGURE 4.4
Characteristic dark eye circles.

Dark eye circles can be black, blue, or pink. Sometimes the discoloration extends completely around the entire eye, so the affected person can have a look that is reminiscent of a raccoon.

Eye wrinkles are typical of allergic children and adults, especially those who have eczema. If you must tip your head or strain to see these wrinkles, you do not have them.

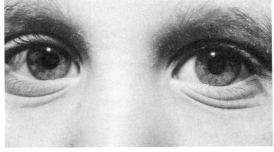

FIGURE 4.5
Allergic eye wrinkles.

Brilliant red earlobes are typical of many allergic children and adults. They provide a red flag at the onset of an allergic reaction. Redness can affect part or all of one or both ears. Sometimes they become so hot that ice is needed to provide relief. This physical change is not always due to foods, chemicals, and common allergenic contacts, however. Sometimes merely being in a hot room will cause the earlobes to become very red and warm, especially in very fair children.

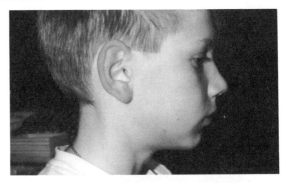

FIGURE 4.6
Brilliant red earlobes.

Abnormally red rosy cheeks can occur in anyone, but they are particularly characteristic of allergic children two to four years old and of adult females who have multiple food or chemical allergies.

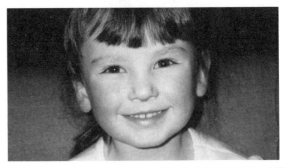

FIGURE 4.7
Red cheeks.

Some physical characteristics are difficult to illustrate visually but very easy to describe and recognize. Teachers and mothers know these "looks," often described as appearing "spaced out," "not with it" or having "glassy, glazed eyes." This type of look seems to come and go for no reason. It typically precedes and accompanies an episode of "impossible" behavior.

In Figure 4.8A you can see the "spaced out" look in a ten-year-old boy's face during an allergy skin test for whitefish.

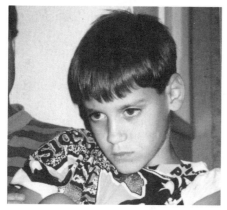

FIGURE 4.8A
Spacey "out-of-it" look.

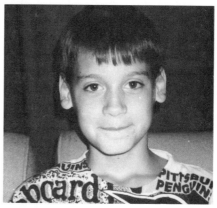

FIGURE 4.8B
A changed expression within 10 minutes of receiving treatment.

A spacey, "out-of-it" look is typical of some children who are sensitive to a food or chemical. Sometimes they truly cannot remember what was said or done during these episodes. This boy's grades dropped markedly

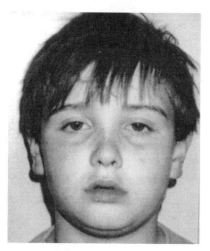

FIGURE 4.9A
Spacey "out-of-it" look.

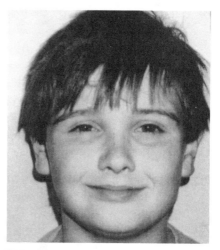

FIGURE 4.9B
Ten minutes after treatment.

and he seemed to exist in a fog during the season when corn was harvested near his home. At the time, he was ingesting a large amount of fresh corn on the cob. His face lost its usual alert appearance, and his ability to learn and remember drastically decreased until he was tested and his allergy treated for corn.

In other children and adults, a frighteningly angry look is seen just before they "totally lose it." Some mothers describe this look as "almost demonic." The children's eyes are half-closed, their lower lip protrudes. At those times, they are capable of putting their heads through a glass window or their fists through a door or a wall. When you confront them, you may feel quite frightened by their inordinately angry appearance. Even three-year-olds can frighten their parents when they look this way. When they no longer have "that look," it means the episode is over. At that time the children often ask what they did that was wrong. It will require all your patience and understanding to believe that they truly do not remember anything that they did or said when they lost control. Reprimanding

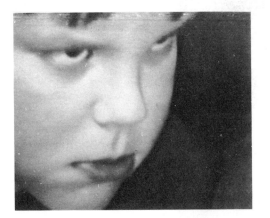

FIGURE 4.10
Demonic look.

these children serves no purpose because they are not able to control or understand their behavior at these times.

Facial twitches or tics, along with rapidly wiggling legs, are very common in some children and adults. Other muscles also can go into and out

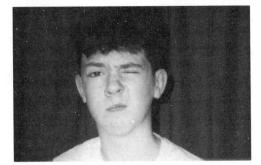

FIGURE 4.11
Facial tic or twitch.

of spasm causing discomfort or pain. Foods, molds, and chemical odors, such as the smell of tar or perfume, are common but unsuspected causes.

Hives, which look like mosquito bites, are often caused by foods, dust, molds, or chemicals. More generalized rashes can be caused by a chronic yeast infection, by contact with formaldehyde in polyester clothing or bedding, or by some chemical found in a laundry detergent or fabric softener.

Eczema causes an itchy skin rashes on the cheeks (see Figure 4.12), in the arm and leg creases, and around the wrists and ankles. Roundish patches scattered over the body are also common. The skin often becomes redder and itchier at the time of some adverse contact, such as while eating a problem food or when reacting to an allergy skin test. The characteristic rash, however, does not appear until the next day. The cause is frequently but certainly not exclusively due to dust, dust mites, molds, and problem foods.

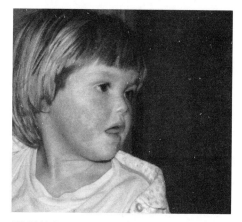

FIGURE 4.12
Eczema or atopic dermatitis on the cheeks.

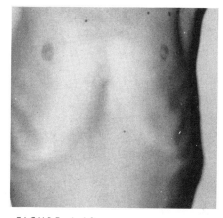

FIGURE 4.13
Asthma.

Mild, early asthma can cause a throat-clearing type of cough. Mild or moderate asthma causes a whistle or squeak when someone breathes out, or exhales. When the asthma is severe as in Figure 4.13, the spaces between the ribs and lower neck can be sucked in, which often indicates difficulty inhaling as well as exhaling.

The four million children who are affected by asthma in the United States[2] usually cough when they laugh, exercise, drink cold liquids, or breathe cold air. These are typical early warning signs that asthma is about to begin. A Peak Flow Meter can help you determine when asthma is imminent. See Chapter 3 for details about how to use a Peak Flow Meter. (For supplies, see Resources.)

Hay fever can cause a drippy or stuffy, itchy nose, as well as nose-rubbing and sneezing several times in a row. If the cause is not found and appropriately treated, recurrent ear, sinus, adenoid, and tonsil infections

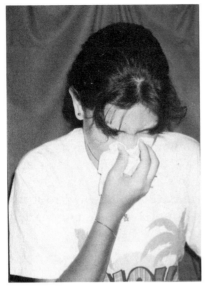

FIGURE 4.14
Hay fever.

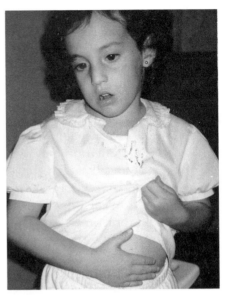

FIGURE 4.15
Abdominal pain.

typically become apparent. All too often, these infections lead to the need for one course of antibiotics after another and repeated, possibly unnecessary surgeries.

Abdominal pain, gas, nausea, diarrhea, constipation, or halitosis are commonly caused by an allergy to your favorite food or beverage. The pain is most apt to cause generalized discomfort in the umbilical area, although other areas can certainly be affected. Localized, fingerpoint pain is more characteristic of an ulcer, which, at times also can be caused by a favorite food.

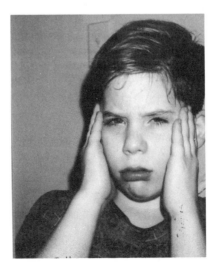

FIGURE 4.16
Headache.

Recurrent headaches are a very common allergic symptom in all age groups (see Figure 4.16). The pain may occur above or behind the eyes or on the sides, back, or top of the head. Favorite foods or beverages are common unsuspected causes of headaches. And if eaten every day they naturally tend to produce daily symptoms. Headaches can occur each day within an hour or several hours after eating certain offending foods. In adults headaches tend to occur during the night, at about three or four o'clock because of what was eaten in the late afternoon or evening.

Adults who have food allergies sometimes resort to eating only once a day, usually at night, so that their reactions will occur while they are sleeping.

Chemicals also can cause a variety of sudden strange feelings in the head, sometimes within seconds. Odors and foods are common unsuspected causes of difficulty speaking or thinking logically. The head may feel "ballooned, dull, or fuzzy."

Sudden unprovoked aggression in both children and adults can be re-

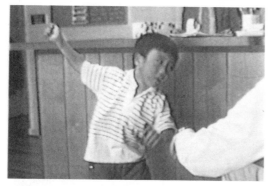

FIGURE 4.17
Aggression.

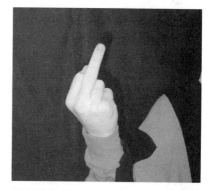

FIGURE 4.18
Vulgarity.

lated to allergy. It is often associated with red earlobes, wiggly legs, dark eye circles, and a special "look." Behavior may include hitting, biting, kicking, spitting, and punching. Sometimes the cause is obvious, especially when the symptoms repeatedly occur after exposure to a particular odor, food, or beverage.

FIGURE 4.19
Withdrawal.

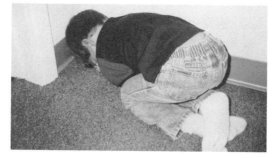

An episode of vulgarity (see Figure 4.18), in which a child or an adult feels compelled to speak, write, or act in a vulgar manner, may be a reaction to contact with a variety of allergenic substances such as a mold or even a food. Such connections can easily be confirmed by Provocation/Neutralization allergy tests.

Some children or adults become excessively withdrawn after specific exposures, foods, or allergy extract tests as shown in Figure 4.19. They hide in dark corners or under chairs. They pull away when you try to touch them and dislike being held or cuddled. They often cover their ears and eyes because they don't or can't tolerate light or ordinary sound. Affected children may grow up to become adults who, at times, inexplicably dislike being touched or being too close to anyone. This obviously can lead to troubled adult relationships.

Scattered pimples on the rounded portions of the buttocks are typical of some food sensitivities. It might also be a reaction to a fabric softener, laundry soap, or synthetic fabric. If there are scratch marks near the anus, however, pinworms are a logical possibility. Check with your doctor. (In infants and toddlers, chemically treated, superabsorbent disposable diapers definitely can cause redness, rashes, and other forms of intolerance.)

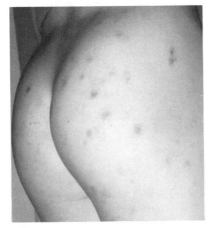

FIGURE 4.20
Pimples on buttocks.

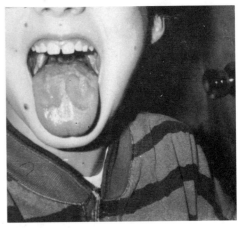

FIGURE 4.21
Geographic tongue.

A typical "geographic" tongue is slightly coated, but islands of denuded pinker areas are scattered over the surface. This type of tongue at times may indicate a food allergy. Once parents are aware of the cause, they can predict exactly when their child's tongue will change. This typically occurs a few hours after certain offending foods are eaten, and it usually lasts for days.

Many allergic children have a yeast overgrowth (see Chapter 14). It is common in children or adults who have taken too many antibiotics, particularly because of an untreated allergy. Adolescents who take antibiotics for acne and females who use birth control pills often develop this same problem. Yeasty individuals tend to have some combination of the following:

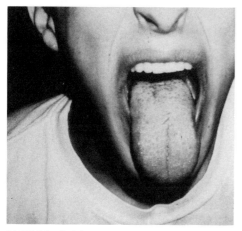

FIGURE 4.22
White-coated tongue.

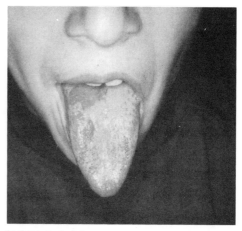

FIGURE 4.23
Mottled food-allergic and yeasty-looking tongue.

- a white-coated tongue (Figure 4.22)
- a red ring around the anus (Figure 4.24)
- a bloated abdomen (Figure 4.25)
- a resistant, chronic, itchy body rash
- a persistent hair or foot odor, not relieved by washing
- an itchy genital area, which can lead to frequent genital touching

These symptoms usually subside quickly after appropriate antiyeast therapy (see Chapter 15).

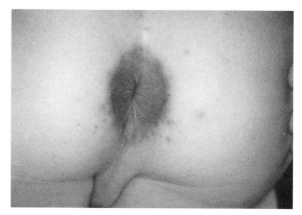

FIGURE 4.24
Red anal ring typical of yeast overgrowth.

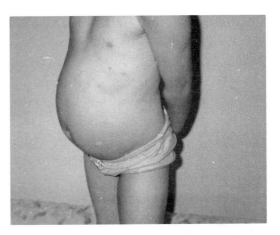

FIGURE 4.25
Abnormally large abdomen.

A white-coated tongue is a common indication of excess yeast. This condition is different from the mottled "geographic" tongue, which suggests a possible food allergy in children or adults. If the tongue is extremely white but also has bald, pink, spotty patches, that person may have a combination of a yeast overgrowth and food allergies.

A red ring around the anus is typical of a yeast overgrowth as in Figure 4.24. It is noted especially in children or adults after the use of too many antibiotics.

A bloated abdomen sometimes occurs with food allergies, but other digestive problems, such as chronic yeast infections and parasites, are also common causes. With appropriate treatment, the abdomen often becomes nice and flat, even in young children.

The symptoms that are illustrated in this chapter do not occur in all children and are not evident every time they are exposed to various offending foods or substances. Each person has his or her own individual pattern of response. Watch your child and yourself. What clues does the body provide to indicate that something is not quite right? Recognizing these clues is the first step back to truly feeling well.

NOTES

1. Doris J. Rapp, *Is This Your Child?* (New York: William Morrow & Co., 1991).
2. Reported on ABC-TV's *20/20*, June 28, 1995.

5 Handwriting and Drawing Changes

Handwriting and drawing changes provide visible clues about what is happening within your child, and what may be provoking it. In this chapter, you will learn how easy it is recognize characteristic changes and to pinpoint the reason behind them. Sudden changes in the writing and drawing of children are often related to specific chemical exposures, to contact with dust, molds, pollen, and/or to allergenic foods or beverages. Individual children and adults may react to some of these substances but not to others. Some severely allergic or environmentally sensitive youngsters respond to all these substances.

With this insight, you can use this component of the ''Big Five'' to see how specific areas of your child's brain are being affected, interfering with writing skills and compromising his or her academic performance. We can gain much insight not only from the way someone writes and draws, but also from the content of the writing and pictures. Whether they are gifted, normal, or slow, children may suddenly show a significant regression or changes in their ability to write or draw during allergy testing.

■ HOW BREAKFAST CAN AFFECT A CHILD'S DRAWING

Figure 5.1 shows a series of drawings made by a six-year-old boy before he ate a breakfast of rice toast, apple juice, egg, and butter. He continued to draw every few minutes over the next half hour. You can see the gradual deterioration of his drawings. Imagine how difficult it would be for him to learn each school day if this were his routine breakfast. It's important to investigate whether a school lunch or snack of these food items could produce similar changes.

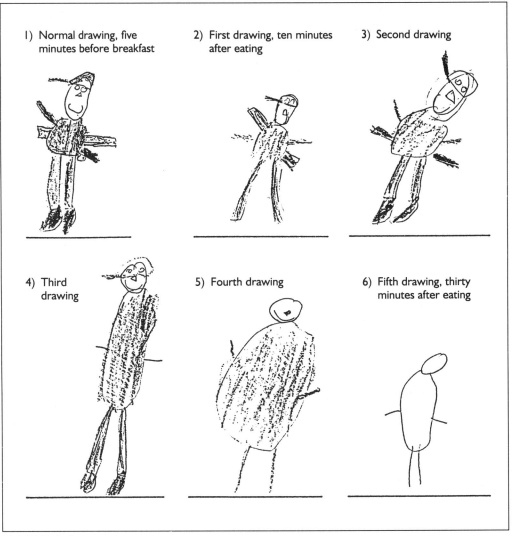

1) Normal drawing, five minutes before breakfast

2) First drawing, ten minutes after eating

3) Second drawing

4) Third drawing

5) Fourth drawing

6) Fifth drawing, thirty minutes after eating

FIGURE 5.1
A six-year-old boy's drawings 5 minutes before breakfast and continuing over a 30-minute period.

■ SPECIFIC CHANGES TO LOOK FOR

Let's consider the significance of some other frequently observed handwriting changes that you may see when conducting the "Big Five":

■ Look for changes in how your child writes early in the morning compared with later, for example, after a midmorning milk break, a lunch, or a snack. Compare writing before with that done an hour after dinner. If there is a significant change, think about what was eaten for dinner.

■ As a teacher, compare how each of your students writes at the beginning and end of each class. Notice whether any students write poorly in a specific room. What is different about that room? Does it have a chemical odor? Does the teacher smell of perfume or tobacco? Or do some of the students? Is the classroom unusually dusty or moldy? Is the ventilation particularly poor? As a parent, check each room in your home the same way.

■ Notice whether your child misbehaves and is unable to write mainly on damp, rainy days. If so, molds may be a problem.

■ Observe whether your child writes backward or upside down after going to the lavatory at school or to the bathroom at home. If this happens, suspect the cleaning agents or other chemical odors in that area, such as scented personal body products.

■ Compare how your child writes his or her name before and an hour after a school or home party. If the writing and/or behavior change tremendously, think about specific foods as a possible cause.

■ Note whether the writing varies before and after a ride on a school bus or in the family car. Is the response the same in both parents' cars?

Once again, the cause often becomes obvious once you take the time to consider the possible causes. Older children, as well as parents and teachers, can become astute environmental detectives, finding causes that others, including professionals, have repeatedly missed.

The variety of changes that can occur in the writing and drawing of children is truly remarkable. They generally reflect how those children are feeling and behaving. Hyperactive children write with large letters. Withdrawn children begin writing small, or they refuse to write at all. Happy children draw upturned mouths; sad children draw tears or downturned mouths. Aggressive children write with obvious hostility and anger, and reflect violence with pictures of blood, skulls, knives, hangings, guns, and tombstones.

As with the other components of the "Big Five," keep detailed records if a child who normally writes well, suddenly and for no obvious reason, makes letters that are too large, illegible, backward, in mirror images, or upside down. Take note when your youngster suddenly scribbles all over a paper and then stabs it. Maybe the cause of this behavior is not simply frustration but an adverse exposure that has affected a specific part of the brain. Take note if your child suddenly reads, as well as writes, from right to left rather than from left to right. Also if he or she suddenly cannot color within the lines. The causes can be embarrassingly evident once you pay attention to the pattern.

Adults also show similar changes in their writing and drawing, but they are generally less frequent and less dramatic than those in children.

■ CHILDREN'S WRITING AND DRAWING CHANGES IN REACTION TO SPECIFIC EXPOSURES

The following illustrations clearly demonstrate the types of changes that occur in children after:

■ eating allergenic foods
■ certain chemical exposures
■ drinking problem beverages
■ smelling offending odors
■ taking medicines that have an adverse effect
■ being tested with a drop or an injection of an allergy extract

Many of these following changes were produced in about ten minutes during "provocation/neutralization" allergy testing, although you certainly can also notice them in your child during ordinary day-to-day activities. As always, during these tests, neither the child nor the parent should know the exact item being tested. To briefly describe the P/N test procedure: a drop of a standard allergy extract is placed in the outer skin layers of the arm or dropped under the tongue. Within a few minutes, children who are sensitive to that substance will show a significant change in their writing, drawing, appearance, and/or actions. This is called the *provocation* or a provoking dose of allergy extract. Then single drops of progressively fivefold weaker (1:5, 1:25, 1:125, and so on) dilutions of the same extract are administered every seven to ten minutes. The writing, drawing, appearance, and behavior of the allergic child will suddenly return to normal. When that happens, the *neutralization* dose—which is a weaker dilution of allergy extract that is able to neutralize or relieve the response—has been found. This dose of allergy extract can be used to treat a child, relieving symptoms in minutes, so that such changes are much less apt to occur in the future. (For more details about P/N testing, and whether it is appropriate for your child, see Chapters 13 and 15.)

Samples of the writing and drawing changes that children experience will be presented according to the type of exposure as indicated below:

■ foods
■ molds
■ dust mites
■ pet hair
■ pollen

- chemicals
- school air
- home air

A few samples of changes in adult handwriting will follow. Then we shall look at the kinds of emotional changes children undergo, regardless of whether the offending substance is a food or chemical. These emotional changes are reflected in changes in the children's writing and drawing:

- immaturity
- aggression
- fear
- depression
- vulgarity
- compulsiveness

■ FIRST CHECK THE NORMAL WRITING

Before you can interpret your child's handwriting changes, you must have a basis of comparison. Ask your child, on a quiet afternoon, to write his or her name and a series of numbers on a piece of unlined paper every ten minutes. Typically, the writing will show very little variation. This will be your basis of comparison. When you have your child perform the same task after exposure to something to which he is sensitive, you may be able to see a distinct difference in his writing. See Figures 5.2a and b on the next page.

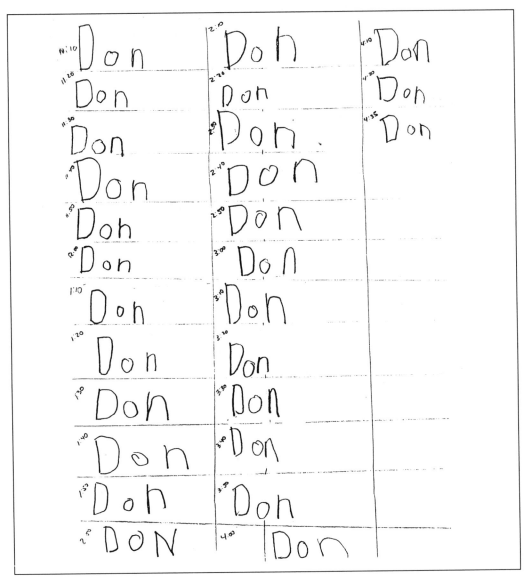

FIGURE 5.2A
Don's normal handwriting, sampled every ten minutes during a quiet afternoon at home.

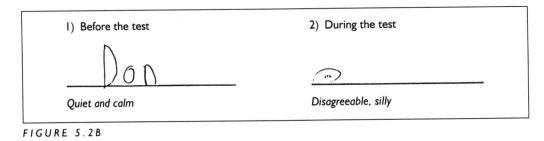

1) Before the test

Don

Quiet and calm

2) During the test

Disagreeable, silly

FIGURE 5.2B

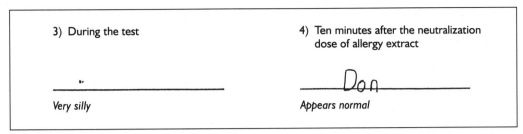

FIGURES 5.3A AND B
Changes in Don's handwriting during testing for allergy to soy.

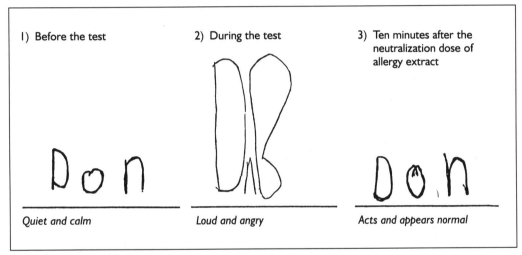

FIGURES 5.4A TO C
Changes in Don's handwriting during testing for allergy to peach.

FOODS

The first three samples show how foods affected the handwriting of six-and-a-half-year-old Don.

Now look at Figure 5.2b, which reveals what happened to Don's handwriting when he was tested for a soy allergy with a soy extract, then given a neutralization dose.

Figure 5.4a shows his response to an allergy test for peach, then to a corrective dose of allergy extract.

It is easy to see that after receiving a provocation dose of soy (Figure 5.3) and then peach (Figure 5.4), Don's handwriting changed. When the neutralization dose of these extracts was given, his writing returned to normal. If Don were to eat soy or peach before or during school hours, he might have difficulty learning, as well as writing. Appropriate food extract treatment should help to relieve this type of problem.

Most allergic children have sensitivities not only to foods but to many other items such as dust, molds, pollen, and chemicals. Any one of these items may cause a handwriting change, either after a routine, everyday exposure or during allergy testing.

Educational experts rarely consider the impact of foods, as well as environmental factors, on sensitive children. In Figure 5.5, six-year-old Sarah not only wrote upside down, she read from right to left during a reaction to

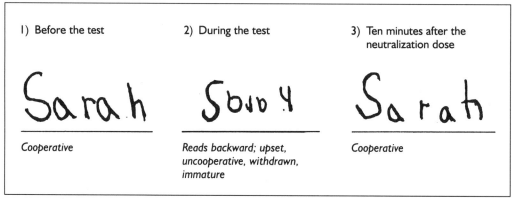

FIGURES 5.5A TO C
Changes in Sarah's handwriting during testing for allergy to strawberry.

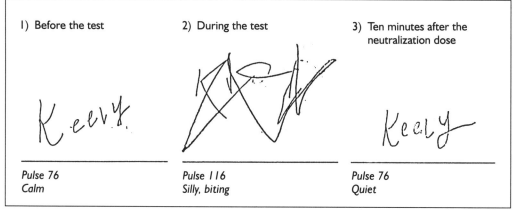

FIGURES 5.6A TO C
Changes in Keely's handwriting and pulse during testing for allergy to food colorings.

a strawberry extract. She also behaved in an uncharacteristically childish, immature manner. The solution to her problem is not a special education teacher or fewer students in a classroom, but the recognition and elimination of the cause.

Seven-year-old Keely experienced significant reactions during a test for allergy to food colorings, then returned to normal after a corrective dose of the extract (see Figures 5.6a to c).

Keely also became silly, hyperactive, and then angry. At that time, her pulse rate of 76 increased to 116 beats per minute, and she tried to bite her mother. After one drop of the right dilution of food coloring, she acted and wrote normally again, and her pulse returned to normal.

In Figures 5.7a to c, ten-year-old Stephanie wrote too large, and the letters were poorly formed during a test for allergy to string beans. The neutralization dose of this allergy extract resulted in improved writing.

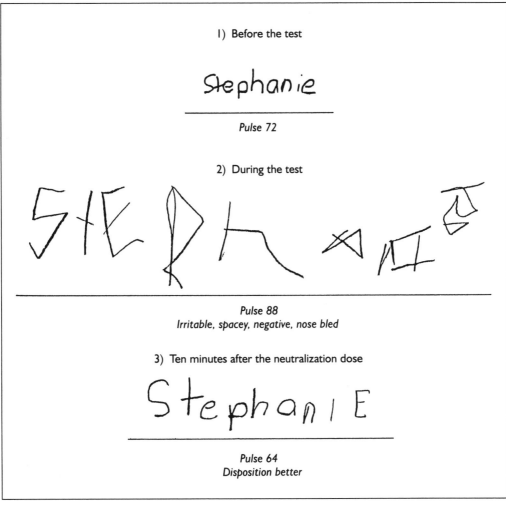

1) Before the test

Pulse 72

2) During the test

Pulse 88
Irritable, spacey, negative, nose bled

3) Ten minutes after the neutralization dose

Pulse 64
Disposition better

FIGURES 5.7A TO C
Changes in Stephanie's handwriting during testing for allergy to string beans.

When Robert was allergy-tested for oats and wheat, his handwriting and behavior changed at the same time. This type of reaction to two different grains suggests that he must be watched closely for a possible sensitivity to other grains and to grass pollen, which is botanically related to grains.

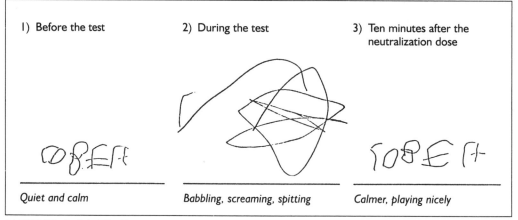

FIGURES 5.8A TO C
Changes in Robert's handwriting during testing for allergy to oats.

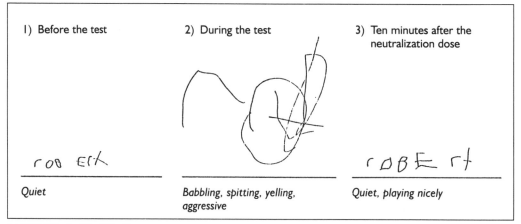

FIGURES 5.9A TO C
Changes in Robert's handwriting during testing for allergy to wheat.

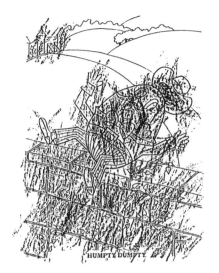

FIGURE 5.10
Coloring before being placed on a diet.

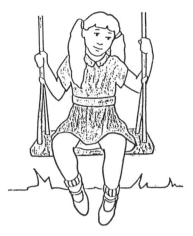

FIGURE 5.11
Coloring after ten weeks of an allergy diet.

The drawing in Figure 5.10 shows how a five-year-old boy colored before he was placed on an allergy diet.

Figure 5.11 shows the same child's coloring five months later, after he had been on an allergy diet for ten weeks. The skeptics will say this improvement merely reflects normal maturity, but such a degree of improvement is most unlikely in so short a period of time. This boy remains well with environmental medical care.

HYPOGLYCEMIA

To be sure, not all changes in handwriting are due to food allergies. For example, sometimes a child's handwriting gradually deteriorates late in the morning or afternoon. If eating eliminates this problem within a few minutes, it might be evidence of a low blood sugar level or hypoglycemia. An **immediate** blood sugar examination will help to verify this diagnosis. A hypoglycemic child often needs to eat every hour or two during school hours, as well as at home, to avoid low blood sugar reactions, which cause recurrent fatigue, irritability, tension, hyperactivity, and aggression. The pattern of each child's symptom response can be very different.[1]

One clue in spotting hypoglycemia is the way your children ask for food. Do they request food—or demand it? The latter suggests low blood sugar. It can happen on and off all day, but it is most apt to occur between 10:30 and 11:30 A.M. and again between 3:00 and 4:00 P.M. Some children are "impossible" when they awaken in the morning *until they eat.* Their

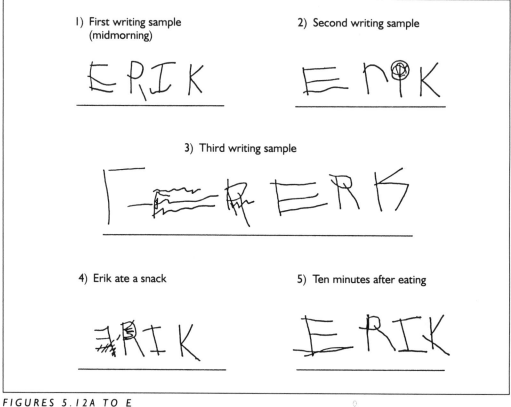

1) First writing sample (midmorning)

2) Second writing sample

3) Third writing sample

4) Erik ate a snack

5) Ten minutes after eating

FIGURES 5.12A TO E
Gradual deterioration in Erik's handwriting, caused by hypoglycemia.

brains may need glucose (sugar).[2] It is a good idea to have a nonsweet snack at the bedside of such a child so it can be eaten upon awakening each morning.

Figure 5.12 shows the deterioration in four-and-a-half-year-old Erik's handwriting late in the morning. Erik was then fed, and within less than ten minutes, his writing returned to normal. His writing change was due to hypoglycemia. Children who have this illness often become a school problem just before lunch every day.

MOLDS

Exposure to molds can be caused by previously flooded basements; leaky roofs, pipes, or sinks; or the use of books after storage in moldy places. Some mold-allergic children will suddenly feel, act, write, or draw differently, particularly on damp days or during the wet seasons of the year. Asthma and/or hay fever tend to be worse during the rainy months, when more molds are in the air. Adults or children who have arthritis or joint problems will also find their problems worsening at these times.

Seven-year-old Shawn's drawings (Figures 5.13a to c) reveal his unhappiness during mold allergy testing. He became visibly sad and angry, drawing a face with a downturned mouth. But as soon as he received the neutralization dose, his drawing showed a happy face.

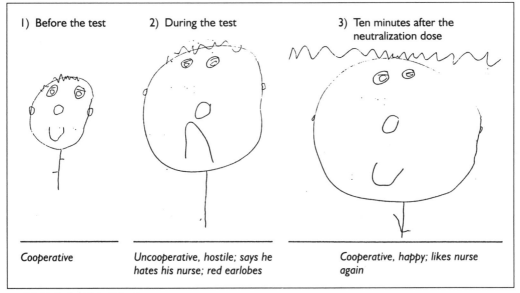

FIGURES 5.13A TO C
Sean's drawing during testing for allergy to mold.

In Figures 5.14a to c, five-year-old Sean wrote backward during his test for mold allergy. His pulse increased, and his ability to breathe easily decreased. As is typical, his writing, pulse, and breathing all returned to normal within ten minutes after receiving the neutralization dose.

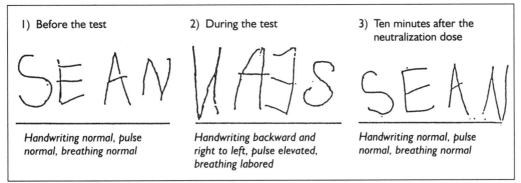

FIGURES 5.14A TO C
Handwriting, pulse, and breathing changes in Sean during testing for allergy to mold.

Seven-and-a-half-year-old Lalena was tested for an allergy to mold. Her writing deteriorated, and she became angry and explosive, complaining that the joints in her fingers hurt. She manifested a range of emotions, beginning with depression, then anger, and then more depression. Ten minutes after receiving the corrective dilution, she was smiling and was her usual happy self again. It is most interesting that ten years later, when she was seventeen, she returned for more allergy tests because of similar mood

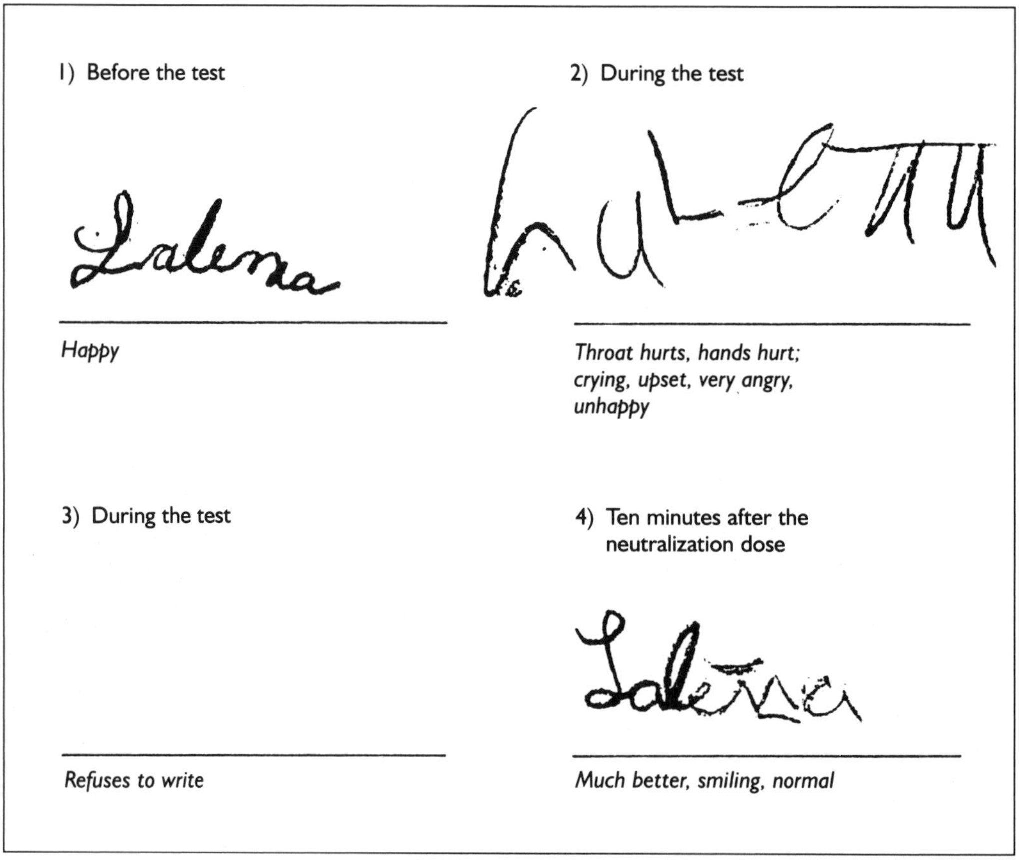

1) Before the test

Happy

2) During the test

Throat hurts, hands hurt; crying, upset, very angry, unhappy

3) During the test

Refuses to write

4) Ten minutes after the neutralization dose

Much better, smiling, normal

FIGURES 5.15A TO C
Lalena's writing changes during testing for allergy to mold.

changes on damp days. Her response to the mold allergy extract again caused her to not "feel right," and she became depressed. The numbness in her finger joints made it difficult to write and shuffle cards. After a different dilution of allergy extract dose was administered, these symptoms again disappeared.

It is rare but possible for allergy testing to precipitate a child or adult's joint pain. When this happens, it suggests that the substance being tested is the cause. We must wonder what this says about the long-term health of Lalena and others who have painful joints. Adults frequently notice that their joints ache more on rainy days. Molds in the air may be the reason, and P/N treatment may help. (In children, it is not uncommon for foods to cause this symptom.)

The drawings in Figures 5.15 to 5.19 were made by the young Lalena, age seven and a half.

Lalena's drawing ability was also affected by the mold allergy testing. Before the test began, she drew the picture in Figure 5.16.

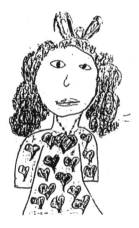

FIGURE 5.16
Lalena's drawing before testing for mold allergy.

She drew the following pictures during the mold test. At the time, she acted unhappy and drew a sad face, as shown in Figure 5.17.

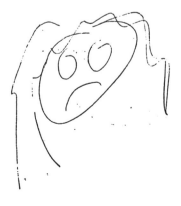

FIGURE 5.17
Lalena's drawing during testing for allergy to mold.

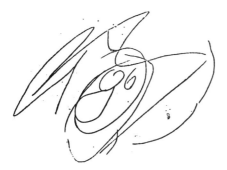

FIGURE 5.18
Lalena's drawing during mold allergy testing.

This picture was drawn after Lalena was given the neutralization dose. Figure 5.19 shows a drawing that Lalena made ten minutes after receiving the neutralization dose.

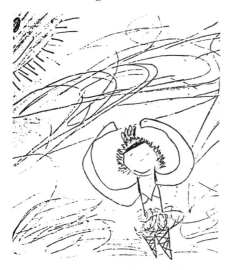

FIGURE 5.19
Lalena's drawing 10 minutes after receiving the neutralization dose.

Remember, children do not react this way to every item that is allergy-tested. Only certain tests appear to affect the writing area of the brain. Robert wrote *normally* when he was tested for allergies to squash, cabbage, peanuts, and histamine. But Figure 5.20 shows what happened when he was tested for mold allergy.

This writing sample certainly suggests that molds can interfere with Robert's academic ability. He should not attend a moldy school or live in an excessively moldy home. He had a number of other sensitivities, but after comprehensive environmental allergy treatment, his health and academic ability improved tremendously. Years later, however, he had a sudden, distinct recurrence of his allergies. His condition did not improve until his astute parents realized that he simply could not live in their vintage "antique" summer home, due to the mold and dust in that area.

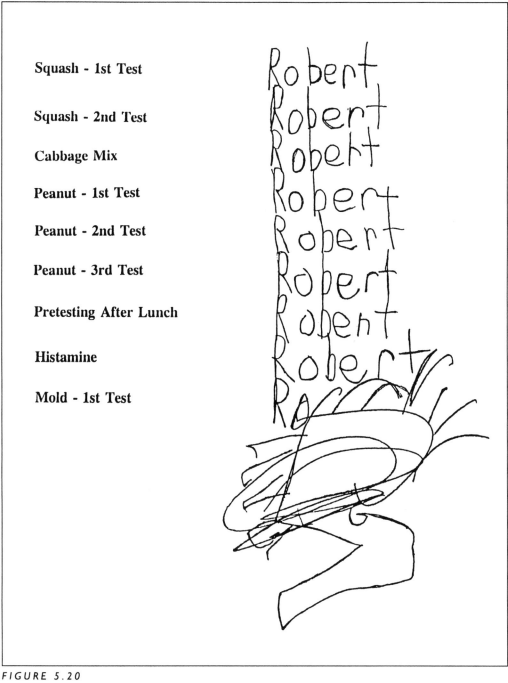

Squash - 1st Test

Squash - 2nd Test

Cabbage Mix

Peanut - 1st Test

Peanut - 2nd Test

Peanut - 3rd Test

Pretesting After Lunch

Histamine

Mold - 1st Test

FIGURE 5.20

Changes in Robert's handwriting during testing for mold allergy.

DUST MITES

Many schools and homes are dusty, mainly because of a poorly maintained ventilation system. The source of the problem is dust mites contained within the dust. These mites are barely visible colorless organisms that thrive in stuffed furniture, mattresses, carpets, and the like. Figures 5.21a to c shows five-year-old Kevin's reaction to a dust mite allergy extract.

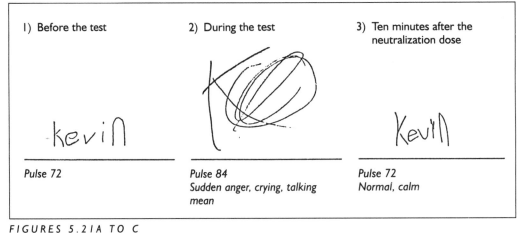

1) Before the test	2) During the test	3) Ten minutes after the neutralization dose
kevin		*Kevin*
Pulse 72	Pulse 84 *Sudden anger, crying, talking mean*	Pulse 72 *Normal, calm*

FIGURES 5.21A TO C
Kevin's handwriting changes during testing for allergy to dust mites.

PET HAIR

Similarly, in Figures 5.22a to c, Dan was tested for an allergy to pet hair. His pulse changes during these tests increased less than 20 beats per minute which is not a significant variation, but the changes in his appearance and manner strongly suggested a sensitivity to pet hair or dandruff.

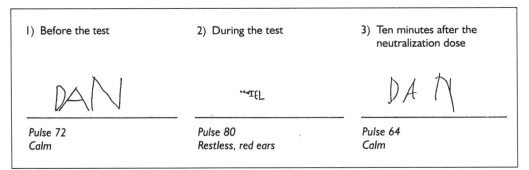

1) Before the test	2) During the test	3) Ten minutes after the neutralization dose
DAN	*IEL*	*DAN*
Pulse 72 *Calm*	Pulse 80 *Restless, red ears*	Pulse 64 *Calm*

FIGURES 5.22A TO C
Dan's handwriting and pulse changes during testing for allergy to pet hair. This extract contains feathers and cat, dog, and rabbit hair.

POLLEN

Pollen can sometimes cause much more than nose and chest allergies. Although less common and less recognized, tree, grass, and weed pollen can cause learning problems in children sensitive to these substances. They commonly become irritable, negative, hyperactive, fatigued, or depressed. Consider whether your child's inappropriate behavior is most evident when the pollen count (which you can find in the newspaper) is elevated. Testing for allergies to pollen can reproduce a wide range of allergic responses. Like the other allergens discussed in this chapter, it can cause some children to write poorly, refuse to write, stab the paper, or throw a pencil at anyone who happens to be nearby. This allergy can be spotted in affected children by checking their handwriting before and after recess or outside gym, especially if a school or home lawn was freshly cut. (If a lawn spray was used, however, similar changes may occur because of a pesticide chemical exposure.)

Figures 5.23a to c shows the changes in the handwriting of a nine-year-old boy, Brian, after he was exposed to freshly cut grass.

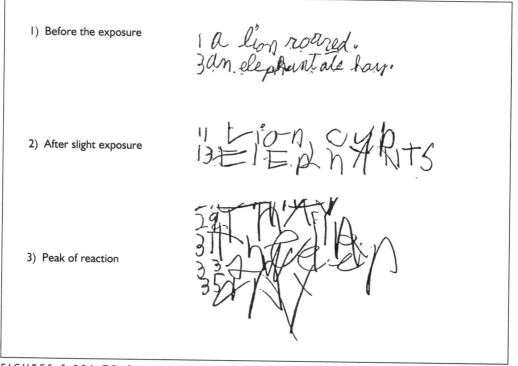

FIGURES 5.23A TO C
Brian's handwriting changes during grass exposure.

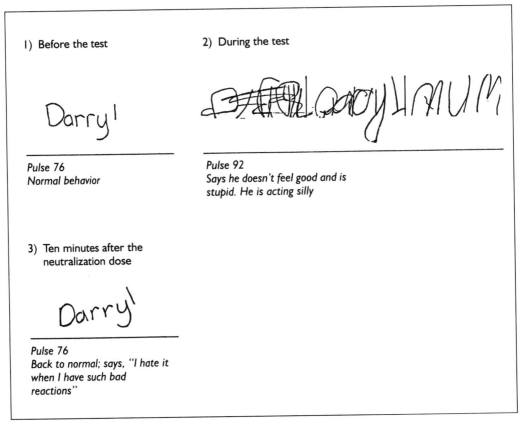

FIGURES 5.24A TO C
Darryl's handwriting changes during testing for allergy to ragweed.

In Figures 5.24a to c, you see the obvious changes in ten-year-old Darryl's writing during a ragweed allergy test. At the beginning of each school year, Darryl would be off to a bad start because ragweed pollen is at its peak at that time of year. If Darryl also happened to be sensitive to molds, *which is certainly typical of most allergic children and adults,* he would be in double jeopardy, since mold levels are also elevated at that time of year.

Because the grass pollen peak corresponds to the time when final examinations are usually given, some children's final term grades do not accurately reflect their year-long academic performance. Unfortunately, the start of each school year in the late summer corresponds to the peak for both the weed-pollen and mold-spore season in many parts of the United States. Some children, therefore, start and/or end the school year with a distinct medical and learning handicap due to their allergies. Chapters 6 and 15 discusses ways to reduce these problems with room air purifiers and allergy extract treatment.

After Darryl's mother made changes in his classroom environment, he could attend school and no longer required home teaching (see Chapter 12).

CHEMICALS

As indicated in Chapter 1, an immense array of symptoms can be caused by a chemical exposure. Chemicals have been associated with memory loss, increased impulsivity, easy distractibility, an inability to concentrate, and difficulty learning. Some children diagnosed as having ADHD may simply have a chemical sensitivity.[3] (Objective documentation can be seen in the brain images shown in Chapter 12.)

Some children, such as four-year-old Ryan in Chapter 1 (Figure 1.1 and 1.2), became tired, limp, and apathetic when exposed to certain chemi-

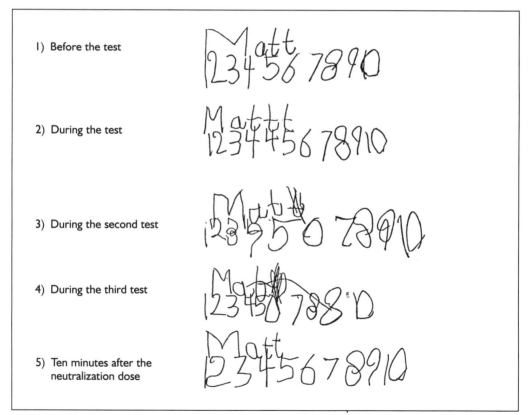

1) Before the test

2) During the test

3) During the second test

4) During the third test

5) Ten minutes after the neutralization dose

FIGURES 5.25A TO E

Changes in Matt's handwriting during tests for sensitivity to hydrocarbons.

cal odors. When he was exposed to a commonly used aerosol disinfectant, he refused to hold a pencil or write. After oxygen was administered, his writing returned to normal. How many other Ryans have problems whose causes are not recognized because educators and parents are not aware of the ways that chemical odors can affect some children?

Another six-year-old, Matt, was tested for a hydrocarbon (gas, oil, etc.) sensitivity. As shown in Figures 5.25a to e, the test initially interfered with his ability to spell; then his letters and numbers deteriorated so much that they became barely legible. Ten minutes after being given a neutralization dose, his writing returned to normal.

In Figure 5.26, you can see a drawing by ten-year-old Marsha, who had been very sad for two years. During that period, she had been taking fluoride tablets. When we tested her with an allergy extract made from these tablets, she drew a face, then started to cry. At that point she added

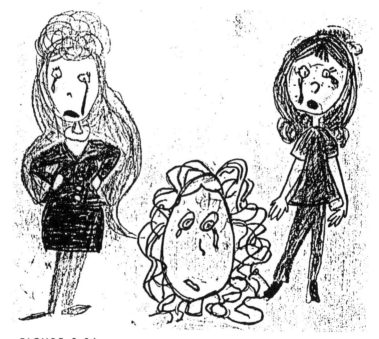

FIGURE 5.26
Marsha's drawing during a skin test for fluoride.

tears to her drawing. As the tears rolled down her cheeks, she said she felt sad. With treatment, her improvement was impressive (as indicated in the discussion of her medical problems, in Chapter 8).

Marsha's pulse increased from 64 to 80 during the reaction and returned to 64 after the neutralization dose was given. This type of pulse

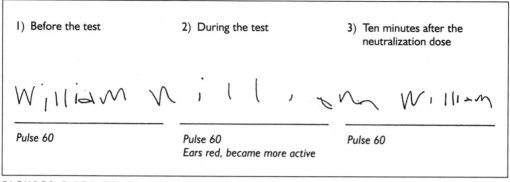

FIGURES 5.27A TO C
William's subtle handwriting change during testing for sensitivity to chlorine.

change is not uncommon during testing, although the change is typically more than 20 points.

In Figures 5.27a to c, an example of eight-year-old William's reaction to chlorine is shown. He was tested for chlorine because his mother said he fell asleep during an exciting dolphin and whale show at Wonderland. (Changes in behavior that occur during visits to aquatic or marine facilities are sometimes due to chlorine or other chemical odors.)

William was one of the first children we evaluated for a sensitivity to carpets and carpet chemicals. Shortly after a new carpet was installed in his school, his grades dropped from 85–90 percent to barely passing. He continuously erased and rewrote. His mother suspected that the new carpet was affecting his classwork. Shortly after he was switched to a different school with plain wooden floors, his grades returned to their original high levels.

SCHOOL AIR

It is very simple to make an allergy extract of the air at a school, home, or workplace. A special machine[4] is placed in a suspect room, such as a classroom, lab, hallway, or lavatory, or any area of a home or workplace. The air is bubbled through a small bottle of saline (salt water) for eight to twelve hours. From this solution, an allergy specialist prepares an allergy extract. After it is checked for sterility, it can be used for P/N allergy extract testing. Sometimes such an extract can be used to treat a child, so he can continue to attend a particular school. You will need written permission from the school to prepare a school air extract.

The writing changes of two children—shown in Figures 5.28 and 5.29—occurred in response to an allergy extract made from the air in their respective schools.

In Figures 5.28a to c, eleven-year-old Marsha's handwriting became very tiny and illegible, and her pulse increased a significant 28 points.

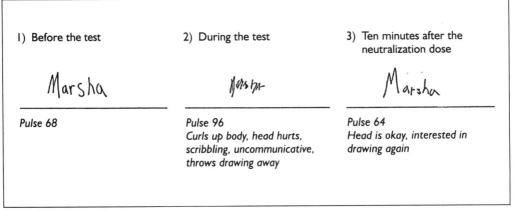

1) Before the test

Marsha

Pulse 68

2) During the test

Pulse 96
Curls up body, head hurts, scribbling, uncommunicative, throws drawing away

3) Ten minutes after the neutralization dose

Marsha

Pulse 64
Head is okay, interested in drawing again

FIGURES 5.28A TO C
Marsha's handwriting and significant pulse changes during testing with school air extract.

In Figures 5.29a to d, ten-year-old Joshua could barely write some of the numbers, and he wrote others backward. He also wrote with his right hand, even though he is left-handed. After receiving a neutralization dose, he wrote correctly again with his left hand.

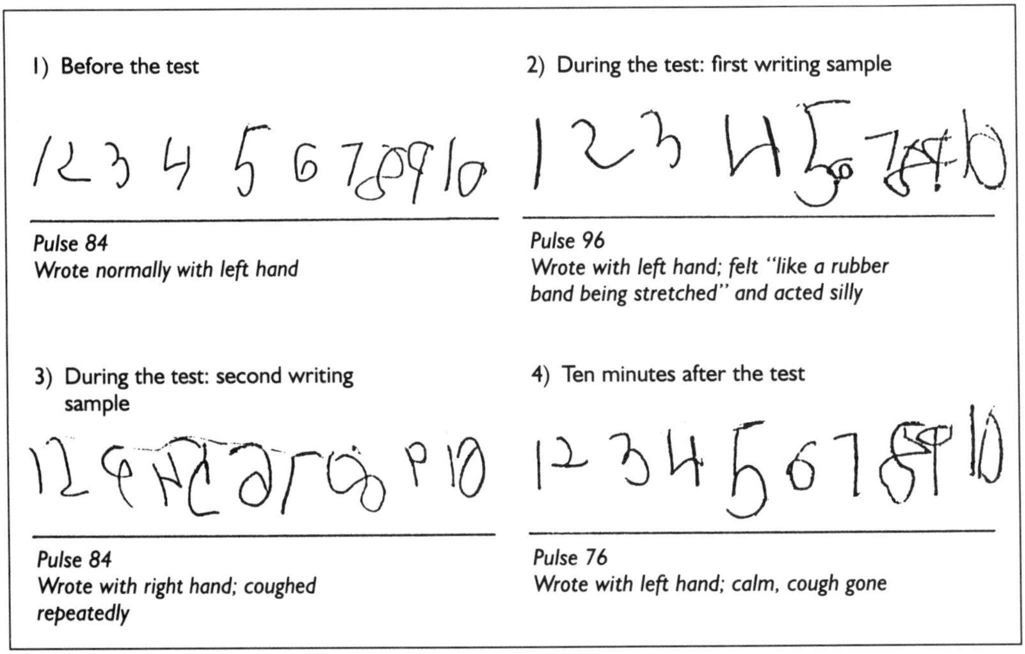

1) Before the test

Pulse 84
Wrote normally with left hand

2) During the test: first writing sample

Pulse 96
Wrote with left hand; felt "like a rubber band being stretched" and acted silly

3) During the test: second writing sample

Pulse 84
Wrote with right hand; coughed repeatedly

4) Ten minutes after the test

Pulse 76
Wrote with left hand; calm, cough gone

FIGURES 5.29A TO D
Changes In Joshua's handwriting during testing for sensitivity to school air.

When Joshua was tested with an allergy extract made from his school carpet, his ability to read diminished and his writing changed as shown in the samples in Figure 5.29.

HOME AIR

Figures 5.30a to c shows how Joshua's handwriting changed after he was tested with an allergy extract made from the air in his home. Once again, the letters are written poorly. This suggests that he could have difficulty doing his homework at home unless environmental changes were made to clean the air there.

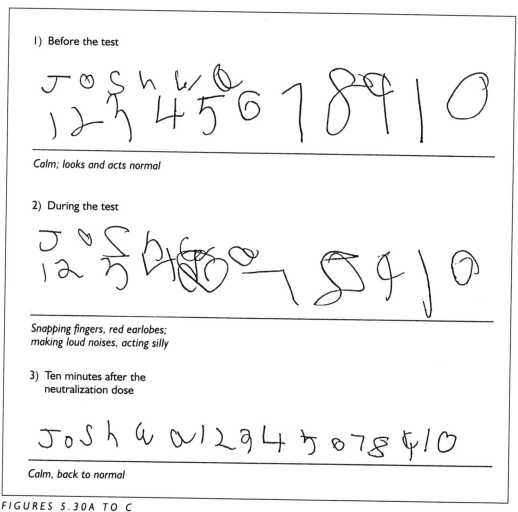

1) Before the test

Calm; looks and acts normal

2) During the test

Snapping fingers, red earlobes;
making loud noises, acting silly

3) Ten minutes after the
neutralization dose

Calm, back to normal

FIGURES 5.30A TO C
Changes in Joshua's handwriting during testing for sensitivity to home air.

▪ ADULT WRITING AND DRAWING CHANGES

The handwriting of adults, in general, changes less often and less drastically than children's; however, at times the changes are equally remarkable. During allergy testing, adults may suddenly write differently, at the same time as they manifest a total change in how they feel, look, and behave. Sometimes they become emotionally labile and feel embarrassed because they cry and don't know why. A few regress and behave or sound childish. When they react to some exposure, they may forget how to spell common words, or they may behave immaturely and refer to themselves by their childhood nickname.

Figures 5.31a to c and 5.32a to e show writing changes on two separate occasions for Kathleen, a mature woman who underwent allergy testing for sugar. On each occasion she responded almost identically. When she was reacting, she wrote her name as Kathy, not Kathleen. Her writing became larger and looked childish. Her writing did not show these changes during placebo testing.

Kathleen's reactions during precise P/N allergy testing for a wide range of substances followed a distinctive pattern. Fortunately, few people have reactions of this severity and intensity, but it can happen. She would suddenly lose her superb sense of humor and her ability to talk; she became unresponsive and eventually unconscious. Her hands and feet clenched, and her joints became rigid. As progressively weaker dilutions of allergy extract were injected into her skin at seven-minute intervals, she gradually improved. First her fingers and joints slowly relaxed; then she was able to answer questions by blinking her eyes. Eventually she could laugh, but she could not speak. Finally, when she was given the correct neutralization

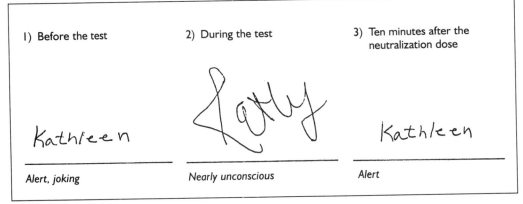

1) Before the test   2) During the test   3) Ten minutes after the
                                                         neutralization dose

Kathleen   [signature]   Kathleen

Alert, joking   *Nearly unconscious*   *Alert*

FIGURES 5.31A TO C
Changes in Kathleen's handwriting during the first test for allergy to sugar.

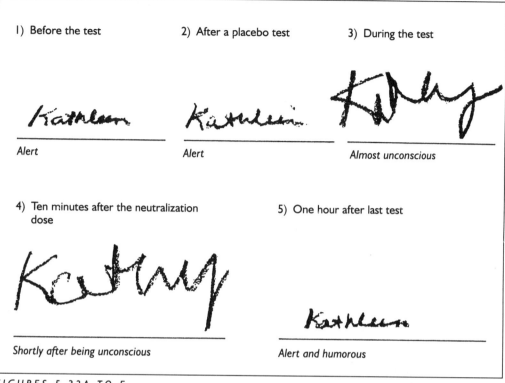

FIGURES 5.32A TO E
Changes in Kathleen's handwriting during the second test for allergy to sugar.

dose of the extract, her writing, muscles, and joints improved, and her ability to communicate and sense of humor returned to normal.

Before Kathy's treatment, the reactions described above occurred whenever she ate sugar. After treatment began, eating sugar caused much less difficulty unless her extract treatment dosage needed to be adjusted.

■ CHILDREN'S EMOTIONAL REACTIONS

The following samples show how environmental reactions producing aggression, depression, vulgarity, and immaturity can be reflected in writing and drawing:

IMMATURITY

Allergy testing can reveal an atypically immature manner in some children when exposed to certain substances. Such changes subside after they receive a neutralization dose.

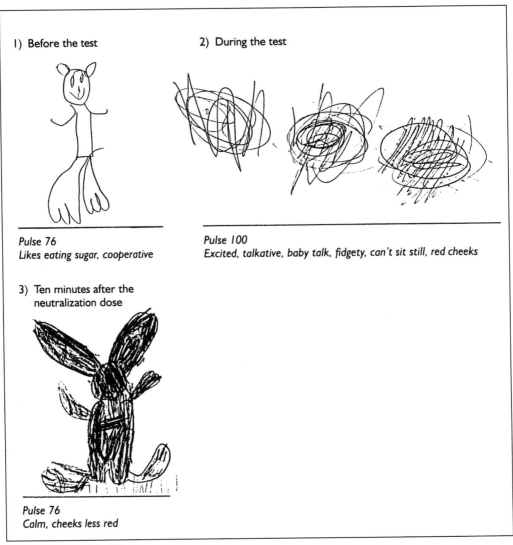

1) Before the test

Pulse 76
Likes eating sugar, cooperative

2) During the test

Pulse 100
Excited, talkative, baby talk, fidgety, can't sit still, red cheeks

3) Ten minutes after the
neutralization dose

Pulse 76
Calm, cheeks less red

FIGURES 5.33A TO C
Betsy's drawing changes during testing for allergy to sugar.

Figures 5.33a to c illustrate immaturity in the drawing of Betsy, a five-year-old, during testing for allergy to sugar. She was fed sugar cubes, then given a neutralization dose of sugar allergy extract. How many other children cannot learn because they start their day with that sugar-flavored grain commonly called a "cereal"?

The coloring in Figure 5.34 shows how Ian, a four-year-old boy, drew under normal circumstances while he was suffering from allergies.

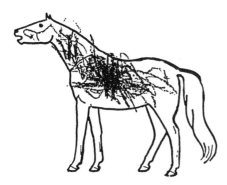

FIGURE 5.34
Ian's coloring while suffering from allergies.

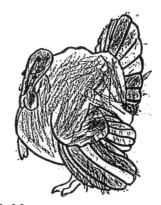

FIGURE 5.35
Ian's coloring after two weeks of allergy treatment.

Figure 5.35 shows Ian's improvement only two weeks after he began comprehensive environmental allergy treatment. The coloring in this figure was done without any assistance from his teacher. His ability to learn improved correspondingly in this same period.

AGGRESSION

Reactions to foods, dust, molds, or pollen, or exposure to chemicals, can also cause aggressive behavior and extreme anger. These feelings are manifested by drawings that depict biting, killing, hanging, knives, tombstones, dripping blood, and bullet wounds.

Ten-year-old Andy became negative toward his mother whenever he drank orange juice. He was tested, treated, and responded well to treatment with an allergy extract for orange. A year later, he again became nasty after he drank orange juice. His mother realized that his treatment dose was no longer helpful and needed adjustment. The first drawing in Figure 5.36 shows how he drew shortly after the allergy test for orange was begun. Clearly he felt aggressive toward his mother, and his handwriting noticeably deteriorated at the same time. Might such reactions help explain some of the unprovoked aggression so pervasive in today's society? This possibility needs intensive, unbiased study.

Similarly, Figure 5.37 shows a picture drawn by Gary, a twelve-year-old boy, during a test for allergy to milk. During this test, Gary became talkative, made funny faces, cleared his throat, and said he felt "blah." He began to cough and become congested. Then he acted aggressive and drew this angry picture. He named the picture "Sharkopolis." Once he was given a neutralization dose, he was again his pleasant self and felt well.

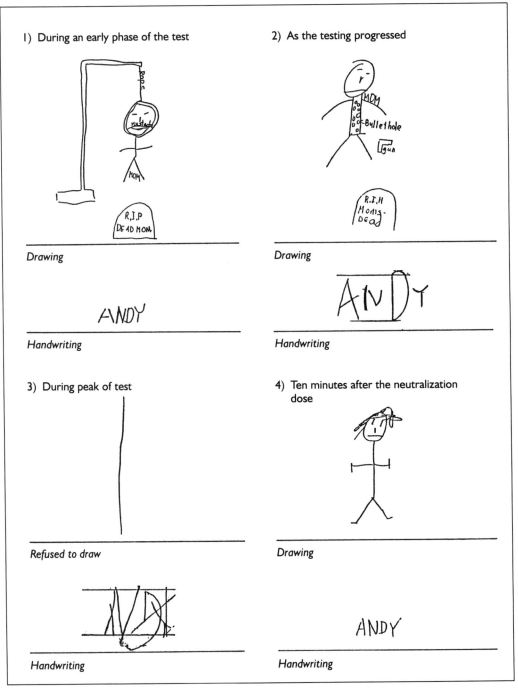

Andy's drawing and handwriting during testing for allergy to oranges.

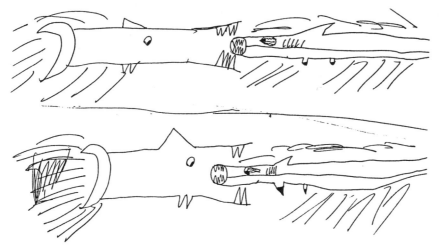

FIGURE 5.37
Gary's aggressive picture, drawn during testing for allergy to milk.

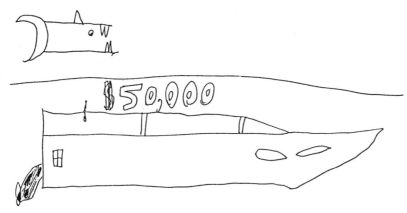

FIGURE 5.38
Gary's mood became more pleasant within ten minutes of receiving the neutralization dose.

FEAR

Figures 5.39a to c show drawings made by six-year-old Cindy while she was being tested for a mold allergy. During the mold reaction, she clearly showed fear. She put the princess in chains, saying "help me." (The other phrase is not legible.)

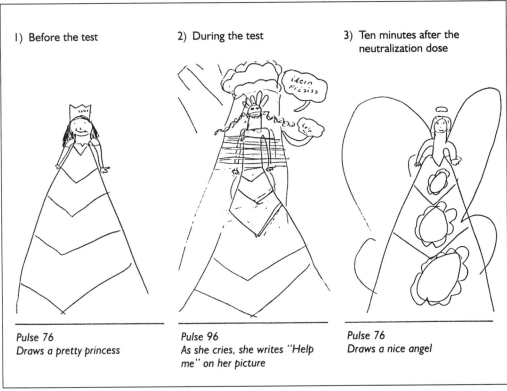

1) Before the test

2) During the test

3) Ten minutes after the neutralization dose

Pulse 76
Draws a pretty princess

Pulse 96
As she cries, she writes "Help me" on her picture

Pulse 76
Draws a nice angel

FIGURES 5.39A TO C
Changes in Cindy's drawing during testing for allergy to mold.

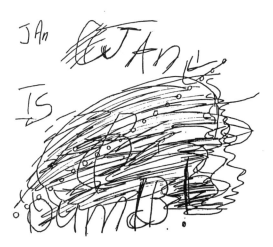

FIGURES 5.40A AND B
Lalena's writing and drawing during the testing for tree pollen.

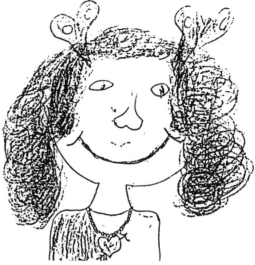

FIGURES 5.41A AND B
Lalena's writing and drawing ten minutes after the neutralization allergy treatment for tree pollen.

DEPRESSION

The writing and drawing of eight-year-old Lalena in Figures 5.40a and b and 5.41a and b reflect how she felt each spring when the trees began to pollinate. On one visit to our center, during the peak of the tree pollen season, she was very depressed and angry. She stated that she "wanted to die" and wrote, "Jan is dumb," Jan being the skin-testing nurse. As soon as she received the neutralization dose of tree pollen extract, she looked and behaved happy and normal, and her drawings reflected the change.

VULGARITY

Some absolutely adorable children write and behave in an atypically vulgar manner after a chemical exposure or eating an offending food. They often manifest similar behavior during allergy testing for these same substances.

Figures 5.42a to c show six-year-old Mike's vulgar reaction to a mold allergy extract. Ten minutes after receiving the neutralization dose, his writing and behavior returned to normal.

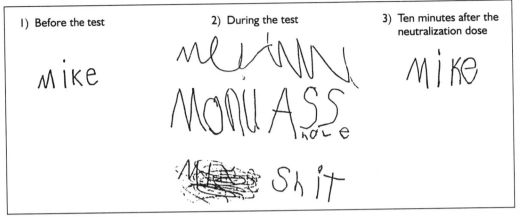

FIGURES 5.42A TO C
Changes in Mike's handwriting during testing for allergy to mold.

COMPULSIVENESS

The phenolic substance called malvin is a compound found in some thirty-five common foods; it is thought by some to be associated with certain neurological diseases, epilepsy, arthritis, and asthma.[5]

These drawings were made by thirteen-year-old Donna when she was tested for malvin. They illustrate how amazingly sensitive individuals can be to even one drop of a chemical.

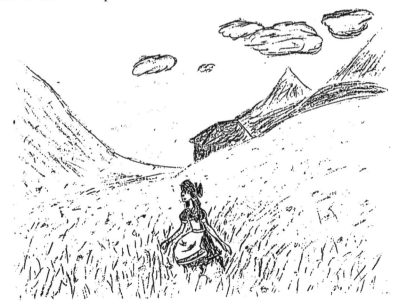

FIGURE 5.43
Donna's drawing before being tested for sensitivity to malvin.

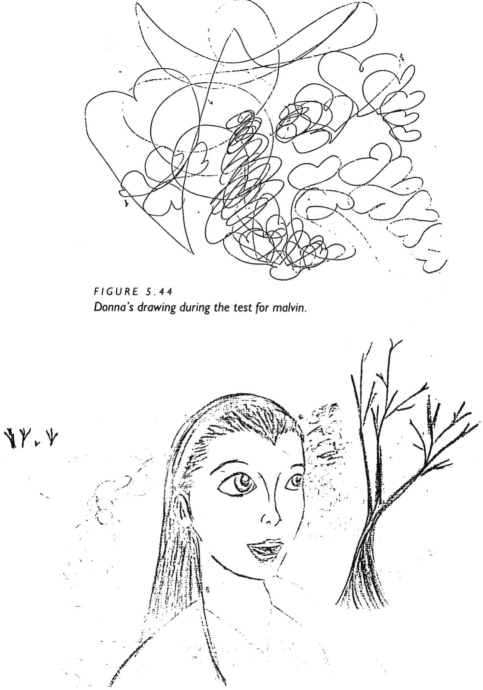

FIGURE 5.44
Donna's drawing during the test for malvin.

FIGURE 5.45
Donna's final drawing after receiving the neutralization dose. After this dose, her symptoms subsided.

■ WHAT SHOULD YOU DO?

In summary, to find answers easily, quickly, and inexpensively as part of the "Big Five," merely ask your child to write and/or draw before and after each class in school, being in each room in your home, each meal and snack, and each unavoidable chemical exposure. Similarly, compare the writing at school versus that at home, before and after going to the lavatory or to bed, or participating in outside play or a school recess. If you notice a significant change in the writing or drawing, note if the change seems linked to moldy places or rainy days. Does he or she inexplicably write well one day and not the next? Check the writing before and after a ride on the school bus or each family car. Is there anything new or different in any classroom or room in your home? With this type of information, you may be able to pinpoint the elusive cause of your child's chronic learning, health, or behavioral problem.[6] Once you find the cause, eliminate it if possible. If that is not practical, many environmentally ill children respond favorably after treatment by a specialist in environmental medicine, so that previous problem exposures cause less or no difficulty (for environmental medical specialists, see Resources).

NOTES

1. Carlton Fredericks, *New Low Blood Sugar and You* (New York: Putnam, 1985).
2. Doris J. Rapp, *Is This Your Child?* (New York: William Morrow and Co., 1991).
3. Ibid.
4. These machines are available from the Practical Allergy Relief Foundation (see Resources).
5. Robert W. Gardner, *Chemical Intolerance* (Boca Raton, FL: CRC Press, 1994).
6. For more information and examples of changes in writing and/or drawing, see Rapp, *Is This Your Child?* (New York: William Morrow, 1991) and *The Impossible Child* (Buffalo: PARF, see Resources).

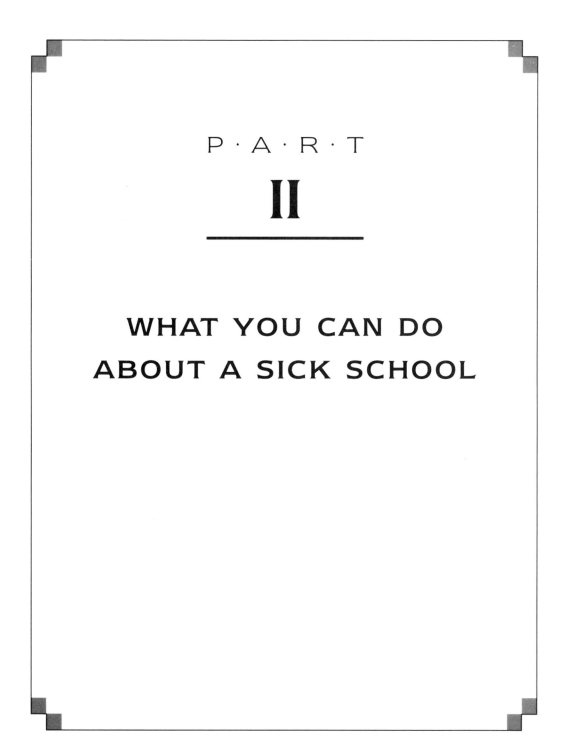

P · A · R · T

II

WHAT YOU CAN DO
ABOUT A SICK SCHOOL

INTRODUCTION FOR PART II

In our schools today, educators address many types of learning problems and misbehaviors such as violence, but they are often totally unaware of the role that environment plays in recurrent health, behavior, and learning problems. About two-thirds of the millions of children diagnosed with Attention Deficit Hyperactivity Disorder (ADHD), for example, simply have an environmental illness and/or a food sensitivity, not a Ritalin deficiency.[1]

The various exposures to substances that make children and adults sick can be either intermittent or constant. Their effect upon your own child's health will depend upon his or her own heredity and sensitivity, as well as the nature, frequency, and amount of each offending contact or odor.

One obstacle that impedes the detection of causative factors is an incomplete appreciation of the following statement:

It is not always *how much* of a substance an individual is exposed to but *how sensitive* that particular individual is to the substance that can cause illness. Sensitivity is what determines whether someone will develop a health or learning problem. For example, one heavy exposure to a pesticide can cause a sensitivity to develop, so that afterward even a minuscule exposure to any chemical in the future can cause an incapacitating illness.

In Table II.1, you'll find a list of key areas and items within schools and homes that adversely affect some students and teachers.

THE NEED FOR PUBLIC AWARENESS

Public awareness of the problems caused by lead, asbestos, radon, and even electromagnetic energy has increased in the past few years. Relatively few

TABLE II.1

Sources of Environmental School Problems

School Area

Art classroom ..	chemicals (i.e., cement, glues, play-putty)
Ceramic classroom	chemicals
Auditorium	dust, molds, chemicals
Biology lab	chemicals
Basement	dust, molds, chemicals
Boiler room	asbestos, natural gas combustion by-products
Cafeteria	food odors, chemicals
Chemistry classroom	chemical odors
Computer classroom	electromagnetic radiation, phenols
Cooking classroom	foods, odors
Gymnasium	dust/molds/cleaning chemicals
Industrial arts classroom	chemical odors
Lavatories	cleaning agents, deodorizers, disinfectants
Library	dust, molds, print odors
Loading docks ..	exhaust fumes
Music room	dust, molds, rosin
Ordinary classroom	dust, molds, chalk, plants, animals, gas heat, fumes
Printing room ..	chemicals
Typing classroom	correction fluid
Shower/locker room	molds, cleaning chemicals, scented products
Swimming pool	molds, pool chemicals, esp. chlorine

Furnishings

- New plywood furniture (emits formaldehyde)
- Synthetic carpets/carpet glues and pads
- Vinyl and/or synthetic space dividers
- Soft vinyl and/or plastic furniture
- Upholstery and furniture stuffing
- Decorations, bulletin boards, etc.
- Odorous plastic shower curtains
- Radon
- Asbestos
- Lead
- Electromagnetic radiation, power lines
- Schools (or homes) built near expressways, over swamps, toxic dump sites, etc.

Construction Materials

- Heating and cooling sources
- Ductwork and filters
- Flooring (tile, carpets, adhesives)
- Maintenance materials (roof and wall insulation, tar, paint, varnish, shellac)
- Pesticides/herbicides/termiticides/fungicides
- Wall paneling (formaldehyde)
- Fountains (germs, lead)

Cleaning Compounds

- Cleaning compounds
- Lavatory deodorizers, disinfectants
- Floor waxes, especially in hallways and gym
- Pool chemicals

Personal Items

- Perfume and other scented body and hair products
- Tobacco
- Freshly dry-cleaned or fabric-softened clothing
- Chlorine bleach and scented laundry detergent
- Mothballs
- Aerosol sprays
- Plastic schoolbags

Personal Items

■ Vinyl notebooks
■ Gum odors
■ Clothing with smelly chemical imprints

Miscellaneous

■ Art supplies
■ Blackboard chalk
■ Bulletin boards

Miscellaneous

■ Chemically treated paper
■ Carbonless paper
■ Newspaper ink or paper
■ Photo and dry paper copiers (toner and developer)
■ Laser printers
■ Crayons
■ Marking pens

individuals, however, are aware of the scope of difficulties caused by common, ubiquitous allergenic substances such as dust, molds, foods, and chemicals. Not only can these substances cause typical hay fever, asthma, or eczema; they can create perplexing illnesses in many different areas of the body. What children and adults inhale, touch, or eat can interfere not only with their health but with their behavior and memory.

Parents should share magazines, books, and videos about environmental illness with their child's principal, teacher, and health office assistants; buy and donate them to your school and local libraries. The more everyone is aware of environmental factors, the safer your school will be for your child and everyone else.

For example, watch the video *Environmentally Sick Schools* (see For Further Reading), and you'll clearly see that some students and teachers routinely become ill when they are exposed to dust or mold (dampness) contamination in schools, homes, and work areas. Similar adverse effects can develop from foods, beverages, and chemicals. Yet not everyone is affected by these exposures. Those who are genetically prone to allergies, however, appear to be particularly susceptible to the development of subtle or obvious illness, or to educational limitations directly related to these environmental exposures. Normal, gifted, and slower-learning children, as well as environmentally ill teachers, experience a wide range of reactions to environmental exposures in schools.

■ PINPOINTING ENVIRONMENTAL PROBLEMS IN SCHOOLS

The chapters in Part II will help you determine exactly what is present in your child's school building that might be causing illness and/or learning problems. Most parents and educators underestimate the prevalence and significance of various environmental factors relative to a child's school performance. They forget that children spend up to 90 percent of their time indoors, much of it in the classroom. The Environmental Protection Agency (EPA) has ranked indoor air pollution among the top five environmental health risks, reporting that indoor pollution levels can be two to five times, and occasionally more than a hundred times, higher than outdoor levels.

When it comes to schools, most of those built prior to 1985 are not very energy efficient—and worse. A 1992 report from the American Association of School Administrators states that five million children are subjected to substandard schools every day.[2] Seventy-five percent of the nation's school buildings are "living" on borrowed time. Twenty-five percent are considered inadequate. Later reports have stated that one-third of American schools need repair or replacement.

To make our schools safer, the causes of environmental problems must be *recognized and eliminated.* The ultimate aim must be cleaner air, less dust and mold, better ventilation, fewer chemicals, purer water, safer lighting, and less polluted foods. Odorous substances must be replaced with those that are less allergenic and environmentally safer. All areas of school buildings, especially classrooms, should be evaluated at regular intervals to determine if they contain elevated levels of dust, molds, and bacteria, as well as other potentially offending particles, gases, vapors, and/or chemicals. Fortunately, diagnostic instruments of varying complexity are available to efficiently identify and measure the levels of problem substances.

Once we recognize and resolve environmental school problems like these—as well as the more familiar ones of lead, asbestos, and radon—fewer students, teachers, or families will have health, activity, or memory complaints. Each chapter in Part II contains practical information about these issues, providing resources and references to help you recognize and resolve your child's specific school-related problems.

■ WHO SETS THE STANDARDS FOR SCHOOL AIR QUALITY?

Although local, state, and federal government agencies have established general guidelines to protect human health and safety, most were established for adult males working in industry, not for children, teachers, or pregnant women in schools. Existing legislation, unfortunately, typically takes the form of suggestions, guidelines, or policies, not mandates or laws that would be much more substantive and require enforcement.

In 1994, the New York State Education Department formulated policies affirming that *every child has the right to a safe and healthful learning environment.* Educators there believe that parents have the right to know about health hazards in schools, and that schools should serve as role models for environmentally responsible behavior. Thus, the state's schools are developing plans to conduct research about current and emerging school environmental and safety issues. For example, New York State schools will be required to report various environmental health matters and actions to the state health department. For details about the policies, contact:

The State University of New York
The New York State Department of Education
Office of Central Services
Albany, NY 12234
(518) 474-3852

THE MARYLAND EXAMPLE

What can states do to reduce school environmental problems? In 1987, the Maryland Department of Education implemented a statewide indoor air-quality program (IAQ), setting an exemplary gold standard for the rest of the nation. A number of Maryland publications describe the state's efforts, including:

- *Indoor Air Quality in Maryland Public Schools*
- *Indoor Air Quality Management Program*
- *Guidelines for Controlling Environmental Tobacco Smoke in Schools*
- *Guidelines for Controlling Indoor Air Quality Problems Associated with Kilns, Copiers, and Welding in Schools*
- *Air Cleaning Devices for HVAC Supply Systems in Schools*

For details about the program in Maryland, write to:

Maryland Department of Education
200 West Baltimore Street
Baltimore, MD 21201
(410) 333-2508

WHERE TO GO FOR MORE INFORMATION

A number of private and governmental agencies can provide additional information, insight, and direction about air quality in schools (as well as in homes and/or the workplace). The Resources section at the end of this book contains a listing of them. Although their various guidelines and standards have similarities, their proclaimed "safe" levels of various contaminants at any one time show a number of discrepancies and sometimes appear arbitrary. In general, these levels have become increasingly liberal. *Unfortunately, such standards appear to be driven more by economic and political considerations than by health concerns.*

As desirable as these resolutions are, however, they do not begin to resolve the most pressing issues: *Who will enforce genuine changes within schools after individuals have become ill? Who will be responsible for the academic and health-related consequences of a child's or teacher's illness resulting from a harmful school exposure?* Here is one example.

COULD YOUR CHILD FALL BETWEEN THE CRACKS?

Christy

During the summer of 1992, a school in the eastern United States underwent renovations and had new carpets installed. However, the remodeling was not completed by the time school started in September, and odors from the renovations and the new carpeting quickly made 12-year-old Christy (and many other students and teachers) ill. At the same time, Christy was also exposed to the foam insulation that was being sprayed onto the school's roof. On one occasion, as she held the door open for a teacher, so much white isocyanate insulation fell into her hair that it had to be washed before she could continue her school day.

Prior to September 1992, Christy had occasional mild headaches that responded well to aspirin. But after she started school that fall, the headaches became an everyday and much more severe problem, and they were not relieved by medication.

To make matters worse, Christy developed other distressing symptoms in the next few weeks: abdominal pain, nausea, bad breath, eye irritation, throat burning, numb and tingling hands, nasal congestion, fatigue/sleepiness, neck and back pain, twitching hands, wiggly legs, a sound/light/cold sensitivity, ringing ears, red earlobes, earaches, and hearing loss.

At first, all of Christy's symptoms would subside when she returned home each afternoon, only to reappear promptly the next school day. During the Christmas holidays, her symptoms subsided, but they returned again after school resumed in January. Her grades began to suffer, and she became worried and depressed. "What's going on?" she wondered. "Why am I so ill? Why am I not feeling better?"

By February, Christy was drinking excessive amounts of water, gaining lots of weight, and sleeping too much. By March, she was simply too ill to attend school. When she received home teaching, she felt better, but she was far from well; her symptoms were less severe but they persisted. Although her grades have improved, they have never returned to their pre-1992 level.

In 1993, Christy had developed the "spreading phenomenon," meaning that the tiniest amount of any chemical odor now caused symptoms. She would become ill from the smell of perfume, hair spray, gasoline, flowers, formaldehyde, or exhaust fumes. She developed a craving for the aroma of candles, but promptly became ill if she smelled them. If she went into a bookstore, within ten to fifteen minutes she would experience a headache, leg aches, and nausea from the odor of the paper and/or the ink. It took several hours before she felt better.

Christy tried to return to school in April 1993, but within thirty minutes, she had developed a headache, and she became so fatigued that she had to sleep the rest of the day. Once again, home teaching had to be resumed. When she was no longer exposed to the inside of her school building, she felt less tired, less irritable, and less nauseated, but these complaints recurred whenever she was exposed to any chemical anywhere.

Christy is presently being tutored at home two hours a day. She has been helped by environmental medical therapy and homeopathic therapy, but she is still not well.

At age 14, more than three years after the harmful environmental exposures at her school, Christy's life is filled with restrictions, limitations, and fears. Her future remains in limbo:

- She is still much too ill to attend school. If her health doesn't improve soon, she may never realize her dream of a college education.
- The family's health insurance isn't paying for the medical care needed to help eliminate the chemicals from her body (detoxification). Her family cannot afford this treatment, and yet the longer she waits, the more challenging it will be for her to reverse her illness and catch up with her academic studies.
- Although further objective brain-image documentation has not been financially possible, it is most unlikely that Christy's brain has recovered. She continues to have constant headaches, and she cannot remember or learn as well as she did prior to her school's renovation in 1992. No wonder she and her parents are worried about her future.

■ CAN THE EPA HELP?

The EPA is well aware that environmental issues influence the health and academic performance of children. It is making strides to raise the nation's general awareness of these factors, but it cannot implement practical solutions within a reasonable period of time without new federal legislation and/or changes in existing laws. For example, before it can recommend that air purifiers be placed in classrooms, the EPA must research the efficacy of such units. Similar studies would have to be conducted on cleaning, maintenance, and remodeling materials. *At present, potentially unsafe materials may be in use for inordinate periods of time because in-depth scientific evaluations have not been conducted. Necessary revisions of federal mandates, however, are far from imminent. If you are concerned, write your state and federal legislators (see Chapter 16).*

Ironically, the EPA's own 1987 new carpet and remodeling guidelines eventually *caused* illnesses in more than 122 of its own employees[3] (see Chapter 10). A survey showed that 40 percent of EPA employees suffered from the Sick Building Syndrome. The agency has protected its own workers by refusing to purchase any more carpets containing the causative toxic agent 4-PCs; but it has *not* similarly advised and protected the public. By early 1995, the EPA had not implemented any substantive solutions for this public risk, even though it had spent millions of taxpayer dollars to remedy its own carpet fiasco and help its sick employees.

■ MAKING CHANGES

Later in this book (Chapter 12), you'll read examples of Canadian schools that have met some of these issues head-on. Some Canadian school districts have resolved their environmentally-related school problems in "scientifically imperfect" but fast, easy, practical, safe, health-beneficial, and cost-effective ways.

Schools in the United States should seriously consider emulating the Canadian solutions. It should not take decades to install air purifiers and use safer cleaning agents and construction materials, nontoxic pest control, and nonharmful floor coverings in schools. These times call for flexibility and common sense. We need an immediate change in priorities.

It took the Occupational Safety and Health Administration (OSHA) seventeen years to issue safety standards for twenty-four toxic substances. In 1984, standards for 484 substances were suddenly issued and implemented. *However, the corporations that produced the toxic substances supplied the information on their safety to the American Council of Governmental Industrial Hygienists; this nongovernmental group, in turn, provided OSHA with the new standards for the threshold limit value of toxic materials. In effect, the fox decided on the design of the hen house.*

Such flexibility shows a lack of little common sense or good judgment. The rules of the game can change quickly for the worse when elusive but powerful pressures intervene. Let us urge some positive changes to be implemented in relation to harmful exposures in schools. In the chapters that follow, you'll get a sense of the pressing problems in our schools, and the urgency to find solutions.

NOTES

1. Marvin Boris et al., "Foods and Additives Are Common Causes of the Attention Deficit Hyperactive Disorder in Children," *Annals of Allergy*, vol. 72 (May 1994), pp. 462–68; C.M. Carter et al., "Effects of a Few Food Diets in Attention Deficit Disorder," *Archives of Diseases in Childhood*, vol. 69 (1993), pp. 546–68; J. Egger, A. Stolla, and L.M. McEwen, "Controlled Trial of Hyposensitization in Children with Food-induced Hyperkinetic Syndrome," *Lancet*, vol. 339 (May 9, 1992), pp. 1150–53; J. Egger et al., "Controlled Trial of Oligoantigenic Treatment in the Hyperkinetic Syndrome," *Lancet* (1985), pp. 540–45; J. O'Shea et al., "Double Blind Study of Children with Hyperkinetic Syndrome Treated with Multi-Allergen Extract Sublingually," *Journal of Learning Disabilities*, vol. 14 (1981),

p. 189; D.J. Rapp, ''Does Diet Affect Hyperactivity?'' *Journal of Learning Disabilities*, vol. 11 (1978), pp. 56–62; Katherine S. Rowe and Kenneth J. Rowe, ''Synthetic Food Coloring and Behavior: A Dose Response Effect in a Double-Blind, Placebo-Controlled, Repeated-Measures Study,'' *Journal of Pediatrics*, vol. 124, no. 5, part 1 (1988), pp. 691–98.

2. Robert Eade, ''Heating, Cooling, and Refrigeration,'' *Engineered Systems*, vol. 12, no. 2 (Feb. 1995); American Association of School Administrators, *Schoolhouse in the Red*. Available from the AASA at 1801 North Moore Street, Arlington, VA 22209.

3. Lynn Lawson, *Staying Well in a Toxic World* (Chicago: Noble Press, 1993).

6 ⊏ Air-Quality Problems

$\mathbf{M}$ajor sources of indoor air pollution include ventilation problems, filtration problems, gases and chemical fumes, dust, pollen, molds, pets, bacteria, and viruses (see Table 6.1). In this chapter, salient aspects of these sources will be reviewed or discussed in detail.

Then, in Chapters 7 to 11, some of the other problem locations and specific substances that typically bother sensitive students, teachers, and families will be considered.

■ VENTILATION PROBLEMS

Ventilation needs attention in the majority of environmentally sick schools in the United States. A 1992 report by the American Association of School Administrators stated that 52 percent of the country's schools had indoor air-quality problems due to "inadequate" ventilation.[1] The problem, however, is much more complex than simply an insufficiency of fresh outdoor air. Improper heating or air conditioning with inadequate filtration and improperly vented noxious gases and exhaust products all play a role as well. Defective heating and cooling units have also contributed to poor indoor air quality and higher energy consumption. Deferred maintenance unequivocally leads to unnecessary and increasing expenditures.[2]

It is generally recommended that school air be exchanged about two to four times an hour. In addition, the air quality should meet the minimum requirement of 25 percent fresh air and 75 percent recirculated filtered air. According to the EPA, it takes three to twelve months before the level of chemicals inside a school, home, or workplace falls to the outdoor concentrations after certain types of construction; for that reason, after major construction of a new building, it is often recommended that 100 percent outdoor air be used for the first six months.[3] Realistically, however, a period longer than six months may be necessary.

TABLE 6.1

Practical Environmental Health Concerns in Schools and Homes

I.	Ventilation problems
II.	Filtration problems
III.	Gases and chemical fumes
IV.	Dust, pollen, molds, and pets
V.	Bacteria and viruses

If your own school has ventilation inadequacies, they may be related directly to inappropriate measures taken in the past to conserve energy. To a large degree, this situation originated and escalated during the energy crisis of the early 1970s. At that time, the recommended fresh-air circulation rate in many schools was lowered to 5 cubic feet per minute (cfm). Some schools vigorously conserved energy by closing their ventilation systems to such an extreme degree that they permitted little or no fresh-air circulation! This measure decreased the need and cost to heat or cool schools. *However, after the energy crisis subsided, many of these ventilation systems were never reopened or properly cleaned because of neglect and/or stressed school budgets.*

More recently, the level of air exchange in many schools was only about 10 cfm in the United States. That's still lower than the following suggested sensible and practical guideline: During times of normal maintenance, schools should provide 15 cfm per person of outdoor ventilation for two hours prior to the students' arrival in the morning, extending until one to two hours after maintenance cleaning is completed at the end of the day. After remodeling or major renovations, this 15-cfm level should be maintained *at all times* for a full year. Again, it takes three to twelve months after the completion of construction before the concentration of chemicals inside a building approaches outdoor levels. Even the 15-cfm level, however, is still not up to other standards; in Canada, for example, the level is presently 16 cfm. In 1989, the American Society of Heating, Refrigeration and Air Conditioning Engineers (ASHRAE) increased the suggested fresh-air circulation rates to 20 cfm for offices. Why should the rates in schools be less?

How does new building construction significantly add to the indoor air-quality problem? In effect, it reduces, rather than enhances, the outdoor-air exchange. For example, windows that don't open and more efficient insulation result in a gradual buildup of allergens such as dust and molds within the building. To make a bad situation worse, ever-increasing amounts of pollution and potentially hazardous chemicals have been and continue to be introduced into our schools (and homes) every day.

Unfortunately, few states have *enforced* their legislation establishing ventilation standards in schools. Recommendations, guidelines, and standards suggested by ASHRAE, for example, are simply inadequate if schools do not comply with them.

The costs of creating a healthy school are more than offset by future savings in maintenance, operation, and reconstruction, as well as in deterring potential legal entanglements. Less tangible but even more important is the associated improvement in the health and academic performance of America's future—the students of today and tomorrow.

CHECK THE VENTILATION SYSTEM

Various studies have shown that at least one-third of buildings have inadequate ventilation, contaminated ductwork, inferior or inadequate filters, and dirty air conditioners.[4] When you discuss possible ventilation problems with your school officials, your approach should be reasonable and should stress cost-effectiveness as well as the health and learning benefits for students and faculty.

A good place to start is by inquiring whether your state has a recommended school air-quality-control policy. Ask when your child's building had its last thorough heating/ventilation/air conditioning (HVAC) evaluation. Some schools have modern, sophisticated computer HVAC programs that have been modified to provide continuous improved air quality. Have licensed professional engineers tested and certified compliance with the standards set in ASHRAE 62–1989? This HVAC evaluation should have included a thorough critique of the efficiency of the ventilation system (ducts, vents, fans, coils, filters, and so on), whether in a single building or in an entire school district.

When licensed HVAC engineers balance ventilation units, they can ensure that an acceptable quality and quantity of air is more evenly exchanged and distributed throughout the building. (For a list of HVAC engineers and consultants, see Resources.) Recommendations concerning maintenance and cleaning of the ventilation ducts, as well as other suggestions, are detailed in the publications by the Maryland Department of Education and the National Air Duct Cleaners Association, listed in the Resources.

You can personally check the ventilation in your own child's classroom. Take a piece of tissue paper, and see if it moves in front of the vents when the blower of a heating system is functioning. Also, are the intake and exhaust vents open or blocked by furniture, files, or boxes? In some schools the only ventilation for years has been the leakage that occurs naturally around light and electrical fixtures.

To make the situation particularly challenging, the quality of the "cleaner" outdoor air is far from ideal in certain locations. Some schools, for example, have intake vents located near exhaust vents, garages, delivery areas, or sites where school buses or other vehicles idle. Other schools are located downwind from nearby industrial and agricultural pollution. These situations can result in poor-quality indoor air being mixed with equally poor outside air. Such factors need to be considered by your school district when new building construction sites are selected.

WHAT SHOULD A VENTILATION EVALUATION INCLUDE?
According to the ASHRAE 62-1989 guidelines, air quality should be monitored regularly for carbon dioxide, carbon monoxide, other gases, chemicals, and particles such as dust, molds, pollen, and bacteria. The levels of total volatile organic compounds (VOCs) and formaldehyde should be checked routinely after new construction. Thereafter, checks should be conducted once or twice a year.

One experienced environmental air consultant firm in Phoenix—Environmental Medicine and Engineering—suggests that the number of particulates larger than 0.5 microns in the indoor air should not exceed 30,000 to 150,000/cubic foot, as measured by a laser particle counter (*see* Resources). For comparison, the level in an operating room should be kept below 10,000/cubic foot of air. These counts are only numbers, however, and do not identify the *composition* of the particles. The 0.5-micron counts include mainly smaller molds, pollen, dust, and tobacco smoke. Counts also can consist of particles larger than 5.0 microns, such as pet hair, insulation fibers, dust, larger mold spores, and pollen, asbestos, and sawdust.

The particulate levels can provide a clue as to whether insulation, such as cellulose, is leaking into ventilation ducts or through wall openings. Oil and grease from equipment can circulate hydrocarbon or other chemical odors throughout a school. Condensation drip pans in refrigerators, for example, need routine monthly maintenance because of slime, molds, and the potential accumulation of a variety of germs.

Ask whether the heating and cooling portions of the school's ventilation systems have been properly cleaned. If the ductwork filters do not fit correctly and are not cleaned frequently, accumulated dust and molds can be circulated throughout the school. Dirt on the heating and cooling coils of HVAC units can reduce their efficiency by 30 percent or more, causing needless additional expense.

Parent and teacher groups can urge that schools take better measures to provide an adequate air exchange, especially in heavily polluted classrooms. All ventilation hoods should be inspected and cleaned annually. When ventilation fans suddenly turn off, accumulated contamination can drift back into the area from which it came. Large ventilation hoods are needed to exhaust contaminated odors from biology and chemistry laboratories, kitchen and cafeteria areas, art and industrial arts classrooms, and rooms where copying, duplicating, and printing equipment are located. Because some printing chemicals are known to cause serious nervous system damage and/or cancer, adequate ventilation in such areas is imperative.

The levels and types of various pollutants permitted are not the only critical questions in schools. We also need to know if the levels of allergenic substances and chemicals inside the building are above or below the levels that cause illness in environmentally sensitive students or teachers.

HOW MUCH WILL VENTILATION CHANGES INCREASE THE SCHOOL BUDGET?

In this era of tight school budgets, school boards must always consider benefit-cost ratios, and decisions are not always easy to make. Sometimes, needed modifications are impractical; certain school buildings are simply too old, poorly designed, and not worth changing. On the other hand, we need to appreciate the ultimate price: chronic health problems and unrealized academic achievement among our children. (School officials in Ontario, Canada, have found some practical and cost-effective answers to these questions, as you'll read in Chapter 12.)

Let your own school administrators and boards know that—contrary to their cursory impressions—improving the air quality in schools can actually sometimes *reduce* expenses. If the air circulation, cleaning, filtration, insulation, and other aspects of the ventilation system need only minor modifications, making those changes often lowers, rather than raises, the school's long-term expenditures. However, some modifications (made in compliance with ASHRAE 62-1989) can cause a slight *increase* in utility costs during both the heating and cooling seasons. To offset this increase, your school can provide comfortable temperatures for a couple of hours before the school day begins, continuing for one or two hours at the end of the day once the daily maintenance cleaning has been completed. Even if a heating/cooling system is not functioning, the ventilation should be continuous. Room temperatures should be maintained between 68° and 75°F.

If your school has major ventilation inadequacies, is dusty and moldy, or smells of chemicals, the initial expenses to remedy the problem can be high. If repairs and maintenance are completed on a timely schedule, however, these expenses will surely be less. Over the long-term, there can actually be immense savings.

Remind school officials that if appropriate changes are made, the need for (and cost of) home teaching, special education for select students, and absenteeism should decrease. At the same time, academic performance should improve, along with the attendance and health of both students and teachers.

Aside from the humane and compassionate issues, it is cost-effective to restore the health of ill students, teachers, and families. Students who complete their education can become resourceful, productive citizens who contribute to society. Well teachers need no health-related compensation. In addition, in today's litigious society, school districts can reduce the possibility of costly legal entanglements if they recognize, acknowledge, and remedy a school's indoor air-quality problems *before* a major crisis develops.

As everyone's awareness heightens, a growing number of school officials and employees are increasingly recognizing and accepting their responsibilities and obligations in relation to environmental issues in schools and workplaces.

FAST, EASY, AND INEXPENSIVE WAYS TO IMPROVE SCHOOL VENTILATION

In Table 6.2, you'll find many possible avenues for improving your child's school's ventilation. Perhaps the simplest and least expensive way would be to open all the windows and doors, but realistically most modern school buildings have windows that do not open. For that reason, they need mechanically controlled ventilation to ensure an adequate air exchange.

More helpful suggestions include: better, more frequent cleaning,

TABLE 6.2

Ways to Improve Indoor Air

To help right away in most cases:

- Clean the entire building more thoroughly and more often. Vacuum heavily used areas often and well.
- Have an HVAC engineer thoroughly evaluate each school or home ventilation system.
- Be sure all ductwork is clean and free of chemicals and molds.
- Filters must fit properly, be clean, and not be laden with molds or germs. Install ancillary ventilation hoods and supplementary exhaust systems in heavily polluted areas.
- Use room air-purifying machines in localized poor-air-quality areas.
- Use central air-purification systems to enhance air quality throughout the building.
- Check for mold and germ contamination in rooms with a high incidence of illness.
- Use only environmentally approved, safer cleaning materials and mold-retardant agents, such as Borax.
- Install and maintain dehumidifiers to eliminate excessive humidity. Check the ventilation system.
- Stringently reduce the use of chemicals.
- Do not allow bus engines to idle while waiting for students to enter or leave the school, or in garages or driveways at home.
- Be sure drain traps contain water to decrease sewer gas.
- Request and read Material Safety Data (MSD) sheets for every chemical used in or around schools and homes. Check for chemical contamination.
- Replace routine pesticide use with safer biological forms of insect and pest control. Do not use pesticide control unless there are pests.
- Offer less pesticide-contaminated, more natural foods and water in schools.
- Stop or restrict the use of perfume, tobacco, fingernail polish, offensive glues, cements, etc.
- Use natural light and full-spectrum lighting.
- Store all flammable materials in OSHA-approved fire cabinets.
- Install exhaust fans in storage closets/rooms where maintenance and art supplies are kept.
- If carpets must be installed, inexpensively check for chemicals and health hazards (see carpeting information in Chapter 10).
- When indicated, carefully raise the temperature to at least 90° F. for a day or two to "bake out" the molds and chemicals.

using safer maintenance materials; routine changing or cleaning of air filters; and complete opening of all intake and exhaust vents, except for intake vents that allow heavily contaminated air to enter the ventilation system. In the latter situation, the intake vents should be sealed and new ones opened in more environmentally sound locations. If there are specific isolated pockets of poor air quality, simple fans and diffusers can improve the distribution of clean air. In addition, inexpensive but efficient floor or ceiling high-efficiency particle arrestance (HEPA) air purifiers can be particularly beneficial and cost effective in schools (see Resources).

MORE EXPENSIVE BUT BETTER WAYS

HVAC MONITORING

Find out whether the school's ventilation system is being monitored properly. Most school maintenance departments can effectively implement the suggestions made by a reputable commercial HVAC company, but *continued professional monitoring is essential*. Controls and dampers must be judiciously regulated to ensure that fresh air circulates well throughout the entire school building. Central air purifiers are costlier than room units, but they can more effectively remove a larger variety of air pollutants.

FURNACE CLEANING

Many HVAC consultants won't clean the inside of a furnace, although they should because a carbon buildup will tend to accumulate there. Also, the evaporator coils and the flue pipe in the heat-exchange unit can become moldy and dusty. In addition, the fan-blade bearings can contaminate the entire ventilation system with grease or hydrocarbon odors.

DUCT CLEANING

I can't overemphasize the need for thorough duct cleaning. Moldy ducts can contain many types of indoor air particles, including germs, which have the potential to cause infection, asthma, hay fever, and other forms of illness in susceptible students and teachers.

The ductwork, coils, and return air plenums in the ventilation system must be closely monitored and thoroughly cleaned when indicated. The ducts should be cleaned according to the standards set by *The Mechanical Cleaning of Nonporous Air Conveyance System Components*, prepared by the National Air Duct Cleaners Association. Independent inspectors can assess the maintenance methods and adherence to standards. The Air Duct Cleaners Association can refer your school system (or an individual) to a local company that has expertise and certification in duct cleaning (see Resources).

Ideally, the ductwork should be constructed of a smooth, nonporous, easily cleaned surface such as sheet metal. The general duct-cleaning technique itself is basically simple. The vents can be vacuumed using powerful motors *when school is not in session*. Holes are drilled in the ductwork every eight to ten feet (depending upon the design) so that high-velocity air (175 psi air pressure) can be injected to dislodge material accumulated in the ducts. While this is being done, at least 4,000 cfm of negative pressure is applied to suck air from the exhaust, intake tributaries, and main duct lines onto a large HEPA filter unit, which collects the debris. The pressure is supplied by a portable inside unit or an outside truck-mounted unit.

Under the best of circumstances, the ductwork should be cleaned every six years. If years have passed since proper maintenance, and special care is not taken, the ducts will discharge large amounts of dust, causing some children to wheeze for the first time. If a cleaning solution is required, a safe and inexpensive substance such as Neolife Rugged Red is recommended (see Resources). When properly done, this process should not further contaminate the school air.

However, here's a note of caution: *Your school should avoid applying surface sealants in ducts. Chemicals should never be sprayed directly into a ductwork system because some can pollute a building to such a degree that it will never again be habitable. School officials should warn duct cleaners well in advance, because some routinely infuse toxic chemicals into the ductwork so quickly that the damage can be done before anyone realizes what has happened.*

INSULATION

Foam insulation looks like shaving cream, and when it is injected into walls, it hardens. Urea foam, which caused so many problems in the 1970s, is no longer used. Even though some forms of foam contain polystyrene, they are usually well tolerated. A new more expensive injected foam called Air-Krete "outgasses" very little, releases no formaldehyde, and appears to cause few health difficulties.

Cellulose insulation is made of recycled newspapers, complete with possible toxic inks. It is treated with boron for fire and insect control. The dry form is blown through holes in the walls into the sides of buildings; once there, it can drift from any wall openings for ducts or electrical wires into the inside of a building, where it can contaminate the air. To prevent this problem, leaks should be sealed and the air purified. If a wet form of cellulose is used during construction, it must be thoroughly dried before it is covered, or a chronic mold problem will be created.

Fiberglass insulation can be applied in a molded form between walls. It is held together with a formaldehyde-based resin, which can release formaldehyde gas in tiny amounts. When the chopped form of fiberglass is used, it is blown into the wall spaces, like dry cellulose; if it leaks into the indoor air, it is more of a danger than cellulose because its particles are very tiny and can potentially lodge in the lungs causing health problems. When it is used to insulate ventilation ducts, *it should be applied only to the outside, never to the inside of the ductwork*. If loose fibers are released as it disintegrates, particularly near the main plenums or ductwork, they can be transported throughout the air in a building.

Cotton/polyester molded insulation is also available. It contains boron, which can irritate the nose if particles are released and inhaled.

Ventilation ducts can become contaminated by odors from tobacco, personal cosmetics, cleaning materials, sprays, cooking, art supplies, and pool chemicals, all of which can be absorbed by porous insulation. Make sure your child's school is entirely "smoke-free"; tobacco residues in teachers' lounges or student lavatories can enter the ventilation system and pollute entire buildings.

A deliberate attempt must be made to increase the use of less odorous and safer furnishings and building supplies, adhesives, vinyl partitions, paint, and pest control, both inside and outside schools and homes, and especially near intake ventilation ducts.

MOST EXPENSIVE BUT BEST WAYS

The best means for improving ventilation in many schools also involve the greatest initial expense. For example, if your school had faulty original construction, it may be necessary to increase the number of intake and return ducts, so that the fresh-air source and turnover can be doubled or quadrupled. In some cases, it may be worthwhile to create supplementary additional access and visual-inspection ports in the ventilation system to ensure adequate cleaning and monitoring. In addition, some buildings were so poorly designed that air from the roof exhaust vents reenters nearby and poorly located intake vents; ideally, intake vents should be located not on the top of a building but on the side that is least exposed to wind-blown pollution.

At times, the construction materials or insulation in ductwork has been contaminated with molds, chemicals, and/or particles from disintegrating insulation. This problem can sometimes be remedied with appropriate cleaning and installation of a quality central air-purification system (see Resources). Some school and other buildings have been so extensively compromised that removal and replacement of the entire ventilation system is required to make them safe and habitable.

■ FILTRATION PROBLEMS

Filtration is a key factor in improving school ventilation. The entire filtration component of a ventilation system must be monitored and maintained closely. Filtration is required both at the outdoor intake and at the indoor return air ducts—relatively simple measures that can be cost-effective and easy to implement.

For educational facilities, section 4 of the booklet *Air Cleaning Devices for HVAC Supply Systems in Schools* (December 1992) should prove helpful; it was published as a technical bulletin by the State of Maryland Department of Education. (For information on obtaining this booklet, see the Introduction to Part II.)

DUCTWORK FILTERS

In general, most ductwork filters remove particles that are 50 to 100 microns or larger in size. Dust mites are about 30 to 40 microns; most pollen is roughly 15 to 30 microns. Ordinary filters may not be effective for the removal of the smaller types of pollen or particles; better-quality filters will more likely be efficient in this regard.

In most buildings with poor ventilation systems, the filtration system can be upgraded easily by using higher-quality, more efficient, properly fitting filters, which then must be maintained on a routine schedule. In some schools, air filters are infrequently or never cleaned or replaced. In a few schools, they have never even been installed!

There are several categories of filters. The inexpensive ones are throwaways that need frequent replacement. The more efficient ones are electrostatic and reusable, but some can be impractical in schools because they need frequent cleaning. Some filters contain charcoal, which helps to reduce odors, fumes, and airborne chemicals.

THE MORE EXPENSIVE BUT BETTER FILTERS

Sometimes a school district's choice of filters is sharply limited, not only by economics but also by the inept design of existing ventilation ductwork. Whenever possible, however, school administrators should select better-quality, pleated, extended-media-type filters, which catch more dust and other particles in their meshlike composition material. Although these filters initially cost more, they last longer and have to be cleaned less frequently. They ultimately reduce heating and cooling expenditures by significantly increasing overall ventilation efficiency.

THE MOST EXPENSIVE BUT BEST FILTERS

High-efficiency particle arrestance (HEPA) filters are the *most* desirable, especially the newer improved types, because they tend not to impede air flow. If air has difficulty passing through a filter because of construction or accumulated dust, the cost of ventilation surely will be increased.

CAUTIONS ABOUT OTHER FILTERS

It is possible to purchase impregnated filters that incorporate the Aegis microbial shield technology chemical substance, which appears to effectively diminish microbial (germ and mold) problems in existing school buildings (see Resources).[5] While theoretically these filters should be beneficial, this chemical product *contains a pesticide in the form of a silane-modified quaternary amine.* Although it is bonded to the filter in a manner that is claimed to avoid any problems, *the bottom line is the way each chemically sensitive child or teacher responds to this type of exposure.* The effective elimination of circulating molds and germs is unquestionably advisable, but unless safety and health monitoring is implemented, it would be easy to miss subtle adverse health effects resulting from this type of chemical exposure in a susceptible group of individuals. On the other hand, it would be impractical to closely monitor the health of all occupants of a building for several months after a germ-retardant filter is installed. Therefore, any filtration product should be checked individually *before installation*, especially if it contains a pesticide. School administrators should ask for the help of an environmentally knowledgeable physician and follow the suggestions in Chapter 5.

Remember, if your child is chemically sensitive, he or she cannot routinely tolerate even minute exposures to certain substances that cause other people no difficulty. I believe strongly that it is unfair to put these growing children, as well as pregnant women and any other adults, at potential risk. Many people don't recognize these obvious cause-and-effect relationships, particularly when they have only vague symptoms such as fatigue, headaches, or a gradual diminution of breathing or brain function. *In fact, an illness caused by contact with a new chemical, such as in a specially pesticide-treated filter, might remain elusive indefinitely if there is little odor and if the exposure is not readily visible or known.*

Another type of filtration is called electrostatic precipitation. In this kind of system, dust and other particles are positively or negatively charged and are collected or deposited on the respectively opposite-charged plates. The problems caused by this type of filtration include the need for continued maintenance to clean the plates, as well as possible lung irritation from the minute amount of ozone produced during its use.

CHECK THE EFFICIENCY OF THE FILTRATION SYSTEM

Certain basic tests, suggested by the ASHRAE 52-76, can be used to evaluate the effectiveness of your school's filtration system. One of them checks the filter's ability to remove a certain percentage of dust particles, which takes into account the weight of the particles. This test is called *arrestance*. Another test, called the dust spot test, measures the soiling of a check spot after filtration.

The higher the arrestance and dust spot numbers that result from testing a particular filter, the better the filter. These findings are usually listed on the data sheets supplied with various types of filters. HVAC firms can conduct this type of testing.

▪ GASES AND CHEMICAL FUMES

A number of gases or volatile fumes unquestionably pose possible ventilation and/or contamination problems in schools. To prevent many of these indoor air-quality problems, your school can use low-level-emission and pest-resistant materials in construction, as well as safe sealers and vapor barriers when indicated (see Resources). By detecting and eliminating gases and fumes early, schools can simultaneously reduce illness while improving the children's academic performance.

CARBON DIOXIDE

Schools need an adequate amount of fresh air to compensate for the carbon dioxide (CO_2) produced during ordinary breathing. Measurement of carbon dioxide levels reflects the amount of fresh air in an area. Good outdoor air contains about 350 parts per million (ppm); excellent indoor air contains 400 ppm; and good indoor air, 600 ppm. If a room has a level of 1,400 to 2,000 ppm of CO_2, both children and adults might be uncomfortable and unable to think clearly, and they may become excessively drowsy. According to ASHRAE standards, even 1,000 ppm is too high, and so the safety level has been lowered to 800. In general, for an area to have ventilation of 15 cfm per person, the differential between the outside and inside air should be about 700 ppm. (So if the outside air has 400 ppm, the inside should have about 1,100 ppm.) These standards, therefore, appear to be somewhat unrealistic.

To resolve the traditional conflict between the cost of providing adequate outside air ventilation and maintaining good-quality indoor air, schools can use CO_2 control sensors. These energy-saving sensors graph the level of CO_2, humidity, and temperature over a period of time to produce what is called *demand-controlled ventilation*. They can stabilize the air quality by recognizing and reducing periods of over- or underventilation (see Chapter 13).

As the concentration of carbon dioxide increases, a child's ability to concentrate, comprehend, and learn decreases. Also, if the concentration of CO_2 rises because of poor ventilation, it is logical to assume that the level of other pollutants is also elevated.

The Gaztech International Corporation manufactures instruments to check various aspects of ventilation efficiency, and these devices range from inexpensive to more costly and complex (see Resources). A fast, easy, and inexpensive way (costing about five dollars) to measure the level of CO_2 is to use a *passive dosimeter tube*; one merely breaks the ends of a glass tube and obtains a direct readout in about eight hours. This indicates the level of carbon dioxide in the area where the tube was exposed. Gaztech also makes a product called Telaire, a monitor that can be used as a hand-held portable unit or be installed in any room permanently. Newer, more sophisticated, computerized ventilation systems can spot-check CO_2 levels routinely and easily make appropriate adjustments.

CARBON MONOXIDE

If your child experiences carbon monoxide poisoning, he or she may develop flulike symptoms, with weakness, headaches, fatigue, dizziness, irritability, visual problems, and difficulty thinking. Carbon monoxide exposures often are not recognized, however, because this gas has neither an odor nor a taste.

You can sometimes spot an odorless carbon monoxide leak if a natural-gas pilot light burns yellow, which indicates that the fuel is not being burned completely and suggests that carbon monoxide is being released. In fact, the presence of carbon monoxide and other gases is commonly due to incomplete combustion and/or to the leakage of natural gas or oil fumes into the ventilation system. This leakage can be caused by poor connections, corrosion, cracks, and gaps; holes in ducts, heat exchangers, chimney flues, or filters clogged with dirt or debris can all contribute to the improper exhaust of these noxious gases. Improper air flow can vent these dangerous combustion gases inside, rather than outside, a school building. For descriptions of the seriousness of this type of recurrent problem, both at school or at home, refer to the many health and learning problems of Liza (in Chapter 2) and the severe behavioral changes of Carl (whose history is discussed in Chapter 15).

Remember, carbon monoxide detectors, like smoke detectors, can save lives (see Resources). Less expensive detectors are chemically treated so they change colors if carbon monoxide is present at dangerous levels at school or at home. These might cost four or five dollars and last for three to four months. More costly detectors can measure levels as low as 5 ppm. (See Appendix for more details about how common gaseous vapors can affect individuals.[6])

OTHER COMBUSTION GASES

A ventilation consultant can quickly pinpoint the location of improperly exhausted combustion products in a school. Using modern instrumentation—which can vary from the simple and inexpensive to the sophisticated and costly—an expert can detect nitrogen, sulfur and carbon dioxides, formaldehyde, nitric oxide, hydrogen cyanide, and various organic chemical vapors. School furnaces, stoves, and hot-water heaters should be examined yearly for gas leaks.

Schools should also be concerned about diesel bus fumes, which can produce carbon disulfide and cause both health and memory problems. Carbon disulfide can be detected when levels reach 0.003 ppm. This very reactive molecule should not be present in the indoor air at *any* level because it is very toxic to the nervous system.

AN UNSUSPECTED SOURCE OF CARBON MONOXIDE AND NITROGEN DIOXIDE: ICE SKATING RINKS

Although ice skating rinks are not directly related to school buildings, the problems they cause might affect the academic performance of students who attend skating practice prior to regular school. Occasionally, a sudden acute medical crisis arises in a skating rink because of an accidental gas exposure. A skater can become ill when he or she exercises for hours on a rink in a building that tends to trap gaseous pollutants. With inadequate ventilation, carbon monoxide and/or nitrogen dioxide from defective gas- or other fuel-powered ice-resurfacing equipment can build up, creating serious health effects.[7] Newer electrically powered resurfacing equipment can alleviate this problem.

VOLATILE ORGANIC COMPOUNDS (VOCs)

Volatile organic compounds (VOCs) will become a household word within the next few years because they are so prevalent and damaging—and at times, even deadly.

Volatile organic compounds include gases such as benzene, toluene, and xylene, which originate from organic sources such as coal, oil, or wood (see Appendix for common names, sources, and health effects). Like tobacco, VOCs can cause immediate mild-to-serious symptoms, which may be subtle or quite obvious. In addition, there could be long-term consequences. Years down the road, exposed students may be more susceptible to various illnesses, while exposed teachers may develop serious health problems in their retirement years.

VOC exposures can be particularly significant during school cleaning and renovation. In poorly ventilated indoor settings, VOC levels can reach 100 ppm or more during painting and cleaning operations.[8] VOC odors can also be absorbed by building materials, insulation, and fabrics, where they can pose potential long-term exposure and subsequent health risks.[9] Typical symptom-causing VOCs—solvents and aromatic chemicals—are found in paints, varnishes, sealants, caulking substances, soft plastics, and adhesives. Synthetic resins may be present in plastics, soft upholstery, synthetic fabrics and carpets, carpet pads, vinyl-coated wallboard or furniture, and plastic floor coverings. Compounds such as formaldehyde are acutely toxic below 1 ppm; benzene is toxic above 1 ppm.[10] *There should be no VOCs in the air we breathe.*[11] The higher the levels, the greater and more obvious the symptoms and dangers.

In spite of the toxicity of many of these substances, they are not detailed on Material Safety Data (MSD) sheets. In fact, they can be deceptively called "inert" ingredients and so mislead the public into believing that they are inactive and harmless. Unfortunately, federal law treats the exact composition of "inerts" as confidential business information and so protected from disclosure. This means government employees who wish to make the information public are subject to various penalties if they do so.[12] Our laws tend to protect big business, not people, and because of the long time delay between the initial offending exposure and the awareness of its health effect, legal recourse by individuals is often impossible.

Your school can check for a variety of VOCs by using air-monitoring badges. After exposure, these badges undergo changes that can identify various compounds within eight hours to three days (see Resources). A number of badges are available from the 3M Company; they are marketed in a sealed can and can be clipped onto any surface in an area that needs an air-quality check. After eight hours of exposure, the badge is resealed and sent back to the company for interpretation. These badges cost between $14 and $90, depending on the number of solvents being detected. Be aware, however, that sometimes these badges indicate there is no problem, simply because a particular badge could not detect the type of VOC that was contaminating a suspect area.

Portable machines are also now available that can detect quickly and "on the spot" which chemicals are in the air in a localized area, whether it's inside or outside (see Resources).

OTHER ODORS

Sometimes an odor in a polluted area will be a clue to a potential problem. Does a given area have the clean odor of ozone, the fishy smell of an amine or bacteria, the sulfur smell of rotten eggs, or a sweet smell because of ketones? Does it smell like a chemical, a mold, excrement, or putrid decay? Those who suffer from chemical sensitivities will be aware of such odors much more quickly than others.

A new "fume" that can cause serious illness is the "artificial smoke" that is used to give a realistic feeling to fire drills and school plays. Needless to say, it can quickly affect chemically sensitive children and teachers, triggering asthma attacks, hay fever, and other health problems, especially in poorly ventilated rooms and buildings.

■ DUST, POLLEN, MOLDS, AND PETS

Everyday substances such as dust, pollen, molds, pet hair, and pet dandruff, as well as foods and chemicals, unquestionably interfere with how some children and adults learn, feel, and behave. Their presence must be analyzed in *every* room or suspect area in your child's school. Repeatedly ask yourself: Is there anything special that appears to be contributing to problems in my child's classroom (or area of our home) at a specific time? Refer back to Chapter 3 for easy and inexpensive ways for older children and adults to determine where and why they are ill.

Obviously, an ounce of prevention is critically important in relieving some children's learning problems. Finding the right ounce, however, requires diligent tracking to detect all the possible sources of a medical complaint.

DUST

If an entire school building appears to be dusty or moldy, you must find out why. Check with the principal, superintendent, and/or school board, and ask what they are willing to do to help reduce the problem.

Dust-related medical complaints can begin early in the school year, shortly after a malfunctioning and poorly maintained heating system resumes operation at full capacity. Dust, molds, and/or germs in the ductwork can be circulated throughout an entire building, adversely affecting anyone who has an allergy or a weakened immune system.

As the school year progresses, some children will become more ill because of the normal, gradual accumulation of dust, molds, and chemicals in a building. To keep children feeling well and learning at their full potential, a school's ventilation and filtration systems and its cleaning routines must be kept up to par. Otherwise, there will be increasing episodes of asthma, hay fever, skin rashes, and infections by December. These problems might flare up, again, when an air-conditioning system is initially turned on in the warmer months, especially if the ventilation system is contaminated with pollen and/or molds, as well as dust. Once again, proper maintenance is the key.

So be particularly attentive to your child's health. Does he routinely feel better during winter vacations, when he is away from school? Does he become ill or change in some other adverse manner shortly after returning to school? Does he feel better when the windows at school are open or when he plays outside? (Recess or outdoor activities, however, can make some children feel worse because of exposure to pollens or to the pesticides used during routine lawn or landscape maintenance. In some areas, aerial agricultural spraying or the escape of toxic chemicals from underground dump sites is an additional potential source of exposure.[13] Contact your local health department for information about this type of problem.)

Asthmatic children, who initially wheeze only when they get infections or during exercise, tend to wheeze for no apparent reason after extended exposure to dust or molds, whether at school or at home. The level of allergenic mites in the atmosphere can now be measured, and provisional standards have been established for the risk level for dust-mite exposures in mite-allergic asthmatic individuals. A risk level for chronic exposure that can cause sensitization is 100 mites per gram of dust, or 2 micrograms of Der pl per gram of dust. (*Der pl* stands for Dermatophagoides pteronyssinus, the dust-mite allergen.) The risk level for acute asthma in dust-mite-sensitive individuals is 10 micrograms of Der pl. To discourage mite growth, the relative humidity in a building should be less than 45 percent.

It is not unusual for a child's in-school wheezing to become more frequent or severe as the school year progresses. Drug therapy often provides temporary but not permanent relief. In addition, the major ingredient in common drugs used to treat asthma such as one finds in certain inhalers can cause some children to feel tired, nervous, and grumpy—and even to wheeze. Some youngsters are also sensitive to the various binders and coatings used in tablets and capsules as well as the aerosol propellants routinely used to relieve asthma.

Until the cause of the asthma is determined and eliminated, your child's breathing problems will persist (see Chapter 3). He or she may be subjected to years of unnecessary drug treatment to help alleviate intermittent or constant, mild or life-threatening asthma because no one stopped the exposure to some offending contact.

More American school officials should emulate the antiallergenic and antidust measures taken in Canada (see Chapter 12). Taking simple measures potentially can help not only the known allergic children or teachers but every potentially allergic individual in an environmentally disadvantaged classroom.

Children in "cleaner" classrooms and homes have fewer allergies and infections, better attendance at school, and improved academic performance.

POLLEN AND MOLDS

Not all school-related medical problems are caused by something generated entirely within a building. Sometimes the cause is outdoor pollen or mold spores that enter a building through the doors, windows, or ventilation system. A combination of both indoor and outdoor pollen and molds will produce even more symptoms.

Mold-sensitive individuals are easy to recognize because they are routinely worse in some way on damp rainy days or during wet moldy times of the year. Molds in schools as well as homes are unquestionably one of the most important unsuspected causes of a wide range of recurrent medical complaints. Most people are unaware of how often these environmental factors can alter the well-being, activity, behavior, movements, and memory of both children and adults.

Typically, pollen-related allergies, illnesses, and/or behavioral or learning problems recur every year *during the same few weeks.* Outdoor pollen allergies cause more symptoms on windy days, but specific pollen symptoms tend to occur at the following times:

■ Tree pollen: in spring, just *before* leaves appear
■ Grass pollen: whenever grass needs to be cut
■ Weed pollen: in late summer
■ Mold spores: in the rainy season or on humid days

If a building is moldy inside, a child can experience symptoms at any time, but they will become most pronounced when outdoor mold levels are also significantly increased. This happens during each rainy season, and especially after a child plays outside on a damp day, or after he is exposed to wet leaves or soil.

In many areas of the country, the grass-pollen season peaks in June. At that time, allergic children routinely become ill and manifest much more than hay fever or asthma. In contrast to their high-quality academic performance during the colder months, they may do poorly on their final examinations. Grass-pollen allergies can alter not only how these allergic youngsters feel but how they learn, remember, and behave. Grass-sensitive teachers might find that they have difficulty preparing lesson plans and teaching effectively when a pollen or mold spore count is high.

Ironically, in some parts of the country, the peak of the outdoor mold-spore and weed-pollen season coincides with the onset of the school year in the late summer. Many allergic youngsters therefore are particularly disadvantaged. *They begin and end each school year with a distinct medical handicap due to their spring, summer, and late-summer pollen and mold allergies. In addition, many mold-sensitive teachers and other adults are perplexed as their productivity and efficiency diminish each year at these times.*

SEASONAL DEPRESSION

Pollen and molds can trigger much more than asthma and hay fever. In fact, one of the most surprising findings in environmental medicine is that pollen and molds routinely cause seasonal depression in some children and adults, not during the dreary winter months but during the warm or rainy times of the year.

Recurring seasonal (spring, summer, and fall) depression is unfortunately quite common. However, its true cause can be completely missed by doctors if depression is the only symptom. Few recognize that mold- and pollen-related brain allergies can cause seasonal depression, even though this was described as far back as 1931 by Dr. Albert Rowe.[14]

Some mold- and pollen-sensitive children and adults repeatedly become excessively sad for one to several weeks at almost exactly the same time each year. Their disposition improves when these allergens are no longer prevalent in the air or after appropriate P/N allergy extract treatment.

The allergy basis of depression can be determined easily by noting a history of recurrent seasonal symptoms[15] and by single-blinded P/N allergy testing and treatment for pollen and/or molds (see Chapters 13 and 15). Mike, a college student, underwent a dramatic change during testing, as is depicted in the videotape *Environmentally Sick Schools.*

MOLDS: ONE UNSUSPECTED CAUSE OF A YOUNG MAN'S DEPRESSION

Mike

In 1993, a 23-year-old college student named Mike suddenly became inordinately sad during the unusually damp late-summer ragweed and mold season. He had no idea why he felt so unhappy; after all, he had no special health, school, financial, or companion problems. His mother, however, suspected that he needed to have his allergy extract treatment adjusted.

When Mike walked into our center for treatment, he was stooped over and barely lifted his head to talk. He avoided looking directly into anyone's eyes and was obviously very dejected. During P/N allergy testing, one drop of mold allergy extract caused him to cry and act totally devastated. One drop of a weaker dilution of the same extract neutralized his symptoms, and he quickly and obviously became much happier. The next day he continued to appear joyful. His health records indicated that he had had similar unexplained episodes of depression during the late-summer months when mold counts were elevated.

DEPRESSION IN VERY YOUNG CHILDREN

As I've written, sometimes very young children, too, show symptoms of seasonal depression. A gifted six-year-old acted sad during the ragweed/mold season. Her mother noted that the girl became exceedingly upset and would scream and kick as soon as she entered the particularly moldy building where her dance lessons were held. This behavior was most evident in the late summer when the high levels of ragweed pollen and outside molds, combined with inside molds, were simply too much for her. Her sadness promptly disappeared, however, after she received P/N allergy treatment for ragweed and molds.

At the tender age of six, this youngster poignantly expressed how she felt during dancing lessons in the moldy building:

DANCING DAY

I was sad, I was crying,
I feel in my tummy like nobody loved me.
I felt like I was gonna cry more.
That made me sadder and sadder.
It feels to be scared,
Like I'm a dumb person that nobody likes.
I felt like I had a nonlistening brain.
I thought I was nothing,
Every time I go dance,
I feel like I want to go home.

Another mother of a chronically ill three-year-old was delighted after her son smiled for the "first time in his life" within minutes of being tested and treated for a dust allergy.

Unfortunately, many children (and adults) feel depressed at times but do not realize they have unrecognized sensitivities to common exposures. Both seasonally and nonseasonally sad, allergic youngsters should be evaluated by a specialist who understands how to test for, recognize, and effectively treat environmentally-related mood and behavioral problems (see Table 14.1). Once these affected individuals are aware of the seasonal nature of their allergy-related depression, their P/N allergy extract treatment should be updated each year *immediately prior to* the mold or pollen season, to help prevent a recurrence. If their problem arises mainly during the colder months, they should consider the possible presence of a dust and/or mold sensitivity, rather than a problem caused by winter dreariness. If it is practical and possible, these children also should have an air purifier at school and in their bedroom (see Resources). Such measures would help reduce their total daily exposure to airborne allergenic substances at critical times of the year. *Psychological counseling during these challenging periods can be much more effective, and at times unnecessary, if possible allergic factors are considered, recognized, and appropriately treated.*

One final note on this topic: Some adult females in particular are routinely diagnosed with an illness called SAD, or Seasonal Affective Disorder.[16] SAD is characterized by lethargy, fatigue, a depressed mood, and a craving for carbohydrates. Scientists have identified the absence of sunlight as one cause of SAD, and light therapy can be helpful. It is possible, however, that a mold and/or dust allergy, plus a food (wheat, corn, milk, sugar) sensitivity, is the cause. P/N allergy testing could easily and quickly confirm or negate such a possibility (see Chapters 13 and 15).

CLEANING UP INDOOR MOLDS

If your school (or home) has a mold or germ problem, much more is required than merely cleaning up the water from a flooded basement, a broken pipe, wet walls, or a leaky toilet or roof. Stagnant water enhances the growth of molds and germs in carpets, walls, ductwork, windows, pipes, radiators, and furnishings. Thus, in schools, measures must be taken to retard and eliminate mold growth in carpets and gym mats, as well as in coatrooms and lockers where wet clothing and boots are kept. (In homes, basements, roofs, and plumbing in particular need to be well-maintained; if humidifiers or vaporizers are used excessively in certain rooms, molds may grow under wallpaper, on windowsills, and elsewhere.) Common sources of increased mold or water in both schools and homes are listed in Table 6.3.

Certain mold-retardant sprays that are commercially available claim to be safe, effective, and nontoxic. They may be, but you can't always believe what manufacturers say about their products' effectiveness. Do they control the growth of molds (yeasts, fungi, and mildew) or of algae and germs (bacteria)? Are they safe when used in or on furnishings or carpets? You need to be seriously concerned about potentially adverse health effects. Prior to using them extensively, you should test to see if a slight purposeful exposure (as suggested in Chapter 3) causes any significant physical change in your child. Watch for delayed changes in his or her well-being.

TABLE 6.3

Common Sources of Mold Contamination in Schools (and Possibly Homes)

- pool/shower areas, locker rooms, damp gym clothing, gym mats
- moldy ventilation ductwork, insulation, filters
- poorly maintained window or central air conditioners
- certain carpets, ceilings, walls (due to moisture from excessive humidity), roof, basement, plumbing or pipe leaks
- water or snow from shoes, boots, or wet clothing
- storage areas for damp sneakers, boots, clothing
- leaky fountains, sinks, toilets
- books and papers stored in damp areas
- unclean refrigerator drain pans and ice machines
- malfunctioning humidifiers and dehumidifiers
- metal window frames
- water accumulations in plugged drains or sump pump areas
- buildings located in humid areas near lakes, rivers, or swampy land

It is also important to have a bioassay test done on mice to see if the spray you plan to use can cause any harmful effects (see Resources). *If the product contains a pesticide, take extreme care to be certain that there is no sensitivity to this or any other so-called "inert" ingredients in antimicrobial preparations.* (Most products contain a main ingredient for which they are purchased plus a number of chemicals such as solvents, stabilizers, or perfumes; the latter are considered "inert" even though they can be more toxic than the key ingredient.)

If these sprays are being used at your child's school, ask for MSD sheets on the product. But realize that these data sheets can be deceptive; they can state that the product has caused no known deleterious effects—but was the safety of the product evaluated carefully and completely? Here's the bottom line: How does it affect *your* child?

Carefully monitored treatment with ozone is one way to effectively reduce mold contamination (and smoke odors) due to the contents or construction of a building but see Chapter 7 because ozone has its pros and cons (see Resources as well).

PETS

One obvious way to relieve a pet allergy is to remove the animal from the classroom or home. Pet hair, dandruff, saliva, excrement, and pet food all can cause illness in certain sensitive individuals. These substances can become part of the "dust" in school buildings.

Most traditional allergists will not treat pet-related problems, but P/N allergy extract treatment can be most helpful for selected individuals (see Chapters 13 and 15). Air purifiers can also help remove pet hair and dandruff from the air (see Resources).

■ BACTERIA AND VIRUSES

Have you ever wondered why students in certain classrooms are more ill with infections than those in other rooms? Why is there more asthma in certain areas of a school or home? Why is attendance consistently lower in one classroom than in another? Why do some teachers fall ill more often than others? Why does one teacher or student after another become sick when assigned to a particular classroom?

Maybe one answer to these questions lies in the level of bacterial or other contamination or pollution in a specific room. In fact, you would expect the levels of bacteria, molds, dust, and possibly chemicals to be higher in rooms where the students and teachers are the sickest.

If your child tends to have repeated infections, as a parent, *you must find the areas in your child's school* that appear to be localized pockets of infections or illnesses (see Resources). With relatively little investigation, most school health personnel can promptly provide you with a global impression about which classrooms, year after year, have the highest absentee rates due to allergies and/or infections. If you're a teacher and tend to become ill too often, submit a written report to the school administration to document your complaint. Check whether the preceding teachers who used your room had similar difficulties. Take a look at the PARF video, where we have filmed a teacher with exactly these problems (see Resources). If you are a parent, talk to school health personnel and tell them which school areas appear to make your child feel ill.

Remember that ventilation inadequacies can be part of the problem. A study by J. F. Brundage et al. found that army recruits had a 50 percent increase in respiratory infections when they were housed in energy-efficient buildings, compared with soldiers housed in older, draftier buildings that had more air exchange. Once again, air quality and quantity are key factors to watch.[17]

DETERMINING HOW MANY BACTERIA ARE PRESENT

An uncomplicated and relatively inexpensive test will provide a *rough* gauge of the level of bacteria and/or molds in specific areas of your school. You will need to obtain petri dishes that contain different types of agar gelatin to detect excessive bacteria or mold contamination. For example, Sabouraud's agar is used to grow molds. These can be obtained from a local hospital or university bacteriology department or from a commercial environmental health supplier (see Resources). (Other types of agar plates are used to grow bacteria, but unfortunately the techniques employed to detect viruses are more complicated.) Open and expose one dish directly to the air for 20 to 60 minutes (the recommended time of exposure varies). Then seal and store the dish in a dark warm place. A few days later, count the number of spots or colonies. In general, one to three mold colonies are acceptable; more than twelve colonies are not.

For specific bacterial and/or mold identification, ask the school administration to provide an analysis and written report on the number and type of colonies found in various areas within the school. If a single bacterium or mold is particularly prevalent, allergy extract treatment for that specific organism might be surprisingly helpful to those who are ill.

One inexpensive and instructive way to perform this test in a school is to make preparing the agar plates and counting the colony growth part of a biology class project. Students can easily conduct this school survey, provided a science instructor carefully ensures that the plates remain entirely sealed after they are exposed. (There should be no direct hand contact with the open mold plates after growth is evident, although, the plates will contain only what is routinely inhaled in the air of each particular area of a school.) This project can provide a practical, educational experience for science students.

If your school has a serious infection or contamination problem, administrators can contact one of several professional groups that conduct environmental evaluations (see Resources). They can do accurate microbial assessment of the room's air for bacteria, molds, viruses, rickettsia, protozoans, and typical allergenic substances. Be sure that their evaluation also considers chemicals. Keep in mind, however, that correcting one problem will not eliminate a health concern that is caused by several factors. Many mold "experts" know how to detect the mold portion of a school problem, but they are sometimes insufficiently knowledgeable about the significant role of offending chemicals.

More sophisticated and accurate testing can be conducted by environmental HVAC evaluation specialists who use the Anderson two-stage air-impact sampler. It uses Sabouraud's dextrose agar to determine the level of microorganisms (cfu/m^3, or colony-forming units per cubic meter) that grow out after school air has been blown over plates of agar. Only rarely do levels as low as 50 cfu/m^3 cause human reactions; in general, levels from 70 to 140 cfu/m^3 are marginal, while those above 350 cfu/m^3 indicate excessive exposure. In contrast, a test that depends only upon gravity to deposit the organisms on the plates will give lower readings: a level of 10 cfu/m^3 usually means no problem, 20 cfu/m^3 is marginal, and 50 cfu/m^3 or above indicates reason for concern (see Resources).

With this kind of test, all excessively contaminated locations can be verified and pinpointed. Then the *cause* of any significant variation in the levels of airborne germs, molds, or particles must be ascertained. Once that cause is removed and the level of molds, bacteria, and particles is dimin-

---

TABLE 6.4

How to Decrease Excessive Bacterial or Mold Growth in Classrooms (and Homes)

- Identify the moldy or germ-contaminated areas.
- Remove obvious mold with cleaning, and/or eliminate moldy furnishings.
- Determine the source of the germs and/or mold in the problem area.
- Clean the problem area with special safer mold retardants or disinfectants.
- Use room or central air purifier to clean air.
- Use room or central dehumidifier to reduce mold.
- Reduce the mold and odors with mold adsorbers.
- Carefully and judiciously use ozone.
- Monitor previously contaminated areas regularly.

ished (as suggested in Table 6.4), previously sick students and teachers should experience a corresponding improvement in their well being.

ELIMINATING GERMS AND ALLERGENIC SUBSTANCES

Chronically ill students and teachers, especially those who are allergic, can unintentionally contaminate schoolrooms with more germs than normal because of their own repeated infections. When that happens, a vicious cycle begins that contributes not only to their own illness but unknowingly and innocently to the illness of other students. Certain rooms, therefore, are truly "sickness-producing" because they are contaminated with high levels of germs.

Simple, relatively inexpensive air-cleaning machines, such as room air purifiers, can definitely decrease some flares of allergy, which in turn helps to decrease secondary infections. A study by Rebecca Bascom et al. indicates that a portable air cleaner significantly reduced, but did not totally eliminate, the upper respiratory congestion and headaches, in both allergic and nonallergic individuals, caused by inhaling tobacco smoke fumes.[18] Anecdotally, teachers have noticed fewer infections and less absenteeism in classrooms where air purifiers have been utilized. More studies should be conducted to evaluate the role of air purifiers in reducing infection by decreasing the amount of contaminants in school air.

Prolonged mold or water contamination is often associated with an overgrowth of various germs. On rare occasions, particularly virulent organisms can multiply within a ventilation system. These organisms can cause illnesses such as Legionnaires' disease, hypersensitivity pneumonitis, and humidifier fever. Although these problems are not common, they can be the result of uncontrolled contamination in the cooling system, humidifier, or tap water of a school or home. Legionnaires' disease organisms, for example, suddenly became evident in the cooling system of one eastern school district; officials there did not want to frighten the community, so they did not inform parents about this potentially serious exposure. Appropriate measures were quickly taken to eliminate the organisms. Later, however, when parents heard about what had happened, they were justifiably upset that they had not been informed. This school system was exceedingly fortunate that no children or teachers became seriously ill.

If Legionnaires' disease is detected in a school, it is imperative to continuously monitor the original source of this contamination to be certain that this potentially lethal health threat has been permanently eradicated. An inexpensive new product called Pool Magic is said to be effective in quickly eliminating Legionnaires' disease organisms for prolonged periods. A similar product (Cooling Tower Magic) claims to be useful for treating contaminated cooling towers and swamp coolers (see Resources).

WHY ARE INFECTIONS SO COMMON IN ALLERGIC INDIVIDUALS?

Allergic individuals who have either been untreated or have responded poorly to treatment are often more prone to develop repeated infections. The classic sequence of events, which is unfortunate but exceedingly common, is roughly as follows:

1. Exposure to dust, molds, pollen, foods, and/or chemicals causes a child's nose, lung, sinus, ear, and/or skin tissues to swell. This edema decreases the blood circulation so that germs that are normally present—for example, in the nose—can enter the body more easily and cause infection.
2. The germs can spread into nearby areas such as the sinuses, the middle ear, and the lungs. These infections are frequently treated with antibiotics, sometimes for weeks, months, or even years.[19] In individuals who become sensitive to germs, asthma or nasal polyps can develop. In addition, some youngsters develop an allergic reaction to the major component of an antibiotic itself, or to the dye, flavor, sweetener, or corn (dextrose) that it contains.
3. Antibiotics routinely disrupt the normal balance of flora in the intestines. They kill off the needed lactobacillus normally found there and allow the level of candida or yeast to increase to an inordinately high level.
4. This imbalance can cause a variety of yeast-related symptoms (see Chapter 14), which often remain unrecognized or are not seriously addressed by some doctors.
5. If a constant upper respiratory allergy and infection persists, some doctors will advise surgery. Many affected allergic children repeatedly have tubes placed through their eardrums to drain recurrent ear fluid (see Chapter 14). Both children and adults may have operations to improve the drainage from their sinuses and/or to remove large infected adenoids or tonsils. But, if the basic cause of these problems—namely, the allergy—can be found and eliminated, such surgery might be totally unnecessary.

This entire pattern of illness can sometimes be prevented if dust, mold, and chemical exposures can be decreased or eradicated. If environmental control or avoidance measures are not adequate, various airborne allergens and food sensitivities might be treated by allergy extracts, diets, and improved nutrition.

There are several ways to approach the problem of recurring infections. (The major steps to decrease bacteria and molds are listed in Table

If the nose, sinus, ear, and lung tissues don't swell in response to an allergen, there will be less infection, less need for antibiotics, less yeast overgrowth, and less need for surgery. Appropriate environmental allergy treatments can frequently diminish or prevent such swelling, by the use of individualized diets, better nutrition, yeast treatment, dust and mold control, avoidance of chemicals, and newer forms of allergy extract therapy.

6.4.) Talk to your doctor about the following general approaches to help your child:

1. Obtain a culture of your child's classroom (as well as bedroom and/or work area) to detect the number and types of bacteria and molds.
2. Use a safer disinfectant in room air humidifiers and vaporizers.[20] Try a mixture of $1/2$ cup Borax, $1/4$ cup vinegar, and 2 gallons hot water. Wash and rinse the humidifier thoroughly. To make the disinfectant stronger, use more Borax. Avoid the common phenol-containing cleaning disinfectants; read labels very carefully.
3. Consider oral or intravenous nutrient therapy, especially vitamin C, which can be helpful for some individuals. Taking higher doses of vitamin C can help decrease infection (see Chapters 14 and 15).
4. Use separate glasses for drinking, and very hot water for rinsing dishes, both at school and at home.
5. Have your child brush his or her teeth more often, and use a new toothbrush each month.
6. Contact an environmental medical specialist for an allergy treatment. Although physicians certainly disagree, a flu and/or bacterial vaccine appears to be most helpful in treating some allergic children who have repeated infections.
7. Try home-remedy preparations, such as Nutrabiotic (Citricidal or grapefruit seed extract) or Australian tea tree oil. These are available in health food stores.
8. Try homeopathic remedies such as echinacea or oscillococcinum; the latter sometimes helps to abort or relieve flu symptoms. (Homeopathic remedies, available from health food stores, either do or don't help. Remember, unlike prescription drugs, the pellet forms usually have no harmful effects and are considered to be safe, providing your doctor approves and you understand that you should call your physician promptly if symptoms persist or worsen. The pellet forms contain a minuscule amount of sugar, which rarely causes symptoms. The liquid

forms can contain ethyl alcohol, which can cause symptoms in some chemically sensitive individuals, such as those who cannot tolerate any exposure to perfume because it contains this chemical [see Chapter 15].)

■ MORE WAYS TO HELP ALLERGIC AND ENVIRONMENTALLY ILL STUDENTS AND TEACHERS

FAST, EASY, AND INEXPENSIVE WAYS

For some fast, easy, and relatively inexpensive ways to help relieve dust, mold, or pollen complaints in your school or home, refer to the list in Table 6.2. Here are some strategies to keep in the forefront of your mind.

MORE EFFICIENT CLEANING
Insist that your child's school be cleaned better, with safer cleaning products (see Resources). Ask school administrators to make sure that maintenance-cleaning personnel are educated *in detail* about how to clean and damp-mop effectively. Classrooms that are less cluttered can be cleaned more rapidly and efficiently. Custodians should know that not only ventilation ducts and filters but also air conditioners and ceiling tiles get dusty. Bare concrete walls and floors increase the amount of irritating, rather than typically allergenic dust within a building; to correct this problem, all concrete should be painted or sealed with a less toxic material (see Resources).

Some parents and teachers have gone directly into their schools, personally cleaned them with safer cleaning agents, and installed quality room air purifiers. These measures can decrease airborne dust, molds, pollen, and to a lesser degree chemicals in the indoor air.

Items that are badly contaminated should be removed. For example, school textbooks may have become moldy during storage and be causing some students to wheeze. Ask if they can be replaced. (Refer to Chapter 3 for help in detecting this problem.) Moldy carpets can be cleansed with safe mold-retardant solutions (see Resources).

Contaminated areas, substances, and items can be cleaned with bacterial- or mold-retardant substances, some of which were mentioned earlier. They include Borax, Australian tea tree oil, citrus seed extract, vinegar, and Purisol spray. These and other products are available from Allerx, AFM Products, and/or health food stores. A dilute solution of zephiran chloride may be appropriate if a stronger disinfectant than Borax is required. Mold-retardant paints, such as Safecoat (available from AFM Products), Benjamin Moore Pristine Low Odor, and Glidden Spread 2000 Low VOC, are also available and at times tolerated well. Casein-based paints are best; rubber-based are the least desirable.

The key is prevention. Once schools are aware of safer, better, and possibly less expensive cleaning agents, most will approve their use. However, reread Chapter 3. Be sure your school is not compounding the problem and creating *more* illness in its attempt to reduce the level of an offending exposure to which someone is sensitive. Some companies claim their effective products are also safe, but are they? How carefully did they monitor the health effects of their product on schoolchildren? We must all become more questioning and critical.

Safer cleaning products are often less expensive and can be equally or more effective than standard brands. The environmentally safest paints, renovation substances, sealants, and pest-control measures should be selected for use both inside and outside schools. Surprisingly, these products can be both cost- and health-effective, on a short- and long-term basis.[21]

Remember, whenever possible, test products that the school is about to purchase in advance on sensitive children (see Chapter 3). For example, in Chapter 14, I'll describe a chemically sensitive youngster who was exposed to a small piece of new carpet to check his response *before* that carpet was installed throughout the school. When the boy had no difficulty, the carpet was installed, and it caused no adverse effects. Canada's environmental program, discussed in Chapter 11, encourages chemically sensitized students who are well enough to be mainstreamed to quickly alert officials when an environmentally offending exposure occurs in their school building. This has proven to be most beneficial.

BETTER VACUUMING

Many routine vacuum cleaners circulate dust as they clean. By using a flashlight around a vacuum cleaner in a dark room, you can actually see how much dust routinely escapes. Ask school administrators if you can check the one used in your school (also examine the one in your home). The typical vacuum cleaner only removes particles greater than 50 microns.[22]

In addition to using electrostatic air filters, HEPA filters, and/or charcoal filters in the ventilation system, some schools use high-efficiency HEPA maintenance vacuum cleaners. These can remove up to 99.97 percent of all particles as small as 0.3 microns found in regular dust, dust mites, mold, pet hair, lead, asbestos particles, and some bacteria. These machines should be used weekly in all classrooms (see Resources).

There are a number of commercial and residential HEPA vacuum cleaners on the market. The prices range from $95 to $1,350, and they were rated in the January 1995 *Consumer Reports* (see Resources). The top six vacuum cleaners contain a HEPA filter or offer it as an option. Talk to your school officials about the type used in your child's school. (If you are interested in a home vacuum system with a HEPA filter, check the phone directory for vacuum-system companies.)

ROOM AIR PURIFIERS

Request that room air purifiers be used in obvious "problem" classrooms. Ideally, they should be used in all rooms. Small, quality portable models, such as Dust-Free, cost from $215 to $375 or more, and they definitely help clean air (see Resources). Room, ceiling, and central air purifiers are available in various sizes. Some can be easily installed into existing ventilation systems.

If your school cannot or will not purchase air purifiers, have a PTA-sponsored bake or rummage sale to earn money to buy them. Use them in all classrooms in which students and teachers appear to be particularly ill with recurrent allergies or infection.

DEHUMIDIFIERS, HUMIDIFIERS, AND AIR CONDITIONERS

If the ventilation system in your child's school is functioning optimally, molds should not be a problem. At times, however, due to unusual circumstances such as floods or leakage, additional measures must be taken to decrease mold contamination.

Dehumidifiers can help decrease mold. They should be used in damp shower areas, locker rooms, basements and near pools, and throughout buildings that are located in humid areas. Basement and roof leaks must be sealed, and moist walls should be damp-proofed from the outside with cement-based safe sealants and plastic sheets.[23]

In dry areas or during cold, dry seasons, humidifiers are typically required. If humidity and temperature are well-controlled, there should be less mold growth and enhanced comfort. Humidity should be kept at about 40 to 50 percent to maintain the comfort level and help control the spread of germs or particulates, including dust mites, that cause illness. If the humidity is routinely above 70 to 85 percent, special measures will have to be taken to reduce mold contamination and improve ventilation. If the level is below 20 percent, the occupants of the building will feel uncomfortable because the air is too dry. A Digital Hygro-Thermometer, available at most hardware stores, inexpensively measures both humidity and temperature.

Dehumidifiers, humidifiers, and air conditioners normally and routinely become contaminated with molds. If possible, avoid swamp coolers, which are used in the Southwest and employ evaporation from wet straw for cooling; they are unquestionably moldy and highly allergenic. In addition, the odor of oil from a fan or motor can cause illness.

Some room and central air conditioners actively circulate moldy air, which can cause a variety of medical problems. At the beginning of each warm season, before they are turned on, all easily accessible parts should be cleaned with a *safe* mold-retardant substance. Unfortunately, many units are so designed as to make proper cleaning both impractical and challenging. Have your school administrators call in environmentally knowledgeable HVAC persons for insight about efficient cleaning; these people should be selected carefully. Most HVAC firms clean air conditioners by blowing out the dust and removing all visible mold, but they must be warned never to spray any toxic or scented chemicals into the unit in an attempt to mask a moldy odor. *Amazingly, chemicals known to damage the nervous system are sometimes used to clean moldy air conditioners in buses and cars.*[24] Caution is strongly advised. Again, ask for and study the Material Safety Data (MSD) sheets before chemicals of any type are used in your school.

Some schools have eliminated obvious mold and improved air quality by using specially designed central or room dehumidification units. Room units such as the MarVent or MarVent Plus, manufactured by the Crispaire Corporation, are available for single rooms with mold problems (see Resources). The latter is designed for use in areas of heavy humidity, such as in the southern United States. Such units help exhaust stale indoor air, pollutants, and harmful gases while bringing as much as 450 cfm of outside air into a building.

A central unit by Semco is also designed to diminish the humidity while increasing the ventilation (see Resources). Once again, try to observe its effect on the children who are routinely ill or known to be mold sensitive (as described in Chapter 3).

REMOVING SMALLER MOLD AND ODOR PROBLEMS
Mold and odor absorbers (or adsorbers) help trap the fumes and odors of mold, must, sewer gases, and chemicals (see Resources). They can be helpful in a school's pool, shower, or gym areas, in locker rooms, and in a slightly moldy basement or roof area. These absorbers also help remove the smells of perfume, tobacco, cooking, lavatory disinfectants, paint, hair spray, exhaust fumes, and polyester in isolated, localized areas. These units are just as effective as the usual dichlorobenzene-based lavatory deodorizers, which primarily mask one odor with another. They are much safer, since some deodorizers contain chemicals that are potentially toxic to the nervous system. Check the MSD sheets, and see Chapter 7.

Zeolite bags absorb moldy odors from damp areas (see Resources). For continued use, place the bag in the sun for six to eight hours every eight to ten months.

Unscented kitty litter (available in pet stores) helps eliminate odors.

Charcoal can be spread in an open container to absorb odors. However, since it is a hydrocarbon, some children may be sensitive to a specific source or type of charcoal.

MORE EFFECTIVE WAYS

OZONE GENERATORS

Ozone generators have been used effectively for limited periods of time to help reduce mold and tobacco odors in hotel rooms, automobiles, and homes. They can be used only when a building, like a school, is totally unoccupied. Ozone is a strong oxidant; it can combine with VOCs and formaldehyde and oxidizes them to carbon dioxide and water.

We are all exposed to varying levels of ozone each day because it is in our atmosphere. In schools and workplaces, it is released whenever photocopying machines are used. The Food and Drug Administration has set a limit of 50 parts per billion for ozone emitted from electronic air purifiers.

The ozone concentration in areas where people are present should not exceed 0.1 ppm. At concentrations between 0.05 and 0.1 ppm, ozone has a distinct odor and can irritate the eyes, nose, and lungs and cause nausea and headaches; elevated levels are therefore easy to detect. Even minute amounts of ozone that are within allowed levels can cause breathing problems in some exquisitely sensitive individuals. Most people, however, notice only that it creates a "clean smell."

Some air purifiers are designed purposely to release a small amount of ozone. A commercial ozone generator that claims to be safe for ordinary room use is called the Tri-O System (see Resources). This air treatment and control system is used to clean and purify air in schools, homes, commercial outlets, offices, and industrial spaces. It eliminates odors; helps destroy bacteria, fungi, molds, and pollen; and eradicates pollutants such as tobacco smoke. It might be ideal for intermittent use in a building located near the water, or in one that is naturally a bit damper than desired. As with other products, check it out personally and make suggestions to your child's school officials (see Chapter 3).

One important note about ozone: *The EPA and OSHA consider ozone to be a toxic and hazardous gas if it is inhaled for prolonged periods, even though to my knowledge no human death has ever been recorded due to overexposure. This warning is somewhat perplexing because these agencies have not made similar proclamations about substances definitely known to be harmful to animals and/or humans. In addition, the Maryland Technical Bulletin regarding HVAC for schools does NOT recommend ozone generators for use in classrooms.*

Ozone generators are obviously *not* routinely advisable, except for an inordinately and unreasonably moldy school or home. Ozonation should be considered only if it can be done carefully by an experienced contractor. Since ozone oxidizes organic matter, no living plant, pet, or person, or anything made of rubber (like an electrical cord), should be in the area when it is used. Ozonation, however, *can* effectively eliminate elevated concentrations of molds and VOCs. For example, for a classroom or isolated home area that is extremely moldy, has a high bacterial count, and smells of chemicals, ozonation might provide a most effective way to remedy all three problems quickly. In certain situations, it can be the only practical choice. In a school, for example, an ozone unit might be set up by a trained person so it can be used for four to eight hours when the building is unoccupied and will remain closed for several days or weeks. After its use, the rooms should be thoroughly aired out. The odor of ozone quickly dissipates, but the smell must be *totally eliminated* before classes can be resumed.

Don't be surprised if ozone machines become less efficient with use. Their ability to release ozone appears to diminish gradually with time, despite claims to the contrary even after critical parts are replaced or repaired.

BETTER BUT MORE EXPENSIVE WAYS

PROFESSIONAL CARPET CLEANING
Many carpet shampoos contain a scent, as well as solvents such as perchloroethylene, naphthalene, ethanol, ammonia, and detergents. These chemicals can cause an array of symptoms (as described in Chapters 10 and 11). A residue of these chemicals left on the carpet can be potentially harmful once it dries, or when it becomes wet during future recleaning.

A basement carpet installed directly onto an unsealed concrete floor is particularly challenging because it can get damp at times. The result can be a heavy contamination with molds. Bare concrete floors should be sealed with a *safe* moisture barrier (see Resources). Some chemical treatments guarantee no mold regrowth for up to three years. You must continue to be vigilant, however, about the health effects of any chemical used in or on a carpet or carpet pad to control mold growth (see Chapter 3).

Proper carpet cleaning requires a steam carbonated water spray, white absorbent pads (on the bottom of the floor-cleaning machine), and a pile lifter and raker. The pads should be white at the end of the cleaning procedure. To kill dust mites, the temperatures must be greater than 130° F. To remove carpet odors, products such as Carpet Guard, Lock Out, and AFM's Safechoice carpet shampoo are said to be helpful (see Resources). Be certain these products are checked *before* use (as suggested in Chapter 3). What is safe for some children can cause problems such as breathing difficulties and headaches in others.

Before selecting a professional carpet cleaning company, your school should consider the following:

■ Be sure the persons who clean the carpet fully understand the equipment and cleaning materials. They must know what should and should not be done and how to do it; some contractors have no idea how to properly use their own equipment.

■ Have carpeting and rugs steam-cleaned on a regular basis with a nonallergenic, nonscented, biodegradable shampoo.

■ A vacuum can be used that blows the exhaust into a truck outside. Such a powerful external extraction process can effectively clean and remove dust mites and other contaminants from indoor carpets.

■ The carpet should be prevacuumed and then rinsed with steamy fresh hot water to prolong its life. High suction is crucial.

■ A fully cleaned carpet and its padding should dry for four to six hours to diminish mold growth, and the room humidity should not exceed 70 percent.

■ Portable and rented cleaning machines are not recommended.

If a new synthetic carpet causes symptoms, the school should air it out thoroughly, steam-clean it with an acceptable soap, suction-dry it quickly (in less than four hours), heavily ozonate the room, and then raise the temperature to at least 90° F for one to two days to help eliminate residual chemicals and molds. Sometimes, however, as chemicals are released, they become sequestered in furnishings, only to "outgas" or reenter the atmosphere at a later date, causing continued illness (see Chapter 10).[25]

BEST BUT MOST EXPENSIVE WAYS

HVAC EVALUATIONS

As discussed earlier in this chapter, your school can hire a local or national professional HVAC consultant firm to check air quality (see Resources). Such a firm should be knowledgeable about school ventilation systems in general and capable of determining exactly what is in the air—including microorganisms, particulates, and chemicals—in every room in the school. Tests for chemicals, radon, lead, asbestos, radiation, and electromagnetic energy levels must be part of this evaluation (see Resources).

Of course, the greater the sophistication of a detection method, the more it costs. School administrators should check with several dealers in your area to find those with the greatest expertise. Firms that conduct thorough environmental evaluations use advanced instrumentation that accurately measures the number and size of biological or other particles within a few seconds (see Resources). Bioaerosol samplers such as the Graseby Anderson, the Rotorod, and the more expensive Met One can measure bacteria, molds (fungi or yeast), dust, and pet hair, but unfortunately they do not specifically identify the source of the various "particles" that they detect (see Resources). Keep in mind that insulation, carpets, and library or book dust can be three major sources of problem particulates in indoor environments.[26]

CENTRAL AIR-PURIFYING UNITS
If an entire school has high levels of molds, dust, and pollen, it is sensible to install a quality central air-purifying unit into the ventilation system (see Resources). This process can be costly, depending upon the size of the school. Many such units contain substances like charcoal in their filters, which helps decrease the chemical contamination of the indoor air.

MAJOR RECONSTRUCTION
If a school is moldy throughout because of extensive flooding, it may be necessary to remove and/or replace walls, ceilings, partitions, and carpets. If the ventilation ductwork is extensively moldy and/or contaminated with potentially toxic chemicals, it might have to be completely removed. Sometimes these forms of pollution make it necessary to remove an entire ventilation system to make a building safe for occupancy.

ALLERGY EXTRACT TREATMENT
A relatively expensive but most effective answer for individuals who have environmental illness is P/N or SET allergy extract testing and treatment for pollen, molds, dust, pets, and foods (see Chapters 13 and 15). The relatively high cost of this effective type of treatment would not be a consideration if insurance companies routinely paid for it (see Chapter 17).

DETOXIFICATION
Detoxification is sometimes required for children and adults who have become extremely ill from exposure to certain forms of pollution in schools. This procedure helps to remove the various chemicals that accumulate in the body after an excessive or prolonged chemical exposure. It can be challenging and expensive, but sometimes there are few other options if an individual's health is to be restored. (See Chapters 14 and 15 for more details about this therapy.)

In general, do not become overly worried about the cost of these methods, since they are rarely required. Remember, your child does not need to attend school in Camelot or Utopia. You merely need to be assured that your child's exposure is below the level that causes illness.

■ SPECIAL CONSIDERATIONS IN RELATION TO HOMES

While the basic information in Table II.1 is applicable for many homes, other considerations may be indicated. Most time is usually spent in the bedroom, family room, and kitchen. Check out each of these areas very carefully for possible sources of contamination. Bathrooms and shower areas tend to be moldy; they also contain many personal product aromas and are subject to cleaning agents, disinfectants, deodorants, and odorous scouring powders.

A moldy basement with a forced hot-air ventilation system that blows mold and dust throughout a home is a common source of allergy and other illness. If a pet is confined to the basement, its dandruff and hair can be circulated throughout an entire house. Pets should never be allowed in the bedroom if someone has an allergy. Cats cause many more serious allergies than nonshedding tiny dogs. Family hobbies also can be associated with special aromas (using art supplies, paint, engine oils) or harmful contacts (fabrics, dried flowers, or wood).

Try to learn more about previous occupants of your home. Did they have any unusual hobbies? For example, did they raise birds in the bedroom that you are planning to use for your asthmatic child? Is there evidence of an oil or gasoline spill in the garage or basement? Is the partition between the garage and the house properly sealed, so that vehicular or garage odors do not drift inside? Are there water lines on the walls of the basement, around chimneys, or in the ceilings of various rooms, suggesting previous water damage? Are the walls textured so that they collect and retain dust? When were the walls and the draperies last cleaned? Years can pass quickly without such routine maintenance. Did the previous owners use or misuse any harmful pesticides or termiticides inside or outside the home? Stringently avoid homes in which previous occupants repeatedly became seriously ill.

HVAC REPORTS

An HVAC report conducted on your home may show the following abnormalities:

AN ELEVATED PARTICULATE COUNT
You must ask why and find the source of the particles. Does your home smell dusty, musty, or moldy? Has it been unused for a while? Is the furniture dusty? Does one room have a higher count than the others? Did someone smoke in the rooms with the highest counts? Look around. Is the clothes dryer properly vented? Is the air different in some manner when the furnace blower is working (indicating a problem in the ventilation ducts)?

Compare the air coming directly from the heating ducts with that in the middle of each room. Is the source from something inside the duct? Does that area need to be professionally cleaned? Take a look and see. If the construction is defective, insulation fibers can leak from the walls into the duct air through poorly sealed ventilation ductwork, through the light fixtures or electric sockets, and through irregularities in the porthole openings. Are the filters dirty, or do they need replacement? Just before the particulate count was taken, did someone vacuum extensively, take down dusty drapes, install or remove or replace carpets, or do anything else that would generate dust and a misleading elevated particulate count?

How does the level of particulates in the inside air compare with that outside? Maybe the source is not within the house but due to a nearby factory. What is the prevailing wind direction? What is located in that direction?

AN ELEVATED MOLD SPORE COUNT
Check the walls for plaster that has bubbled. Look for stains and water lines on walls, ceilings, under windowsills, and around skylights and chimneys, indicating possible mold contamination. Look carefully for leaks near the plumbing or near sump pumps. Think about vaporizers and aerosol chambers. If they were used, the molds could be under the paint or wallpaper. Is the roof flat? Are the drains off the roof open, or is there a backup on the roof and possibly into the walls?

AN ELEVATED CARBON DIOXIDE LEVEL
A school may need better ventilation because many individuals routinely breathe carbon dioxide into its air. But this should not be a factor in a home. Check for faulty ventilation vents.

AN ELEVATED CARBON MONOXIDE LEVEL
Carbon monoxide has no odor but notice where you can smell natural gas. People who have chemical sensitivities can easily pinpoint a problem area because of their enhanced perception of smell. A gas odor may indicate a leak from a gas appliance, such as a kitchen stove, furnace, hot-water heater, or clothes dryer. Defective furnaces for some reason appear to cause recurrent problems, in spite of attempts to make obvious repairs. (See the stories of Liza in Chapter 2 and Carl in Chapter 15.)

AN ELEVATED CHEMICAL LEVEL
Find the source of the chemical. Could it be smokers, pesticides, new carpets, carpet pads or glue, paint, or plywood furniture? Were the draperies or bedspread recently dry-cleaned? Were the carpets recently cleaned? Was

any reconstruction done, inside or outside, to the roof, basement, or garage? Is the furnace okay?

Most homes need only an air purifier, cleaning with more natural products, and the stringent avoidance of chemicals inside the home. If this provides relief, do no more. If it does not, some of the measures mentioned in this chapter will have to be implemented.

NOTES

1. American Association of School Administrators, *Schoolhouse in the Red*. Available from the AASA at 1801 North Moore Street, Arlington, VA 22209.

2. See W.C. White and R.A. Kemper, *Building-Related Illness: New Insight into Causes and Effective Control* (Cincinnati: Kemper Research Foundation, 1989).

3. L.S. Sheldon et al., *Indoor Air Quality in Public Buildings*, EPA project summary, no. EPA/600/S6-88/009a (Sept. 1993), p. 3. The requirements of ASHRAE 62-1989 are more stringent.

4. James E. Woods, "Cost Avoidance and Productivity in Owning and Operating Buildings," *Occupational Medicine: State of the Art Reviews*, vol. 4, no. 4 (Oct./Dec. 1989), pp. 753–70.

5. White and Kemper, *Building-Related Illness*.

6. See also Nicholas Tate, *The Sick Building Syndrome* (Far Hills, NJ: New Horizon Press, 1994), pp. 80–81, 163.

7. On health risks in skating rinks, see K. Hedberg et al., "An Outbreak of Nitrogen Dioxide-Induced Respiratory Illness Among Ice Hockey Players," *Journal of the American Medical Association*, vol. 262, no. 21 (Dec. 1, 1989), pp. 3014–17.

8. See David Rousseau and W.J. Rea, *Your Home, Health and Well-Being* (Vancouver, B.C.: Hartley and Marks, 1989).

9. See Tate, *Sick Building Syndrome*, and Hedberg, "Outbreak of Nitrogen Dioxide."

10. See Rousseau and Rea, *Your Home*.

11. Personal communications with Dr. John Laseter of AccuChem Labs and Dr. Ralph Herro of Herro Environmental Care.

12. *Rachel's Hazardous Waste News*, no. 250 (Sept. 1991).

13. See Joan Dine, "Toxic Reduction," in chapter 8 of Naomi Friedman's *Greening Synagogues and Community Centers* (Takoma Park, MD: Shomrei Adamah, 1995); and Marion Moses, *Designer Poisons* (San Francisco: Pesticide Education Center, 1995).

14. Albert Rowe and Albert Rowe, Jr., *Food Allergies* (Springfield, IL: Charles Thomas, 1972).

15. D.J. Rapp, *Is This Your Child?* (Buffalo, NY: Practical Allergy Research Foundation, 1989), pp. 278–81.

16. Norman E. Rosenthal, "Diagnosis and Treatment of Seasonal Affective Disorder," *Journal of the American Medical Association*, vol. 270, no. 22 (Dec. 8, 1993), pp. 2717–20; Robert M. Cohen et al., "Preliminary Data on the Metabolic Brain Pattern of Patients with Winter Seasonal Affective Disorder," *Archives of General Psychiatry*, vol. 49 (July 1992), pp. 545–52.

17. See J.F. Brundage et al., "Building-Associated Risk of Febrile Acute Respiratory Diseases in Army Trainees," *Journal of the American Medical Association*, vol. 259 (1988), issue 14, pp. 2108–12.

18. Rebecca Bascom et al., "Nasal Inhalation Challenge Studies with Sidestream Smoke," *Archives of Environmental Health*, vol. 47, no. 3 (May–June 1992), pp. 223–30.

19. On nonantibiotic treatments, see Michael A. Schmidt et al., *Beyond Antibiotics: 50 (or So) Ways to Boost Immunity and Avoid Antibiotics* (Berkeley, CA: North Atlantic Books, 1994).

20. On safer disinfectants, see A. Berthold-Bond, *Clean and Green* (Woodstock, NY: Ceres Press, 1990), p. 34.

21. See Carolyn Gorman, *Less Toxic Living* (Texarkana, TX: Optima Graphics, 1993); David Steinman and Samuel Epstein, *The Safe Shopper's Bible* (New York: Macmillan, 1995); Janet Marinelli and Paul Bierman-Lytle, *Your Natural Home* (Boston: Little, Brown, 1995); Debra Dadd, *Nontoxic, Natural and Earthwise* (Los Angeles: Jeremy P. Tarcher, 1990).

22. Roger Maurice, ''HEPA Vacuum Cleaners,'' *Human Ecology Study Group*, vol. 5, no. 2 (June 1994); available from P.O. Box 360, Winnetka, IL 60093.

23. See Rousseau and Rea, *Your Home*. Safer sealants are available from AFM Products (see Resources).

24. Rapp, *Is This Your Child?*

25. Glenn Beebe, *Toxic Carpet III* (Cincinnati, OH: Glenn Beebe, 1991).

26. See NEA Professional Library, *Healthy School Handbook* (Washington, DC: National Education Association, 1995), p. 106.

7 ⦃ Indoor and Outdoor Chemicals

Many people have been or are now being adversely affected by the abundance of chemicals found in and around schools. Because this phenomenon is so infrequently recognized and poorly investigated, we have no estimate of the scope of chemically related illnesses. It seems logical, however, to conclude that more individuals are becoming sensitized to chemicals every day, unaware of the inherent danger of certain common, even ubiquitous exposures.[1]

Each day, most of us, including our schoolchildren, routinely come in contact with more than five hundred chemicals, because of the markedly increased use of these substances in every aspect of daily life. In 1945 the United States produced 10 million tons of chemicals; today we produce 110 million tons. In 1991 an estimated five billion pounds of chemicals were released into our air every day. *Over a lifetime, the average American will be exposed to an estimated 54,000 of the 70,000 chemicals in commercial use today. Unfortunately most of the technologically advanced chemicals in use today have not been fully evaluated for safety by any federal, state, or local agency. Only a relative handful have been investigated in relation to human health—just 2 to 10 percent have been studied for their effect on the nervous system, even though the human body has no natural way to eliminate many of them. To make matters worse, nothing is known about the combined effects of the many chemicals to which we are exposed every day.*[2]

▩ RECOGNIZING THE PROBLEM

True, a few dangerous chemicals have been recognized and restricted. But others have remained elusive for years because no one has recognized cause-and-effect relationships between them and various physical ailments. If the time period between a harmful exposure and the onset of a serious illness is inordinately long, it is even harder to identify, let alone prove, a relationship. Those delays have been exacerbated by purposeful deceit and misrepresentation on the part of those with vested interests. For example, it took years for the public, and even longer for our government, to acknowledge the obvious harmful effects of tobacco, asbestos, and formaldehyde. It will take many more years for the government to properly address the effects of chemicals found in carpets, mattresses, foods, water, clothing, perfumes, and personal body and baby-care products—many of which find their way not only into our houses but also into our schools.[3] (See Chapter 10 for a more detailed discussion of carpets, pesticides, and formaldehyde.)

Gandhi once said, "One of the things that will destroy us is science without humanity." Unless our governmental monitoring agencies begin to protect the people rather than big business, we and future generations are truly in jeopardy.

In general, Americans lack awareness of the potentially deleterious health, behavioral, and academic effects of the routine use of chemicals in schools as well as homes. Yes, there are some progressive school administrators who are anxious to recognize and correct chemical problems. Much more common, however, are the poorly informed school officials who prefer to ignore or deny these risks. Unfortunately, far too many school districts lack the knowledge, guidance, mandates, and finances to overcome their inertia. If your child's school has asbestos, lead, and radon, and an improperly designed, malfunctioning, or poorly monitored ventilation system with dirty ductwork, inadequate filters, and excessive dust, molds, chemicals, and/or germs, expect major troubles.[4] It is only a matter of time before these combined factors erupt into a medical crisis that will finally force the school administrators to improve the quality of the indoor air and the learning environment.

Remember, your family's health depends on your awareness that chemicals can affect you. Because we lead such busy lives, most of us pay little attention to potential chemical problems until an illness actually occurs, at which time we regret we did not learn about possible harmful effects much earlier. But in reality, it is much easier than you think to make your home more healthy. Try to use natural products, and bring no chemicals into your home unless you have at least checked the MSD sheets first. And in your school, follow the guidelines you'll find in this chapter. You will be light-years ahead of most families if you take a few precautions and make a few simple changes.

■ THE RISKS OF SICK BUILDINGS

You've probably heard the term *Sick Building Syndrome.* It is a condition that can occur in an older building, due to the factors just discussed; but more commonly, it refers to chemicals used in constructing a new building. Initially, the occupants of a sick building experience transient health problems that subside after they leave the harmful exposures. Sometimes improved ventilation resolves the problem. However, if the air quality in the building remains poor—as it did for Christy described in the Introduction to Part II, and for the two teachers discussed in this chapter—people can and do develop an illness called Multiple Chemical Sensitivities (MCS) which affects many body areas. Unless they are knowledgeable about this illness and are financially secure, those who are severely afflicted frequently become progressively more debilitated because, over time, the slightest exposure to any number of chemicals can precipitate a flare-up. At the same time, an estimated 80 percent of chemically affected persons also develop food sensitivities.

These severe sensitivities can drastically restrict the lives of those affected. We must not allow this problem to continue to develop in students, teachers, or anyone else.

It is not uncommon for students and teachers to become ill in the same classroom, but each individual's symptoms can be different. Nancy and Sister Martha typify many of the most seriously ill teachers who have sought help from environmental medical specialists. Their trials and tribulations clearly demonstrate why everyone must become more knowledgeable about indoor and outdoor chemicals. At present, few people are as ill as they are, but their numbers are growing. If you take a few simple precautions and learn as much as you can, however, you and your loved ones are at considerably less risk. Both of the teachers, as well as Marsha, the student in Chapter 8, were assigned to the same classroom at different times. All three required environmental medical care for similar allergies and multiple chemical- and food-related symptoms.

A TEACHER MADE SICK BY HER CLASSROOM

Nancy

Nancy is a young, vibrant, well-trained special education teacher whose symptoms—from fatigue to muscle aches—became progressively more evident over a period of about eight years. At first, she wondered why she felt so bad; why she was unable to control her behavior at certain times. Although her complaints were particularly apparent when she was teaching in her classroom, years passed before she realized that excessive chemical exposures there were part of her problem. For example, because her classroom was located next to the students' lavatories, she was unknowingly inhaling the odor of disinfectants. She had no idea that the combination of chemicals used during school renovations, the aerial pesticide spraying nearby, and fumes from the fresh paint in her new apartment, along with molds at her school and in her waterbed at home, were creating havoc on her immune system. This array of exposures exceeded the level that her body could tolerate, and she developed a severe debilitating chemically related illness.

Nancy saw one physician after another, but none of them recognized the true cause of her sickness. After "every imaginable test" was conducted, she was told that she was stressed and that her health problems would go away if she would just calm down. At one point a psychiatrist told her to "tough it out" when she felt dizzy. Her extreme exhaustion, muscle weakness, constant ear ringing, and severe depression finally forced her to take a leave of absence for ten weeks in the spring of 1991. At that point, she was too tired to get out of bed, take a shower, or prepare a snack. She cried most of the time and became so ill that it took twenty minutes for her to crawl the few steps from her bedroom to the bathroom. She lost her self-confidence, convinced that she was a weak or "bad" person because she couldn't control her moods or regain her physical health. Little did she realize that her depression had a biochemical origin and could be helped by dietary restrictions, nutrients, and environmental changes.

Eventually, the Right Diagnosis

When Nancy was finally seen by an environmental physician, Kalpana Patel, M.D., of Buffalo, New York, she was complaining of the following symptoms:

- extreme fatigue
- mood swings, excessive crying
- numbness of fingers and face
- irritability
- headaches, a heavy head
- nausea, abdominal pain

- muscle aches and spasms
- leg cramps and pain
- ringing in the ears
- dizziness and blackouts
- difficulty concentrating
- an inability to focus

Most physicians have been taught that patients with multiple complaints of this type have a psychological problem; but this variety and number of symptoms are typical of many chemically sensitized adults and children.

Under Dr. Patel's care, Nancy underwent P/N allergy extract testing, during which many of her symptoms were reproduced. (The details of this testing method are described in Chapters 13 and 15.) A single drop of standard allergy extracts provoked symptoms within eight to ten minutes. Then these reactions subsided significantly about ten minutes after Nancy received one drop of the neutralizing dilution of the same allergy extract that had caused the responses. A placebo (a mock injection) caused no change in how she felt or acted. Testing was conducted so that she was usually unaware of which item was being tested at any given time. A few of her responses to these tests are listed on next page.

Substance Tested	Symptoms Caused by One Drop of Allergy Extract
Dust/dust mites	Facial numbness; heaviness in her head; fatigue; swelling of her mouth and cheeks; itching and burning of her eyes; pressure in her ears; and pain and tightness in her jaw.
Molds	The above symptoms, plus cramping of her hands and feet; facial pain; a hot feeling in her face; dizziness; and vertigo.
Phenol (found in lavatory disinfectants)	Symptoms similar to her response to dust, plus numbness in her hands and feet; difficulty talking; a rapid heartbeat; extreme fatigue; and a metallic taste in her mouth.
Her school air	Strange spasms in her face and mouth; numbness in her right arm, knees, and hands; tightness of her arms and legs; nausea; a heavy head; hot face and tight jaw; backache; trouble thinking clearly; depression; crying; and anger.

Nancy's responses to two of the allergy tests, perfume and phenol, are shown on the videotape *Environmentally Sick Schools* (see For Further Reading). At the end of the last test—involving an allergy extract prepared from her school air—Nancy had a frightening response, similar to one she had previously had at school. She suddenly ran wildly from the doctor's office into the parking lot, screaming and using vulgar language. Her car keys had to be taken from her because when this happened in the past, she had driven at a reckless speed.

After a thorough clinical evaluation, Nancy was found to be sensitive to foods, dust, molds, pollen, and chemicals. She also lacked some of the essential nutrients that will be discussed in Chapter 14. By the time she was seen by her environmental specialist, her multiple chemical exposures had raised her sensitivity to such a high level that she had developed the "spreading phenomenon." A nuance of almost any chemical odor now made her ill. At times scented body preparations or hair spray would make her so confused that she could not recall the names of her students or even tell the time. A whiff of perfume could cause uncontrollable laughter and terrible tics and twitches. School bus fumes sent her "into orbit" with a heavy head, depression, and difficulty thinking. Even the odor of chemicals in treated paper and the ink in newspapers and new textbooks bothered her.

Getting Proper Treatment

After Nancy received allergy extract treatment for the various substances to which she was sensitive, her symptoms improved markedly. Her comprehensive environmental medical therapy was combined with detoxification, which included exercise, massage, saunas, and frequent intravenous nutrient therapy. For a year she also drank a formulation called Ultraclear for oral detoxification (see Resources). During these detoxifying procedures her closet, car, bed, and air purifier reeked, from the many chemicals being released from her body.

After two years of this therapy, she stated, "I feel so well that it is a foreign feeling for me. I honestly look forward to what is yet to come. It's all up from here!"

Nancy was fortunate in that her family gave her positive support during her ordeal.

Once they realized that she had a genuine illness, they also learned how to detect the causes of her extremely unusual responses to inadvertent exposures. For her and her family, it was a relief to finally detect what had caused her reactions.

In September 1994, however, Nancy lost her job and with it her health insurance. But she did not want to expend her energy fighting for individual coverage, Social Security, Workers' Compensation, or disability aid (see Chapters 16 and 17). Instead, she decided to investigate alternative methods of help for her condition, which would be less expensive. She tried shiatsu, a form of finger acupuncture, and energy balancing. Shiatsu was so beneficial that in time she was able to discontinue her allergy extract therapy, her extremely strict Rotation Allergy Diet (see Chapter 3), and all nutrients except vitamin C. However, she found that she needed to continue to avoid chemicals, drink purer water, and eat organic foods, while limiting or avoiding certain major food offenders.

At times, Nancy now finds that she can tolerate certain exposures that previously caused devastating and debilitating effects. If she is very cautious, she can go to church and shop in a mall for about ten minutes, something she had dared not even consider for many months. She can visit friends, have a real Christmas tree, and even cautiously attend a concert. Even so, she rarely goes anywhere without a charcoal mask, and she is constantly fearful that she will inadvertently be exposed to something that will cause a setback. If her symptoms flare because of an exposure, especially if she is stressed, she uses vitamin C, alkaline trisalts (see Chapter 15), shiatsu, and meditation. Although certain exposures are still impossibly challenging and incapacitating, she is encouraged because she continues to gradually improve. At first, she was able to tutor students in her environmentally safer home. Now she is back at school, in a different classroom. By using good judgment, extreme caution, and avoidance, she has adjusted to a different, far more normal, and reasonable lifestyle.

ANOTHER TEACHER MADE SICK IN THE SAME CLASSROOM

Sister Martha

Sister Martha had typical allergies, and so did many of her relatives. She knew, for example, that when she ate certain foods, she would break out in hives, but she didn't realize how severe and incapacitating a combined environmental/allergic medical problem could be. At one point Sister Martha became so ill in school from certain exposures that she believed she would never feel well again. She was unable to work for two months, becoming so incapacitated that she could barely walk or talk. She had diarrhea, extreme thirst, fatigue, and dizziness. She sat at home wearing dark glasses. In desperation she finally called Nancy, the teacher described above. They had shared the same classroom, and she had heard that Nancy had similar complaints, such as fatigue and problems walking. She wondered why they both developed similar medical problems at about the same time.

At their school, Nancy and Sister Martha had been assigned to a small converted tutoring room that had originally been a custodian's "broom closet." It was located between two lavatories, whose pipes and vents entered their classroom, as did the odors of the disinfectants and deodorizers. At one time, there had been an overflow of sewage into this classroom; the carpets had subsequently been cleaned, but the walls remained stained and moldy. In addition, the room contained a dirty "old slop" sink and a large electrical panel. The room had a well-earned reputation: Neither teachers nor students wanted to be assigned there. But amazingly, in spite of its many now-acknowledged shortcomings, this room continues to be used for teaching at the present time!

As if the specific problems inside Sister Martha's classroom weren't enough, streams of polluted, oily water (caused by underground leakage) oozed onto the basement floor of her school each spring. The resulting mix of noxious pollution and allergenic substances permeated the entire school building.

Her Condition Worsens

Beginning in September 1992, Sister Martha experienced a major flare-up of her symptoms, shortly after workers removed asbestos by carrying it through her poorly ventilated classroom. Following this "clean-up," she would feel ill after only ten minutes in her classroom. Each day, she developed some combination of headaches, swelling of her tongue and throat, a weak voice, irritability, impatience, ringing in the ears, hearing loss, dark eye circles, tight chest, rapid breathing, easy bruising, fatigue, lethargy, apathy, difficulty concentrating, diarrhea, poor balance, and excessive thirst. And what was the diagnosis from her doctor? She was told she had an emotional or "functional" problem.

In December 1992, Sister Martha began to cough, and she developed joint stiffness with pain and swelling, tight muscles, and numb fingers. The left side of her body often fell asleep. She had spasms of her face muscles, and she complained of dizziness. Light bothered her eyes, and she had visual problems and dark eye circles. She also had excessive mucus and saliva.

Because of her numerous medical complaints, Sister Martha eventually insisted on being switched to another classroom in the school. However, after only about half an hour in the different room, similar symptoms developed. To help delay and diminish these symptoms, she would arrive ninety minutes before class to open the window and air out the room. This strategy might have been beneficial if the basic problem had been only a lack of clean indoor air; the outside air, however, was polluted by a nearby store that ground corn, sold fertilizer, and supplied propane.

Pinpointing the Problem

Finally, Sister Martha underwent P/N allergy extract testing, during which she was found to be sensitive to many substances, including chlorine, glycerine, histamine, and ethyl alcohol. When Dr. Patel tested her with an allergy extract prepared from the school air, many of her classroom-related symptoms were reproduced. During a single-blinded provocation allergy test with molds, one drop of extract caused the left side of her body to become numb, and she could hardly move and barely walk. This particular response had previously been diagnosed as a cardiac problem and treated unsuccessfully with several medications. Once her sensitivity to molds was recognized and treated appropriately with a neutralizing allergy extract dosage, her "heart" problem disappeared.

In April 1993, as part of Sister Martha's treatment by Dr. Patel, she started a Rotation Allergy Diet. At this writing, she must continue to adhere strictly to her diet and avoid chemicals. Also, if she does not receive neutralizing treatment doses of her mold and dust allergy extract every two to three days, she becomes light-headed and can't think or remember as well as usual. Inhaling certain allergenic substances such as dust and molds continues to cause asthma and dizziness, but fortunately these complaints can be relieved within a few minutes by her allergy extract. (This treatment provides more rapid and effective relief than her previous asthma drugs.) Overall, she has responded very favorably to comprehensive environmental/allergic medical therapy. Her symptoms and general well-being have improved. In 1994, she said she had once thought she "would never feel this well again."

Although there is no doubt that Sister Martha is better, her life is still filled with limitations and restrictions. She cannot eat fruit more often than every two or three days; she can drink only pure water and must sharply limit milk and wheat. She must not remain in a shopping mall longer than forty minutes, although that is far better than previously when she could not tolerate such an exposure for more than a minute or two. She needs her allergy extract every other day on school days, but she does not require an injection on weekends at home. We anticipate that she'll continue to improve so that in time she can relax her restricted lifestyle even more.

MAKING CHANGES IN YOUR SCHOOL

To help minimize problems in your child's school, here are some general considerations to discuss with school officials and the PTA. (They are also applicable in your own home.)

- *Urge your school to purchase a portable air purifier for each polluted classroom or school area, to remove dust, molds, pollen, and certain chemicals (see Resources).*
- *Choose furnishings made of metal, solid wood, or waterproof exterior grade, not of vinyl or plastic that smells of chemicals. On pressed wood, plywood, or particle board that emits chemical odors, use a safe sealer (see Resources).*
- *Your school should use 100 percent outdoor-air ventilation twenty-four hours per day for at least two full weeks after any major remodeling or construction work, to help rid the building of chemical odors.*
- *Help identify the presence and the source of a large number of harmful gases by using a Combustible Gas Detector (see Resources). It lights up and makes a sound as it approaches a gas. It does not specifically identify the gas, but it helps direct you to its source. The TIF8800A Combustible Gas Detector can detect methane, ethane, propane, benzene, butane, acetylene, hexane, gasoline, toluene, and naphtha in a range of 50 to 1,000 parts per million (ppm); it is also said to detect halogenated hydrocarbons, alcohols, ethers, ketones, and industrial chemicals including formaldehyde. Using the Combustible Gas Detector may help convince a reluctant school to investigate complaints.*
- *Consider using plants that absorb odors.[5]*
- *Urge your school and county libraries to obtain reference books and videos about environmental issues related to chemicals (see Resources). If no money is available for such items or for air purifiers, consider holding a bake or rummage sale to raise the money.*

WHAT TO DO IF CHEMICALS ARE MAKING YOUR CHILD SICK

Nancy's and Sister Martha's symptoms are typical of those that can develop after indoor environmental exposures. To get started on reducing those exposures, use the information in Table 7.1 as a guide to making changes in the school environment.[6] At the same time, it is important to try to discern which items are causing your child's specific medical complaints. This can be a difficult process because a wide variety of substances that can adversely affect the nervous system are used during routine school (or home) maintenance and renovations. Even so, pinpointing the offending chemicals is crucial because of the possibility, however remote, that your child may truly never be the same after exposures to certain substances (see Chapter 3). For documentation, videotape how your child looks, acts, and writes before, during, and after school. Also, videotape ''before and after'' responses in specific classrooms after certain exposures. This documentation may help convince a skeptical school principal, physician, psychologist, or insurance company of the seriousness of your child's special needs. Sometimes, specially trained neuropsychologists can provide help in documenting the role of chemicals in your illness (see Chapter 13).

One easy and inexpensive problem-solving approach is to obtain written permission from the school to prepare an allergy extract of the school air.[7] You can also do this at home, too, if your home air is involved. With this extract, an environmental medical specialist can test and possibly treat

---

TABLE 7.I

Chemical Reduction in a Nutshell

To reduce the level of chemicals in schools and homes:

■ Use environmentally safer cleaning agents.
■ Avoid chemical-laden cleaning materials, furniture, and construction materials.
■ Use safer sealants for doors, furniture, and cement.
■ On floors, use hard vinyl or ceramic tile with safer glues, not carpets or chemical-laden carpet pads.
■ Monitor airborne chemical levels with badges or tubes.
■ Eliminate the sources of chemical contamination and/or bake out and ventilate the affected room or building very well.
■ Allow no tobacco, and strongly discourage the use of perfumed or scented items.
■ Use room or central air-purifying machines, which help remove chemicals.
■ Take measures to diminish mold contamination.
■ Use safer pesticides inside and outside the building.
■ Do not allow cars or buses to idle nearby.

your child so that school attendance, living in a certain home or apartment—and your youngster's well-being—will no longer be a problem. Although a school-air allergy extract will not identify which component in the air is causing symptoms, it can show the health effects caused by the air that students and teachers routinely breathe. If something inhaled into the lungs is a problem and there is enough of it, both in the school air and in the air extract, a single-blinded P/N allergy extract testing can pinpoint specific cause-and-effect relationships.

In the remainder of this chapter, I'll discuss specific details about where your efforts at minimizing health problems in your school would be most effective.

■ MAINTENANCE AND CLEANING CHEMICALS

To prevent illness, you must learn what chemicals are safe to use and why. Whenever a school decides to use a new odorous chemical for cleaning or maintenance, teachers and parents of children who become ill from chemicals should be notified in advance. Ask to be informed about when, how, and exactly where any chemicals will be applied or used. The school administration must provide you with MSD sheets for every chemical used, especially for those used in known "problem" areas. These MSD sheets, at times, will provide simple and obvious answers to your questions. But unfortunately, they are often needlessly complicated, incomplete, deceptive, difficult to interpret, grossly misleading, and inaccurate. (For more information, see Chapter 10.)

If you have concerns about a certain exposure, request a sample of *every* suspect item being used. Date them, label them, and store them in a tightly covered glass container. Keep them in a safe place *in your home*; you may need them for future analysis and/or testing.

TYPICAL MAINTENANCE AND CLEANING CHEMICALS

School officials and knowledgeable adults should conduct research into the types of cleaning and maintenance supplies being used. Schools must stop using any "typical" detergent soaps, disinfectant aerosols, polish, floor wax, and floor strippers that contain dangerous solvents that can possibly damage the nervous system. Here are some specifics to keep in mind:

■ Lavatory disinfectants and room-air fresheners usually contain a number of potentially toxic chemicals such as phenol, ethanol, xylene, cresol, ammonia, chlorine, formaldehyde, and naphthalene. These chemicals can potentially damage many major body organs, as well as the nervous system, in susceptible individuals.

■ Xylene is found not only in air fresheners but in bus and automobile fuel exhaust. It is used in biology laboratories for the preparation of glass slides. When inhaled at levels too low to produce a noticeable odor, xylene sometimes causes confusion, balance problems, a slow reaction time, birth defects, and miscarriages.[8] Air fresheners commonly contain agents to "deaden" nerves so you can't smell, plus a perfume to cover up the odor of the chemical. (Refer to the story of Ryan in Chapter 1; his illness was caused by a commonly used disinfectant aerosol.) These air fresheners should be replaced with safer, less expensive products such as Borax (sodium carbonate) and water. Zephiran is tolerated by some, but not all, sensitive children and adults.

■ Floor cleaners and waxes often contain potentially offending petroleum derivatives or hydrocarbons. Higher-quality, safer floor waxes need stripping less often, which not only reduces the expense but also lessens everyone's exposure to toxic chemicals.

■ Carpet cleaners and deodorizers contain perchloroethylene, chlorine, naphthalene, ethanol, ammonia, and detergents.

In Chapter 10, you'll find more details about the types of chemicals in common cleaning supplies used in many schools.

SAFE MAINTENANCE AND CLEANING AGENTS

Suggest to your school officials or to the individuals who do your school cleaning that they consider using less expensive, nontoxic, safer cleaning agents (also see the list in Table 7.2 and Resources). For additional practical information, refer to these books: *The Nontoxic Home and Office; Clean and Green; Nontoxic, Natural, and Earthwise; Designer Poisons;* and *Less Toxic Living.* They discuss common products that cause illness, as well as safer substitutes.[9]

TABLE 7.2

Nontoxic Cleaning Agents

■ **Baking Soda:** air freshener, mild abrasive scouring powder
■ **Vinegar and lemon juice:** dirt and grease removers; reduce mineral buildup
■ **Vegetable-oil-based detergents and soaps:** cut grease, remove dirt
■ **Borax:** deodorizer, cleaner, stain remover; decreases mold and bacteria

---

To be sure these cleaners are well-tolerated, follow the suggestions in Chapter 3. Basic nontoxic cleaning agents are listed in Table 7.2. You may also follow these instructions for using them:

1. An inexpensive general cleaner can be made by combining ¼ cup baking soda, ½ cup vinegar, 1 gallon water, and 1 cup ammonia. This cleaner will help diminish mold and mildew on walls, floors, and ceilings.

2. For general cleaning, use an all-purpose 100 percent organic and biodegradable product such as Neolife Rugged Red or Shaklee Basic H (see Resources).

3. For toilet bowl cleaning, try ½ cup each of baking soda and vinegar. Carolyn Gorman, the author of *Less Toxic Living*, has suggested using 1 cup Borax mixed with ¼ cup lemon juice or vinegar, or 1 denture tablet, Sol-V-Guard or DeScale It, to remove lime or scale.

4. Stop using chlorinated, odorous scouring powders; instead use Bon Ami polishing powder or bar, which is effective and safe for removing grease and oils.

5. To clean glass, use 3 Tbsp. ammonia, plus 1 Tbsp. vinegar and ¾ cup water.

6. For plugged drains, cautiously pour 1 cup baking soda and ½ cup white vinegar down the drain, then cover it tightly for one minute. The chemical reaction causes pressure in the drain that helps dislodge obstructive matter. Rinse with hot water and repeat as needed. Use 3 Tbsp. washing soda in the drain once a week to prevent such problems.

7. To inhibit mold growth, try:
   - sunlight and increased ventilation (open windows)
   - straight Borax paste (Borax and hot water), applied to walls; leave it on the walls for a number of days, and then vacuum to remove the powder when it is completely dry.
   - a Borax solution for cleaning (¼ cup Borax per 2 cups hot water)
   - full-strength distilled white vinegar
   - spraying with Purisol (see Resources)
   - deodorant-free kitty litter (from pet stores)
   - mold adsorbers or silica gel (see Resources)
   - cornstarch for books that smell of mildew
   - heat, which kills molds, "baking out" moldy areas.

8. For a deodorizer, try lemon juice, baking soda, unscented kitty litter, and/or Zeolite bags to help absorb molds and pollutant or smoke odors (see Resources).

9. For a disinfectant, use ½ cup Borax, ¼ cup vinegar, and 2 gallons hot water. An expensive alternative is Australian tea tree oil, an essential

oil that is a natural germ and mold retardant, available in health food stores. Use 2 tsp. to 2 cups water, applied from a spray bottle. Similarly, citrus seed extract (Nutrabiotic or Citricidal), also available in health food stores, is well-tolerated by some.

10. Certain plants can help remove chemicals. Aloe vera and potted chrysanthemums help eliminate toxins. The latter, however, can flare ragweed allergies. English ivy is said to help remove benzene. Fig trees and spider plants may eliminate formaldehyde.[10]

ODOR-EATING SUBSTANCES

A number of substances, mainly plants, appear helpful in removing specific gases or chemical smells, absorbing odors or pollution in general.[11] They include: (a) spider plants, (b) philodendron, (c) pothos, (d) peace lily, (e) mother-in-law's tongue, (f) English ivy, (g) bamboo palm, (h) gerbera daisy, (i) Warneck's dracaena, (j) *Ficus*, (k) pot mum, (l) mass cane, (m) granular charcoal, and (n) Chinese evergreens.

Here is a list of some chemicals these plants can positively affect (the letters after each chemical name correspond to the plants listed above):

- *formaldehyde (plywood, pressboard glue, permanent press clothes): a, b, e, f, g, h, i, j, k, l*
- *carbon dioxide: a, b*
- *trichloroethylene (dry-cleaning solvent): d, f, h, i, k*
- *benzene: d, f, h, i, k, j*

For more information, see Resources. Note that some plants can also help remove electromagnetic energy and reduce static electricity.

▪ CONSTRUCTION MATERIALS[12]

Surprisingly, the materials used in floors, walls, and ceilings can create health difficulties. Check each of the following items (using the guidelines in Chapter 3) if you suspect they are causing a sensitivity in you or your child:

FLOORS

▪ Very hard vinyl tile flooring seems to be tolerated by most individuals. However, the polyvinyl chloride used in softer vinyl tiles and linoleum can bother some chemically sensitive persons. Cushioned rubber tile can emit odors for many months. French scientists claim that asbestos fibers may be released from heavily used floors. Again, check it out.

▪ Safer sealers for wood, plywood, and tile are essential (see Resources).

■ Plain concrete is economical, but it must be sealed with a safe sealer or paint.[13]

■ Hardwoods, such as oak, maple, ash, beech, and birch, make excellent but expensive floor coverings. Odorous woods like pine and conifer should be avoided. An individual can be sensitive to the odor of one type of wood but not another.

■ Ceramic tile and terrazzo (which is concrete with marble or granite chips) are usually well-tolerated, but they are costly, and some of the grouting materials used with them cause symptoms. Also, be careful of the glazes, which can contain lead.

Not only do most flooring materials already contain chemicals, but they are routinely installed and/or finished with even more chemicals. Synthetic carpets and their installation materials can cause serious medical problems in some students and teachers (as discussed in Chapter 10). Prior to purchase, be sure to individually check new flooring material, plus every substance used for installation and maintenance. Even when floor products are advertised as "safe," they may not be tolerated by everyone. Refer back to Chapter 3 to find out how you can help document that a particular product is causing your child to become ill. Also, *The Healthy School Handbook* has an excellent chapter on this topic, written by Mary Oetzel;[14] see also For Further Reading.

WALLS AND CEILINGS

Inexpensive types of wood, like plywood and particle board, often emit formaldehyde, which can cause symptoms. Solid natural wood such as oak, poplar, and birch are more expensive but are definitely preferable. Certain woods are less odorous than others.

Room dividers are made from layers of particle board (formaldehyde) covered with plastic fiber. When they are new, the chemical odor can be more than offensive; it can be harmful to health.

An attempt was made to ban urea–formaldehyde ceiling insulation in 1982 but it was unsuccessful. Nevertheless, be warned that some scientists believe this product carries risks. I would not purchase a home if its ceiling or walls contain this potentially harmful substance.

(Also, see the section on plastics on page 183 for other furniture problems.)

PAINTS

Paints often contain toluene, benzene, xylene, naphtha, fungicides, and/or hydrocarbons or kerosene (see Chapter 7). Benjamin Moore Prestine or Low

Odor, Safecoat by AFM, and Glidden Spread 2000, are safer, but each must be checked because even less odorous "safer" paints can cause illness in some sensitive individuals. Again, use the "Big Five" discussed in Chapter 3 for possible insight about the effects of a particular product upon your child.

PLASTICS

Plastics are a smorgasbord of potentially harmful and at times cancer-causing chemicals. A plastic that has an odor and is soft, such as in a book bag, a lunch box, a pencil container, or a toy, can cause more difficulty than the harder, less smelly forms of plastic (that is, the kinds used in the construction of furniture). Sometimes it helps to soak the product in a solution of one cup of baking soda and a quart of water for a long period.

You may notice that you or your child cannot refrain from wiggling while sitting on vinyl-covered furniture or a hard plastic chair. By contrast, you sit contentedly on wooden or metal furniture. Once again, use the "Big Five" in Chapter 3. If plastic furniture at school makes your child wiggly, ask for the chair to be changed. A wooden beaded or an inexpensive Mexican-leather seat-cover might resolve this problem.

Latex and nylon are somewhat less toxic forms of plastic, but they too can cause illness in some children who are sensitive to petrochemicals and/or hydrocarbons (substances derived from oil, gas, or living organic matter). In addition, the minute amount of phenol and benzene in nylon can affect those who are sensitive.

Here are some other important points about plastics and their chemicals. (For more details about these chemicals, refer to Chapter 10.)

■ Many plastics contain phthalates.
■ Polyester in cloth can release a minute amount of formaldehyde.
■ The polyurethane so commonly used in upholstered furniture and mattresses can release toluene diisocyanate, potentially causing chest, eye, and skin symptoms in some individuals.
■ Lucite/Plexiglas is an acrylonitrile or acrylic plastic substance that is suspected of causing cancer. It can cause intestinal and breathing problems, weakness, headache, and fatigue.
■ Teflon is a fluorocarbon plastic or tetrafluoroethylene, which can cause eye, nose, throat, and lung irritation.
■ Less harmful forms of plastic are cellulose, Formica (melamine), and Bakelite. Bakelite is a phenol/formaldehyde resin form of plastic that "outgases" quickly with use.

■ Polyvinyl pipes are said to be safe, but toxic and potentially cancer-causing substances can leach from these pipes into the water.[15]

FURNITURE
Chairs are often padded with polyurethane foam (a form of phthalate) and covered with polyester, acrylic (acrylonitrile), and polyvinyl chloride plastic. Stain-resistant fabric contains formaldehyde.

ROOFING

Health problems such as tics, twitches, headaches, and breathing and memory problems can be caused by tar odors. Isocyanate insulation can cause medical illness too. (See the story of Christy in the Introduction to Part II.)

Unless the need is imperative, roof repairs should always be made *at the end rather than at the beginning of the school year.* If possible, do it only when school is not in session. If the roof of your home needs repair, try having it done when you are not there.

PROBLEMS FROM TARRING A SCHOOL ROOF

Jerry

Jerry is a 17-year-old with many allergies and environmental health problems. Even so, he generally got through his school day fairly well, except for developing tics or twitches when he was exposed to molds or chemicals. In everyday life, however, it is exceedingly difficult to anticipate and prevent chemical exposures.

That's what happened to Jerry in August 1993, when hot tar was used to repair the roof of his school. As the school year began in early September, the odor was horrendous while the roofing work continued. By September 13, Jerry was becoming pale and nauseated with headaches that lasted all day. He made strange, embarrassing noises (vocal tics) and had facial, chest, and shoulder muscle twitches or jerks. On several occasions, his father had to pick him up at school because he was so ill.

At the same time, approximately seven teachers at Jerry's school also experienced symptoms. They were told by their physicians to stay home. One student had to be hospitalized because of breathing problems, and many other students and staff complained of burning eyes, breathing difficulties, or headaches. In addition, there appeared to be more fights and disruptive behavior than usual among the students. The onset of these various problems seemed to be directly related to the intensity of the tar odor.

Meanwhile, during each school day, Jerry's problems became progressively worse, and at night he had difficulty falling asleep. By September 30, his symptoms were so severe that he could no longer attend school. He was placed on temporary home tutoring until the roofing was completed. While he was at home, his school-related twitching subsided. In November, Jerry tried to return to school but again experienced tics and irritability. At the end of November, his migraines recurred, and when his parents investigated, they found that the roofing contractor had started working at lunchtime, rather than waiting until school was out for the day. Jerry had to stop attending school again.

In time, even after his teachers could no longer smell anything, Jerry complained of a faint odor once he was back at school, and his severe symptoms recurred. In January 1994, he actually was unconscious in class for fifteen minutes.

Despite his doctor's requests to install an air purifier at the school, along with other measures, school officials refused to comply. They tried to assure the staff and students that the roofing material was nontoxic and that their symptoms were only temporary. The administrators did, however, finally agree to arrange for the contractor's crew to work on weekends and overtime.

You may well ask why the roof tarring was not done at the onset, rather than at the end, of the long summer vacation. Why didn't the school officials know or acknowledge that the odors could constitute a potential health problem? Because of their inaction, not only did Jerry miss six weeks of school, but his exposure caused serious, distressing *chronic* health effects. Ever since his repeated exposure to the tar odor, his sensitivity to other substances has heightened. Exceedingly minute amounts of numerous other chemical odors that previously caused him no difficulty now produce embarrassing tics within just a few minutes—and we have no idea how long this will last.

■ RISKS IN THE WATER SUPPLY

WHAT ABOUT CHLORINE?

Some individuals cannot drink ordinary tap water from school drinking fountains, take a shower, or tolerate prolonged baths or swimming because of problems associated with chemicals like chlorine used for water "purification." Most of us think of chlorine as normal and safe because it is purposely added to our water supply, along with as many as sixty other chemicals. Some of these chemicals help decrease germs and algae to arbitrarily chosen "safe" levels. Chlorine has a taste and can irritate the eyes, nose, and skin. In some sensitive individuals, however, even a small trace of chlorine can cause much more difficulty. Surprisingly, just the odor of chlorine, as well as pool bromines and dental fluorides, can produce physical illnesses. A few children act tired, wild, or depressed after such exposures, while others are unable to think clearly or act appropriately (see Liza in Chapter 2, and Karen, Marsha, Mary, and Marlene in Chapter 8).

Breathing chlorine fumes can unquestionably precipitate or worsen asthma in some youngsters, especially if they swim for long periods of time in a heavily or recently chlorinated pool, whether at school, at home, or in a community. Profound symptoms can even be provoked by a single prolonged excessive exposure. Sometimes, an exposure can cause so much difficulty that future swimming in chlorinated pools is no longer possible. *To reduce lung irritation and possible chemical sensitization, avoid any pool contact shortly after chlorination.*

How can you tell if your child is affected by chlorine? Look for obvious changes in how your child feels, behaves, or learns shortly after a swim in a chlorinated pool. If these same complaints are not evident after a swim in fresh, nonchlorinated water, chlorine may be a problem. Surprisingly, once sensitization has occurred, even the minute amount of chlorine found in a glass of tap water can cause illness (for more discussion of water, see Chapter 8).

If your child experiences relatively minor irritation of the eyes, nose, and skin after chlorine exposure, merely rinse the affected areas with clear nonchlorinated water. To cleanse the front of the eyeballs, open the eyes in a sink or use an eye cup. Similarly, rinse the nose by placing the face in a sink or tub of non- or less-chlorinated water (don't hold the nose while doing so). To rinse the skin, shower in water that contains no chlorine. Special devices can be placed on shower heads at school and at home to help remove chlorine and other chemicals. Water purifiers should be placed at the intake water source to improve the quality of water throughout the school (see Resources).

Chlorine can become a potentially significant health hazard in other ways. Combined with organic material such as decaying leaves or plants, for example, it can change to chloroform and trihalomethanes. The latter is a common precursor to a wide range of substances known to be harmful and dangerous; chlorine products have caused cancer in animals, and possibly in humans, as well as damage to the liver, kidneys, and nervous system. Chlorine, chloroform, and other halogenated hydrocarbons tend to concentrate in the bladder and rectum prior to excretion or elimination from the body; chlorine breakdown products are thought to be possible factors related to cancer in those areas of the body. In one medical study, 9 percent of bladder cancer, 18 percent of rectal cancer, and possibly other forms of intestinal and liver cancer could be attributed to the long-term consumption of chlorinated water.[16]

An antichlorine (as well as an antifluoride) movement has arisen, which investigates the possible need to reduce, limit, or prohibit the use of chlorine. Our governmental protection agencies should decide *within a reasonable period of time* whether to continue the use of chlorinated water. The EPA is presently investigating safer ways to disinfect our water supplies. In the meantime, chlorinated chemicals are also routinely found in pesticides, refrigerants, air conditioners, and dry-cleaning fluids.

POOL CHEMICAL SUBSTITUTES

Your school may want to learn more about the newer pool chemical substitutes that are alternatives to chlorine.[17] Bromine and fluorine are not the answers; they are so similar chemically to chlorine that they can cause health problems identical to those caused by chlorine.

Then there's ozone, which is known to kill bacteria, algae, and viruses and to oxidize organic material; for ozone to be effective, however, it must be adequately mixed with pool water before it naturally breaks down to oxygen. Even when ozone or oxygen is used, a small amount of chlorine is usually needed.

There are other new possibilities that reduce—*but do not eliminate*—the need for chlorine in commercial or residential pools.

Some newer products include Baquacil and Dioxychlor (see Resources). A variation using oxygen radicals to kill algae and bacteria is the Boss Oxygen Purification System, which claims to need 90 percent fewer chemicals for pool care. Nevertheless it requires about 0.4 ppm of chlorine. Similar products are often recommended for spas, cooling towers, fountains, aquariums, and swamp coolers (see Resources).

Another possible substitute for chlorine is ionization with electrodes made of copper and silver alloys (see Resources). The copper kills algae and the silver is antibacterial. In general, all these products claim to reduce the cost of pool maintenance by decreasing the need for both chlorine and algaecides. However, most patients with chemical sensitivities react to such minute amounts of many chemicals that any residual chlorine may cause symptoms.

Some of these newer pool cleansing methods have been used for only a short time and thus may not have been adequately evaluated for effectiveness and safety.[18] School officials must fully investigate any substitutes so that an old problem is not simply replaced with a new one. As a parent, you should study the product literature, check with your physician, and follow the suggestions in Chapter 5 to decide whether a new pool chemical substitute is well-tolerated by your child or yourself.

■ PESTICIDES USED INSIDE SCHOOLS

A New York State survey found that 87 percent of the state's schools use pesticides containing substances that can cause immediate and long-term health problems.[19] This is unconscionable, since natural substitutes are available. Moreover, the safer substances can reduce the cost of pest control for school districts by 20 to 80 percent. Some 50,000 pesticides that are already on the market have yet to be evaluated or reassessed to determine their safety. About six thousand new chemicals are identified each week. At the rate the EPA is conducting its evaluations, they will not be completed until well into the *twenty-second century*! Can we wait that long? It appears that dangerous pesticides have been allowed on the market for many years, in part because the EPA simply has too many duties and responsibilities. Determining the health risks of pesticides must be given a much higher priority.

If your child's school system insists on using toxic pesticides that can potentially damage the nervous systems of not only insects but also children, then parents, teachers, PTA groups, and others who are aware of the dangers must insist that school administrators learn more about totally natural pest-control substances called biocides.[20] Biocides can *safely* and effectively deter or eradicate certain insects or vermin (see Chapter 10). One pest management advisory group called Praxis provides Biotool Kits for all types of pests, gypsy moths, and odors in drains and septic tanks, for schools as well as businesses. These kits use *no* pesticides in any form (see Resources).

Schools can also purchase a product called the Bug Banisher, available from Earthtek Corporation. It is basically a negative-ion electron-field generator that is guaranteed to repel certain insects, so that most but not all are gone in four to ten days (see Resources).

The state of Michigan (and probably other states as well) has some surprisingly dangerous termite-control laws, which apparently insist that the soil beneath a building must be impregnated with large amounts of a pesticide such as Dursban. This treatment must be done prior to construction, to prevent termite infestations. It would be safer and less expensive to use large amounts of biologically safe diatomaceous earth instead. Yet because of intertwined bureaucracy involving federal and state governments, common sense has become lost in the shuffle, effectively impeding safer termite-control measures.

If your child's school becomes infested with termites, a combination of borates, nematodes (worms that eat termites), and predatory (entomophagous) mites will safely and effectively eradicate this problem. First, school officials should check on what your state recommends or mandates. *Must* unsafe chemicals be used rather than safer products? If the answer is yes, ask why. Do those who insist on the use of harmful neurotoxic substances do so because they are merely uninformed or apathetic, or do they have vested interests that need further discussion or investigation?

LAWN CHEMICALS

Ask school officials to use the safest possible natural lawn chemicals and see that they are applied only on weekends or after school hours. (Also, help educate your landlord and those who maintain your lawn at home.) Request MSD sheets for *all* preparations used. Sometimes only part of a company's natural lawn care is actually "natural."

Refer to Chapters 10 and 18 for more detailed information about the potentially serious problems inherent in the use of certain pesticides and herbicides. Also read *Cleaning Up America the Poisoned, Poisoning Our Children: Surviving in a Toxic World, The Poisoning of Our Homes and Workplaces,* and the newest, most informative books, entitled *Designer Poisons* and *Our Stolen Future.*[21]

Another excellent book, *Chemical Intolerance* by Dr. Robert Gardner, is a source of scientific and technical biochemical information about the physiology of common illnesses related to these kinds of chemicals.[22]

Herbicides are pesticides. They can kill more than weeds. Some chemicals in herbicides, as well as pesticides, can be neurotoxic or potentially harmful to the brain, nervous, and hormonal systems of insects, pets, and humans. When safer ways to control weeds and pests are available, why tolerate brain-damaging substances in or near schools, or anywhere else?

▪ CHEMICALS USED IN THE CLASSROOM

Marking Pens

A student at a small private school suddenly began to act in an inappropriate manner. His mother investigated and discovered that the chalkboards in the school had recently been replaced by white boards. Instead of chalk, dry-erase acetate markers, which contain methyl isobutyl ketone, butyl acetate and various esters, were now being used. Shortly after the new boards were installed, the boy developed pallor, dark eye circles, listlessness, unusual irritability, coughing, stomach cramps, and repeated sore throats. Other children in the same classroom developed similar symptoms, as well as headaches. Even so, the principal was reluctant to investigate this issue or replace the markers—that is until a group of parents pointed out that the manufacturer stated explicitly that its markers were *not designed for classroom use*!

If you have suspicions like these, confirm them in an organized manner (see Chapter 3). If your child is suddenly different in some way, investigate as the parents did in the above example. Were any changes made in the classroom (or at home) shortly before your child became ill? Permanent-ink pens and markers *can* cause symptoms. See if the school will use water-based ink markers, ballpoint pens, and odorless crayons instead. The solution to a problem like this is often obvious and easy to find, but someone like you must take the time to find it.

In *The Healthy School Handbook*, William Rea, M.D., of Dallas recounts a study he conducted with a group of dentists. He asked them to write a few lines with a pen, which they did easily, without errors. Then he had them sniff a board marker containing the solvent toluene. After doing so, 50 percent of the dentists could no longer write with accuracy. They experienced short-term memory impairment, shaky hands, and difficulty with hand-eye coordination.[23]

Parents must insist that only safe markers be used in schools, and that our government protect its citizens more fully from harmful chemicals.

TYPEWRITER CORRECTION FLUID

Correction fluids can contain trichloroethylene, cresol, ethanol, and naphthalene. Some foolish children who purposely inhaled the vapors to feel "high" have stopped breathing, had cardiac arrest, and died. Your school should use only the safer forms of water-based correction fluid.

GLUES

Adhesives such as epoxy and rubber cement emit volatile chemicals. The vapors of naphthalene, phenol, ethanol, vinyl chloride, acrylonitrile, and formaldehyde can be toxic.

PRINTING MATERIALS

Ordinary paper used in schools often contains many chemicals. It can emit odors that affect how some children and adults think, act, and remember. While reading certain books, magazines, and newspapers, these individuals may feel sick, develop headaches or skin rashes, or become fatigued, upset, confused, or unable to concentrate, because of the contents of the paper or ink.

Certain paper products, such as "carbonless" carbon paper, may contain polychlorinated biphenyls, acetone, ethanol, phenol, toluene, xylene, and cresol. In addition, the odors of duplicating machines, copy machines, laser printers, toners, and developers have chemicals that can cause medical and memory complaints; they can contain ethanol and ammonia, and the dry-copy forms may emit ozone and other fumes. Adequate ventilation, with direct venting to the outside, can help diminish this problem in print or copy areas.

Chemicals like benzene are commonly used in schools that print newspapers and teaching materials. These chemicals have the potential to damage the nervous system and possibly cause cancer. Ask for the MSD sheets on every chemical used in printed material that your chemically sensitized student will read. Unfortunately, however, some dangerous chemicals are classified as "inert" and won't be listed on these sheets (see Chapter 10).

As a parent, you should insist that the school district's printing presses *never* be housed in a building that contains classrooms. The classroom of one kindergarten student in New York was located directly across the hall from a room containing the school district's printing shop. In September, the boy could count to one hundred and easily catch a ball. By December, he could count only to ten and could no longer catch the ball. His brain image (see Chapter 11) showed a pattern of the type seen following mild neurotoxic damage. After spending about six months in a different school and undergoing allergy extract therapy and detoxification measures, this child regained his previous levels of knowledge and coordination. A follow-up brain image has not been performed, however, due to a lack of insurance coverage and funds. By the way, others in his classroom became similarly ill from the same exposure, and some continue to have symptoms. *In spite of this knowledge, this school district's printing shop has NOT been moved to another building.* (The district did, however, replace the louvered door with a solid one, and it installed better ventilation in the printing room.)

If you suspect this kind of chemical sensitivity, and if it has been documented by using the suggestions in Chapter 3, ask your physician to confirm the health or learning effects of certain exposures (as indicated in Chapter 13). A special allergy extract can be prepared from various types of paper so that specific challenge testing can be performed. Once you know that something is making your child ill, the best treatment is to judiciously eliminate future exposures to that item.

Here's another approach to try: If a book, newspaper, or magazine has made your child ill, try opening it and spreading the pages apart. Then bake it or dry it out in the oven for about five hours at 100°F. Your objective is to heat the paper just enough to release the chemicals without burning the pages.

If printed matter is a major ongoing problem for your child, you can purchase or create a glass reading box with openings for the hands so he can turn the pages. Encasement boxes can also be purchased to reduce computer odors and exposures to electromagnetic fields (see Resources).

■ PERFUMES AND SCENTED PRODUCTS

Many children and teachers have difficulty in classrooms (and at home) because of exposure to scented body and hair products such as soaps, hair sprays, body lotions, creams, shampoos, deodorants, perfumes, and aftershaves. Perfumes can contain formaldehyde, phenol, chloroethylene, cresol, and artificial fragrances. Some scented hair sprays contain the chemical polyvinyl-pyrrolidine (PVP), which has the potential to cause enlarged lymph nodes, changes in the lungs and blood, and possibly cancer. Clothing can smell of perfume, dry-cleaning fluid (perchloroethylene), fabric softeners, mothballs (paradichlorobenzene), formaldehyde, or polyester (formaldehyde). In addition, many schools routinely use scented cleaning agents, disinfectants, or deodorant aerosols that can emit pleasant but, at times, illness-producing aromas. Even if your child is initially affected by only one specific type of perfume, innumerable scents can eventually cause reactions, especially if the exposure is continued over time.

Controlling the use of perfumes and scented substances, in both schools and homes, can be an immense challenge. Asking for voluntary cooperation sounds fine, but is it really a viable option? Much as they have attempted to do with cigarettes, schools eventually will have to enforce specific rules for those who refuse to comply in relation to scented items. By some means, those who insist on using scented products will have to be separated from those who become ill from exposure to them. If some teachers, for example, want to use highly scented products, they can be urged to apply them *outside*, as they leave for the day.

Our bodies can respond in only a limited number of ways to offending exposures (see Table 1.1). Thus, perfumes cause the same symptoms that are typical of other chemical exposures. A sensitive child could easily fail an examination simply because a nearby youngster has used Dad's aftershave or is wearing some new unwashed polyester or freshly dry-cleaned clothing. *A gradually increasing number of children now require home teaching solely because they cannot think or act appropriately after such exposures.* Similarly affected adults often cannot work outside their own home because of these types of aromas.

In Chapter 15, you'll read about another child, Carl, who had significant problems related to perfume. Sandra, a teacher, has similar difficulties (see Chapter 11). A whiff of a student's perfume can dramatically and quickly alter her voice and health. (Her response to an allergy extract from a school carpet is shown in *Environmentally Sick Schools*.) Another video shows that sudden hoarseness and breathing problems can develop within seconds after a single-blinded allergy test with a drop of ethyl alcohol, a common component of many perfumes. However, one drop of the correct dilution of an ethyl alcohol extract quickly and completely relieved Sandra's symptoms (see Chapters 11, 13, and 15).

For children with asthma, the problem can become even more serious. Approximately *70 percent* of asthmatics react to perfume. Their lung capacity can decrease by 20 to 60 percent within minutes or even seconds of a

A GIRL WHO CAN'T ATTEND SCHOOL BECAUSE OF PERFUME

Alice

Let us consider 14-year-old Alice, who unfortunately represents a rapidly growing number of chemically sensitized children. Her reactions are extreme, but they demonstrate how severely some children can be affected.

Alice's allergies became evident early in her life. By the time she was three, her parents were aware of her food sensitivities. Not until she was ten years old, however, were the chemical aspects of her medical and learning problems suspected or treated. The intervening years were "lost" in many ways, and her condition probably worsened because her environmental sensitivities were not recognized earlier.

Alice is presently so sensitive to perfumes and other smells that it is impossible for her to attend any school. In addition, scented detergents and fabric softeners, moldy books, ink or paper in certain new books, mimeo or photocopy paper, lighter fluid, soft plastic, lawn chemicals, and asphalt can all cause Alice to babble incoherently, become giddy, make strange sounds, talk like a baby, and/or walk and act in an inappropriate manner. These exposures cause her to speak and think unclearly, and they certainly interfere with her ability to learn and remember, even though she is gifted intellectually.

In order to help others understand the cause and severity of these problems, Alice has shared her reactions to an allergy extract for peas on the *Environmentally Sick Schools* video. Her footage shows what actually happens to some children who have this type of environmental illness. A variety of similar distressing reactions were provoked when she was tested for molds, egg, garlic, phenol, and formaldehyde.

Is it fair that this intelligent young lady must receive home teaching because her school cannot provide an environmentally "clean" classroom? Should parents of such children have to pay for computer-taught courses, private schools, or tutors? Will she ever be able to fulfill her academic potential if her formal education consists of only ten hours or less per week of professional personal instruction? Will one year's education in a three-year period, which is all the time that home teaching provides, prepare her for college?

Alice is not the only child whose future is fractured due to our reluctance as a society to face school chemical issues head-on. What price will we pay as a nation if this bright young woman, and the rapidly growing number of others who are similarly affected, are not given an opportunity to learn at a level commensurate with their abilities? Put yourself in the position of Alice and her parents. Would you not be justifiably dismayed, disheartened, and discouraged? She is presently improving, but whether her recovery will be sufficient and soon enough to allow her life to get back on course, we simply do not know at this time.

brief exposure to perfume. It is possible to develop such severe asthma that a child might need to be rushed to a hospital.

How do perfumes cause such potentially severe symptoms in just seconds? One answer lies in the olfactory nerve in the nose, which provides a direct line to the brain. One whiff, and it immediately transports some chemicals to the critical thinking and behavior areas, often triggering a headache. This is particularly important because so many scented products are applied directly to the face or hair, providing a more prolonged and closer exposure that can increase both the intensity and duration of the symptoms.

With advanced technology and ingenuity, the chemical industry has created a vast number of totally synthetic aromas. They are often made from hydrocarbons or organic compounds derived from coal tar or petrochemicals (gasoline, oil, and natural gas). According to the National Institute for Occupational Medicine, the cosmetic and perfume industry uses more than eight hundred chemicals, and a single perfume might contain as many as two hundred of them to create its unique pleasant aroma (see Appendix). But as you've already read, the slightest smell can cause perilous illness in many chemically sensitive individuals, even if only one classmate wears a scented shampoo or if a teacher wearing perfume passes them in the hallway.

THE NEED FOR ACTION

Unfortunately, these difficulties with perfume will not simply go away on their own, any more than those associated with tobacco did. At some point, this issue will have to be faced head-on.

Many schools and workplaces will soon be faced with difficult and challenging questions: Should scented personal products be allowed in schools, workplaces, and public buildings if only a small number of individuals are adversely affected by minute exposures to them? Will a progressively larger number of students eventually develop similar but more pronounced chemical sensitivities to scented items? We simply don't know the answers at this time.

It took years to eliminate tobacco from the workplace and airlines, but

The perfume and cosmetic industry is *not adequately regulated*. Our government has exempted fragrance manufacturers from listing the ingredients in their products. If some of these are so neurotoxic that the brain can be damaged, the thinking public must ask, "Why?" and "What can be done about it?"

it has been done. As impossible as it seems at this time, perfume and scented items should be discouraged and eventually banned from all areas of all schools, as well as public places. If not, even those who are not presently affected can potentially become sensitized in the future.

IF A SCENTED PREPARATION BOTHERS YOUR CHILD

If your child is not feeling well because of some preparation that someone at school uses, the best treatment is to remove the offending substance, or separate your youngster from the source of the odor. It might be necessary to wash a child's body and hair. At times, the clothing will have to be changed and cleaned.

For your own child's use, choose hypo- or less-allergenic hair and body preparations, available at health food stores. These are better tolerated by most people, but check each one as suggested in Chapter 3. Some individuals who can't tolerate natural floral scents have no difficulty with certain citrus or herbal aromas. If you can find one that does not have an adverse effect, use it instead.

If someone else's personal body products are at fault, avoid close contact. Ask that the location of your child's seat in the classroom be changed if the source is a nearby youngster's perfume. Sometimes you or your child need only to ask an "offender" nicely to voluntarily discontinue the use of a scented product. Most will cooperate if you explain that an odor is causing illness. If needed, videotaping such a response can be persuasive, providing it does not cause an alarming reaction. Check with your physician to find out how to safely document mild perfume sensitivities. If all else fails, request a change to another classroom or a transfer to a different school.

In your own home, it is often, but certainly not always, easier to control the use of perfumes. Sometimes when grandparents, relatives, and friends visit, their aromas stay behind after they leave. It requires tact and diplomacy to request that the sources of these scents not be brought into the home, but if a child or adult becomes seriously ill from perfume, continued exposure simply cannot be tolerated.

Charcoal masks are helpful (see Resources), but most children and even some adults are embarrassed to use them. One clever environmentally ill child (Alice, who was mentioned earlier) partially filled a soda-pop can with special charcoal. It allows her to breathe filtered air through a straw without needing a mask—and no one knows she is not drinking a beverage.

Some perfume-sensitive individuals must have a source of oxygen readily available both in school and at home, so that they can be treated as quickly as possible after an unavoidable routine chemical exposure. If oxygen is administered quickly, the effects of the exposure can be markedly decreased. Doctors usually prescribe oxygen for about ten minutes at the rate of 4 liters per minute every half hour, until the symptoms subside. Small portable units are available for school, home, work, or car use. Check with your doctor and use the yellow pages of your phone book.

RESTRICTING SCENTED SUBSTANCES

A few schools now recognize the role of odors in causing illness and impairing school performance. They routinely purchase and use only nonscented, safer cleaning and maintenance products. They also request that specific teachers voluntarily discontinue using certain scented products. Some teachers have been compliant and have graciously discontinued the use of scented preparations that bother a student. For those who do not, either the affected student or the teacher has had to be transferred to a different room or school.

The challenge has been met head-on by the University of Minnesota's School of Social Work, where 250 students volunteered to prohibit perfume, cologne, and scented products. The other students in this four-story building also were urged to stay "scent free."[24] The Maryland House of Delegates, for its part, is debating designating fragrance-free zones for its work and public space.

In 1994, the progressive state of New York recognized that scented products could prevent some children from learning at a level commensurate with their ability. On page 10 of a report entitled *Recommendations to Improve the Environmental Health and Safety of School*, the state education department stated, "Schools shall develop guidelines to reduce exposure to chemical fragrances which can cause possible adverse reactions in some individuals." Recognition of a problem is the first step in solving it. It took years for illnesses related to tobacco and asbestos to be acknowledged and definitive corrective measures instituted. In time, stringent effective measures will have to be taken, not only to control the ingredients in scented items, but to curtail their use in schools and elsewhere.

THE WORST POSSIBLE EFFECT OF PERFUMES

I've already discussed some of the symptoms (such as headaches and breathing problems) associated with exposure to perfumes. The disconcerting news is that a few very chemically sensitive adults have had visible changes *in their brains*. These changes have been documented. SPECT test images have shown changes related directly to an offending perfume exposure in both the blood flow and function of the brain after such exposures[25] (see Chapter 13).

The good news is that some of these documented brain-tissue and IQ changes appear to be reversible. This is especially true if the affected individuals completely avoid further exposure to odors and offending chemcals. Prompt, comprehensive environmental medical and nutritional therapy appears to be at least partially helpful.

To more fully understand the effects of scented items, beauticians and workers employed in the production or sale of perfumed items (and pesticides) should be thoroughly evaluated and studied.[26]

■ OTHER SUBSTANCES THAT CAN POSE PROBLEMS

FINGERNAIL POLISH

Both nail polish (containing phenol, toluene, xylene, and formaldehyde) and nail-polish remover (acetone) can cause wheezing, congestion, headache, fatigue, hyperactivity, confusion, and dizziness in some children and adults. The acetone and acetates in nail-polish removers can potentially damage the kidneys and the liver. While most people show no effects from these products, chemically sensitive individuals can become ill in seconds from minimal exposures. It is easy to spot who is bothered because some form of illness, or a change in appearance, actions, thinking, or handwriting, occurs quickly (within minutes) after an offending exposure.

DRY-CLEANED CLOTHING

Freshly dry-cleaned clothing can emit the following chemicals: trichloroethylene, trichloromethane, perchloroethylene, and tetrachloroethylene. Merely sitting next to someone who is wearing a freshly dry-cleaned item, or standing near recently dry-cleaned drapes, can cause serious illness in sensitized individuals. If possible, such items should be well-aired before they are worn (see Chapter 15). Instead of keeping them in a bedroom closet, dry-cleaned clothing should be thoroughly aired out until no odor is perceptible.

TOBACCO

Although most people are aware that tobacco can cause irritation of the eyes, nose, and throat, as well as cancer, many do not realize the other effects that the odor of secondhand tobacco smoke can have on sensitive individuals. Tobacco or the odor of it on clothing or hair can cause an increased tendency to develop respiratory infections, bronchitis, pneumonia, asthma, and especially middle-ear infections. Some sensitive youngsters become hyperactive or misbehave after smelling tobacco, and some adults develop headaches, eye irritation, an increased heart rate, an irregular pulse, high blood pressure, and lung cancer. Pregnant teachers, in particular, should be very cautious.

School lavatories should be closely monitored and controlled because this is where youngsters gather and smoke. Some sensitive children cannot use the toilets in school because of the tobacco odors (and the perfumed cleaning products used there). High-quality air filtration of contaminated areas is helpful.

What's the ideal solution? *No one* should be allowed to smoke on school property or on school buses.

ALCOHOL

Alcohol is a problem in many schools and homes in our country. At least five environmental medical books are available that discuss food sensitivities and alcoholism.[27] These books suggest that most alcoholics are allergic to grain and that this allergy can be the major factor in their addiction to alcohol. Their grain sensitivity can cause an intense craving, and in some individuals this leads to obesity or alcoholism. Without a doubt, some alcoholics feel and act drunk after only their *first* drink or after eating a food that contains the same grains as those in their favorite alcoholic beverage. In the 1940s, Dr. Theron Randolph reported this finding, and he found it to be particularly true for allergic individuals. Although it is not true of all alcoholics or all allergics, this observation is certainly valid for some.

AEROSOLS

In some schools, aerosol abuse is presently more common than abuse of cigarettes, marijuana, and alcohol. The acute and chronic effects caused by such behavior in your children and others can be devastating and permanent. Aerosols release not only the component in the spray for which they were purchased but also a variety of propellants, some of which can be harmful. This can be true even for some asthmatic aerosol medications.

In some schools, especially in Texas and the Southwest, an inordinate number of adolescent youngsters disregard their bodies and brains by purposely sniffing the chemical solvent vapors found in various room fresheners, cooking and hair aerosols, marking pens, correction fluids, gasoline, glue, paint thinner, shoe polish, spray paint, lighter fluid, and freon (fluorocarbons).

One survey revealed that in one area up to 17 percent of 14-year-olds tried inhaling or sniffing aerosols during 1993. John Laseter, Ph.D.,[28] has detected these solvents or their breakdown products in the blood and urine of many of these children.

The responses to inhaling such vapors can include hallucinations, confusion, an inability to concentrate, slurred speech, slowed movements, and a temporary or permanent loss of memory. Other responses include damage to the kidneys and liver, heart irregularities, and serious mood and behavioral changes. *The most serious of these potential effects, however, are permanent brain damage or death.* Some of these children will be institutionalized for the rest of their lives because they are no longer capable of thinking or functioning in a normal manner.

Teachers, parents, or school janitors who suspect aerosol or chemical odor abuse should watch for telltale debris in children's wastebaskets.

> Some thoughtless youngsters will be institutionalized for the rest of their lives because of the extensive brain damage caused by sniffing aerosols. Others will end up in cemeteries.

▪ OUTDOOR CHEMICALS

Chemicals used outside a school can enter ventilation ducts and contaminate the inside of the school, causing adverse health effects among individuals in these buildings (see Table 7.3).

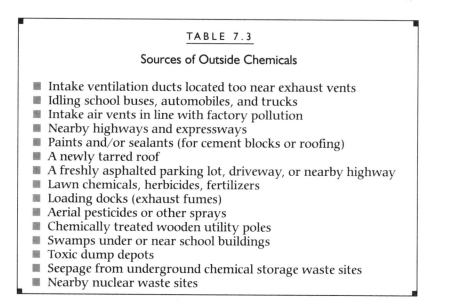

TABLE 7.3

Sources of Outside Chemicals

- Intake ventilation ducts located too near exhaust vents
- Idling school buses, automobiles, and trucks
- Intake air vents in line with factory pollution
- Nearby highways and expressways
- Paints and/or sealants (for cement blocks or roofing)
- A newly tarred roof
- A freshly asphalted parking lot, driveway, or nearby highway
- Lawn chemicals, herbicides, fertilizers
- Loading docks (exhaust fumes)
- Aerial pesticides or other sprays
- Chemically treated wooden utility poles
- Swamps under or near school buildings
- Toxic dump depots
- Seepage from underground chemical storage waste sites
- Nearby nuclear waste sites

BUS AND AUTO FUMES

Ask your child how he or she feels after the bus ride to school or a ride in the family car.

Some children feel ill every time they go on a trip in a car or on the school bus. In Chapter 3, I discussed how to evaluate your child's well-being before, during, and after a bus or car ride. Do headaches, nausea, vomiting, asthma, dizziness, poor coordination, poor vision, and/or memory problems occur between the time the child leaves home and arrives at school? Most schools have areas where buses routinely line up in neat rows as they arrive and leave. The idling engines heavily pollute the atmosphere with exhaust fumes, including carbon monoxide. These odors routinely trigger health problems for some children and teachers as they enter or exit their schools each day.

Some students become ill whenever a bus driver stops because the idling engine allows exhaust fumes to enter their bus. The contamination of exhaust fumes and fuel odors can be present in both the front and rear of a bus. Each bus is different, so ride with your child and determine where your child is most comfortable. Another option is to request that a less odorous school bus be assigned to your route. Sometimes the route itself can be altered, or maybe your child can be picked up later so the ride is shorter. Some parents create a carpool so several children can ride to school in an automobile rather than in a school bus. Some schools in Canada provide clean vans for chemically sensitized children who would otherwise have to be taught at home (see Chapter 12).

Also, evaluate how your child (and how you yourself) feel in *each* of your own family's cars. Sometimes a child will do well in one car but not the other. The answer can be simple: Use the car that causes the least difficulty. To improve the interior environment, car air purifiers are available that can be plugged into the automobile cigarette lighter socket (see Resources). In addition, a charcoal mask can be used. Charcoal under the seat might help to reduce odors, too. A baking soda paste on the vinyl seats may help reduce the smell of plastic; it can be vacuumed or brushed off after it is dry. Then cover the seats with aluminum foil and several heavy cotton blankets.

The more you know about indoor and outdoor chemicals at school, at home, and elsewhere, the better chance your child and family will have to remain healthy.

NOTES

1. L. G. Regenstein, *Cleaning Up America the Poisoned* (Washington, DC: Acropolis Books, 1993).

2. National Research Council, Commission on Life Sciences, Board on Environmental Studies and Toxicology, Committee on Neurotoxicology and Models for Assessing Risk, *Environmental Neurotoxicity* (Washington, DC: National Academy Press, 1992).

3. For more information on these chemicals, see Marion Moses, *Designer Poisons* (San Francisco, CA: Pesticide Education Center, 1995).

4. See *Indoor Air Pollution*, publication no. 523/217-81322 (Washington: Government Printing Office, 1944); available from EPA Indoor Air Division (see Resources).

5. Joan Dine, "Toxic Reduction," chapter 8 in Naomi Friedman, *Greening Synagogues and Community Centers* (Takoma Park, MD: Shomrei Adamah, 1995).

6. See *Indoor Air Quality in Schools*, available from the EPA Indoor Air Division (see Resources).

7. Change Shim and M. Henry Williams, "Effects of Odors on Asthma," *American Journal of Medicine*, vol. 80 (Jan. 1986), pp. 18–22.

8. C. Wilson, *Chemical Exposure and Human Health* (Jefferson, NC: McFarland and Co., 1993).

9. For information on nontoxic cleaning products, see A. Berthold-Bond, *Clean and Green* (Woodstock, NY: Ceres Press, 1990); Carolyn P. Gorman, *Less Toxic Living* (Dallas, TX: Environmental Health Center 1993); Debra Dadd, *Nontoxic, Natural and Earthwise* (Los Angeles: Jeremy P. Tarcher, 1990); Debra Dadd, *The Nontoxic Home and Office* (New York: Jeremy P. Tarcher, 1992); and Moses, *Designer Poisons.*

10. On the chemical-removing properties of plants, see Nicholas Tate, *The Sick Building Syndrome* (Far Hills, NJ: New Horizon Press, 1994), pp. 80–81, 163.

11. See Dine, "Toxic Reduction."

12. See J. Bower, *Healthy House Building: A Design and Construction Guide* (Bloomington, IN: Healthy House Institute, 1993); D. Rousseau, W. J. Rea, and J. Enwright, *Your Home, Your Health and Well-Being* (Vancouver, BC: Hartley and Marks, 1989); Janet Martinelli and Paul Bierman-Lytle, *Your Natural Home* (Boston: Little, Brown & Co., 1995).

13. Bower, *Healthy House Building.*

14. NEA Professional Library, *The Healthy School Handbook* (Washington, DC: National Education Association, 1995).

15. Dadd, *Nontoxic, Natural and Earthwise.*

16. See R.D. Morris et al., "Chlorination, Chlorination By-Products and Cancer: A Meta-Analysis," *American Journal of Public Health*, vol. 82, no. 7 (July 1992), pp. 955ff. See also Regenstein, *Cleaning Up America.*

17. For more on chlorine-free pools, see C. I. Noss et al., "Water Chlorination Impacts Health Effect," *Chemical Abstracts*, no. 98–212722K (1983); J. D. Berg et al., "Growth of Legionella-Pneumophilia in Continuous Culture and Its Sensitivity to Inactivation by Chlorine Dioxide," *Chemical Abstracts*, no. 101–20407V (1984); R. W. Bradford et al., *Oxidology* (Chula Vista, CA: Bradford Foundation, 1986); and R. Bradford and H. Allen, *Exogenous Oxidative Mechanisms in Combating Infectious Agents* (Chula Vista, CA: Bradford Foundation, 1986), which contains forty-three reference articles.

18. See Morris, "Chlorination."

19. D. I. Volberg et al., *Pesticides in Schools: Reducing the Risks* (New York: State Department of Law, Environmental Protection Bureau, 1993). See also Regenstein, *Cleaning Up America*, and Moses, *Designer Poisons.*

20. Rachel Carson Council, "Breast Cancer and Pesticides," *Rachel Carson Council News*, no. 82 (Mar. 1994); the publisher's address is 8940 Jones Mill Road, Chevy Chase, MD 20815. See also Regenstein, *Cleaning Up America*; and Moses, *Designer Poisons.*

21. Regenstein, *Cleaning Up America*; N. S. Green, *Poisoning Our Children: Surviving in a Toxic World* (Chicago: Noble Press, 1991); J. Thrasher and A. Broughton, *The Poisoning of Our Homes and Workplaces* (Santa Ana, CA: Seadora, 1989); and Moses, *Designer Poisons.* Theo Colborn, Dianne Damanoski, and John P. Meyers, *Our Stolen Future* (New York: Dutton, 1996).

22. Robert W. Gardner, *Chemical Intolerance* (Boca Raton, FL: CRC Press, 1994); the publisher's address is 2000 Corporate Boulevard N.W., Boca Raton, FL 33431.

23. Rea, *Healthy School Handbook.*

24. *Buffalo News*, Nov. 2, 1994.

25. G. Heuser, A. Vojdani, and S. Heuser, "Diagnostic Markers of Multiple Chemical Sensitivity," *Multiple Chemical Sensitivities: Addendum to Biologic Markers in Immunotoxicology* (1992), pp. 117–38; G. Heuser, "Diagnostic Markers in Clinical Immunotoxicology and Neurotoxicology," *Journal of Occupational Medicine and Toxicology*, vol. 1, no. 4 (1992); Thomas J. Callender et al., "Three Dimensional Brain Metabolic Imaging in Patients with Toxic Encephalopathy," *Environmental Research*, vol. 60 (1993), pp. 295–319; and T. R. Simon et al., "Abnormalities in Scintigraphic Examinations of the Brains of Desert Storm/Desert Shield Veterans," presented at the twelfth annual international symposium on Man and His Environment in Health and Disease, Feb. 24–27, 1994.

26. See Moses, *Designer Poisons.*

27. Billie Sahley and Katherine Birkner, *Breaking Your Addiction Habit* (San Antonio, TX: Pain and Stress Clinic, 1990); Joseph D. Beasley, *Wrong Diagnosis, Wrong Treatment* (New York: Creative Infomatics, 1987); Marshall Mandell, *Dr. Mandell's 5-Day Allergy Relief System* (New York: Pocket Books, 1981); Theron Randolph and Ralph Moss, *An Alternative Approach to Allergies* (New York: Harper & Row, 1989); Richard Mackarness, *A Little of What You Fancy* (Great Britain: Fontana Paperbacks, 1985).

28. John L. Laseter, "Solvent Abuse Monitoring in Juveniles," *Treatment Centers* (Apr. 1993).

8 ⊏ Food and Water

Food and water, and the chemicals in or on them, can certainly affect learning, behavior, and health. Some of the problem items are commonly recognized; they are the so-called junk foods, such as candy, cake, cookies, soft drinks, chocolate, pizza, and popcorn. Surprisingly, however, there are also some major *unsuspected* offenders, including "good foods" such as milk, bread or wheat, corn, orange juice, and eggs. Of all the foods that can cause chronic unrecognized illness, milk and other dairy products (cheese) are unquestionably the most prominent.

As a parent, your challenge is to detect which specific foods or beverages may be affecting your youngster, both at school and at home. A major clue is the repeated onset of sudden, troubling changes in how your child feels, behaves, or learns shortly *after* lunch, snacks, or parties. Sugar, red dyes, and artificial sweeteners and flavors all can cause hyperactivity, and they're plentiful in the diets of many children. Each year, the average American consumes 147 pounds of sugar, for instance, and drinks 22 gallons of carbonated beverages. In 1950 each person drank less than 16 ounces of soda pop during a year; in 1980 the average individual drank more than that *every day*—or about 500 twelve-ounce cans per year. Most of us don't drink enough water even though this beverage is so healthful.[1] To make matters worse, even common medications can contain enough dye, sugar, corn, and other offending flavors, additives, and binders to impair normal brain and body functions in some sensitive individuals. *And, remember, it is not how much but how sensitive someone is to a food ingredient that determines whether a reaction will occur.*

■ FOOD

When Do Food Reactions Occur?

Food-related problems are often easy to detect in children. Again, you and your child's teachers should be particularly alert for changes occurring fifteen minutes to an hour *after* he eats or drinks. Some affected children simply do not feel, look, behave, or remember normally at these times. Most commonly, they develop a runny or stuffy nose, asthma or coughing, abdominal complaints, and headaches, as well as changes in mood, temperament, and the ability to learn. If their sensitivity is extreme, even the slightest *odor* of a food such as peanut butter, fish, or eggs can cause a dramatic change, such as asthma, hivelike swelling, or hoarseness.

Some children may experience delayed food sensitivities, which commonly cause symptoms such as eczema, canker sores, recurrent fluid behind the eardrums, joint tenderness, arthritis, bladder spasm (bed-wetting), or bowel disease (irritable bowel, colitis, or Crohn's disease). In these individuals, their food-related symptoms may not occur until eight to forty-eight hours after a problem item has been ingested. This inordinate delay can make detection of the specific offending food items very challenging. In many instances, cause-and-effect relationships are overlooked for years. (I am ashamed to state that even though I am a board-certified pediatric allergist, I missed detecting these types of sensitivities for eighteen years because I did not know or appreciate that both immediate and delayed food reactions can occur, or that *any* part of the body can be affected by what is ingested.)

RELIEF FOR FOOD SENSITIVITIES

To help prevent or treat immediate and delayed food responses, you can use an alkali such as Alka Aid (see Chapters 3 and 15). If it is taken *prior to* eating, it can prevent symptoms; if it is taken *after* a food reaction has begun, it can help stop the response. Alkalies appear to relieve reactions in about 66 percent of children in about fifteen minutes.

WHAT TYPES OF REACTIONS CAN FOODS CAUSE?

As life-disrupting as food sensitivities can be, these problems can be identified and successfully managed—but first a proper diagnosis must be made.

Matthew, Scott, and Paula were helped easily and quickly—in less than a week—with the Multiple Food Elimination Diet (which is detailed in

Chapter 3).[2] As you read their medical and behaviorial complaints, notice the obvious similarities among them, and consider how their lives would have been changed if food sensitivities had been suspected earlier and the correct diagnosis and treatment had been given at that time.

A DIET HELPED MATTHEW IN FOUR DAYS

Matthew

Matthew, a 12-year-old boy, was extremely hyperactive, but he was not on drugs to control his behavior. He had been overactive since infancy, and for the first two years of his life, he slept only three hours a night and napped only two hours a day. As a toddler, he frequently complained about leg aches and abdominal pain. He had been treated successfully for hay fever and an allergic cough with typical pollen and dust allergy extract therapy ever since he was seven years old, but the hyperactivity persisted.

His mother described Matthew's typical day this way: In the morning he was stuffy and tired. He was cranky, would get upset over the homework he had not done, cry, call himself stupid, and pester his sister. Then he would go to school. When he arrived home, he immediately removed his shoes and did somersaults through the house. He thumped and jumped from room to room. When he watched television, he tapped and banged his hands and feet constantly. At dinner he rapped his fork and knife on the plate, picked up and handled one thing after another, turned the salt shaker upside down, and repeatedly kicked either the table or his sister. Intermittently throughout the meal, he jumped up to do somersaults in the living room.

After supper, Matthew would try to do his homework but would get upset because he forgot some books at school and would repeat aloud that he was stupid. He'd write two or three words, and then rip up the sheet because of an error, doing this about five to six times. He'd cry and become terribly upset. At bedtime he would complain that his muscles and belly had ached all day. It would take ninety minutes for him to fall asleep. He said his mind was speeding and he could not relax. He'd roll and toss all night, talking and experiencing bad dreams.

The next morning he would either lose his homework or leave it at home. During the day he talked constantly and would not listen to teachers or anyone else. He never had an appetite, nor ate more than half a meal.

Eventually, food sensitivities were suspected, and Matthew went on the Multiple Food Elimination Diet. After just four days, he was obviously much better; after seven days, his improvement was remarkable. His mother reported he was less active, less easily aggravated, friendlier, and happier and had lost his aches and chronic cough. His appetite was much better.

When foods were reintroduced to Matthew's diet, his mother discovered that milk caused him to become depressed and irritable and to talk excessively. Chocolate caused a runny nose and bellyaches but did not affect his activity. Corn provoked light-headedness, bellyaches, excessive talking, and insomnia. Red dyes caused irritability and nose stuffiness and made him "spaced out" and forgetful of what he was saying. On the other hand, eggs and sugar caused no obvious symptoms.

To confirm his milk sensitivity, Matthew was given unmarked capsules that contained either milk or sugar. He became depressed and developed a bellyache from the milk-filled capsules, while the sugar-filled capsules had no effect.

In time, Matthew's mother also observed that when he drank chlorinated water, he developed a stomachache, and when he consumed soy oil or foods packed in the oil (such as tuna fish), he became cranky and complained of muscle aches. Wheat made him hyperactive, irritable, and depressed.

Matthew's mother rechecked his wheat sensitivity at five-day intervals by feeding him wheat crackers at 10:00 A.M. after he had avoided wheat for four full days. On one occasion after eating the crackers, he argued with his sister and was sent to his room by 10:45. He felt listless and fidgety and then became hyperactive. He used paper and matches to start a fire on the basement floor; then he turned a hose on the flames, and after spraying the floor, he slid and played in the water. He was giddy all day, aware of his happy feelings and saying that it sure beat being depressed. During dinner, he threw down his fork and started doing somersaults again. Although he became more reasonable by 9:30 P.M., he remained hyperactive.

One week after Matthew had started the Multiple Food Elimination Diet, his Conner's hyperactivity score had fallen from an abnormally high 18 to a low normal 1 (see Chapter 3). Five months later, while he continued to avoid milk, chocolate, corn, wheat, and food coloring, his score was still 1. His teacher commented that Matthew acted better in school, and after just four weeks on the diet, his grades had already definitely improved. By then, he could also relax, watch TV without wiggling, eat calmly, and sleep quietly. He would awaken refreshed and happy in the morning, and his homework was no longer a source of exasperation for him and everyone else.

A DIET CHANGED SCOTT'S LIFE IN SEVEN DAYS

Scott

Scott was 11 years old when I first saw him in my office. Born into a family with a history of allergies, he was a very active infant. He broke his leg after he learned to walk because he charged uncontrollably into walls and furniture. Almost every day since he was a toddler, he experienced excessive gas after eating, and at times he had abdominal pain. He tended to have leg cramps at bedtime. His behavior was unpredictable and inappropriate; at various times he was irritable, grouchy, clumsy, restless, and/or hostile. He talked and cried too much. He rarely gave or received affection.

Once Scott began school, he was placed in a special class for children with learning disabilities. He had many school problems because he was so easily distracted. He simply would not mind the teacher, and he could not conform like other students. He fought with his brother and his schoolmates, and he had no friends. On one day, his mother received nineteen calls from neighbors complaining of his behavior. He was sassy and tended to rave on and on in a senseless manner. At times he almost acted "insane." He was seen by a neurologist and a psychologist for six months of therapy, but without any obvious improvement.

Finally, Scott was placed on the Multiple Food Elimination Diet, and within a day, his leg cramps were gone; after two days his activity level had improved. By the end of the week, his mother said her "bananas kid was gone." He still got into about one fight a day, but in the past, he had fought all day long. He was able to play amicably with the neighborhood children for the first time in his life. He talked less and even napped. He became loving and kissed his parents. He no longer had belly gas, and he stopped sucking his lower lip. He didn't cry all the time. Whereas going to church had once been a hassle, now he was quiet during the entire service.

Two teachers called Scott's mother to comment on his marked improvement in school. After the one-week diet, his Conner's hyperactivity score fell from an abnormally high 19 to a normal 1. Fourteen weeks later, his score was zero, and at the six-month point, it was only 2. His mother was delighted with his improvement. She discovered that he had a nice, pleasant personality that had previously been completely hidden.

A CHANGE IN DIET HELPED PAULA IN FOUR DAYS

Paula

Paula, whose parents had allergies, was initially seen at our center when she was five years old. She had experienced typical nose, eye, and chest allergies since she was two or three, and her symptoms were evident throughout the year. Her parents complained that she seemed unusually emotional and was frequently so depressed that she cried for hours. Paula was also hyperactive and irritable. She frequently experienced bellyaches, diarrhea, and headaches. She could not play, learn, or adjust to school.

Paula is the only youngster I have ever seen whom I could not examine during the first visit; she was impossibly restless and wiggly. I was perplexed by this and sincerely believed she had suffered brain damage at birth, but a detailed history revealed nothing to confirm my suspicion. I felt sorry for her parents, so instead of asking them to make their home allergy-free for two weeks—and then place Paula on the Multiple Food Elimination Diet for the next two weeks—I asked them to do both at the same time. It was obvious that both the child and her parents needed help as soon as possible for her allergies.

Just three days later, Paula's mother called and said she was extremely pleased. I assumed her youngster's hay fever and asthma had improved, but her mother said no; instead, it was Paula's disposition and her behavior that were remarkably better.

This child had shown me what I had not been taught during either my pediatric or my allergy and immunology training. At that time I was certain that it was ridiculous to think that food allergies could affect a child's behavior. Nevertheless, I was amazed (and perplexed) by this youngster's dramatic improvement. She had provided the first key insight that has culminated in this and several other books over the past twenty years.

After Paula had gone on the diet she was so much better, her teacher called me because she assumed the improvement was due to some new drug the child was taking. She explained that Paula now played normally, joined in school activities, and listened to stories. Relatives noted that she climbed onto their laps for the first time and liked to be kissed and cuddled. Her parents said they could now take her for a car ride; in the past, within five minutes, she had been climbing throughout the car, making short rides a hassle and long rides impossible. And for the first time, Paula slept all night long.

Two weeks later, during her second visit to my office, Paula proved to be a joy. She was pleasant and cooperative and allowed me to conduct a complete physical examination without objecting. She even permitted needle allergy skin testing without a whimper. Her mother had ascertained that after the diet, Paula experienced irritability, hyperactivity, and throat-clearing in response to milk. Corn caused diarrhea, abdominal pain, and disposition problems. Chocolate, blueberries, and mint triggered eye circles, temper flares, hyperactive behavior, crying, and even a different way of talking. The smell of specific perfumes caused extreme hyperactivity within a few minutes.

Three years later, Paula's schoolwork was excellent, and she had no difficulty except when she ate too much of the foods that caused her original symptoms, although she could even eat and tolerate small amounts of these foods on special occasions without problems. However, she must still continue to avoid certain types of perfume.

IS BREAKFAST OR LUNCH YOUR CHILD'S PROBLEM?

Sometimes a child's early-morning inattentiveness is not related to the toothpaste used after breakfast or to fumes on the school bus. Instead, the cause could be a food item that was ingested for breakfast. As already noted, many illnesses and behavioral and learning problems are the direct result of eating sugary, dyed foods—perhaps a breakfast cereal or beverage, milk, bread (with wheat, yeast, and preservatives), eggs, or juice. These items commonly have caused changes in certain children by the time they arrive at school.

To help determine the amount of sugar a cereal contains, look at the list of ingredients, which appear on the package in descending order by weight. If a cereal is mostly sugar, this ingredient will be listed early— either before or immediately after the grain. Some cereals that contain 80 percent sugar have healthful-sounding names and slick advertising, but they are really grain-flavored candy, not sugar-flavored grain! I find it so disappointing that many parents allow their children to make such a poor food choice to begin their day, and even more disconcerting that many schools serve foods that are not nutritious. Some school breakfast and/or lunch programs even sell junk foods in vending machines, even though school officials know full well that these items can interfere with some students' ability to learn or act appropriately. (See Table 8.1 for a typical school lunch menu.)

TABLE 8.1

Typical School Lunch Menu

Monday	Tuesday	Wednesday	Thursday	Friday
Hot dog	Pizza	Hamburger	Hot dog	Spaghetti
Bacon cheese-burger		Chicken sand-wich	Pancakes with syrup	BBQ chicken wings
Nachos w/ cheese		Caesar salad	Hot ham and cheese bagel	Mozzarella sticks
Ham, egg, and cheese English muffin		Junior Frosty	Pretzel	Applesauce
			Dessert	Turkey/cheese sub and chips

Many children are quickly conditioned to vigorously demand the foods they want from their parents, knowing that their dietary desires will be granted. Parents often accede to their children's demands in order to achieve temporary peace, not realizing that the food being most vigorously requested is typically the very one causing so much unrest, disharmony, and disruption in their child and family.

If school or home lunches are a problem for your child, it is usually obvious. Affected children typically feel differently from normal, experiencing behavioral changes within an hour after eating.

You (and to a degree, teachers and school health personnel) can check your child before and again after eating (as suggested in Chapter 3). If time is limited, merely have your child write before lunch or a snack and half an hour afterward. If your child writes poorly only after certain meals, it is possible that her brain was affected by what was eaten.

WHEN ARE SNACKS A CONCERN?

Midmorning milk snacks, whether at home or at school, can cause havoc in youngsters who are sensitive to dairy foods. Yet few parents recognize that dairy products cause behavior and activity problems, even though it becomes blatantly obvious after they pay closer attention. Notice whether your own child begins to sniffle, rub her nose, clear her throat, sound congested, make clucking sounds, cough, or wheeze within an hour after ingesting a dairy product. The congestion from dairy foods also makes certain children prone to repeated nose, sinus, ear, and chest infections, as well as leg aches and bed-wetting at night. Remember, however, that *different* foods and beverages affect *different* youngsters in *different* ways. Each child (and adult) requires individualized observation and monitoring.

CAN "PARTY TIME" CAUSE DIFFICULTIES?

During birthday parties or school celebrations (Christmas, Halloween, and Valentine's Day, for example), watch your child for marked changes and ask teachers whether he has become totally "impossible." Specifically, look for significant changes in how he acts, feels, looks, behaves, and learns.

LOOKING FOR CLUES AND PINPOINTING THE PROBLEM

As I've already pointed out, in less than an hour, a child with a food sensitivity may react to eating a particular food by feeling sick or speaking and acting inappropriately. He may suddenly exhibit telltale clues such as dark puffy eye circles and bright-red earlobes or cheeks (see Chapter 4). A few children begin to wiggle their legs rapidly, speak unclearly, talk too much or too loudly, write poorly, or even be unable to walk as well as usual because specific areas of their brains or muscles have been altered (see Part I). Other youngsters will put their heads on their desks and promptly fall asleep; still others will hide in corners and act untouchable.

Some children suddenly develop bad breath, bloating, belching, rectal gas, coughing, asthma, or congestion. Others need to rush to the lavatory because some food item has caused nausea or a bladder or bowel spasm; a few will have accidents because they can't reach the lavatory in time. The mood changes can include negativity, irritability, and anger, vulgarity, aggression, violence, as well as depression and sudden fatigue.

These changes are typical of unsuspected environmental/allergic illness. Of course, there can be other reasons for these responses, but too frequently, parents, teachers, psychologists, and medical advisors do not even consider foods as a possible cause. If no one tries to find and treat the source, the problems can persist and disrupt normal living for years or even a lifetime.

THE RISK OF MISDIAGNOSIS

If your child eats and suddenly becomes inattentive or impulsive, can't concentrate, and is hyperactive, your doctor could easily misdiagnose him as having Attention Deficit Hyperactivity Disorder (ADHD). More than two million youngsters are presently diagnosed with ADHD, and many are treated with activity-modifying drugs such as Ritalin. In 1990, 750,000 children were receiving these drugs. In the United States, we use five times as much Ritalin as the rest of the planet.[3]

Teachers often encourage this drug use because it can turn an unsettled, disruptive child into a calm and quiet one. A fast "drug fix" can certainly provide temporary relief, but this can be far from the best solution over the long term (see Chapter 16). Parents and teachers who prefer Ritalin for a child should learn about its many side effects and the early-warning danger signs associated with its use.[4] Some children complain they simply don't feel the same or normal on the drug. In addition, a rising number of children are using Ritalin, a class 2 narcotic, for drug abuse because it is so readily available compared to other street drugs.[5]

Keep in mind that allergies can certainly cause ADHD-like symptoms. In fact, as many as two-thirds of hyperactive youngsters have a food-related cause for their inability to concentrate and sit still.[6] In repeated studies, a simple hypoallergenic diet has been shown to help significantly, often within three to seven days (see Chapter 3). Why shouldn't a dietary change be tried before Ritalin?

Fortunately, a growing number of parents vigorously resist drug therapy and work hard to find and eliminate the real cause of the problem. They might find help from a specialist in environmental medicine (see Resources), who can help them choose the form of available therapy they want.

ARE PESTICIDES TO BLAME?

Sometimes a child's school problems are directly related to the pesticides and preservatives routinely found in many fresh or packaged grocery-store foods.[7] For example, a child might be able to eat organically grown, less-contaminated fresh fruits or vegetables *without* difficulty, but *identical* products from an ordinary grocery store might cause illness. The difference is probably due to the chemicals in or on the food. Some parents find that their children have no symptoms if they make their own bread and rolls with organic grains, using a bread-maker, while well-preserved regular baked goods repeatedly cause illness or misbehavior. (Bread-makers are available at large electric-appliance stores.) These parents obviously should prepare a bag lunch for their child to take to school.

If pesticides are a problem for your child or other family members, eat, buy, and/or grow organic or less-contaminated foods. Wash and/or peel the skin off apples and other fruits. Most of the pesticide is on the surface, but some is certainly inside. Buy only *lean* meat, because the fat contains stored pesticides and chemicals (For details about the individual components of pesticides, see Chapters 10 and 11). Use only filtered spring or glass-bottled water. And do not buy, drink, or send liquids to school in either plastic or Styrofoam.

DO YOU SUSPECT PARTICULAR FOODS?

If you or a teacher has observed that one or more specific foods are a problem for your child, this can be checked easily. After your child has not eaten suspect foods for four to seven days, purposely feed each of the possible suspect food items to him, one at a time, at two-hour intervals. Reaching a definite answer is truly easy, providing your child has not ingested a problem food in any form for at least four days before this challenge feeding.

For example, you can feed your child a *single* suspect food or beverage on Monday and Friday, or Tuesday and Saturday, to see what happens (see the Single Food Elimination Diet in Chapter 3).

Carry out such challenge feeding at a time when you can watch your child very carefully, such as after school or on a weekend. If you attempt this kind of purposeful food challenge in the morning before school, you will miss your youngster's reaction if it occurs on the school bus or at school.

Remember, the key is to add a *single* suspect food or beverage back into the diet after avoiding that item in all forms for at least four days. Be sure to check "before and after" each suspect food is ingested (see Chapter 3).

With this technique, perplexed parents are often pleasantly surprised to find how easily they can pinpoint exactly which foods cause specific complaints. Once they begin to recognize cause-and-effect relationships, they find it difficult to believe that they missed the obvious for such a long time. Then, once the offending food is identified, a food allergy that is not life-threatening (the vast majority) can be treated with an allergy extract, so the previously offending foods can be eaten again and cause less or no difficulty.

HOW TO MANAGE EXTREMELY DANGEROUS FOOD SENSITIVITIES

Caution: Your child should never purposely ingest any food or beverage if it is suspected of causing an alarming or life-threatening reaction.

Sometimes a child (or adult) has to be hospitalized for an emergency after eating or even smelling just a speck of egg, fish, peanut butter, or some other allergenic food. In such a situation, you have no need to verify what you already know with an elimination diet. If your child has had a frightening allergic reaction, ask your physician for an IgE RAST test for that suspect food (see Chapter 13). If you're unsure about the safety of a particular food or diet, ask your doctor. If there is skepticism, share the facts in Chapter 15.

Older children or adults who have had potentially serious food reactions *must* receive instructions about using both inhaled and injectable adrenaline. They should carry this life-saving drug with them at all times unless a school nurse or someone else is immediately available to administer this medicine.

Extremely serious life-threatening food allergies can be very difficult, even dangerous, to test or treat with allergy extract. This is sometimes possible, however, in special hospital units, like the Environmental Health Center in Dallas, Texas (see Resources). If an allergy extract treatment dose for an offending food can be found, future accidental exposures should be less potentially dangerous (see P/N allergy testing in Chapters 13 and 15). However, you must always consider the health benefit-risk ratio of any form of medical treatment. For example:

- *Possible Benefit:* It may well be better for your child to have a purposeful challenge under the best possible medical conditions, than to be faced someday with an accidental food-related medical crisis that will be treated by well-meaning individuals who probably have little training in the correct medical treatment for severe food-allergic reactions.
- *Possible Risk:* Allergy extract testing and treatment, even under the best of conditions, always carries an element of inherent danger.
- *Possible Hope:* It is too soon to be certain, but preliminary studies suggest that it may be possible to treat alarming food allergies with the new EPD (Enzyme Potentiated Desensitization) method, which uses homeopathic dilutions of allergy extract, or with other alternative methods (see Chapter 13). Continued research should provide more definitive and hopefully safe answers shortly.

■ WATER

At your child's school, the tap and shower water, as well as the pool water, can affect the health of students so that they cannot learn, and the health of teachers so that some cannot teach. Similar difficulties can arise from the water used in homes.

DOES INSUFFICIENT WATER CAUSE ILLNESS?

Our bodies are primarily water, and most children and adults need to drink more of it each day. Dr. F. Batmanghelidj's *Your Body's Many Cries for Water* stresses that the brain and body require water, not some other beverage, to function optimally.[8] The kidneys need enough liquid to excrete bodily wastes. Many conditions, such as asthma, arthritis, stress, ulcers, and low back pain, he claims, can be helped by drinking more pure water (for adults, two quarts per day). A dry mouth and tea-colored urine are late

A YOUNGSTER WITH DAILY HIVES

Karen

In May, six-year-old Karen began to have hives, which continued until October, when she became very ill and had to be given cortisone. The medication helped for about two weeks, but then, in spite of continued steroid therapy, the itchy hives spread over her entire body.

At that point, Karen's physician stopped all her previous medications except the cortisone, changed her antihistamines, and tried various diets. All were ineffective. In desperation, the doctor admitted Karen to the hospital, where she was allowed to drink only spring water and caramelized brown sugar—and this approach seemed to work. Within two days, the hives gradually disappeared, and as new single foods were added slowly to her diet, her dosage of steroids was tapered. She had no further outbreak of hives for five days—but they recurred after she was accidentally served a regular hospital breakfast, although at the time no one could determine the cause.

Upon her release from the hospital, Karen's parents were told to give her spring water and caramelized sugar, along with the few foods that had not caused her difficulty in the hospital. The hives subsided gradually and did not recur with the addition of new single foods—that is, until she ate a gelatin dessert prepared with tap water. Over time, a few other foods such as orange juice, eggs, and corn caused repeated flare-ups. But once all the offending items were excluded from her diet, the cortisone therapy could finally be discontinued. Her hives did not recur, until she was given tap water again several months later. Today, hives are no longer a problem for her, provided that she avoids tap water and drinks only glass-bottled water. We never determined what in the tap water caused her hives.

Karen's experience clearly illustrates that the best solution to a medical problem is not necessarily administering a better drug, but finding and eliminating the cause of the symptoms. This solution can be challenging, but it is certainly possible and well worth the effort. Parents can provide many answers if they observe their children closely and keep detailed records.

indicators that the body is dehydrated. It helps to drink more water a half hour before eating.

WHAT IN WATER CAUSES ILLNESS?

The most common contaminants in water are germs (sewage), chemicals (industrial and agricultural), and possibly radiation and lead. Industrial chemicals are the source of about 45 percent of the major pollution in water. If these chemicals enter the body and cannot be eliminated, they tend to be stored in body fat. In time, and under certain circumstances, they can cause serious illness in some individuals (see Chapter 14).

For an extensive discussion of the many aspects of problems caused by water, refer to volume 1 of *Chemical Sensitivity* by William Rea, M.D.[9] In 1965, only 4 percent of the patients seen at Dr. Rea's Environmental Health Center in Dallas had a sensitivity to water. By 1994, the incidence was 98 percent.

Here are just some of the substances in water that can cause your child to become ill:

CHLORINE

Chlorine is added to water to reduce the number of germs, but in fact, it becomes a potential source of illness. Many individuals (like Liza, described

---

DEPRESSION CAUSED BY FLUORIDE

Marsha

Ten-year-old Marsha was initially seen at our center in January 1992 because of classic allergies and chemical sensitivities. Her symptoms included depression, fatigue, difficulty concentrating, easy crying, muscle aches, headaches, intestinal complaints, and extreme walking problems.

But that hadn't always been so. Until the age of eight, Marsha had been a vivacious, curious youngster who learned easily. However, when her family moved to a town that did not include fluoridation in its water treatment, her doctor immediately placed her on fluoride tablets. Within a few days, she began acting very differently, and during the next several weeks, she developed extreme depression. She became so tired that she would often lay her head on her school desk. As time passed, she became progressively more ill and lost all desire to learn. Before long, she could not attend school or even leave her home. She had no interest in anything.

Marsha's parents sought treatment from pediatricians, psychologists, psychiatrists, and neurologists. One doctor prescribed a psychotherapeutic medication, imipramine (Tofranil), which apparently worsened her condition. Later, it was determined that this medication was one cause of her unusual walk and peculiar hand, leg, and body movements.

Although Marsha's parents informed all her doctors of their concern that her illness might be related to the fluoride tablets, this information was repeatedly and summarily discounted. The doctors insisted that fluoride tablets could not cause her type of illness. Each specialist also ignored her parents' pleas to temporarily stop the use of imipramine.

Prior to coming to our center, Marsha had been confined to a psychiatric hospital for almost two months at a cost of $750 per day. One psychiatrist at the hospital recommended therapy for "an indefinite period of time." Her parents eventually removed her from the hospital because they did not feel that she was improving. They realized that the counseling therapy had been totally ineffective, and they strongly doubted that her problems were psychological. They continued to believe that she had a physical illness, possibly due to the fluoride tablets.

At our center, we immediately prepared an allergy extract from her fluoride tablets and tested Marsha with it. We videotaped her response to this test. During her reaction to one drop of the extract, she hid behind her stuffed animal and said she felt sad, as tears ran slowly down her cheeks. She had been drawing faces before the test, but when she began to have feelings of sadness, she added tears to the faces. After we properly treated her with a better dilution of the fluoride-tablet allergy extract, she stopped crying and was obviously less depressed. Her pictures now had happy faces.

In time, we found that Marsha also suffered from Allergic Tension Fatigue Syndrome and had unusual responses to mold allergy skin tests. We evaluated her sensitivity to other common inhaled allergenic substances, as well as some foods and chemicals. We investigated and documented the deleterious effects of the two drugs, fluoride and imipramine. Her improvement was unequivocally remarkable, as the video *Environmentally Sick Schools* clearly illustrates.[10]

Part of Marsha's diagnostic evaluation included using the more precise P/N allergy testing with regular allergy extracts. She improved either during or shortly after each testing visit, but her symptoms tended to recur every few weeks because her mold allergy extract treatment doses needed adjustment. Comprehensive allergy treatment gradually enabled her to resume a normal life, but she has needed counseling because of the difficulties that her previously unrecognized chemical and environmental sensitivities caused her.

How is Marsha two years later? She has perfect school attendance, outstanding schoolwork, and beautiful handwriting. She is a happy, bubbly, energetic young lady who enjoys dancing, running, and living a normal active life. She is on the honor roll and president of her class.

Table 8.2 shows the changes that took place in Marsha's IQ. In June 1991, while receiving fluoride tablets, her IQ was 71; when she was in a children's psychiatric hospital in New York City in December 1991, it was 57; and by July 1993, 19 months after comprehensive allergy treatment, it was 125. Although this kind of immense improvement is not commonly seen, it clearly is sometimes possible when the principles of environmental medicine are correctly applied: Find and eliminate the cause, and the patient will improve.

TABLE 8.2

Marsha's IQ Changes

Date		Verb	Perfrm	Full
		Before Environmental Medical Treatment		
6/91	School	97	71	83
12/91	Hospital	73	57	63
		After Environmental Medical Treatment		
3/92	Home	97	65	80
8/92	Home	106	90	98
7/93	Home	117	125	122

in Chapter 2) are so chemically sensitive that they experience health problems from chlorine whether it's in drinking water, a shower, a pool, or a spa. (See Chapter 7 for more details about the possible harmful effects of this substance, and about possible safer substitutes.)

FLUORIDE
Fluorides are chemically similar to chlorides (or bromides) and are presently found in many urban water supplies. A variety of popular articles and books discuss the potential adverse effects of fluorides. At present, it does not appear to decrease dental cavities.[11] The account on pages 215 and 216 discusses one child's sensitivity to fluorides and the many health problems they created.

If you want to see if the fluoride in your toothpaste, or that which your dentist wants to use on your child's teeth, might be a problem, do the "Big Five," discussed in Chapter 3.

PESTICIDES
You need to be aware of the many other water contaminants, including lawn and aerial herbicide sprays, that eventually can find their way into groundwater, wells, cisterns, and reservoirs. In a diluted form, these pesticides and herbicides eventually can come out of home faucets.

In many areas of the Midwest, where there are large tracts of farmland, most of the wells and groundwater are badly contaminated. Water-treatment plants do not usually remove chemicals from tap water; rather, they add more of them. One preliminary report suggests that lawn sprays can cause a four-fold increase in cancer in children.[12] In addition, when yards are treated with pesticides, children are more apt to develop tumors called sarcomas; even no-pest strips are associated with increased risks of leukemia.[13]

COPPER AND LEAD
Water sitting in copper pipes and in galvanized pipes containing zinc can leach these metals into itself. Because of the potential presence of copper and zinc, along with the lead used for soldering, it is essential to check the levels of these metals in the blood or hair of sick children (see Table 15.1). Unless the ratio of copper and zinc is properly balanced, illness can result (see Chapters 14 and 15).

Chemicals from vinyl chloride pipes are known to be related to heart disease and cancer. In some parts of the country, harmful asbestos cement pipes are still being used.

PLASTIC AND STYRENE

Ideally, all water should be stored in glass. If liquids are stored in plastic or styrene instead, these chemicals will be leached into the contents of the container. With each swallow of a liquid that has been stored in plastic or styrene, more of these chemicals will enter the body. In fact, when you are in the hospital and are administered intravenous treatment that has been stored in a plastic bag, you receive not only your prescribed medication but also a dose of plastic that your body will have to store and hopefully, eventually eliminate (see Chapter 15).

DISTILLED WATER

Surprisingly, some distilled water, in contrast to hard water, can create health difficulties. In the process of distillation, valuable minerals are typically lost while chemicals are retained. Older distilled water units evaporate and then recondense the vapors of these chemicals back into the water. This action is diminished in newer units.

Thus, distilled water may lack minerals, especially magnesium and calcium. Magnesium in particular is very important because it is frequently deficient in persons who have heart attacks or muscle problems (see Chapter 14). If your family uses distilled water, nutrient supplementation may be required. Check with your doctor.

"SOFTENED" WATER

"Softened" water may contain a chemical that, on rare occasions, can cause joint tightness and swelling. Few people appear to be affected this way, and doctors rarely consider sensitivity to a chemical in "soft" water as a possible cause of a chronic health complaint. Mary was sensitive to a component in one brand of water softener.

"SOFTENED" WATER AS A CAUSE OF BODY SWELLING AND HIVES

Mary

At the age of ten, about a week after she had received treatment with penicillin, Mary experienced an episode of hives and swollen joints. She subsequently had hives intermittently about every three months until she was 12 years old. At various times, her hives became a daily problem.

Mary was tentatively diagnosed as having a collagen disease, because of her tender swollen joints and body swelling associated with extreme fatigue. At times she could not walk up a flight of stairs because her knees were so swollen. Treatment with cortisone and antihistamines was ineffective. Eventually, her family recalled that they had installed a "softened" water unit in their home about a month before she developed her daily symptoms. They immediately discontinued use of this water, and within a week Mary was the best she had been in months. Then she accidentally drank "softened" water a month later, however, and developed joint swelling that persisted for about fifteen days.

Mary was hospitalized later that year for study. During a single-blinded challenge with gradually increasing amounts of her home's "softened" water, nine tablespoons caused definite finger and joint redness and swelling within about ten minutes. Regular tap water did not have this effect. Various brands of "softened" water from "new" tanks caused no swelling. But "softened" water from "used or older" tanks that had to be exchanged or recharged caused obvious symptoms.

At the age of 14, Mary drank some well water. Within three hours her hands began to ache and within five hours her face, shoulder, fingers, and legs had become swollen. She could not walk, and one fingernail fell off because of the extreme swelling. This body swelling lasted one and a half months. The cause was never determined.

For the next few years, Mary had intermittent swelling that usually could be attributed to the accidental ingestion of "softened" water. Now, at 21, joint swelling and hives are no longer evident. She has no desire to purposely challenge herself with "softened" water, but she doubts that her previous sensitivity is still present.

HOW TO CHECK YOUR OWN WATER

To find out the status of your own home or school water supply, start by calling your water and health departments and requesting current reports. Inquire about which chemicals (chlorine or fluoride) are added to the water, and what kinds of pipes transport water in your city. Ask for a map of the toxic dump sites in your area. Are they near the municipal water supply source?

The EPA monitors only eight inorganic and ten organic chemicals in water supplies. That leaves at least 30,000 potentially hazardous pollutants entirely without regulation. Therefore, much can be missed. In addition, some water supplies can contain parasites such as Giardia or the organisms that cause Legionnaires' disease. Careful monitoring is essential, and if you are concerned, you can obtain an independent analysis. (See Table 13.1; for chemical contamination, contact a laboratory such as Accu-Chem, an environmental evaluation company listed in Resources; for germ or parasite contamination, contact a university bacteriology or parasitology department or your health department.)

Unfortunately, you may have to test your school or home water supply repeatedly because a sample might cause symptoms on one occasion but not on another. Contaminants and pollutants in any water supply change day by day. Some industries, for example, purposely empty their chemicals directly into nearby water sources (or the atmosphere) on weekends, when their chance of being detected is reduced. Others store their waste in chemical dump sites that gradually leak or seep into the groundwater.

Dr. John Laseter at AccuChem has found that certain water supplies have a characteristic "fingerprint" or pattern of chemicals. These patterns can be so specific that his lab can sometimes recognize the source of a water sample solely from its chemical printout. The Mississippi River, for example, becomes progressively more contaminated with pollutants and potentially cancer-causing agents as it flows toward the Gulf of Mexico.

HOW TO PURIFY YOUR WATER

There are several steps to proper water purification:

- *One step is to remove particles and dissolved solids. For this process, a school can use distilled water or reverse osmosis. The latter process passes the tap water through a membrane that separates the water from its pollutants.*
- *To remove volatile chemicals, another step, activated charcoal can be used. The carbon particles help trap the chemicals, but this is effective only when the charcoal is not saturated. The filters can become contaminated with germs, so they should be changed at recommended times. To remove the germs, distillation seems the best procedure. Water purification systems for individual faucets or entire building or home water supplies are available (see Resources).*

HOW TO TELL IF YOUR WATER SUPPLY BOTHERS YOUR CHILD

Why wouldn't you immediately know if water was making your child ill? As with illness-causing foods and beverages, *the connection may not be obvious.* Check to see if your child is sensitive to your water supply by using only *glass-bottled* filtered or pure spring water for all drinking and cooking for a period of four days prior to testing. This means you must pack lunches for your child, and make sure he doesn't drink tap water at school or at home.

To detect a sensitivity to water, do the "Big Five" (see Chapter 3). It should be done twice: before, and then about ten minutes after you place a teaspoon of tap water under your child's tongue. It is best if he eats nothing for about four hours before the test. Then, notice what changes occur during the next half hour or so.

This simple test can cause definite changes in some chemically sensitive individuals if something in the tap water is a source of their illness. However, this type of test will not be helpful if the water caused an illness (such as diarrhea) because of germs, parasites, or other organisms.

Keep in mind that water can cause a vast array of symptoms, some of which are mentioned not only in this chapter but throughout the book. In chapter 7 of volume 2 of Dr. Rea's book *Chemical Sensitivity*, he describes adults who had severe intestinal problems, including bleeding in the esophagus (food tube), heart disease, and severe arthritis, from chemically contaminated water supplies.

Here is the story of an allergic adolescent named Marlene who experienced fatigue, in part because of her sensitivity to water.

WATER SENSITIVITY AND FATIGUE

Marlene

Seventeen-year-old Marlene had received allergy injection therapy for dust, pollen, and molds for several years. But she was still always tired, and her referring physician could not determine why. She lived about a hundred miles from our center and slept during the entire drive to our office.

At that time, I doubted that Marlene or anyone else had Allergic Tension Fatigue Syndrome (see Chapter 1). She was admitted to the hospital for a urinary problem, and she stated she had headaches every day of her life. She had frequent bellyaches and muscle aches, too, especially near her back and shoulders. Her eyes felt "granular." She had no energy, and on weekends she would sleep sixteen hours a day.

In the hospital, Marlene was not allowed to eat because a minor surgical procedure was scheduled for the day after her admission. Surprisingly, by the next day, she felt better. She said that in the past, she'd often felt healthier about 11:00 A.M. and seemed worse again by 1:30 P.M. This history strongly suggested that she was sensitive to something she ingested for lunch.

While Marlene was in the hospital, I requested that she drink only distilled water and eat only honey and carrots for three days. At the end of that time, she had no aches, was energetic, and felt the "best" she had in years. We then tested individual foods and beverages, one at a time, to uncover the problem items. The findings: If she drank three glasses of tap water, she developed a headache, but well water from her home, distilled water, and spring water caused no problems. Also, as single foods were reintroduced into her diet, she was told to eat only a tablespoon of each suspect food, wait at least a half hour, and then eat the remaining portion if she continued to feel fine. She found that certain foods—potatoes, milk, and chicken, for example—caused a headache or bellyache within half an hour; she could consume others without difficulty. She could eat gelatin made with filtered water, but when the same dessert was made from the filtered water that had been used to cook potatoes, she experienced symptoms. (This helped document that potatoes caused her to become ill.) During her hospital stay, we also found that the odors of perfume, tobacco, warm plastic food trays, and cleaning solutions caused symptoms.

After Marlene's hospitalization, her mother was delighted with the changes that had already occurred in her child and everything we had learned. Marlene herself was so happy that she sang songs during the long ride home. She had never been so vocal or alert.

During the subsequent weeks, Marlene's family realized for the first time that she was naturally talkative. The family actually began to complain that, in contrast to her previous tendency to say very little, now she was rarely quiet. Marlene wanted to go to parties and began to act like a normal teenager. She no longer slept twelve to eighteen hours a day.

Clearly, something in ordinary tap water affected how this young woman felt. Remember, chemicals are not removed at most city water treatment centers. Rather, chemicals are added.

WHAT WATER SHOULD BE AVAILABLE IN SCHOOLS?

Whether at school or home, I strongly recommend that your family drink only *glass*-bottled or filtered water, or use a water purifier *without plastic parts*, either under the sink or at the intake water source (see Resources).

The children described in this chapter clearly could not learn at a level commensurate with their ability because of the intensity and type of their medical symptoms. To avoid the kinds of problems these youngsters had, school cafeterias, water fountains, and showers should provide pure, non-polluted water. In addition, water coolers should be sanitized safely and regularly (for a discussion of water in swimming pools, see Chapter 7).

Urge your legislators not only to pass but to fully enforce more laws to protect our water supplies. Even when pollution regulations are passed, these laws are not always enforced. Is it fair to the public that the government purposely allows some factories to continue to pollute our water for grace periods that can last years? If the government and factories themselves know about the terribly harmful effects of the chemicals they release into the water and the air, why shouldn't this activity stop immediately?[14]

The essence of this dilemma is how we choose to spend our tax dollars. Should our government protect our economy or the health of its constituents? Some government officials do not find this an easy decision, but their unfortunate compromising attitudes have led to an environment that is literally gasping for breath.

■ AN EDUCATION GAP NEEDS CORRECTION

Food- and water-related learning and behavioral problems, unfortunately, are not presently part of the routine curriculum in regular teacher or medical colleges (see Chapter 14). Fortunately, an expanding number of individual progressive educators, psychologists, and physicians are gaining expertise in these problems. They are in an enviable position to help the many children and adults who routinely cross their paths.

However, the general lack of medical acceptance of the possibility of a food or water basis for behavioral problems is discouraging and totally unwarranted. In the medical literature itself, entire textbooks have been devoted specifically to food allergies, dating back to the 1920s, and about water sensitivity, dating back to the 1940s. In addition, there is an abundance of articles, books, and videotapes confirming the role of food and water in causing many behavioral and learning problems.[15]

About eight million of the 53 million Americans under the age of 18 now suffer from some kind of emotional, behavioral, or mental disorder.[16] Does it not seem sensible to find out whether food and water are factors and whether a dietary change is indicated? Is this not better than merely masking symptoms, often only on a temporary basis, with better and more expensive drugs?

NOTES

1. F. Batmanghelidj, *Your Body's Many Cries for Water* (Falls Church, VA: Global Health Solutions, 1995).

2. See D. J. Rapp, *The Impossible Child* (Buffalo, NY: Practical Allergy Research Foundation, 1989), and Doris J. Rapp, *Is This Your Child?* (New York: William Morrow, 1991).

3. Merrow Report, PBS, South Carolina ETV, Oct. 20, 1995.

4. Rapp, *Is This Your Child?*

5. Merrow Report.

6. Marvin Boris et al., "Foods and Additives Are Common Causes of the Attention Deficit Hyperactive Disorder in Children," *Annals of Allergy,* vol. 72 (May 1994), pp. 462–68; C. M. Carter et al., "Effects of a Few Food Diets in Attention Deficit Disorder," vol. 69, *Archives of Diseases in Childhood* (1993), pp. 546–68; J. Egger et al., "Controlled Trial of Oligoantigenic Treatment in the Hyperkinetic Syndrome," *Lancet I* (1985), pp. 540–45; J. O'Shea et al., "Double-Blind Study of Children with Hyperkinetic Syndrome Treated with Multi-Allergen Extract Sublingually," *Journal of Learning Disabilities,* vol. 14 (1981), p. 189; D. J. Rapp, "Does Diet Affect Hyperactivity?" *Journal of Learning Disabilities,* vol. 11 (1978), pp. 56–62; Katherine S. Rowe and Kenneth J. Rowe, "Synthetic Food Coloring and Behavior: A Dose Response Effect in a Double-Blind, Placebo-Controlled, Repeated-Measures Study," *Journal of Pediatrics,* vol. 124, no. 5, part 1 (1988), pp. 691–98.

7. L. Mott and K. Snyder, *Pesticide Alert: A Guide to Pesticides in Fruits and Vegetables* (San Francisco, CA: Sierra Club Books, 1987).

8. Batmanghelidj, *Cries for Water.*

9. William Rea, *Chemical Sensitivity,* 3 vols. (Boca Raton, FL: Lewis Publisher, 1991–95).

10. You can see Marsha's reaction in the video *Environmentally Sick Schools* (see Resources).

11. On fluoride, see the *ICRF Newsletter,* P. O. Box 97, Ardsley, NY 10502, especially the issue from October/November 1995.

12. See "Study Cites Child Risk of Cancer," *Philadelphia Inquirer,* Feb. 27, 1995. See also Jack Leiss and David Savitz, "Home Pesticide Use and Childhood Cancer," *American Journal of Public Health* (Feb. 1995), pp. 249–52.

13. Ibid.

14. Gordon K. Durnil, *The Making of a Conservative Environmentalist* (Birmingham, AL: Indiana University Press, 1995).

15. Albert Rowe and Albert Rowe, Jr., *Food Allergy* (Springfield, IL: Charles C. Thomas, 1972); Katherine S. Rowe and Kenneth J. Rowe, "Synthetic Food Coloring and Behavior: A Dose Response Effect in a Double-Blind, Placebo-Controlled, Repeated-Measures Study," *Journal of Pediatrics*, vol. 124, no. 5, part 1 (1988), pp. 691–98; H. J. Rinkel et al., *Food Allergy* (Springfield, IL: Charles C. Thomas, 1951); J. B. Miller, *Relief At Last!* (Springfield, IL: Charles C. Thomas, 1987); J. B. Miller, *Food Allergy: Provocative Testing and Injection Therapy* (Springfield, IL: Charles C. Thomas, 1972); F. Speer, *Allergy of the Nervous System* (Springfield, IL: Charles C. Thomas, 1970); Jonathan Brostoff and S. J. Challacombe, *Food Allergy and Intolerance* (London: Bailliere Tindall, 1987); Jonathan Brostoff and Linda Gamlin, *The Complete Guide to Food Allergy and Intolerance* (Westminster, MD: Crown Publishing, 1989); T. G. Randolph and R. W. Moss, *An Alternative Approach to Allergies* (New York: Harper & Row, 1989); and T. G. Randolph, "Human Ecology and Susceptibility to the Chemical Environment" (questionnaire), *Annals of Allergy*, vol. 19 (May 1961), pp. 533–38.

16. *USA Weekend*, Oct. 27–29, 1995.

9 ¬ Lead, Asbestos, and Other Factors

In this chapter, some other commonly recognized, significant factors that can cause illness and interfere with your child's ability to learn and feel well will be discussed. Unfortunately, these factors are often given more consideration than the equally and, at times, much more significant environmental issues discussed in Chapters 6, 7, and 8. They include:

- lead
- lighting
- electromagnetic energy
- asbestos
- radon

■ LEAD

Lead is the major recognized indoor health hazard. An estimated one and one-half million children are affected by exposure to lead and can have learning problems as a result. I believe that chemical pollution is a far greater hazard, but lead is certainly a significant, unrecognized problem in some homes and schools.

No amount of lead should be tolerated in any school or home water supply. Unquestionably, it can interfere with a child's ability to learn. It is a greater potential problem for your child than for you because in children the barrier between the blood and the brain is not yet as developed as it is in adults; lead, therefore, is more apt to cause brain damage in children, while in adults it is more apt to damage the nerves.

LEAD POISONING

There is no demonstrably safe level for lead. Unfortunately, most Americans have gradually accumulated lead residues in their bodies from previous exposures to contaminated air, food, or water. When lead poisoning occurs, early symptoms can include any combination of the following: abdominal pain, anemia, nausea, vomiting, loss of appetite, constipation, headaches, dizziness, poor coordination, memory loss, clumsiness, muscle pains, muscle weakness, cramps, irritability, depression, problems in seeing or hearing, numbness and tingling, a metallic taste in the mouth, excessive thirst, insomnia, lethargy, and seizures.

Lead can also cause a permanent decrease in IQ, short attention span, hyperactivity, and difficulties in walking or writing. A child who is subjected to chronic low-level exposures may develop permanent nervous system damage, psychological problems, and behavior disorders, as well as kidney, liver, intestinal system, heart, and blood problems. The immune system can be damaged. Lead can cause malformed sperm and low sperm counts.

Lead poisoning is frequently misdiagnosed because both a chemical sensitivity and Attention Deficit Hyperactivity Disorder can cause similar symptoms. All of these conditions must be considered if a child has the types of complaints described above.

SOURCES OF LEAD CONTAMINATION

Lead can contaminate water that flows through lead-soldered pipes or fountains. The longer the water sits in those pipes, the more lead will be leached into it. You can reduce this problem, however, by flushing the water system in the morning, prior to drinking.

The water in your child's school can be checked for lead contamination through your local or county health department. Mail-order laboratories that provide private water testing are listed in Resources, at the end of this book.

The EPA recently proposed to intensify the monitoring and analysis of drinking water and to place more restrictions on chemical discharges into surface and groundwater. Suggestions and guidelines are not enough, however; enforceable laws must be in place.

Most lead poisoning results from lead in paint chips, paint dust released during renovations, and solder used in water pipes or food cans. Unfortunately, it does not require much contact with lead to cause illness. Water isn't the only potential source of lead poisoning. Glassware and dishes, as well as paint applied to buildings prior to 1980, should be checked for lead content, too (see Resources).

HOW TO CHECK YOUR CHILD FOR LEAD POISONING

If you or your doctor suspects that your child may have lead poisoning, he or she can order an inexpensive blood screening FEP (free erythrocyte protoporphyrin) test. If the results are abnormal, more specific blood testing can be performed to verify whether lead is a problem or not. A simple blood serum test for lead can more accurately detect whether your child's lead level is elevated.

The acceptable lead reference level is 0 to 10.0 micrograms per deciliter (mcg/dL), and without a doubt, levels over 10 mcg/dL can be harmful. Hair analysis and abdominal X-rays can also help detect lead.

The next challenge is to find and remove the sources of lead exposure in both your home and your child's school.

And what about treatment for lead poisoning? Your doctor can decrease a body's lead contamination by using a drug called EDTA (ethylene diamine tetracetate), which combines with the lead so that it can be excreted in the kidneys.

The National Lead Information Center can provide you with further information about lead contamination and hazards (see Resources).

■ LIGHTING

The type of lighting in your child's school—and the light fixtures in the classroom—can pose health concerns for your youngster. Here are some important facts to keep in mind.

FLUORESCENT LIGHT AND OTHER SENSITIVITIES

The best lighting for schools (and elsewhere) is natural light. But in many classrooms, students spend about six hours a day beneath fluorescent lights. These ordinary fluorescent lights can emit X-rays, radiation, and radio waves—emissions that can decrease productivity and cause fatigue, confusion, eyestrain, irritability, depression, and hyperactivity in some sensitive children. A few youngsters fare even worse, experiencing serious atypical reactions. In one environmentally ill ten-year-old boy, for example, his eyes roll back whenever he walks under fluorescent lights.

The most common adverse reaction to light is a photo- or light sensitivity. When it is extreme, the affected persons must wear sunglasses indoors and outdoors, even on overcast days. They can't see clearly, and some complain that their eyeballs hurt, or they feel pain directly behind their eyes when they are exposed to any type of light. (That's different from a sinus infection, which is more apt to cause tenderness when you touch or tap the bones that surround the eyes.)

Under what circumstances can a light sensitivity develop? Some children suddenly become intolerant of light during a reaction to an environmental exposure or to a challenge allergy skin test. One young woman who was tested for allergy to ragweed pollen developed such an increased sensitivity to both light and sound that she ran to a distant, dark corner of our office, covered her ears, and curled her body into a ball. Other children have also assumed this fetal position, with their heads down, their legs pulled tightly against their abdomens, and their arms wrapped around their legs. Some have inexplicably huddled under a chair or behind a piece of furniture, making themselves untouchable. Or they have covered their eyes with their hair and their ears with their hands, vigorously objecting to the sound of ordinary speech. Then, when the environmental exposure or allergy skin test is over, they return to looking and acting normally, and ordinary light and sound are no longer a problem.

So what are the solutions to these light-related problems? Some can be relatively inexpensive. For example, school buildings should be constructed so that the maximum amount of natural light is utilized. A hyperactive child's seat may be moved so it is not directly beneath the fluorescent tubes—or the school can get rid of the fluorescent lights in problem classrooms. A study of one classroom concluded that hyperactivity decreased by 33 percent when full-spectrum lighting replaced fluorescent lighting.[1] So why do we not use full-spectrum lighting all the time, but instead encourage drug therapy with Ritalin? Germany banned fluorescent lights in both schools and hospitals years ago; maybe German health officials know something that we don't.

To learn more about the possible health effects of light, read John Ott's books about how different light wavelengths can affect all living organisms.[2] Ott photographed spectacular changes in the cells of plants, animals, and humans related to various types of light exposures. His time-lapse videos of children clearly demonstrate that some students become hyperactive under fluorescent lights, and his books and studies confirm his observations.

If fluorescent lighting must be used, it should be full spectrum and properly shielded to reduce radiation emanations from the cathode end of the fluorescent tubes. Ultraviolet light should also be available. (See Resources for information on sources of full-spectrum lighting.) Dr. Ott showed that shielded lighting or regular incandescent lightbulbs cause less difficulty, but they are not presently used in most of our schools. (Also refer to Irene Wilkenfeld, who discusses many aspects of light in *The Healthy School Handbook*.[3]

Researchers have also discovered that different parts of the eyes can react adversely to various types of environmental exposures. Satoshi Ishikawa, M.D., dean of a medical school in Japan, heads a team of prominent research ophthalmologists who have published extensively on how electromagnetic radiation and various chemicals (such as organophosphates or malathion) can affect vision.[4] (For more details, see Chapter 14.)

LIGHT FIXTURE AND BLIND MAINTENANCE

Can miniblinds affect your child's health? Surprisingly, the answer is yes. Miniblinds can be dusty and therefore cause classical dust-related allergic symptoms. They should be cleaned regularly ultrasonically, which is relatively inexpensive.

School light fixtures, ceiling grilles, and walls can also be sources of dust; they should be cleaned with compressed air when school is not in session and prior to carpet cleaning.

■ ELECTROMAGNETIC ENERGY

High-tension wires, electrical line transformers, radio and television transmitting antennas, and electrical power stations all emit an immense amount of electromagnetic energy. Yet surprisingly, emissions from regular telephone power lines can be greater, at times, than emissions from certain high-power lines. Your child can also be exposed to varying amounts of EMF energy emitted by computers, lighting fixtures, television sets, microwave ovens, refrigerators, and electric dishwashers. Localized electric fields can even be found around certain small electrical appliances at school and at home (like clocks, stoves, hair dryers, and electric razors) *even when they are not in use.* In certain individuals, this minor degree of exposure can cause symptoms.

Presently, however, not much is known about the health effects of EMFs. Most school systems have *no* regulations about EMFs in or near schools (and usually no established standards exist for the workplace, either). We know that 60 hertz (cycles per second, which are generated from electrical power systems in the United States) can affect human hormone levels and other important biological systems. It is also clear that the health of some very sensitive individuals can be changed significantly by energy emissions. In some exquisitely sensitive people, seizures have been produced repeatedly from exposure to beepers, microwave ovens, computer screens, and fluorescent lights. There are also reports, especially from Sweden, of higher-than-normal rates of leukemia in families located near high-voltage electrical lines; sometimes as low as 2 to 3 mG (on next page). These tip-of-the-iceberg patients certainly indicate that electromagnetic energy can dramatically and adversely affect the human body.[5]

There is even increasing evidence that EMFs can increase the toxicity of chemicals by allowing them to more readily access the sensitive nerve cells in the brain. Research shows that low-level magnetic fields and even microwaves can increase the permeability of the blood-brain barrier in rats and humans; this allows particles to enter the brain that can disrupt normal function.[6]

CLUES TO POSSIBLE ELECTROMAGNETIC ENERGY ILLNESS

Until more is known, you should be alert for signs that your child may have developed an illness in reaction to exposure to EMFs. If he experiences any of the following symptoms at school or home, EMFs might be the cause.

■ Chest pain, headaches, blurry vision, or any unexplained discomfort while sitting directly in front of a standard upright computer. (By contrast, laptops cause fewer health difficulties.)
■ Looking, feeling, or behaving in ways other than normal after exposure to a computer, television set, or microwave oven
■ Feeling ill or different just before or during a thunderstorm or certain other weather changes
■ Not feeling right near high-power electric wires
■ Tics or seizures

We now know that smoke detectors can be potential sources of radiation. To avoid risks, replace yours with ionization-type smoke detectors, which have a "photocell," or with photoelectric-type detectors—and ask your child's school to do the same.

HOW AND WHAT DO YOU MEASURE?

Is your child being exposed to potentially dangerous levels of electromagnetic energy? You can find out by using relatively inexpensive instruments called gaussmeters, which measure and quantify EMFs (see Resources). EMF emissions are greatest a few inches from the source, and they diminish with distance; but in general, a level of about one milligauss (mG), measured about two feet from the item being checked, is considered safe, while levels over 10 mG are cause for concern. Although the acceptable level in Sweden is 2.5 mG, scientists there have warned that as little as one or two mG can produce adverse health effects in very sensitive individuals. The background magnetic fields in most homes varies from about 0.5 to 4 mG, while the level might be 50 to 500 mG directly under a high–voltage line.

CAN STATE OFFICIALS MAKE A DIFFERENCE?

Officials in New York State are recognizing, investigating, and evaluating the importance of electromagnetism issues in some schools located near high-power lines. Experts in this field suggest that schools should be located no closer than one mile away from powerful EMFs. New York State utility companies have cooperated with the initiative and have attempted to reduce the power emissions near certain schools. Maybe you can encourage similar action by your own state in relation to your child's school.

WHAT CAN YOU DO ABOUT ELECTROMAGNETIC ENERGY?

Here are some practical applications concerning electromagnetic fields to keep in mind:

- *Measure the electromagnetic fields in various areas inside and outside your child's school. If your youngster is bothered by EMFs, insist that she avoid localized "hot spots." If there is a generalized elevated level of electromagnetic energy throughout the school, talk about it with school officials and your state education or health department.*
- *Urge your child to spend as little time as possible within a few inches of anything electrical. Unlike a magnetic field, an electric field can exist due to leakage even when the power to a plugged-in appliance is turned off. It is best to disconnect electrical items when they are not in use. If you are in doubt, measure the electromagnetic field and consider taking corrective action if it is over 10 mG. Remember, below 1 mG is supposed to be safe; 2.5 mG to 10 mG is the "gray" area.*
- *Have your child sit more than nine feet from the front of a television set, even when it is turned off, because of the electrical discharge.*
- *Remember, you can't guess the intensity of EMF emissions from an electrical appliance or source. Each one has to be measured. The amount of electricity an appliance uses does not reflect the size of the EMF it generates.*

The bottom line is that we simply don't know how harmful electromagnetic energy might be. We don't know the effects of prolonged low- or high-level exposure to electromagnetic fields. Until we have more information, it seems prudent not to build new schools (or homes) near significant sources of electromagnetic power.

Meanwhile, more and more books are being written about the health effects of electromagnetic energy. Yet this topic is still not a regular part of the curriculum in most medical schools. To find physicians who have in-depth expertise with patients who have EM symptoms, contact the American Environmental Health Foundation in Dallas, Texas, or the Breakspear Hospital in England (see Resources).

COMPUTERS:
THEIR SPECIFIC ELECTROMAGNETIC PROBLEMS

Computers have revolutionized the lives of millions of people—but at what price? They generate ozone, positive ions, static electricity, and EMFs that can bother some individuals. The cathode ray tube behind the video display terminal can cause eyestrain, eye irritation, double vision, irritability, fatigue, stress, itchy skin, and chest, head, neck, and back pains. For those sensitive to chemicals, the odor of volatile organic chemicals (VOCs) emitted from computer printers can cause symptoms.

Minimize problems by making sure there is adequate ventilation in the area around your computer, which will help reduce the ozone to tolerated levels. Also, to reduce exposure to electromagnetic energy, you and your child should type as far away from the screen as you can, and take a ten- to fifteen-minute break every hour.

CHOOSING A COMPUTER SHIELD

Here is a sampling of the various computer shielding products that are available:

- *A computer-screen mesh shield, or the protective computer screen called the Clarifier (see Resources).*
- *The Ultra 7000, a low-radiation CRT (cathode ray tube) display, claims only 0.1 mG electric field at 20 inches in front of the monitor.*
- *Your computer can be encased in glass and vented to the outside. The cord can be wrapped in foil tape.[7] Safe Reading and Computer Box Company makes a galvanized steel enclosure with a glass front (see Resources). It has its own exhaust fan and window exhaust tube. This box can also be used for televisions.*
- *Microsoft Windows makes a Finish Line program that can control a glass-encased computer and enter data with a point-and-click mouselike device that has an on-screen keyboard.*

The liquid crystal display (LCD) screens on portable computers also emit radiation, but it is less powerful and does not extend as far as that of a regular computer. If a rechargeable computer is causing symptoms, use it when it is disconnected, then recharge it in a different room, preferably at night. If this does not resolve the problem, try to find a computer that meets the Swedish standards. (On May 5, 1994, the European Parliament passed a resolution to combat the harmful effects of nonionizing radiation.)

Additional precautions can be taken by using special grounded glare-free screens to diminish eyestrain. These screens also help block radiation.

They can be attached to any properly grounded computer. If you prefer, you can wear a special protective chest cloth to reduce radiation-associated symptoms.

ARE COMPUTERS SAFE FOR PREGNANT WOMEN?

There are ongoing debates concerning the safety of computers for pregnant women. Some reports indicate isolated increases in rates of miscarriage and/or birth-damaged babies among women working in areas with multiple computer terminals. Certainly not everyone is affected, but disturbing scattered reports of this type keep reappearing. Remember, the cathode ray tube from computer terminals can emit energy at the same level as nearby high-tension power lines.

> **M**ore magnetic radiation is emitted from the sides and back of a computer than from the front. Students should stay at least 40 inches from the back and sides of a video display terminal and about 30 inches from the front. EMFs are strongest close to a computer but drop off rapidly at arm's length.

The consensus among the agencies that try to protect us (the Food and Drug Administration, the National Institute for Occupational Safety and Health, and the National Academy of Sciences) is that the amount of radiation emitted by computers is too small to pose a significant health threat during pregnancy. While this is probably true *for most women* under ordinary circumstances, some reports have reached a far different conclusion.

ELECTROMAGNETIC ENERGY AND MALE FERTILITY

Studies, some dating back more than twenty years, have indicated that the offspring of men

- *who work near electromagnetic energy,*
- *who work in nuclear plants,*
- *who have undergone eleven or more X-rays, or*
- *who smoke tobacco,*

have an increased susceptibility to leukemia, lymphoma, and brain cancer.[8] We must wonder, if these exposures affect adult fertility, whether they can also affect children before or after puberty and their future fertility. This is another reason for giving the location of schools a high priority, avoiding the various types of EMF pollution as much as possible.

The book *Computer Health Hazards* by Marija Hughes has fifty pages listing references and short summaries on this topic.[9] This publication is a must if you are concerned and pregnant. Once again, it appears that we simply do not yet know enough about the health effects of computers. Until more is known, concerned pregnant women would be well advised to avoid spending long periods of time in front of a computer.

■ ASBESTOS

Asbestos has become a matter of widespread concern. It was used for many years in construction, fireproofing, thermal and acoustic insulation, and reinforcement of roof and floor tile products, and as insulation around pipes in homes and schools. The loosely bound, sprayed-on asbestos insulation found in asbestos cloth, asbestos cement, or vinyl asbestos tile-flooring materials can gradually disintegrate, releasing asbestos particles that float in the air. Any of these sources can be potentially harmful, and thus immense caution is required to protect both the skin and lungs from their harmful effects, in particular from a chronic lung disease called asbestosis. The EPA has stated that *no* level of asbestos exposure is safe. Nevertheless, with asbestos, cause-and-effect relationships can easily be missed for years because the lag time between an exposure and the onset of illness (such as lung cancer) may be as much as forty years.

Consider these facts: EPA studies have shown that nearly all the school buildings in the United States (107,000) contain some level of asbestos in the building materials, insulation, or fireproofing. One-third (35,000) of those buildings may contain loose, friable (readily crumbled) asbestos, which poses a risk to some 15 million children and 1.4 million staff workers.[10] Why haven't steps been taken to minimize the risks associated with these substances? The deterrent is cost.

Unfortunately, our laws typically fail to protect individuals from injuries that occur years after an exposure, even when there is no question about why someone has developed a specific illness. I believe there is a bias in our country in favor of industry and our economy, in preference to the health of single individuals or the American people.

It is true that many states, including New York, passed legislation as early as 1979 to annually inspect for friable asbestos in public schools and make plans to abate any imminent hazards. In 1986 Congress passed the Asbestos Hazard Emergency Response Act, which was made more comprehensive in scope and depth in 1991. But laws are a mockery if proper enforcement is lacking, and if knowledge of a wrongdoing is followed by years of approved inaction.

If asbestos is properly managed and maintained, its risks are relatively small. If it is necessary to eliminate it from an existing building, however, or if the building is to be demolished, the dangers of its improper removal must be fully appreciated. Removal must be done *carefully and cautiously* and only by those who have complete expertise in this area. (See the experience of Sister Martha in Chapter 7.)

■ RADON

Radon is a colorless, odorless, tasteless radioactive gas. It is produced by the decay of uranium, which is naturally found in the soil, rocks, and water in certain scattered areas of the United States. *All* schools must be individually checked for radon because high levels have been found in every state, and radon problems can vary markedly from one area to another.

Radon enters a building from the soil, through cracks and holes in the foundation—that is, through expansion floor joints, crawl spaces, and ventilation conduits, and around pipes, joints, drains, windows, and/or doors. As a result, radon levels can vary greatly from room to room in the same school or home. It is not normally found more than two stories above a foundation. If the foundation of a building is tight, little or no radon will enter.

The indoor concentration of radon can vary considerably. The outdoor air averages about 0.4 picocuries per liter (pCi/L), in contrast to 1.3 pCi/L or much higher indoors. To put this in perspective, an exposure to 4 pCi/L per day for a lifetime is roughly equivalent to smoking four cigarettes a day; about three smokers out of a thousand would get cancer in their lifetime from that amount of exposure. In a study of sixty schools by the New York State Health Department, 85 percent had room levels less than 4 pCi/L, while one percent had rooms with a level higher than 20 pCi/L. In an informal telephone survey of ninety-one school districts, almost 25 percent (twenty-two) reported finding levels exceeding the 4 pCi/L level. In 1992, EPA studies based on a sampling of nine hundred schools projected that 20 percent of them contained unsafe radon levels. They also estimated that 70,000 classrooms in 15,000 schools have radon levels exceeding the EPA's safety standards of 4 pCi/L of air, while 10,000 classrooms have "excessively high" radon levels.[11]

The indoor radon level is partially dependent upon the adequacy of ventilation. The better the ventilation, the lower the radon level. In addition, the balance between the air pressure outside and inside the building is critical; if it is not correct, pressure differentials can either suck more radon into the school or cause a backdraft so that combustion fumes or hydrocarbons are also not properly exhausted. These pressure inequities also can cause excessive condensation on the outside walls, leading to an inordinately rapid deterioration of the exterior of the building.

Once radon enters a building, it spreads freely through the indoor atmosphere. Radon is inert, so it does not chemically bind with other materials in the environment. But as it decays, small bursts of radioactive particles are released that can attach to dust. When these dust particles are inhaled, they can damage lung tissue, at times leading to cancer. For this reason, it is crucial that high-efficiency air filters in the ventilation system or portable room air-purification units, as well as HEPA vacuum cleaners, be used in schools. These will diminish the amount of dust in the air, reducing hay fever, asthma, and other forms of allergy, while decreasing the possibility of radon attachment to dust.

The harmful effects of chronic low-dosage radon exposure were not fully recognized until recently. We now know, however, that there are no safe radon levels. Radon presents a *substantial health risk* even though no short-term effects have been reported. Children are possibly more at risk than adults. In the United States, 5,000 to 15,000 people develop lung cancer each year from radon exposure. The rate of cancer increases with rises in the amount and duration of the exposure.

Your child's school, as well as all other public buildings, work areas, and homes, must be monitored for radon. Even though radon is easy and relatively inexpensive to detect, no federal or state laws or regulations enforce radon testing in most schools. State health departments do issue *guidelines* and *suggestions*, however, which should be followed by education departments. Check with your school officials to determine if and when adequate radon testing has been performed.

Mandatory federal regulations for school radon testing are pending; some states are also considering setting their own regulations. Once again, *asking* is not enough to protect the public. We need laws that are enforceable.

WHAT CAN *YOU* DO TO DETECT RADON?

Scanning or preliminary radon testing kits are available as alpha track detectors and activated charcoal canisters (see Resources). Detailed information about charcoal radon-detector kits can be obtained from your local health department. The National Safety Council's detection kit has met the EPA's requirements under the Radon Measurement Proficiency Program (see Resources).

With these kits, school and office personnel or parents can determine whether rooms or entire buildings are contaminated. All frequently occupied rooms in contact with the ground should be checked. If the test results indicate a level above 4 pCi/L, short- and long-term monitoring should be conducted. For more information on radon testing, see Resources.

If your child or another family member has an environmental illness, you must be careful not to replace one problem with another in an attempt to limit radon exposure. For example, you might want to repair thin wall cracks that are allowing radon to enter a school building, but certain poly-urethane sealants can emit harmful toxic fumes of their own. Although silicone sealers are less toxic, they are less effective in excluding radon from a building. The answers are not simple. For less toxic sealants, see Resources.

> The solutions to asbestos and radon problems are not always available and sometimes are simply not known. At present, we're aware of the dangers, but our current laws do not adequately protect us.

NOTES

1. Marilyn Painter, "Fluorescent Lights and Hyperactivity in Children: An Experiment," *Education Digest*, vol. 42 (April 1977), pp. 36–37.

2. John Ott, *Light, Radiation and You* (Greenwich, CT: Devin-Adair, 1982); John Ott, "Influence of Fluorescent Lights on Hyperactivity and Learning Disabilities," *Journal of Learning Disabilities*, vol. 9 (1976), pp. 417–22.

3. *The Healthy School Handbook* (Washington, DC: NEA Professional Library, 1995).

4. Satoshi Ishikawa et al., "Aggravation of Allergic Conjunctivitis Possibly Due to Electromagnetic Waves," *Current Aspects in Ophthalmology* (1992), pp. 214–18; Doris J. Rapp, *Is This Your Child?* (New York: William Morrow, 1991), pp. 70, 279. Williams, Reals, *Chemical Sensitivity*, vol. 3, (Boca Raton, Fla.: Lewis Publishing, 1996), chapter 27.

5. R.O. Becker, *Cross Currents* (Los Angeles, CA: Jeremy P. Tarcher, 1982); Cyril W. Smith and Simon Best, *The Electromagnetic Man: Health and Hazard in the Electrical Environment* (London: Robinson Publishing, 1989).

6. F. Prato et al., "Extremely Low Frequency Magnetic Field Exposure from MRI/MRS Procedures: Implications for Patients (Acute Exposure) and Operational Personnel (Chronic Exposures)," *Annals of the New York Academy of Sciences*, vol. 649 (1992), pp. 44–58.

7. See *The Human Ecologist*, no. 62 (Summer 1994), p. 10, available from Human Ecology Action League (HEAL) (see Resources).

8. *Clinical Pearls News*, vol. 2, nos. 1–2 (Jan. 1992).

9. Marija Hughes, *Computer Health Hazards*, 2 vols. (Washington, DC: Hughes Press, 1993).

10. See Nicholas Tate, *The Sick Building Syndrome* (Far Hills, NJ: New Horizon Press, 1994), pp. 80–81, 163.

11. Ibid.

10 Pesticides and Carpet Chemicals

$\mathbf{T}$wo major areas of chemical concern, pesticides and carpet chemicals, deserve in-depth discussion in relation to the school and home environment because contact with or exposure to them can potentially cause long-term, serious health and memory problems in students, teachers, and families.[1]

The books listed in this chapter and in For Further Reading provide additional discussions of the frightening adverse effects that can be caused by these particular substances. Also, the tables in the Appendix furnish basic essential information about chemicals frequently found in schools, homes, and workplaces.

To begin, here is one youngster's story, which illustrates the types of health problems that such exposures can cause.

A PESTICIDE AND CARPET SENSITIVITY

John

John, a 13-year-old boy, had a personal and family history of classical allergies. At the start of the school year in the fall of 1992, he returned to his newly remodeled and carpeted middle school—which also used pesticides. He soon developed many health problems, including nasal symptoms, a tight chest and chest pain, headaches, dizziness, nausea, flushing, and hives. Also, his knuckles, toes, and feet ached, and his ears felt full. By October of that year, he experienced mood swings, extreme fatigue, tingling fingers and lips, a weak voice, a funny mouth taste, and hot flashes. He also complained of itchy skin, muscle aches, puffy dark-circled eyes, severe abdominal cramps, diarrhea, and flulike symptoms. He was so nauseated each day that he could not eat lunch. By January 1993, his arms and fingers were numb and tingling. At the end of the school day, he sometimes had double vision.

Most of John's symptoms subsided within one to four hours after he left school and while he was on vacation. However, the symptoms promptly recurred as soon as he entered the school building for any reason. Finally, in late January 1993, his family transferred him to another school.

John's symptoms subsided until March 1993, when he returned to the original, remodeled school. But after only fifteen minutes, he developed a tingling upper lip, began to gag, and thought he would vomit. His eyes swelled, and he was forced to leave the school again. On that same day when visiting the school, John's father developed asthma, itchy eyes, and shortness of breath. For the next few days, his father's muscles ached severely.

In April 1993, John happened to enter a newly painted and carpeted store. Within fifteen minutes, he had cramps in his right leg and thigh and was forced to leave the building.

What Was Happening to John?

Clearly, John's multiple chemical sensitivities had their onset when the original school building was remodeled. Unfortunately, his chemical sensitivity not only persists today, it has become more extreme because the odors in many buildings or places with poor air quality now bother him.

When John was tested with an allergy extract prepared from his problem school's air, he developed droopy eyes, extreme fatigue, and abdominal pain. A mock placebo allergy injection did not cause symptoms (see Sick School Video in Resources).

John's blood showed that changes had taken place in his immune system. His protective white blood cells, called T cells, had decreased in number. His level of IgE was elevated, as is typical of allergic children. He also had formed antibodies against the fat (myelin) coverings of his own nerves.

John also exhibited some problems with the transmission of nerve impulses to and from his brain. His brain-image (SPECT) test showed mild changes that are typical of the damage caused by a neurotoxic exposure. Unfortunately, these tests have not been repeated due to a lack of funds and insurance coverage.

John's Condition Twenty Months Later

How was John twenty months after these evaluations were conducted? He continued to be bothered by a wide variety of chemical odors. A whiff of perfume could cause him to develop abdominal pain, nausea, stiffness in his neck and joints, and a severe headache. At times he stated that he felt as if the top of his head would "blow" off. His eyes still burned and watered. He continued to need daily naps and was too tired to play soccer with his friends. He felt discouraged. His new school was better for his health, but he missed his many friends and teachers at the other school.

Even though some of John's symptoms were less severe, others were just developing, in what is known as the ripple effect. For example, he was starting to have trouble with his eyes. He could read for about five minutes, then the words started to blend together and/or appear backward. An eye examination revealed no obvious cause. The day after he swam in a chlorinated pool, he was very tired and had trouble concentrating and thinking clearly. Sometimes his mind simply went blank. His neck tended to crack frequently; this was never a problem in the past, and for some unknown reason it was most evident when he was in a mall.

What About the Future?

The prime question, of course, is related to John's future. Will his nerves, brain, muscles, vision, digestion, and immune function return to normal after comprehensive environmental or other care such as homeopathy? He should be detoxified so that more chemicals in his body can be eliminated (see Chapter 14), but this takes several weeks; who will pay his travel and living expenses? How long will it take before he can casually go with his friends into public places, such as a mall, church, restaurant, or movie theater, without worrying about who will be near him or how the area was cleaned? Even if he appears to be well again, can a sudden accidental, unavoidable exposure to a chemical at some future time lead to an even more serious environmental illness?

Unfortunately, we don't have the answers at this time. We only know that John appears to be improving. He is far from being over his illness and he is unfortunately not alone in his struggle with this kind of illness.

▪ PESTICIDES

The term *pesticide* means "something that kills pests." The most common pesticides include fungicides for use against fungi and molds, rodenticides for rats, herbicides for vegetation, bactericides for bacteria, nematocides for worms, and termiticides for termites. They are often similar in composition. They are also difficult to avoid in our society because they are present in chemicals that contaminate food, water, soil, air, homes, and schools.

Pesticides are known to damage the nervous system, genitals, heart, lungs, intestines, blood, liver, and kidneys. Many pesticides have been shown to cause cancer and birth defects in animals and humans.[2] Chlorinated compounds repeatedly have been linked to cancer and to sexual changes, due to their estrogenlike effect (see Chapter 14).[3] However, ascertaining the real scope of the illnesses related to pesticides is a major challenge. Health and learning problems have become so prevalent and pervasive that it is virtually impossible to pinpoint the many individuals whose problems are related to direct or indirect pesticide exposure. The symptoms tend to begin shortly after a major exposure, but chronic long-term illnesses can begin with subtle symptoms, so that the cause-and-effect relationship is not readily apparent.

Of the millions of pounds of pesticides sprayed on crops each year, only 1 to 3 percent ever actually reach pests, some of which are becoming pesticide-resistant. Thirty years ago, 7 percent of preharvest crops were insect-damaged in spite of the use of 50 million pounds of pesticides; today, 13 percent of crops are insect-damaged, even though 600 million pounds of pesticides are used. Meanwhile, in one report, nearly 80 percent of the cancers in 20,000 patients were thought to be caused by ten pesticides found on fifteen different foods.[4] Washing and peeling foods helps, but pesticides routinely permeate the insides of foods, too. These include common foods which our children eat in school.

In its own research, the Food and Drug Administration (FDA) found 108 different pesticides on twenty-two fruits and vegetables. Meat and dairy products, as well as fish and eggs, can be even more heavily contaminated than fruits and vegetables. The DDT levels in some human breast milk (even though the chemical was banned in 1970) is so high that it can exceed the levels that the FDA permits in cow's milk.

ACTIVE VS. "INERT" INGREDIENTS

Pesticides are a combination of the active ingredients, the ones used to kill pests, plus the substances in which they are dissolved or blended. The latter are erroneously called "inert" substances. They include solvents, binders, enhancers, propellants, and fillers which sometimes cause more serious health effects than the active ingredients.

The 50,000 pesticides on the market today contain about 600 active ingredients and 1,200 or more "inert" substances. Of these 600 pest-killing

---

RISK FACTORS IN CHILDREN

Young children are at greater risk from pesticide exposure than teachers or their parents. The reasons are several:

- *Children eat more food, drink more water, and breathe more air in proportion to their weight than do adults. Children incorporate more pesticides into their bodies than adults because they are still growing.*
- *Their immature and developing physiological systems, such as the immune system, can be more sensitive to the adverse effects of pesticides and other toxins than these same systems in mature individuals.*
- *Children are physically shorter, therefore are closer to the ground, where pesticides are usually applied. They tend to roll on sprayed lawns and play ball on pesticide-treated athletic fields, increasing the amount that they touch and breathe into their lungs.*
- *They often forget to wash their hands. Little children tend to put "everything" into their mouths, increasing the amount of pesticide that is actually ingested.*
- *They play directly on carpets, which contain lawn pesticides from contaminated shoes. Children spend more time on the floor than do adults. The level of pesticides found indoors is usually higher than that outdoors.*
- *They don't know that they should run inside for cover during aerial chemical spraying. Most people are totally unaware of the potential dangers of some chemical sprays. If pesticides such as malathion are so potentially harmful, do you think your small child, vegetable garden, or sandbox should be directly exposed?*

ingredients, the EPA can provide safety assurance for only about six. Of 400 pesticides on our foods, only twenty-seven have safety data.[5]

The "inert" substances, which can be just as dangerous as the active ones (or more so), make up as much as 50 to 99 percent of the pesticides sold. Their chemical components are "trade secrets," and the U.S. government requires no toxicity evaluations or public disclosure of their composition. Yet they include some of the most dangerous substances known to man: asbestos, benzene, xylene, DDT, and Chicago waste sludge.

Several years ago, a woman on the East Coast was given a dental adhesive to use over a six-month period to repair her partial plate, which kept breaking. The MSD sheet for the adhesive listed its active ingredients as 2-butanone and toluene; both are known to be neurotoxins. These toxins resulted in damage to her brain, and in addition, 75 percent of her lower jawbone died. However, this effect was thought to be due not to these neurotoxins, but to an "inert" ingredient in the adhesive called beta chloroprene, *which our government does not require to be listed on the MSD sheet.* When beta chloroprene is absorbed, it can cause bone and tissue death. This indicates that people should be cautious not only because of the obvious toxic active components in dental adhesives but also because of the unlisted inert components.[6]

Some studies suggest that increased aggression, learning disabilities, serious eye changes, and/or lower IQ scores in students are related to pesticide exposures. Some forms of childhood brain cancer have definitely been linked to consumer pesticide use.[7]

HOW ARE INDIVIDUALS ROUTINELY EXPOSED?

In our nation's schools, pesticides are used outside on lawns, athletic fields, trees, and shrubs. These outdoor chemicals are then tracked into school buildings, homes, and work areas in amounts capable of causing illness. As many as forty-four pesticides are applied to lawns; thirteen of these are found in the groundwater and four are considered to be potential carcinogens. Is it any wonder that cancer is becoming more and more widespread?[8]

To make matters worse, nearby aerial spraying of parks and farmlands can potentially cause illness if the prevailing winds blow toward schools and homes. These pollutants can enter intake ventilation ducts and become part of indoor air. Similarly, pollution from incinerators and paper mills, and other nearby aerial factory waste, can cause significant contamination inside and outside nearby buildings.

Pesticides are also routinely applied inside school buildings to control roaches, ants, fleas, and termites in places like kitchens, lavatories, walls, and basements. Indoor pollution is a hundred times higher than it is outdoors, according to the EPA; pesticides linger indoors, especially in buildings with inadequate ventilation. Although chemicals are usually sprayed in classrooms when the building is vacant, sometimes an oily residue is left on the children's desks and classroom tables, and it can cause symptoms.

The health office at your school should notify all parents and teachers exactly when pesticides will be applied, and which ones. A log should be kept in the health office to record any illness, misbehavior, or atypical learning difficulty that begins or worsens within a few hours, days, or weeks after these chemicals are used. Student records should be analyzed to see if the onset of health, emotional, or learning problems is associated with the use of pesticides. You should make similar observations when pesticides are used inside or outside your home or on your lawn or the neighbor's. Also, be sure you close the windows when the lawn spray trucks approach your street if you don't want these chemicals inside your home.

Chemical manufacturers make unusual claims to justify keeping their products on the market. For example, they may point out that there has been a decrease in the incidence of some virtually nonexistent health problem (for example, equine encephalitis) and attribute this decline to a particular type of pesticide. This was the reason a health official in a city in upper New York gave when asked why they continued to use toxic pesticides as herbicides in a residential area of a city in New York.

The For Further Reading section at the end of this book lists books and articles with helpful and specific information on pesticides in food and elsewhere, and they offer safer ways to control common indoor pests. The Resources section will direct you to suppliers of safer, natural forms of pest control.

PESTICIDES IN THE PLAYGROUND

Wooden playground structures are preserved with chemicals that protect them from molds, insects, and bacteria. Creosote, pentachlorophenol (PCP), and arsenicals have been used for this purpose, but they are not safe for either children or adults.

Here are some important points to consider:

■ PCP specifically is no longer available "over-the-counter" in the United States. PCP-contaminated wood was once used *inside* buildings, particularly in Germany, where it caused severe, permanent neurological damage in exposed children and adults. Its vapors, which can be released for seven years, are easily absorbed through the skin. Children are more sensitive to it than adults. The toxic contaminants in PCP include dioxins, dibenzofuran, and hexachlorobenzene. PCP poisoning can cause headaches, dizziness, nausea, vomiting, chest pain, fever, rashes, and eye, nose, and throat irritation; chronic exposure can cause liver, kidney, neurological, and blood diseases.

■ Arsenicals can cause rashes, intestinal upsets, cancer, and nerve damage, as well as increased skin pigmentation.

What are the alternatives for outdoor playground equipment? Schools can use metal, or wood that naturally resists decay—such as redwood, Douglas fir, ponderosa pine, western red cedar, or cypress. Safe wood preservatives are also available.[9]

PESTICIDES IN SCHOOL CAFETERIAS

The EPA allows four hundred pesticide ingredients to be used in our foods. Not surprisingly, then, most purchased cafeteria foods and beverages, as well as those used at home, contain a wide range of pesticides.[10] Many schools now provide indigent and other students with low-cost, government-subsidized foods for lunch (and sometimes for breakfast). These meals may include dairy products, for example, especially milk and cheese, which certainly can be contaminated with pesticides. To compound the problem, a significant number of children and adults also have allergies or lactose intolerance to dairy products. These allergies may be related to a wide range of illnesses as well as learning and behavior problems in children.

Many parents and teachers are not aware of the health, emotional, behavioral, and learning problems that dairy and other so-called "good" foods can create. But, as discussed elsewhere in this book, common problems they can cause include recurrent nose and eye congestion and asthma, as well as the less common recurrent ear fluid, leg aches, intestinal upsets, constipation, halitosis, hyperactivity, unacceptable behavior, learning problems, prolonged bed-wetting, and increased need to urinate. Keep in mind that contrary to popular opinion, *if a diet is well-balanced or if nutrient supplements are given,* most children do not need milk after about eighteen months of age.[11]

Peanut butter is another food that is often generously supplied to schools—but it contains pesticides and is potentially highly allergenic. A few children not only cannot ingest it but develop severe asthma attacks from even the slightest aroma from a nearby child's peanut-butter sandwich. The slightest touch can cause hives or itchy, swollen skin. Even so, peanuts and raisins are staples for many children, although they are listed in the FDA's Total Diet Study as two of the most pesticide-saturated foods in this country. Safer peanut-butter preparations from organically grown peanuts are available at most health food stores, as are organically grown, unsulfured raisins.

We must therefore conclude that if free or government-subsidized foods are contaminated, they are certainly not gifts. We need to think more about supplying wholesome foods and pure water to youngsters, both at school and at home. Our nation cannot remain healthy and productive if the next generation is nourished with polluted foods and beverages.

SCHOOL FOODS AND FEDERAL LAW

Aren't there laws to protect our schoolchildren from contaminated foods? There's the Delaney Clause, found in Section 409 of the federal Food, Drug, and Cosmetic Act. (However, this clause applies only to processed foods.) It states, *"No substance found to cause cancer in man or animals may be added to food."* Because pesticides are considered to be food additives, this law clearly forbids our food supply to be contaminated with pesticides that are known to cause cancer. This law was upheld in 1992 by the Supreme Court, *but it has not been enforced.* In the past, the EPA apparently used a loophole in such a way that allowed processed foods to be considered safe if they contained pesticide residue levels no higher than the levels tolerated for raw foods. Even though that interpretation was rejected by the Supreme Court, the clause has still not been enforced. (In fact, further efforts are under way in Congress to weaken it.) So dangerous pesticides continue to contaminate our foods and families.

Does the government want to protect us or doesn't it? Why should it weaken or not enforce the law when it knows that pesticides are so harmful? Some believe that the government's action (or lack of it) is related to misconceptions about the level of harm pesticides can cause. Is the EPA underestimating the potential harm that can be caused by carcinogenic substances in foods? Is it overestimating the benefits of blemish-free food that is less nutritious? (Pesticides are actually used more often to prevent insects from blemishing foods than from destroying them.) Maybe the EPA should think more about the long-term benefits of a healthy population and less about the short-term economic gains of big business. How valuable is a healthy economy in a nation of sick children and adults? Are the vested interests of some legislators taking precedence over simple common sense?

At the present time, chemicals are allowed in and on our food unless it can be proven *conclusively that the harm outweighs the benefits.* The EPA has the obligation to protect the health of all Americans. The present risk-benefit assessment philosophy is certainly not fulfilling that obligation. We need not only to enforce the Delaney Clause but to enact more stringent laws that forbid the distribution of substances that can seriously harm humans and animals. We as well as people in other nations need to be protected

TABLE 10.1

Where to Write About Your Concerns

■ Write to your own congressperson or to Christopher Shays, chairman of the Subcommittee on Human Resources and Intergovernmental Affairs, Washington, DC 20515. The subcommittee members include Bernard Sanders* (VT), Edolphus Towns (NY), Mark Souder (IN), Steven Schiff (NM), Connie Morella (MD), Tom Davis (VA), Dick Chrysler (MI), Bill Martini (NJ), Joe Scarborough (FL), Mark Sanford (SC), Tom Lantos (CA), Thomas Barrett (WI), Gene Green (TX), Chaka Fattah (PA), and Henry Waxman (CA).
■ Regarding the Delaney clause, write to Carol Browner, Office of the Administrator, Environmental Protection Agency, 401 M Street, S.W., Washington, DC 20402.

*Bernard Sanders's accomplishments have greatly helped to increase awareness of health-related environmental issues in Congress.

from further contamination of our bodies, schools, homes, work areas, and planet.

It's important to write to government officials and legislators to let them know how you feel. See Table 10.1 for their addresses. If you would like to learn more about the problem of pesticides in foods, see For Further Reading and Resources.

One recent report helps explain why Congress is moving so slowly in this area. After the Delaney Clause was upheld in court in 1992, a political action committee (PAC) that favors the use of pesticides was formed and contributed $3.1 million to members of Congress. Significantly, more of the pesticide PAC cash is said to have been given to the members who oversee pesticide legislation. For a copy of this report, contact the Environmental Working Group (see Resources).

WHY IS PESTICIDE TOXICITY FREQUENTLY NOT RECOGNIZED?

Surprising as it may seem, the true extent of pesticide contamination in American schools and homes does not appear to have been thoroughly investigated or evaluated.[12] No studies, for example, have been conducted to compare the health, intelligence, and pesticide levels in the blood or urine of exposed students and teachers with those of unexposed individuals.[13] Detailed health records after pesticide use are not collected and analyzed. Most physicians have had little formal training in recognizing, diagnosing, and treating chemical sensitivities. When pesticide toxicity is routinely recognized, it is done so mainly by toxicologists, or by occupational physicians or physicians working in the field of poison control.

The toxic effects of pesticides, however, are not identical to the symptoms of chemical sensitivities. Some of the symptoms overlap, but others are entirely different.[14] The health problems that develop vary from chemical to chemical in both children and adults. (For details about the effects of specific chemicals, see Appendix.) And while environmental medical specialists are educated to recognize, document, and treat these health problems, this specialty is a part of the curriculum at only a few medical and osteopathic colleges.[15]

A CLOSER LOOK AT PESTICIDES

In general there are three major types of pesticides:

■ chlorinated hydrocarbons or organochlorides
■ organophosphates
■ carbamates

Let's look at each type more closely, and then at some particularly deplorable individual pesticides.

ORGANOCHLORIDES
Organochlorides linger for long periods in the environment and are acknowledged to cause serious illnesses.[16] They have been repeatedly linked to cancer and reproductive problems, for example.[17] You've probably heard of some of the more common organochlorides, which include DDT, dieldrin, chlordane, dioxin, heptachlor, endrin, mirex, benzene hydrochloride (BHC), lindane, aldrin, pentachlorobenzene (PCB), and toxaphene.

There are regulations and restrictions on only a few of these chemicals, and by the time the EPA finally banned the use of some of them, 97 percent of humans, and most fish, animals, and even breast milk, had been contaminated. Ironically, some of the banned chemicals were replaced by even more toxic ones.

Other chlorinated chemicals commonly used in schools and homes include the chlorofluorocarbons, which are used as refrigerants and in air conditioners. Even the amount of chlorine in the bleached paper used in most textbooks can bother some very sensitive students. The answer is to use books made with unbleached paper.

ORGANOPHOSPHATES
The organophosphates include malathion (it acts like a nerve gas), parathion, leptophos, and the cancer-causing flame retardant called Tris, which

was used in children's sleepwear in the early 1970s.[18] The consequences of the Tris tragedy are about to be seen: according to Sierra Club estimates, more than half a million children who were exposed to Tris will develop cancer in adulthood or sooner![19]

And then there's malathion. In 1981 California allowed 160,000 gallons of it to be sprayed over thirteen hundred square miles *each week*, even in residential areas in and near Los Angeles. The protection of industry and crops from the Mediterranean fruitfly took precedence over the health of the public. There is no doubt that chemicals like malathion can affect the brain, nervous system, muscles, eyes, reproductive system, and other body areas. The possibility of long-term brain damage from continued exposure is realistic cause for concern.

CARBAMATES

The final category of pesticides is the nerve gas type called carbamates, such as carbaryl (Sevin). Carbaryl is used in clothing, medicines, and plastics. It is known to cause intestinal, respiratory, visual, memory, nervous system, and muscle problems. In addition to its harmful human health effects, it kills bees. Bees pollinate crops. No bees means no crops. Think about it.

FIVE DEPLORABLE PESTICIDES

To give you a sense of some of the specific pesticides that have threatened our health, here are descriptions of just a few.

CHLORDANE

Chlordane, an organochlorine insecticide, poisons the nervous system and damages the immune system. It causes birth defects and reduced fertility and is a probable cause of cancer. It is particularly harmful for pregnant or breast-feeding women and young children. Almost all uses of chlordane were banned by 1988, yet it continues to contaminate our food and water and to make some of our foods and fish unsafe to eat. Why? One reason is that it lingers in soil fourteen years after its use, and we do not know how to decontaminate that damaged soil.

Chlordane residue is found in a wide range of imported products such as fish, rice, mushrooms, beef, and squash. Could the fact that the United States continues to produce and export chlordane each year be a factor? Ironically, some of it comes back to our shores in the products that these foreign countries export to the United States.

HEPTACHLOR

Heptachlor is a chlorinated hydrocarbon found in DDT and aldrin. Like chlordane, it contaminates soil and poisons nerves. Its so-called "safe" alternative chemical is Dursban (chlorpyrifos), an organophosphate insecticide *that is used as a wartime nerve gas.* It inhibits proper transmission of impulses through the nerves of the body. (For more about Dursban, see the box on page 252.)

The EPA allows a loophole for heptachlor (as well as chlordane) by *conditionally* registering them. Again, the thinking public must ask whose vested interests allow these toxic substances to continue to be produced. There must be much that we need to know and are not being told. (See For Further Reading).

DIOXIN

Dioxin is another chlorinated hydrocarbon.[20] Dioxinlike chemicals include PCBs (polychlorinated biphenyls) and, in dioxin's most lethal form, TCDD (2,3,7,8-tetrachlorodibenzo-p-dioxin), used in Agent Orange. Common sources of dioxin are pulp and paper mills, industrial and incinerator wastes, and factories that make or use chemical pesticides or plastics, cosmetics, detergents, solvents, and dyes. Dioxin enters the atmosphere and water from these sources, and then contaminates the soil, the air, and much of the food that we eat, particularly meat, fish, and dairy products. It is even found in breast milk.

The risk of cancer increases with dioxin exposure, ranging from one in a thousand to one in ten thousand. Dioxin is believed to be a factor in the recent doubling in rates of breast, prostate, and testicular cancer. Other studies suggest that liver and blood cancers are related to dioxin exposures (see Chapter 18). In addition, dioxin can cause immune defects, diabetes, thyroid disease, and a wide range of reproductive problems (lowered sperm counts, decreased testosterone, testicular atrophy, small penis size, and birth defects).[21]

The sperm count in healthy males has dropped approximately 50 percent in the last fifty years. Also, about five million women in the United States now have endometriosis, a painful pelvic menstrual disorder that causes sterility; 80 percent of monkeys exposed to daily low levels of dioxin also developed this problem.[22] Is there a connection?

For more information about the potential estrogenic and other hormonal effects of pesticides in animals and humans, see Chapter 18 and Appendix. We urgently need more research to find out if our next generation of girls and boys are at risk or have already been harmed.[23]

XYLENE

Xylene is not an active ingredient in pesticides but is used as a solvent for them, as well as in drugs, dyes, and gasoline, and in lens cleaners for microscopes. Because it is a solvent, xylene might be unlisted and lumped into the "inert" category on an MSD sheet. It can adversely affect human health if its fumes are inhaled or if it touches the skin. It can cause eye, nose, and throat irritation, headaches, nausea, fatigue, stomach discomfort, dizziness, and a light-headed feeling. On a long-term basis, xylene exposure can cause liver, kidney, and blood disease.

The legal exposure for xylene, established by OSHA, should not be higher than 100 ppm in an eight-hour period. It should not exceed 150 ppm in a fifteen-minute period.[24]

DACONIL

Daconil 2787 is the brand name for chlorothalonil, a lawn-care chemical that is a wettable powder capable of irritating the skin and mucous membranes of the eyes and respiratory tract on contact.[25] The following admittedly extreme story demonstrates why it may be important to know what is being used on your child's school's lawn or in nearby parks.[26]

In 1982 a healthy vacationing navy lieutenant became very ill with flulike symptoms while playing golf at the military base. He developed a headache and nausea. He soon became atypically irritable and began "blowing up" at his fellow officers for no apparent reason. By the third day, he was seriously ill. A quickly spreading rash on his stomach prompted him to check into a naval hospital. His rash turned into baseball-size blisters. When the blisters broke, the skin all over his body began to peel.

Doctors were unable to diagnose his problem. His internal organs failed, and his condition rapidly worsened. Less than two weeks later, this previously healthy young lieutenant died of a heart attack.

Because a military officer in top physical condition had died under mysterious circumstances, an investigation was launched. Using infrared photography, it was discovered that the golf course had been saturated with Daconil 2787, a lawn fungicide. When the young lieutenant's shoes, golf clubs, and golf balls were viewed under ultraviolet light, they were found to be coated with Daconil, too. This chemical had been thought harmless, so it was routinely sprayed on the golf course each week. Further investigation revealed that ten years earlier, four people had died in a similar manner after a comparable chemical had been used as a fumigant. The Navy's forensic pathologist concluded that an allergic reaction to Daconil was the probable cause of the lieutenant's death.

As mentioned before, this Daconil story is extreme. Yet herbicides have become a routine (some might even say mindless) part of lawn maintenance in schoolyards, parks, golf courses, and around homes. One reason for their ubiquity is their heavy promotion by petrochemical manufacturers, plus the premium our society places on keeping lawns and parks lovely with "labor-saving" products. Many communities and school districts apply lawn pesticides recklessly. Certification of commercial pesticide applicators is suggested but it is certainly not always well-controlled or properly monitored.

By our thoughtless loss of priorities, we are threatening our children's present and future, as well as our own. Children, especially toddlers and sports-minded teenage boys, naturally run, play, and roll around in grass. Surely they deserve something better than the opportunity to accumulate and store dangerous chemicals in their little bodies. Perhaps in these times, when job creation is such a major issue, we could create employment by replacing chemical use with nonchemical lawn care and manual weed clipping.

TERMITICIDES IN SCHOOLS AND HOMES

Dursban (chlorpyrifos) is a termiticide that is commonly sprayed around buildings.[27] Dursban can cause nausea, dizziness, diarrhea, anxiety, and seizures.

Natural termite control is effective and safe—it should be used near schools and homes instead of Dursban.[28] There is no reason not to use common sense and safer methods when they are available. Some governmental regulations insist that homes be termiticided with toxic substances when they are sold; unless the next occupants are alerted, they could be placing themselves in danger.

HOW CAN YOU DETECT CHEMICALS IN THE AIR?

To determine which gaseous chemicals are being emitted in the air near your child's school or your home, urge an "on the spot" analysis (see American Environmental Health Foundation, in Resources). For a discussion about such chemical emissions and exposures, contact the Citizens Clearinghouse for Hazardous Wastes (see Resources).

IS OUR GOVERNMENT FOR THE PEOPLE OR FOR BIG BUSINESS?

There are countless examples of the U.S. government's failure to protect the health of citizens. For instance:

■ The Department of Agriculture insisted that California fumigate its fruits with ethylene dibromide, another potential cancer- and birth-defect-producing substance.

■ By law, a product that kills 50 percent of the laboratory animals exposed to it through ingestion or inhalation can still receive the federal regulatory designation "nontoxic"![29]

■ An insect repellent called DEET has unquestionably caused innumerable health problems and even deaths. Yet the state of New York recently rescinded its ban on insect repellents containing over 30% DEET.[30] The information about "inert" ingredients may not appear on those sheets—*even though this information is critical to the health of everyone at the school*. Again, our laws unquestionably and repeatedly protect industry rather than the public.

■ PEST MANAGEMENT

WHAT SHOULD YOUR SCHOOL DO?

To evaluate your school's pest-control program, begin by finding out exactly which pest problems exist in your school. At the same time, if you feel the students and teachers are less healthy after pesticide applications, study the Material Safety Data (MSD) sheets, which list the active ingredients in all the products that were used (see Appendix).

As part of your assessment of your school's program, keep these common causes of pest problems in mind:

■ overwatering of lawns and landscape beds
■ poor sanitation
■ leaky faucets
■ broken screens
■ improper food storage
■ ineffectual pesticide sprays
■ indiscriminate killing of insect predators, parasites, and disease pathogens

If your school's present pest-control program is not effective, entirely safe, and cost-effective, you should consider urging the school board and school administrators to implement a biologically safe form of pest control.

Organizations that can help you with safer pest management are listed in Resources. Integrated Pest Management (IPM) programs incorporate safer, cost-saving control measures for ants, fleas, roaches, lice, termites, weeds, plant diseases, and vectors such as mice and rats.

Urge your school administration to request an IPM evaluation. IPM experts can evaluate the extent of your school's problems and the effectiveness of current pest-control methods, and then make suggestions concerning what is needed.

IPM stresses prevention, but unfortunately there are times when some least-toxic methods of pest control must be used. Only if it is absolutely necessary, and only as a last resort, should *ANY* possibly toxic substance be used in or near a school. Pesticide spraying in school buildings (or home areas) on an arbitrary schedule, *regardless of the genuine need for pest control*, is not only not sensible, it can be dangerous.

To carry out an IPM program properly, *everyone concerned* must be educated. Key maintenance employees must learn exactly how to eliminate a pest problem and keep it in check. The initial improvement is only the beginning, however, and ongoing maintenance and monitoring are essential. Policies and procedures must be routinely implemented to eliminate any existing pest problems and to prevent future ones. This approach, in the long run, provides cost-effective pest control.

Overall, IPM programs can vary a bit, but they usually include the following:

- Excluding pests from their food supply
- Trapping and monitoring various pests
- Teaching custodians and food-service and garbage-management personnel exactly why, when, and how to do what is needed.
- Using pest-management tools
- Educating all teachers, parents, and older children about pest control.

Some school systems end up *reducing* their pest-management costs by as much as 80 percent, while successfully and safely eliminating most pests, using IPM. One school district in Arizona that implemented IPM reduced its pest-control budget from $46,000 to $14,000 in the first year. No wonder these programs are now being mandated or initiated in school districts in Maryland, Florida, Texas, California, Illinois, Pennsylvania, New York, Oregon, Michigan, and Arizona. Their suggestions are practical and sensible, as indicated below.

OTHER OPTIONS

A number of other nontoxic pest control measures are available for schools, homes, and businesses.

TAKING ACTION

Here are a few practical, commonsense aspects of integrated pest management programs:

- *Store foods in designated areas, not in drawers, lockers, or buses. Immediately remove food scraps and empty wastebaskets.*
- *To eradicate rats, let them sip some Miller Lite beer. The carbonation produces gas. Rats cannot belch, so they die. (This is very cruel; cage traps are more humane.)*
- *To kill ants, set out a bowl of cornmeal and a bowl of water. The ants will swell up and burst. Use plain boric acid as bait.**

Another way to kill ants is to mix 3 cups water with 1 cup sugar and 4 teaspoons borax. Soak cotton balls with this mixture, and place them in a jar with tiny holes in the cover. The ants will find the mixture in the jar and be killed.

For anthills, pour boiling water or 1/2 tablespoon cornmeal with 1/4 tablespoon soy oil and 1/4 tablespoon boric acid over the area.

- *To eradicate roaches, use boric acid near the floor edges, sink drains, and structural cracks and crevices where roaches tend to walk. Use sticky traps, and caulk and seal obvious cracks.*
- *To detect fleas, wear white socks. You can easily see the fleas on the socks as you walk in a contaminated area. Vacuum thoroughly, and use flea traps or sticky paper.*
- *To get rid of flies, use nontoxic biodegradable sticky tapes or traps.*
- *To eradicate termites, use harmless nematodes.*
- *To eliminate meal moths, use Biolure, which contains a pheromone sexual attractant in a sticky container.*

* Avoid using boric acid near children or pets. It is very poisonous.

- Praxis, Pest Management Advisory Group, has a number of specific controls for pests, gypsy moths, as well as drain and septic tanks odors.
- Earthtek Corp. repels ants, ticks, roaches, scorpions, moths, flies, aphids, etc. with negative ions using their "Bug Banisher."

For more information about these control measures, see Resources.

■ CARPETS

THE EPA LEARNS ABOUT CARPET SAFETY THE HARD WAY

In 1987, after the EPA installed synthetic carpets in its main offices in Washington, painted the walls, and replaced the furniture, some employees collapsed and were rushed to the hospital with symptoms typical of chemical sensitivities. The building had to be evacuated a number of times. Initially, this medical crisis affected more than 122 employees. For many months, the EPA repeatedly denied any cause-and-effect relationship. As a result, more than a thousand frustrated EPA employees rallied in front of the building in 1988 because the carpet had not been removed.

Improved ventilation measures and carpet cleaning failed to resolve the problem. Finally, in 1989, the EPA took out 27,000 square yards of the carpeting. The EPA provided alternative work space in other buildings for some of the most severely affected individuals. A few employees were placed on permanent disability.

The EPA's own carpet problem ironically raised the agency's awareness of the actual and potential health hazards of some carpets. In 1989 William Herzy, an EPA union official and senior scientist, said that the problem was related to 4-PC (4-phenylcyclohexene), a key component in the styrene butyl rubber used to bond carpet fibers to their backing. At some point the EPA decided it would never again install carpets on its premises that emit this chemical. *We must respectfully ask: If carpets containing styrene butyl rubber and 4-PC are not safe for EPA employees, why are they safe for the rest of the American public?*

Over eight years have elapsed, yet the EPA has still issued no official statement on the potential risks associated with the chemicals that were thought to be factors in this health crisis. The EPA staff continues to be protected from certain suspect chemicals in carpets, *but the agency has not, as yet, completed the comprehensive scientific evaluation that is necessary to assure the safety of Americans in regard to common carpet-chemical exposures.*

In 1990 the EPA held a dialogue with carpet industry officials, during which the agency apparently promised to restrict its evaluation to the total volatile organic chemical emissions and not to the health effects! If the EPA did make such a promise, why would it agree to such a stipulation? Who is it protecting?

In 1996 the chronic toxic effects of carpet chemicals continue to be inadequately evaluated, even though there has been an *immense* number of health complaints related to carpets. These complaints have been lodged with federal agencies, including the EPA and the Consumer Product Safety Commission, as well as with the carpet industry itself. One must ask why there has still been no definitive action when ever-increasing numbers of people appear able to trace the onset of their acute or chronic, potentially permanent health, memory, and mood problems directly to the installation of synthetic carpeting in their school, home, or workplace. The public deserves to know which carpets and carpet products are safe and which are not.

HOW A NEW CARPET CHANGED ONE FAMILY'S LIFE

The Sands Family

In March 1985 the entire Sands family—including three children and a pregnant mother—became ill shortly after they were exposed to 130 yards of common carpeting. Little did they know that that experience would dramatically and permanently change their lives.

The carpeting was removed three weeks later, but the family had to leave their home for several more weeks. Each time they tried to return, all the family members became very ill again. Their home had changed so dramatically that it was no longer habitable. They did not really begin to improve until they permanently moved from this house four years later.

By 1995, ten years later, the Sands family had lost their original home, fought the medical establishment, been called crazy by doctors, friends, and family, and endured an exhausting, costly legal battle with a corporate giant. The health and well-being of the Sands children continues to be tenuous, causing daily concern, worry, and challenges.

The Evolution of the Illness

Let's go back and look more closely at the plight of this family. Immediately after the installation of carpeting in their home, a strong odor seemed to cause all the children and both parents to experience severe headaches. The odor was initially thought to be formaldehyde, but an analysis showed it contained 4-PC and dimethylformamide. The carpet installers only laughed when the mother, Linda Sands, questioned them about the safety of the fumes.

Because of the intensity of the family's headaches, their physician advised, them to "Air out the house." In a frigid winter, however, that was impractical. The state health department did not respond to the family's calls for more than six weeks, so they contacted an environmental lab on their own.

Even after the carpeting was removed, and after they had lived away from the house for several weeks, the family's health problems continued. The residual chemicals that permeated their house—including their home furnishings, and even the walls—continued to bother them. They had all become chemically sensitized.

While the Sands family were getting sicker and sicker, Linda realized she was pregnant. Her fear for her unborn child was enormous. It was a mother's worst nightmare. At that time, her own health was terrible. Shortly after the carpeting was installed, she had felt that her lungs were on fire. She had developed body aches, nausea, unexplained body bruises, double vision, frequent urination, diarrhea, knifelike headaches, tender painful skin, sinus infections, extreme body tremors, facial numbness, burning skin, short-term memory loss, difficulty walking, and burning pain in the right shoulder, throat, and chest. Her skin became so sensitive that she cringed at the slightest touch. But as with her other symptoms, her skin did not become painful until shortly after the carpet was installed.

Linda's concern for her unborn child turned out to be justified. The baby girl was born prematurely and was very unhealthy. She seemed extremely lethargic and developed chronic ear, sinus, and respiratory infections shortly after birth. Her voice tended to be hoarse, and she choked frequently. When she tried to learn to walk, she fell more than was normal. Her parents recognized that something was terribly wrong.

In addition, Beverly, the older daughter, developed bronchitis, respiratory problems, chronic headaches, fatigue, sores in her mouth, twitches, and chronically chapped lips. She still coughs for weeks at a time, even when not exposed to carpeting.

Lois, her younger sister—who was three years old when all this started—developed excessive throat and ear infections, dizziness, headaches, asthma, burning and spasms of her throat, and lost the bladder control she had had for eighteen months. She began to sleep in a curled-up fetal position with clenched fists, and at times she would awaken trembling and shaking. She had to leave preschool because she was so tired; since then, regular schooling has been impossible because of her chemical sensitivities. Her white-blood-cell count became so low—only 1,800 to 2,000—that I urged the family to receive chemical detoxification immediately. (A normal count is 5,000 or above.) A seven-week detoxification program helped the entire family, but ten years later, Lois still becomes ill when exposed to chemicals.

The younger boy, Jeremy, slept all the time and was unable to do his schoolwork. He almost seemed to be in a trance. He would come home from school, and within twenty minutes he would fall asleep on the couch, sleep through dinner, and have to be carried to bed. He was too tired to play soccer and complained of nausea, burning airways, severe headaches, asthma, memory loss, and weak legs. Ever since the carpet exposure, he has had chronic neck aches and extreme fatigue whenever he is exposed to chemicals.

His older brother, Charles, had to quit track because of extreme fatigue. He also wheezed so badly after he ran that all his sports activities had to be sharply curtailed. He experienced headaches and nausea. He had allergies as a young child, but had been well for many years prior to the new carpet exposure. After the exposure, however, he developed a burning throat, headaches, fatigue, chest pain, and bronchitis. Since then he has had immediate breathing problems—and his arms and legs occasionally become numb especially when he is exposed to chemicals in stores, cars, or buildings.

The father, Phil, had a history of migraines as a child, but he had suffered few attacks as an adult. After the carpet was installed, however, he had daily headaches, accompanied by a burning nose and throat. (When the family finally moved out, Phil cleaned the house. Then he suddenly developed prostate problems with bleeding. Maybe it was unrelated, but he had had no previous history of this problem.)[31]

Taking Steps Toward Healing

Three years after the new carpet was installed, an occupational health specialist advised the family to move out of the house. Anderson Laboratories performed a bioassay test (described in detail in Chapter 13), which proved that a three-by-twelve-inch piece of this carpet was extremely toxic to mice. During the test, the mice tended to cower in the corners, crying in pain if a single tiny puff of air was blown on them. (Linda Sands's skin pain was similarly sensitive.) This carpet was found to be the most toxic that that laboratory had ever examined. The test could not be completed because none of the mice lived beyond the third hour of exposure.

After weeks of detoxification, the family had to spend their limited remaining resources on building a low-toxicity home. The children's health became more stabilized in the new environment, and Linda felt that she finally had her children back after six long years.

Then it happened again. Jeremy suddenly became so tired that, he again seemed to be in a trance. The family learned that a new carpet had been installed in his school in August. His new flare-up of symptoms subsided as soon as he stopped attending that school.

An Update

The Sands family are all much better now, but ten years later, the symptoms of the chemical sensitivity still continue to plague each of them. The two youngest children are not allowed to attend school because their parents fear the effects of accidental or purposeful chemical exposures. The children continue to have problems in some stores and from other inadvertent exposures.

Charles and Beverly are now adults. Charles moved into a ten-year-old condominium, and within a week, he experienced the same fatigue, chest pain, and shortness of breath of the type he had manifested a decade before. Even though the carpet in the condominium had no obvious odor, when the rest of the family came to visit him, they could stay for only about forty-five minutes. They all developed muscle pain or illness within minutes, and one of the girls developed a swollen face, nausea, and a headache. She remained ill for two weeks. Lois screamed and went totally out of control for about ninety minutes, then began to cough and became exhausted. Interestingly, the condominium carpeting had been installed at about the same time as the type in their original home, and it appeared to be remarkably similar.

Providing they remain extremely careful and avoid being exposed to chemicals, the Sands family remain improved due to a second detoxification program and their commitment to eat organic food, drink pure water, and stay away from chemicals. They have totally changed their lifestyle. Linda remains so fearful, however, that her younger children have remained on home teaching. Each time they try to return to school, some random chemical exposure causes a recurrence of their respective illnesses.

Linda is writing a book, *God's Answer to a Mother's Plea,* in which she discusses how she was spiritually helped, bit by bit and day by day, to cope with her family's tragedy. Injustices and illnesses kept happening to this family as they struggled to restore their lost health. And although everyone is presently better, their individual symptoms quickly return after any inadvertent chemical exposure. We must be concerned about other families who are similarly ill but have no idea what is causing their illness.

SYNTHETIC CARPETS—HOW IT ALL BEGAN

Problems associated with carpeting are nothing new. In the 1970s, the Consumer Product Safety Commission first began receiving calls about illnesses related to new carpets. Acute and chronic health problems would often begin within a few hours or days after the installation of a synthetic carpet. At that time, formaldehyde was thought to be the major offender.

By 1982 a rapidly increasing number of mild to extremely serious health and emotional problems were reported as a possible result of exposure to new synthetic carpets. The padding and adhesives used in installation were also suspect. From the beginning, however, many "experts" have either ignored carpet problems or have chosen to deny them aggressively. Literature from the Carpet and Rug Institute (CRI) has stated that those who are ill have merely chosen to believe that they are breathing something noxious and that anxiety is causing their health problems.[32] The CRI might want to talk with Nancy Harvey Steorts, former chair of the Consumer Product Safety Commission, who was forced to temporarily abandon her home after a new carpet made her extremely ill.

THE 4-PC QUESTION

There are two prime suspects in carpeting problems, and they are found in about 95 percent of all synthetic carpets: styrene and butadiene. These two chemicals combine to form a latex adhesive that locks carpet fibers in place on their backing. Their union creates the by-product called 4-PC (4-phenyl-cyclohexene), the chemical that was identified with the EPA's carpeting problems. 4-PC is apparently one cause of the distinctive, unpleasant odors given off by some new synthetic carpets. It is thought to pose a potentially serious health threat to susceptible individuals, although this suspicion requires more in-depth study.

Unfortunately, once an individual is sensitized to it, any item containing this styrene-butadiene latex combination may cause symptoms. *Some latex-based wall coverings, certain indoor and outdoor paints, caulk, sealants, tires, and a wide variety of rubber products and clothing, can contain this combination, and produce the same complaints associated with exposure to a synthetic carpet.*

This carpet-bonding agent is only one of many potentially toxic or neurotoxic (nerve-damaging) substances found in some carpets (see Table 10.2). Many of today's carpets contain a smorgasbord of chemicals capable

---

TABLE 10.2

A Few Common Carpet Chemicals

acetone	undecane	decane
bis (2-ethylhexyl) phthalate	caprolactam	toluene
benzene	diethylene glycol	diisocyanate
ethylybenzene	formaldehyde	vinylcyclohexene
12-propylbenzene	hexane	4-phenylcyclohexene
p-dichlorobenzene	styrene	xylene

of causing a variety of adverse effects in sensitive individuals.[33] Some carpets contain forty or more chemicals that have *not* been evaluated for safety. In nineteen carpets that have been evaluated by the EPA, a total of sixty-four neurotoxic chemicals have been found.

Other chemicals are intended to make carpets mold- and stain-resistant and waterproof. Collectively, all these chemicals, plus those used for carpet installation and in carpet pads, can number as many as 120. Some are toxic, carcinogenic, or known to lead to abnormalities in newborns. For example, many synthetic carpets contain benzene, a known cause of leukemia in children. Others contain toluene, formaldehyde, styrene, dichlorobenzene, phthalates, and xylene. All of these have been reported to cause neurological damage and/or emotional problems (see Appendix).

THE FORMALDEHYDE PROBLEM

An authoritative health or government agency has its own criteria for "acceptable" levels of chemicals that nonetheless cannot be tolerated by sensitive children or adults. Such levels generally refer to *what appears to be tolerated by most individuals.* Unfortunately most chemically sensitive people typically tolerate levels that are *considerably lower* than what is officially "acceptable."

For example, the acceptable indoor level of formaldehyde is 0.1 ppm.[34] This level is well-tolerated by *most* individuals and is far below the recognized toxic level. An indoor formaldehyde level that is ten times the "acceptable" level, however, or 1.0 ppm, is clearly recognized by government agencies as hazardous. The problem is that people who are extremely sensitive to formaldehyde cannot tolerate even the minute amounts found in cosmetics, toothpaste, facial tissues, soft drinks, and beer. The larger amounts found in polyester clothing, wallboard, plywood furniture, and many synthetic carpets and cotton mattresses definitely can cause illness (see Chapter 7). This is true even at levels much lower than 0.1 ppm.

A person's ability to tolerate formaldehyde, therefore, is not always dependent upon the *level* of formaldehyde but on how *sensitive* that person is to the level to which he or she is exposed. As more and more people are becoming sensitized and ill when they are exposed to the present "acceptable" level, this level should be lowered to afford these individuals more protection.

PROVING THE EXISTENCE OF A CHEMICAL PROBLEM

There are easy ways to measure the level of specific chemicals in indoor air, as well as in the bloodstream (see Resources). Your doctor can order tests to confirm whether your blood contains too much of a given chemical (see

Chapter 13). You can contact the American Environmental Health Foundation has a portable machine to accurately ascertain if the level of a specific chemical is too high in a particular location (see Resources).

Here are the key ways to evaluate whether a person's health problem is caused by exposure to a chemical:

History and Physical Examination

Note whether:

1. The onset of symptoms coincided with the time of a new or large exposure to a certain chemical.
2. The physical examination revealed evidence of allergies or nervous system and/or other organ damage. (Be sure to see a doctor who knows about chemical sensitivities for the necessary documentation.)
3. The health problems are typical of those associated with the specific chemical exposure.

Air-Quality Testing

Note whether:

4. An excessively high level of the chemical in question is found in the air in an area where the person was exposed.

Blood and Urine Testing

Note whether:

5. An excessively high level of that same chemical is found in the blood, urine, or tissues (such as fat) of that person (see Chapter 13). Other evidence of damage to the nervous system may include a decrease in an enzyme called cholinesterase. The blood should be examined *as soon as possible* after an exposure. Evidence of damage to the immune system can be documented by certain laboratory tests, but the time of the exposure in relation to the time of the blood and/or urine collection can be critical.

This advice, however, is not always practical because ailing individuals might not suspect that a certain exposure was the cause of their illness for several weeks. Many do not want to become ill again through a purposeful reexposure. It is possible that your health providers might not know exactly where to have certain tests performed or what to test. They might have the correct blood or urine collection materials or tubes (see Chapter 13). The laboratory can advise you concerning the best times to collect blood and urine samples.

Allergy Testing

6. Note whether a single-blinded challenge skin test, using an allergy extract made from the carpet or room air and conducted with appropriate placebo or mock controls, reveals a sensitivity.

   An open challenge can be done with a specific suspect substance using a chemical testing booth at an environmental medical facility.

   All such challenges and their associated responses should be videotaped (see Chapter 13). Even if such testing is stringently controlled and blinded, skeptics will tend to attribute the person's symptoms to emotions.

Brain-Image Testing

Note whether:

7. Brain-imaging techniques (qEEGs or SPECT tests) show that the blood flow or function of the brain is altered shortly after a chemical exposure (see Chapter 13).

Mouse Testing

Note whether:

8. Bioassay challenge testing, which purposely exposes mice to suspect chemical vapors from carpets, for example, further documents cause-and-effect relationships. During such testing, the effects on the mice are objectively and scientifically monitored (see Chapter 13).

   Do not be swayed by the negative opinions of others concerning this type of scientific evaluation, unless you have checked into any possible vested

---

WHO PROVIDES CARPET SAFETY INFORMATION?

Fortunately, a number of resource aids are available to help keep the public informed about carpet concerns. The National Center for Environmental Health Strategies is a public advocacy clearinghouse that collects data about reported carpet problems and provides information and direction toward solutions. Pertinent information is also available from Environmental Education and Health Services, and in Glenn Beebe's *Toxic Carpet III*. (For sources of all these aids, see Resources).

For the other side of the issue, the carpet industry has its own 1995 report, which in essence states that vinyl tile, with installation and maintenance, is dustier and more expensive than carpets; according to the industry, their data suggest that tile may "outgas" more chemicals than carpeting.

interest on the dissenters' part. (These methods are undoubtedly scientific, reliable, honest, and urgently needed, not only for carpets but for the many other potentially dangerous substances to which we are all exposed on a daily basis.)

Neuropsychiatric Examination

Note whether:

9. A neuropsychiatric examination helps to differentiate a true physical illness from a purely emotional problem (see Chapter 13).

CARPETS IN SCHOOLS

Now let's talk specifically about schools. From the environmental medical point of view, carpets should *not* be placed in schools. The benefit of noise reduction in no way compensates for the introduction of potentially harmful chemicals, some with such serious risk sequelae. We cannot ignore the animal studies. A large percentage of synthetic carpets seem to produce adverse effects in mice—particularly carpets that have an SBR (styrene-butadiene rubber) backing. Wooden flooring or hard vinyl tile would be a better choice (see Resources). Another good choice would be a carpet that has unquestionably been *proven* to be environmentally safe (see Resources).

LEARNING AFFECTED BY CARPETS

Warren

Eleven-year-old Warren always did well in school. His grades were continually in the ninetieth percentile. But shortly after his public school installed a new carpet, Warren developed multiple ear infections—and his grades progressively declined. He scribbled and erased so much that he could not complete his assignments. He found it impossible to sit still. His mother suspected that molds or chemicals, such as phenol, in the new carpet were at fault. She had her son transferred to an older Catholic school, which had wooden floors. In a few weeks, his grades dramatically improved and returned to their previous high level.

Warren's phenol-related sensitivity was confirmed during P/N allergy extract testing (see Chapter 13). One drop of a phenol extract caused him to repeatedly erase, and he could not draw or write as well, or as quickly, as usual. Then, after one drop of the correct weaker dilution of phenol allergy extract, he wrote and drew without any hesitation or difficulty. Changing schools resolved his problem, but it was not without a price. He had to leave all his school friends, and his parents now have to pay for his education in a private school because he cannot tolerate any other local public schools in his area.

Remember, chemically contaminated carpets pose a much greater potential health problem for children than for adults. All carpet pads and installation glues also must be critically evaluated for safety. All carpets retain dust and molds, so they present an obvious potential risk for allergies. In today's world (carpeting also has been shown to contain as many as ten thousand germs per square foot![35]) Nose bleeds, bowel or bladder accidents, or vomited material on a carpet can pose a risk for serious communicable illnesses such as hepatitis and AIDS. Tracked-in pesticides, lead, heavy metals, and cleaning chemicals retained in carpets compound the risks. Studies have indicated that pesticides tend to accumulate in carpets; in fact, more and higher concentrations of pesticides have been found in carpet dust samples than outdoor soil, where the elements and microbial action can break them down.[36]

CARPETS ARE A UNIVERSAL PROBLEM!

Rossella

One mother in Italy wrote to our center to tell us what happened after new carpets were installed in her daughter Rossella's school. Approximately half of the installation took place during school hours. Shortly after the carpets were laid, Rossella had a recurrence of asthma while other children in the classrooms developed nausea, vomiting, respiratory infections, and breathing difficulties. The response of the school officials was similar to many educational facilities in the United States: "It's just a cold or flu." They refused to check the school's ventilation.

Four weeks after the carpet installation was completed, Rossella's mother sat on the newly carpeted floor with her kindergarten child, and her own eyes stung from the "sickening new carpet smell." The windows were shut tightly, and the heat had been turned on. A local environmental hygienist assured her that Rossella's neurological and respiratory symptoms were temporary and no serious health problems could arise from the exposure. However, the chemicals in that carpet and/or adhesive were later found to include hexane, toluene, ethyl alcohol, and methyl alcohol. This mother's concern that continued exposure to the new carpet could possibly hurt Rossella was certainly justified.

WHO CHECKS SCHOOL CARPETS FOR SAFETY?

The Vermont laboratory of Rosalind Anderson, Ph.D., evaluates the safety of carpets using a Bioassay technique. This means that air is blown over suspect items, such as carpeting, and into a glass chamber which contains four mice. She can observe obvious and subtle changes that occur in the mice and objectively measure the degree of airway irritation or spasm, muscle, skin, and nose changes, as well as difficulty learning a maze. Hundreds of carpets, varying in size and age, have been studied at her facility. Some of the carpets have had no effect on mice; others have caused rashes, bleeding, congestion, and paralysis in some mice. Some have even died within fifteen minutes.

Approximately three hundred consecutive carpet samples were sent to Anderson Laboratories by clients who indicated that the samples had made them ill. When these samples were tested, all but three caused the test mice to become ill. In fact, about 80 percent of randomly purchased carpet samples cause illness of varying severity in the mice.

(In addition to carpets, Anderson Laboratories tests a wide range of common items, such as plywood furniture, tile, common cleaning agents, disinfectants, and even samples of air. Similar studies should be conducted on mattresses, pillows, shower curtains, and items that are in direct and prolonged contact with infants, such as plastic baby bottles, baby mattresses, and disposable diapers.)

As you do your own research into this subject, you may encounter a number of carpet producers with safe-sounding names who *claim* their carpets are natural and harmless. Some say that the safety of their carpets has been evaluated, but their supporting data does not include any animal studies. We called a number of such manufacturers and urged them to send a sample to Anderson Laboratories. Of the very few who did submit a sample for *a preliminary evaluation*, only two received a favorable report (see Resources). The video *Environmentally Sick Schools* clearly demonstrates the effect of a year-old piece of nonodorous school carpet on test mice (see Resources). Many of the children and teachers remain ill four years after they were initially exposed to this carpet. The bottom line is obvious: we need to know if the chemicals found in carpets or pads, or the products used for their installation, can cause difficulty in infants, toddlers, children, adults, or pregnant women.

Skeptics of this type of Bioassay testing will say that if a mouse rolls over, twitches, shakes, and develops a serious nervous system problem after exposure to a carpet, it is only a mouse. They are entirely correct. *What happens to a mouse certainly is not equivalent to what happens to a child. If, however, an exposure causes similar medical symptoms in both the mice and children, the situation certainly needs careful and immediate consideration.*

A mouse is not a child, but if the odor given off by some item causes obvious illness, paralysis, or the demise of a mouse, do you want your child exposed to it?

Concern about carpets is not limited to the United States. In their book *Chemical Children*, doctors Peter Mansfield and Jean Monro discuss carpet problems in England, and doctor Klaus Runow has written about problems with carpets in Germany.[37] Clearly, the issue of pollution in our schools, homes, and workplaces has become a universal consideration.

THE CARPET INDUSTRY RESPONDS TO THE PROBLEM

Even though the carpet industry has supposedly received thousands of complaints since 1972, none were documented until 1980.[38] In the past, the Carpet and Rug Institute (CRI) denied the need to "warn" the public and insisted that carpets do not present a potential health hazard. But it now recognizes the public's concern and is doing research to identify harmful substances in carpets. The industry also has several teams of its own "investigators" who respond to consumer complaints. However, it is difficult to understand how these complaints can be conscientiously handled if the organization which employs the investigators does not acknowledge the potential health hazards, including possible toxic effects on the nervous system, caused by the highly dangerous chemicals in many types of carpets.[39]

The industry also independently implemented a "Green Seal" program, affixing green seals to carpets that are considered safe. *But the industry sets its own safety standards, and it requires only one piece of a specific line of carpet to be evaluated per year.* Of course the standards for carpets must be set by others. "Safe" carpets should not produce symptoms in mice or allergic or chemical sensitivity in any other individual.

In November 1993, the CRI voluntarily faced some of these issues, ironically even those not addressed by either the Consumer Product Safety Commission or the EPA. Carpets are now labeled with "consumer information" which includes an owner's manual and precautions about proper installation. But the labels can be tiny, at times lost in promotional material on the back of carpets, and lacking in critical information. How often do carpets that cause illness slip through the system without identification numbers? Nor do the warning labels list the specific chemicals found in the carpets, or explain the potential long-term health effects of those chemicals. For example, while some chemicals are thought to be expelled from a carpet within seventy-two hours, many others certainly are not; some carpets appear to pose potential health hazards for years, even when there is no obvious odor.

The "warnings" on carpets are somewhat reminiscent of the warnings about cigarettes and cancer, about lawn pesticides and their effect on hormones, and about sugar and food dyes in relation to hyperactivity. The opinions of those with vested interests must be taken with a bit of reserve and caution. In fact, supervision and cautions should be the duty of an impartial federal agency whose function is to protect the American public. Its gold standard in relation to carpets should be a simple one: To achieve a truly high level of safety, carpets must not cause illness. If individuals develop health problems from a carpet, the pad, or the installation materials, research is needed to provide meaningful answers *as quickly as possible.* The ultimate effects may not be inconsequential or insignificant. Remember, few things are of more importance than the brains and nervous systems of the present and next generation. When the stakes are so high, let us err on the side of caution until we have more unbiased data on carpet safety.

The ultimate concern cannot be the carpet industry's financial bottom line. The carpet industry certainly can produce entirely safe carpets if it earnestly desires to do so. We must do everything in our power to urge carpet manufacturers to make the changes that are necessary to protect our children and everyone else as soon as possible.

OTHER PROBLEMS RELATED TO TOXIC CARPETS

When dealing with the potential health risks of carpets, here are some other issues to keep in mind:

- *The impression that a toxic carpet can be left in place and "treated" if it no longer causes illness is not always valid. It is true, however, that time and increased ventilation, cleaning with very hot water and fast drying, heavy ozonation, and elevated temperatures or "baking" for prolonged periods all can sometimes help to a degree. But for some carpets and some individuals, these processes are simply not enough. Sometimes using "treatment chemicals" on carpets only adds another factor to the original problem (see Chapter 11).*

  In certain situations, the only answer is to remove the carpet. But even this can be potentially hazardous for those who do it. In addition, the strong initial odors and/or the removal process can leave a "residue" in the air that can permeate the furnishings (furniture, walls, drapes, and so on). This "residue" can make the contents of a school or home unsafe for habitation. Glenn Beebe observed that many spiders had normally been seen in his building, but only dead ones were found after he installed a new synthetic carpet that permanently ruined his own health, finances, and life.[40]

- *Many physicians are unaware of the possible health effects of carpet chemicals. They do not recognize, diagnose, or treat chemically related illness or sensitization caused by such exposures. Even some toxicologists do not recognize sensitivities due to low dose exposures to chemicals in spite of the many patients and papers that discuss this illness (see For Further Reading).*

CARPET MAINTENANCE

Unfortunately, the carpet dilemma goes beyond choosing the right carpet, pad, and adhesives; carpets need to be cleaned, and the cleaning agents must be chosen with care. For example, one ingredient found in most carpet and upholstery cleaners is perchloroethylene. This solvent is a commonly used spot remover and is a known cancer-causing agent. Other components of cleaners that can cause illness are naphthalene, ethanol, ammonia, detergents, and perfumes (see Chapter 7). (For safe carpet cleaners, see Resources.)

CARPET CLEANING CAN CREATE A HEALTH PROBLEM

Wallace

Nine-year-old Wallace, who was feeling and learning well while receiving comprehensive environmental medical care, suddenly became worse in school on a particular Monday morning. He realized that his vision was not right, and his eyes hurt. He could see small letters but not large ones. He experienced double vision and problems in differentiating colors. He complained of nausea, stomach pain, and headaches during school hours.

His mother noticed that his ears were abnormally red immediately after school. She knew that this clue suggested a possible harmful exposure. Her son's complaints began within fifteen minutes after he entered school that day, and they persisted for several hours after he returned home. When she checked with the principal, there was only one new variable: The school had cleaned its carpeting the weekend before. Fortunately, his symptoms gradually subsided during the next week.

About two years later, however, the identical problem recurred. Wallace suddenly developed similar visual problems. Again, they subsided in a few days. When his mother checked with the school, she found that the same carpets had been cleaned again in the same manner. The MSD sheet indicated the product used for cleaning contained mineral spirits, polyalkyl methacrylate, and a perfluoroalkyl ester.

We have no definitive proof, but it appears that some factor related to carpet cleaning triggers Wallace's visual problems, nausea, and headaches. How many other children might have similar symptoms, but no one spent the time investigating the cause?

Wallace's story clearly indicates that every time a child's symptoms recur, parents must attempt to find out why so that future flare-ups may be prevented. If you are suspicious, acquire MSD sheets for all the chemicals used to clean and maintain your child's school. Ironically, the chemicals used for maintenance and care of a carpet can sometimes cause more health problems than the chemicals in the carpet itself. Existing safe carpets in the school and home need to be cleaned safely and frequently. (Chapter 7 discusses how to do this.) Vinyl tile also must be maintained, but a review of the literature in the Carpet and Rug Institute's 1995 report states that there are no published assessments regarding chemical emissions from tile.[41] It is obvious, however, that freshly manufactured tile must be well-aired prior to installation, certainly before school sessions are resumed.

LEGISLATORS RECOGNIZE THE PROBLEM

Several U.S. representatives, particularly Bernard Sanders (I–Vermont) and the late Mike Synar (D-Oklahoma), as well as former New York State attorney general Robert Abrams, have been instrumental in increasing everyone's awareness of potential problems related to carpets. The carpet industry has responded, on its own initiative, more responsibly in some ways than our own protective governmental agencies.

Until more basic research is completed, it appears that no mandates or recalls of carpets are possible. Nevertheless, the public is increasingly recognizing the problems with carpets, and a solution must be forthcoming. Because of the many vested interests, however, it will probably not be resolved quickly. In the meantime, when it comes to carpet safety, everyone is on his or her own. The public, legislators, and the carpet industry must ultimately resolve this issue. The stakes are unbelievably high.

THE BEST WAY TO CHOOSE AND INSTALL CARPETS

If carpets are the only option in your child's school, their potential health hazards should be determined *prior to their purchase and installation*. Save your school system money and possibly some heartache by urging that synthetic carpets not be installed unless the selected carpet has been thoroughly investigated in advance by *an independent unbiased laboratory*. If a carpet is not "mouse safe" per Anderson Laboratories' standards, consider the possibility it might not be "child or adult safe." Unless a school administrator is absolutely positive that a specific carpet and installation materials are perfectly safe, they should not be purchased.

"Safer" linoleum, cotton area rugs, hard vinyl tile, and "safer" woolen carpets (and less allergenic adhesives), which have fewer chemicals and no waterproofing, are all available as alternatives (see Resources). Even the so-called "safer" alternatives, however, must be evaluated by an impartial laboratory. If your school is willing to pay an enormous amount of money to install carpets, it should also be willing to spend a relatively small amount to send a sample to a laboratory like Anderson Laboratories (see

Resources). An *impartial* scientific evaluation is important. Natural carpet materials may not be as safe as their advertising implies.

Care should also be taken with hard tile, although it has been used for many years without repeated reports of major illness after installation. In my opinion, an outstanding impartial evaluation by Mary Oetzel indicates that vinyl composition tile (VCT), rather than carpets, is definitely cost-efficient in school buildings.[42] Oetzel concludes that hard tile costs about half as much for installation, maintenance, and replacement. Whereas carpets need replacement approximately every eight years; hard vinyl tile needs replacing only once every thirty-three years.

In twenty years, the savings from using tile instead of carpets can run into the millions, Oetzel says. In one school system, the cost for 250,000 square feet of vinyl tile over a twenty-year period was estimated at $2.7 million, versus $5.4 million for carpeting. This is a savings of over $2 million for that school district alone.

However, these figures are at distinct odds with those listed in the Carpet and Rug Institute's 1995 report. In *Floorcovering Products for Schools*, CRI's data indicate that carpets last ten to twelve years, while tile lasts twenty to twenty-two years, and both need daily maintenance.[43] CRI concludes that it costs $88 more per year, over a period of twenty-two years, to install and maintain tile in comparison to carpets. The CRI report also states that tile is dustier and "outgasses" more chemicals than carpets. As mentioned earlier, the institute also implies that symptoms caused by new carpets are "perceived," not real; it claims that some chemicals in carpets are not emitted and therefore do not present a health risk. It further maintains that if carpets do "outgas" chemicals, they pose no risk of cancer. The CRI's bottom line: The low levels of toxicity from carpets present no risk to health.

I suggest that you read both reports and decide for yourself which seems most plausible: Mary Oetzel's study, or the information supplied by the carpet industry.[44]

CARPET ADHESIVES AND PADDING

Carpets should not be installed when school is in session, and several weeks should elapse before students and faculty are exposed (see Chapter 6). Of course, similar precautions should ideally be taken if carpet is installed in your home.

Urge that school administrators choose carpet padding and adhesive with extreme caution. The installation materials can be a potential health hazard, depending on the composition of the carpet padding and the adhesive used to hold the carpet in place. Little quality control exists for carpet padding, which is a serious problem since it is possible for each pad produced to vary slightly in composition.

In one school, at least 30 percent of both teachers and students became ill shortly after a new synthetic carpet was installed (see Chapter 11). The carpet was installed while school was in session, and the label on the adhesive read as follows:

> Use only with adequate ventilation. Notice: Reports have associated repeated and prolonged occupational overexposure to solvents with permanent brain and nervous system damage. Intentional misuse by deliberately concentrating and inhaling the contents may be harmful or fatal. Keep out of reach of children.

WHERE DO WE GO FROM HERE?

We are all exposed to carpets every day in schools, work areas, and homes. Until we can verify the safety of carpets, are we wise to allow millions of people of all ages to be exposed to them?

To repeat, more scientific studies are needed *as soon as possible*. While the existing reports are neither completely consistent nor conclusive, abundant evidence certainly shows that some carpets can cause serious, prolonged adverse health effects in some people. The carpet industry states that it wants to produce safe carpets, but it has given us little or no assurance as to which specific carpets are safe and which are not. This inordinate delay in scientific evaluation is unfair both to the public and to the carpet industry.

For years, the EPA, the Occupational Safety and Health Administration (OSHA), the National Institute for Occupational Safety and Health (NIOSH), and the CRI have tried to evaluate the complex variables and factors that must be fairly interpreted. The enormous political and financial ramifications of their decisions may jeopardize their ability to give full and fair consideration to the pressing health issues. The ultimate challenge must be to consider the following questions:

■ What are the health and learning effects of each one of the immense number of chemicals, including the "inert" substances (listed, in part, in Chemicals in Appendix), found in and on carpets, carpet padding, and carpet adhesives?
■ How do these chemicals affect infants, toddlers, children, pregnant and nonpregnant women, men, and the elderly?

If these questions constitute too great a challenge for fair federal evaluation, then *independent* private funding is essential and urgently needed.

We cannot continue to ignore the many schools that have had to be closed temporarily, and the many homes and buildings that can no longer be occupied, because of the sudden onset of "strange" illnesses *at the exact time that new carpeting was installed.*

The many children and teachers discussed throughout this book illustrate the immense suffering from health and memory problems caused by environmental exposures. There is too much evidence for us to continue to ignore that their bodies and brains can be damaged, especially their immune and nervous systems. The critical issue is not mice but humans, and the stakes are so awesome that we cannot wait any longer for the answers. The bottom line is that chemicals are making some children ill and adversely affecting their health and intellectual capacities. We must do something about it, and we must do it now.

NOTES

1. See Lewis Regenstein, *Cleaning Up America the Poisoned* (Washington, DC: Acropolis Books, 1993); and Marion Moses, *Designer Poisons* (San Francisco: Pesticide Education Center, 1995).
2. Ibid.
3. Joan Dine, "Toxic Reduction," chapter 8 of Naomi Friedman, *Greening Synagogues and Community Centers* (Takoma Park, MD: Shomrei Adamah, 1995); J. R. Davis, R. L. Brownson, R. Garcia, D. J. Bentz, A. Turner, "Family Pesticide Use and Childhood Brain Cancer," *Archives of Environmental Contamination and Toxicology* (Jan. 1993), pp. 87–92.
4. See Cindy Duehring and Cynthia Wilson, *The Human Consequences of the Chemical Problem* (Sulphur Springs, MT: TT Publishing, 1994); Regenstein, *Cleaning Up America*; and Moses, *Designer Poisons*.
5. Russell Jaffe and M. Hoffman, *16 Million Americans Are Sensitive to Pesticides* (Reston, VA: Health Studies Collegium, 1990).
6. See Duehring and Wilson, *Human Consequences*; C. Wilson, *Chemical Exposure and Human Health* (Jefferson, NC: McFarland and Co., 1993).
7. Moses, *Designer Poisons*; Allan Lieberman, Patricia Hardman, and Patricia Preston, "Academic, Behavioral, and Perceptual Reactions in Dyslexic Children When Exposed to Environmental Factors—Malathion and Petrochemical Ethanol" (Tallahassee, FL: Dyslexia Research Institute, 1981); "Family Pesticide Use."
8. See Dine, "Toxic Reduction," and "Family Pesticide Use."
9. EPA, *The Recognition and Management of Pesticide Poisonings*, 4th ed. (Washington, DC: Government Printing Office, 1989), number EPA-540-9-88-001, p. 73.
10. See Jaffe and Hoffman, *16 Million Americans*; G. Cannon *The Politics of Food* (London: Century Hutchinson, 1987); and C. Walder and G. Cannon, *The Food Scandal* (London: Century Hutchinson, 1987).
11. Frank A. Oski, *Don't Drink Your Milk* (Syracuse, NY: Mollica Press, 1983).
12. See Moses, *Designer Poisons*.
13. William Rea, *Chemical Sensitivity*, 4 vols. (Chelsea, MI: Lewis Publishers, 1996).
14. Nicholas Ashford and Claudia Miller, *Chemical Exposures: Low Level and High Stakes* (New York: Van Nostrand Reinhold, 1991).

15. For information on colleges that offer a specialty in environmental medicine, contact the American Academy of Environmental Medicine, listed in Resources.

16. William J. Rea et al., "Study on the Critical Reference Value from the Regression Equations Between Chlorinated Pesticides and Immune Parameters," *Environmental Medicine*, vol. 9, no. 1 (1991) pp. 10–16; and David Steinman and R. Michael Wisner, *Living Healthy in a Toxic World* (New York: Putnam, 1996).

17. See "Family Pesticide Use" (note 3).

18. Regenstein, *Cleaning Up America*; and Moses, *Designer Poisons*.

19. See Steinman and Wisner, *Living Healthy.*

20. Susan Kashner, "Dioxin: In the News and in Our Food," *New York Coalition for Alternatives to Pesticides News*, vol. 5, no. 3 (Summer 1995), pp. 1–2.

21. Ibid.; see also Marguerite Halloway, "Dioxin Indictment," *Scientific American* (Jan. 1994), p. 25; and Theo Colborn, Dianne Dumanoski, and John Peterson Myers, *Our Stolen Future* (New York: Dutton, 1996).

22. See Steinman and Wisner, *Living Healthy*; and Halloway, "Dioxin Indictment."

23. *Rachel's Environment and Health Weekly*, no. 432 (Mar. 9, 1995).

24. New Jersey Department of Health, *Hazardous Substances Fact Sheet* (Apr. 1989), pp. 1–6.

25. See EPA, *Recognition and Management of Pesticide Poisonings.*

26. "A Golfer's Mysterious Death Suggests That Lawn Care May Be Hazardous to Your Health," *People* (June 1986), pp. 105–09. See also "Family Pesticide Use" (note 3).

27. See *New York Coalition for Alternatives to Pesticides* (note 20).

28. Dine, "Toxic Reduction"; and "Family Pesticide Use."

29. Ibid.

30. Steinman and Wisner, *Living Healthy.*

31. See Rea, *Chemical Sensitivity*; and Rea, "Study on the Critical Reference Values."

32. *Floorcovering Products for Schools* (Dalton, GA: Carpet and Rug Institute, 1995).

33. *Informed Consent*, vol. 1, no. 1 (International Institute of Research for Chemical Hypersensitivity Nov./Dec. 1993), pp. 6–33.

34. See Carpet and Rug Institute, *Floorcovering Products.*

35. Roger L. Anderson, "Biological Evaluation of Carpeting," *Applied Microbiology* (1969), pp. 180–87, and Rosalind Anderson, "Toxic Emissions from Carpets," *Journal of Nutritional and Environment Medicine* (1995), pp. 5, 376–386.

36. R. G. Lewis et al., "Evaluation of Methods for Monitoring the Potential Exposure of Small Children to Pesticides in the Residential Environment," *Archives of Environmental Contamination and Toxicology*, vol. 26 (1994), pp. 37–46.

37. Peter Mansfield and Jean Monro, *Chemical Children* (London: Century Hutchinson, 1987), and Klaus Runow, *Klinische Ökologie* (Stuttgart: Hippokrates Verlag, 1994).

38. Beebe, *Toxic Carpet III.*

39. By Mary Oetzel of Environmental Education and Health Services (see Resources).

40. See Beebe, *Toxic Carpet III.*

41. See Carpet and Rug Institute, *Floorcovering Products.*

42. Mary Oetzel, *The Comparative Cost of School Floorcoverings* (Austin, TX: Environmental Education and Health Services, 1992, 1994). See Resources for publisher's address.

43. Carpet and Rug Institute, *Floorcovering Products.*

44. See also "Clean Schools, Safe Schools: An Operations Manual for Maintenance and Custodial Services," Texas Association of School Administrators; John W. Roberts et al., "Chemical Contaminants in House Dust: Occurrences and Sources," *Proceedings of Indoor Air '93*, vol. 2; J. Ratoff, "Home Carpets: Shoeing in Toxic Pollution," *Science News*, vol. 138, no. 6 (Aug. 11, 1990), p. 86.

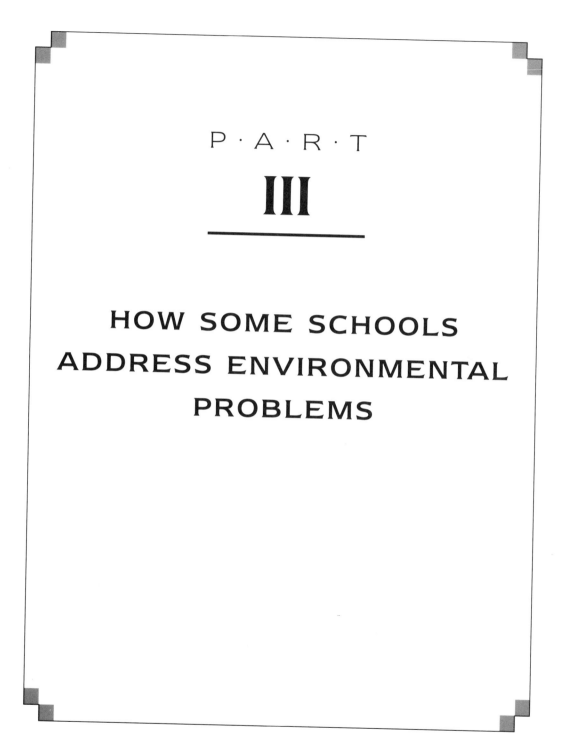

P · A · R · T

III

HOW SOME SCHOOLS ADDRESS ENVIRONMENTAL PROBLEMS

11 Lessons Learned from Sick Schools

Once problems develop in a sick school, they must be identified and corrected as soon as possible. In this chapter, I'll describe two sick school cases, and the lessons that can be learned from them. How did students, parents, teachers, and administrators face the problems? What did they say and do? The experiences of these schools illustrate how typical problems develop and either are sensibly resolved or are allowed to persist. The irresponsibility of some school administrators and other decision-makers, when it occurs, is most regrettable, particularly because the health of both our children and teachers is at stake.

■ GENERAL OVERVIEW

It is really quite easy to spot an environmentally contaminated school. Suddenly, many students and teachers develop similar symptoms at approximately the same time. If over 20 percent of students, teachers, and other school personnel are affected, the chances are excellent that environmental exposure is at fault. The major common symptoms are outlined in Chapter 2. They should not be summarily passed off as mass hysteria or a persistent, highly contagious flu.

Just before a sudden health crisis occurs, there is almost always a new factor that tips the balance, causing a tenuous situation to suddenly cause illness. Always look for a significant recent change in or around the school building. For example, poor air quality caused by excessive dust and/or molds might ordinarily be bearable; however, during renovation, when the air is further contaminated with chemicals, the combination of old and new pollutants can create an intolerable and even potentially health-damaging situation.

A school-related illness, like an environmental illness that occurs at home, is most apt to be noted shortly after a new school has opened or after an existing school has completed some major remodeling or renovation. The root of the sudden problem is usually much more complex than a slight inadequacy in a ventilation system, for example. Commonly, the problem begins shortly after a long school holiday or summer vacation, during which major repairs were done.

■ A SICK SCHOOL IN THE SOUTH

During the 1989–90 school year, students at a school in the southern part of the United States began experiencing unexplained multiple fainting episodes. The frequency of these episodes and the number of students affected grew rapidly and finally peaked in the spring of 1991. They experienced other significant health problems which included headaches, fatigue, and asthma. A few children were misdiagnosed as having appendicitis because of abdominal pain, but this can also occur in youngsters who have food and chemical sensitivities.[1] As parental concern mounted, the school system and the parents joined forces to find and eliminate the cause of the problem.

Initially, however, no one was equipped to handle this type of crisis effectively. Slowly, but surely, this changed. The parents' three-year struggle climaxed with the creation of a final report, written by their school's Advisory Committee which included school officials, to help others facing similar school-related problems. By sharing their own school's challenges and solutions, they hoped that other communities might avoid the unnecessary problems they experienced in their attempts to resolve their school's environmental crisis.

The sequence of events for this particular school was roughly as follows:

5/89 to 9/90:	Major renovations are made in the school building.
2/90:	One child faints.
9/90:	Another child faints.
10/90:	The office of risk management is contacted.
11/90:	The PTSA (Parents, Teachers, and Students Association) and the school administration begin monthly meetings. The number of fainting episodes increases each month.
12/90 to 6/91:	An indoor air-quality evaluation is made and reported on in January. A few minor problems are detected and corrected.

1/91:	As more students are affected and the frequency of fainting increases, concern about the health of the students intensifies.
2/91:	School officials contact representatives of governmental agencies, and attendance at monthly meetings increases.
4/91:	One student suddenly and mysteriously dies. This teenager's death spurs additional interest, urgency, and unity in the entire community. An indoor air-quality (IAQ) evaluation consultant is chosen.
5/91:	Until this time, most parents were totally unaware that other students, besides their own, were experiencing similar symptoms. At a community meeting, held fifteen months after the first child fainted, they finally communicate adequately with one another and realize they have a serious problem. Mothers and fathers form a parent group that begins meeting weekly. The school prepares a questionnaire for parents, to which about 50 percent respond. Of that group, 46 percent state that shortly after the renovations, their children developed complaints that interfered with their learning and/or health. Consultations are held with epidemiological and occupational health experts.
6/91:	The indoor air-quality report is released.
8/91:	A private environmental service inspects the school, and successful corrective measures are finally implemented.

It took much more than a year for the unsatisfactory conditions to be detected and corrected. The major problems were more than a combination of dust and molds associated with improper ventilation. New factors included outdoor and indoor chemicals associated with major renovations, as well as some plumbing irregularities. All were possible contributing factors, the apparent last straw that overwhelmed the health-safety tolerance level.

The renovation project had started in 1989, and was not completed until September 1991. Walls were torn down, and classrooms were created in an open space in the center of the building. In addition to the presence of many indoor chemicals, such as paint strippers and disinfectants, outside chemicals, such as pesticides, were entering the building. Air-intake grilles were covered with garden mulch. Not only did this decomposing organic material reduce the amount of fresh air in the building, but it introduced methane gas and molds into the ventilation system. In one building, the intake grilles on the outside wall had been mistakenly installed upside down, preventing rainwater from escaping through the "weep" holes. This stagnant water had made the ductwork moldy. The ventilation system was neither balanced nor fully functional for more than a year after the renovations were completed. This imbalance meant that different areas of the school had different levels of heat and even fresh air. Other significant problems included:

- The ductwork was disconnected in one large section of the ventilation system.
- One large connecting ventilation duct between floors was entirely missing.
- Sixty dry traps allowed sewer gases to infiltrate the building (enhanced by a negative air pressure inside the building).
- Natural gas plumbing was improperly installed.
- Bathroom sewer pipes were improperly capped.
- Paints and solvents were improperly stored.
- Fuel was leaking from the ground behind the school.

9/91:   As the various unacceptable conditions are corrected, the fainting episodes finally diminish markedly. Some problems persist, however, because the air quality is still not uniformly adequate throughout the building. However, the use of chemicals within the school has been sharply limited. Parents, teachers, and administrators are much more aware of the potentially harmful health effects of indoor pollutants.

10/91: One last fainting episode occurs in a known problem area that still has a "fishy, moldy" smell. Mold is found in the insulation of pipes in that area. Once that is corrected, the fainting finally stops.

11/91: The final health department report is issued.

2/94:   The parent group's final report is completed.

SUMMARY OF THE SOUTHERN SCHOOL'S EXPERIENCE

The lesson to be learned from this experience is that everyone's awareness and knowledge of environmental health problems must be heightened, so the sources of a school's crisis can be eliminated as quickly and effectively as possible. In addition, groups in affected schools should help other schools avoid similar problems by explaining what they did, what worked and what didn't, to help resolve their own schools' challenging environmental concerns. Students should not be used as "canaries in the coal mine" to determine that a new or remodeled building is safe or not safe. Environmental factors should be taken into account *before*, as well as during and immediately after, any construction of school buildings (as well as houses and offices) prior to their occupancy.

The health of the students at this southern school should be closely monitored in the future. How are they doing now, several years after the problems began? How will they be in the future? Follow-up studies should be conducted at regular intervals to compare those who were exposed and became ill with those who had no symptoms.

SUGGESTIONS FROM THE PARENT GROUP

Here are some of the recommendations made by the parent group in its final report. They may be applicable to managing problems within your child's school:

1. Screen and identify responsible consultants who can comprehensively assess a school building, its indoor air quality, and the students' health as soon as possible. At the southern school, *parents became increasingly concerned about the evaluation techniques and methodologies used by consultants to investigate the obvious environmental conditions.* Fortunately, in most middle-class school systems, at least some parents are professionals who have the expertise and background to fairly assess the competence of some experts. Ask them to help evaluate the recommendations of consultants, to determine if they are truly capable of recognizing, preventing, and resolving their school's problems.
2. Consult an experienced environmental health physician without delay. Most medical-school educations do not presently include the recognition and treatment of environmental allergies and chemical- or food-related illnesses. The health problems triggered by conditions in schools are often due to chemical sensitivities, not to a chemical toxicity. Physicians who evaluate ailing students and teachers must be well aware of this distinction.[2] Without such understanding, they can easily miss the correct diagnosis.
3. Arrange meetings of parents, teachers, and school officials, and properly moderate them to maintain control. Without a general meeting, where input from many people is solicited, it is impossible to determine the scope or seriousness of a problem. In the case of the southern school, a general meeting finally showed parents that their children's health problems were much more extensive, serious, and complex than they had anticipated.
4. Inform the school district and state education departments, as well as the local, county, and state health departments, of any localized, potentially serious school health problem and its ramifications.
5. Create advisory boards to address the many aspects of the problem. Each board should include parents, teachers, and school officials. Students should also have some input.
6. Keep everyone informed. In the southern school, people from

throughout the community were upset because school and health officials had initially addressed the problem in a manner perceived as arrogant rather than with compassion and understanding. These "experts" had interpreted the situation as arising from mass student hysteria rather than an indoor air-quality problem. They neither recognized nor addressed certain health problems associated with the fainting episodes—such as headaches, fatigue, and asthma—at any point during their evaluation. As parents and school personnel became more informed, they recognized the need for a clear-cut comprehensive approach to the health crisis.

7. The various agencies which are knowledgeable about sick schools must communicate with one another, as well as with the public. At the southern school, some agencies did not share data with others, nor did they contact consultants who might have had more expertise. This resulted in potentially harmful delays, as well as inadequate corrective measures and needless expense.

8. Each school must have adequate facilities and personnel to care for ailing students and faculty. School officials must keep detailed, accurate health records of attendance and health complaints. When asked to do so, they should promptly provide definitions of specific health problems so that symptoms can be compared and the degree of illness quantified. This southern school had only one clinic aide in its health office who was responsible for more than two thousand students, she simply was unable to assess the scope and significance of everyone's health problems.

9. Take measures to prevent future crises. Know who is responsible for procedures related to the building and its air quality, and for attending to the health concerns of those in the school. Precheck all new furnishings and all maintenance, construction, remodeling, and cleaning materials for possible safety and health risks. Conscientiously monitor all aspects of indoor air-quality compliance.

10. Compile and maintain a reference library of books, videos, and audiotapes about environmental issues so that everyone can become better informed (see For Further Reading).

11. Parents, teachers, and school officials should write articles for journals, discussing these serious school issues and providing insights to aid other school districts.

12. Obtain pro bono help from graduate students in health-related fields, and technical support from appropriate firms or knowledgeable individuals. One generous, caring expert who helped this southern school detected previously missed, significant sources of problems within half an hour. Caring, knowledgeable individuals who are willing and eager to help others do exist.

■ A SICK SCHOOL IN THE EAST

During the 1992 summer vacation, a school in the eastern part of the United States began making renovations. Because of unanticipated delays, carpets had to be installed within a few days after manufacture, while they still smelled strongly of chemicals. This carpet installation continued in certain areas of the school for a few weeks after classes were back in session. In addition, questions arose about the type and amount of glue used to install the carpet in certain heavily used areas. The glue later proved to be a major potential source of difficulty for both children and teachers.

What else happened at this school? Isocyanate insulation material was sprayed on the roof while students and teachers were in and around the building. This substance drifted through open windows onto students' desks, and equipment in the computer room, music room, and other areas. Staff members were asked to move their cars, but students were allowed to play on the school grounds, where some were accidentally sprayed. According to one young student, she had to wash the particles from her hair after holding open a school door while a worker, *who wore protective clothing*, was spraying the roof above her. Three years later, this girl reports continuing to have daily headaches, being unable to attend school, and, while previously an excellent student, now having memory and learning problems. Her account unquestionably makes her one of the sickest of the affected children. The seriousness of her exposures must be acknowledged and cannot be summarily dismissed, as some officials are prone to do.

Within two weeks after the school session began, other children began to develop many health problems (of the types listed in Tables 1.1, 1.2). These problems became progressively more apparent in both students and teachers each day. For the first time in their lives, some of them developed asthma and hay fever symptoms; those who already suffered from these symptoms tended to worsen. Some children experienced easy bruising, nosebleeds, or fainting. Some had such extreme fatigue that they could not remain awake and alert in class; several adolescent boys broke into tears because they were simply too tired to play ball. An increasing number of children and teachers also complained of various *combinations* of symptoms: headaches, recurrent flulike congestion or aches, fatigue, coughing, burning eyes and throat, hoarseness, rashes, loss of appetite, nausea, abdominal cramps, easy crying, and/or numbness or tingling of the toes, fingers, or face.

As time passed, the grades of some affected students gradually fell to lower levels than they had ever experienced. Increasing numbers of children and teachers had more and more difficulty remembering and concentrating. Behavioral problems, irritability, negativity, depression, and mood changes became increasingly evident. A few girls and female teachers developed unusual menstrual problems.

Most of these complaints surfaced within a few minutes to an hour after each school day began. Those affected often became progressively sicker toward the end of each day. Many children complained of burning eyes or throats, particularly early in the day; a few also developed blurred or double vision by the late afternoon. At first, the condition of most of the students and teachers improved one to four hours after leaving the school building, but later, the more seriously ill found that their symptoms did not subside until late Sunday afternoon. In time, the very sickest needed a long school vacation or holiday before they felt better. *Three years later, whenever the most seriously ill students and teachers entered that same school building, some of their original warning health and memory complaints recurred within minutes.*

Despite the many health problems in this school from September to December 1992, the school administrators introduced additional chemicals into the building over the Christmas holidays. New plywood cabinets were installed; this type of wood routinely "outgasses" chemicals such as formaldehyde. Odorous vinyl partitions were placed in other classrooms. A room with a poor architectural design was newly created in an alcove that had little ventilation. These additional exposures caused a fresh flare-up of symptoms in the previously affected students and teachers, as well as in others who had appeared to be well until that time.

Although the school administration acknowledged that there was a problem, the actions taken were unfortunately insufficient and the inadequate ventilation seemed to persist. For example, the administrators tried to use fans to better circulate and balance the air quality in certain areas. The sickest teachers and students routinely sat near windows that could be opened during the winter months, so they could intermittently put their heads outside to breathe cleaner but frigid air for a few moments.

HOW DID THE COMMUNITY REACT?

Let's now examine, in turn, how the school officials, school employees, health departments, teachers, parents, school nurses, and physicians dealt with these problems.

SCHOOL OFFICIALS
Initially, the school officials adamantly refused to transfer some of the students and teachers whose illnesses seemed directly related to being in the school. They ignored the medical warnings and directives of board-certified environmental medical specialists about the risks to specific children and

teachers who had become too ill to attend that school. Administrators continually tried to reassure everyone that the school was safe, asserting that sick children and teachers merely had a prolonged flu, mass hysteria, psychological problems, or some other preexisting condition. They did, however, admit that allergylike reactions that "are not too serious" could develop from products such as carpets.[3]

In March 1993 the school issued a report that said there were no indications that the air quality in the building was a problem. In July of that year, officials stated that there were no major problems with the heating, ventilation, or air-conditioning systems. All their subsequent reports indicated that the school was essentially safe. They stated:

> We recognize some people have been truly ill as a result of their level of sensitivity to the changes in the school environment. A few of these people have become more ill than most. . . . Some have become frightened and perhaps ill due to this, or exaggerated reports, misinformation, and rumors.[4]

SCHOOL EMPLOYEES

Cafeteria personnel admitted to using pesticides to control ants in the kitchen area. Custodians were aware of a natural gas leak near the intake of the ventilation system, and they admitted to parents that some of the gas was being sucked into the building each night. They also had to suction an unidentified liquid that routinely leaked onto the carpet in one particularly busy school area.

HEALTH DEPARTMENTS

County and later state health officials were asked to evaluate many of the early and subsequent health problems at the school. The initial report by the county health department revealed a number of deficiencies in the ventilation system. The indoor air was analyzed for certain gases and chemicals, and one office, for example, was found to have a higher-than-recommended level of trichloromethane (see Appendix). Inspectors reported "two very minuscule" natural gas leaks but said these leaks did not significantly alter the indoor air quality. A water heater sporadically leaked carbon monoxide, and they acknowledged that in several classrooms the carbon dioxide levels were generally above the accepted limits. The ventilation dampers were open to only 15 percent of their capacity. The dampers were adjusted, and recommendations were made to lower the carbon dioxide levels to below 1,000 ppm, but the health department repeatedly failed to respond to requests to provide explicit data about the specific carbon dioxide levels in the school.

Ironically, some of the ventilation intake and exhaust ducts were located at the ceiling level, which meant that that area was well-ventilated. The students, however, were at the floor level, which contained new carpet and adhesive chemicals and which was subject to an inadequate air exchange. In time, the air quality in some poorly ventilated areas was improved, thanks to the judicious placement of diffusers and exhaust fans, which helped distribute the inside air more effectively.

One air-quality evaluation had reported the presence of volatile organic chemicals "just above the detectable limits" in the air. These chemicals included trichloromethane, benzene, toluene, and methylene chloride (for details, see Chapter 7). So on several occasions in the fall of 1992, the school was closed while the building was "baked out" or heated to 85°F, which helped eliminate the chemical odors. Intensive heat can increase the "outgassing" of chemicals by 400 percent. The school building was then well-aerated after each baking to expel the released chemicals. Such an exchange of air can reduce the overall indoor chemical levels by 25 percent.[5]

The chemical used in the school roof was polymeric-diphenylmethane diisocyanate, a form of polyurethane (see Chapter 7). In low concentrations, it can cause nose, throat, lung, eye, and skin problems. Health department officials said they could not find this chemical in the air when they finally did their evaluations. Just before they made their inspection, however, parents noted that the doors and windows were opened wide, which would lower the CO_2 and chemical levels.

(As a parent, you should watch for any day or nighttime flurry of unprecedented activity in and around a possibly sick school, especially, immediately prior to a scheduled state health department inspection. Don't be surprised by a hasty, massive purge of possible suspect items just before an inspection. If any unusual school activities occur, you or another parent might want to videotape them.)

When the eastern school building was initially closed in October 1992, the smelly new carpets were sprayed with a water-soluble herbal deodorant. A liquid bacterial digestive enzyme was applied—which caused the carpets to feel slimy. Subsequently, the carpets were thoroughly cleaned. After these remedial changes, however, the health of some of the originally affected students and teachers became even worse once they returned to school. Their previous symptoms not only recurred, but a burst of new health problems became evident. In addition, other children and teachers who hadn't been symptomatic before now had various medical complaints related to the new aromas caused by the multiple chemical substances in and on the carpet. Eventually, one carpet was removed from a room, and some water-damaged tiles were repaired.[6]

In July 1993 a teacher was notified that some of those original materials collected from the school and stored by the health department had been ruined by a fire caused when a transformer blew out. Surprisingly, ten days later, an underground cable electrical problem damaged another stash of original school samples. Meanwhile, subsequent reports from health and school authorities consistently reassured everyone that the school air was improved and presented no significant health problem.

(At your own school, if it's legally possible, obtain permission to date, label, and save samples of all suspect school items. Keep them in glass jars in your own home. Accidents happen, and sometimes valuable "originals" are lost or destroyed.)

TEACHERS

Within a few hours after returning to school in September 1992, some of the teachers became ill. In early October an informal survey conducted by the teachers indicated that 43 percent (34 out of 78) of them were sick in some way; by the end of that month, 82 percent (64 out of 78) described having some of the symptoms listed in Table 1.3.

One teacher complained of headaches caused by the sickening-sweet enzymatic deodorant that had been used to reduce the new carpet's chemical odor. She said that one of her students had fainted. A few teachers reported they were repeatedly told by the school administrators that their illnesses were purely psychological.

One teacher noted a warning on the can of carpet adhesive that had been used to install the indoor carpets. This product's MSD sheet cautioned that this "petroleum process oil is considered a suspect animal carcinogen by the IARC. It contains aromatic hydrocarbons which may cause cancer based on animal data. Risk to your health depends on level and duration of exposure."[7] (Carpet adhesives can take a month to dry unless the ventilation is adequate. Adhesives often contain benzene, a hydrocarbon known to damage the nervous system and cause cancer. Because benzene is present in such a tiny amount in the mineral spirits used in adhesives, however, it is considered to be an "inert" ingredient. For this reason our government does not require the manufacturer to list it on the label. Ethylene glycol is commonly found in some school carpets also.[8] It can break down to ethylene, another hydrocarbon that can cause cancer or nervous system damage. Hydrocarbons and alkyd-aromatic thermoplastic solvents are also frequently present in carpets, but certain governmental agencies do not require MSD sheets to state that these are hazardous. Formaldehyde is another potentially harmful chemical in carpets. See Chapter 10 and Appendix for details about carpet chemicals and adhesives.)

Despite their health concerns, some teachers at this school reported they were repeatedly and strongly warned not to discuss the situation with anyone, or they would be "punished for insubordination." Many said they feared they would lose their jobs if they discussed, even with their own physicians, what was happening to them or what they had observed. Some also reported they received anonymous, threatening phone calls. (If you have such a problem, be sure to request Call Trace from the phone company. You simply dial a special "key" number after such a call, and for a small fee, the phone company will trace the call and turn the matter over to its Annoyance Bureau. Contact your local telephone company for more information.)

When sick teachers requested transfers to other schools, they were not always granted; *two years later, some teachers were still not having their illnesses taken seriously and were being told they could not switch to another school.* Several were forced to remain in the original building that had caused them to become sick, even though their illnesses became progressively more severe. They realized their health was probably being jeopardized, but their greater fear was the loss of a job and income. Nevertheless, one teacher became so concerned about the potential health risks that she refused to continue teaching; she told school officials that her classroom was unsafe both for herself and for her students. Another teacher eventually lost his job *and* his home and was forced to move back with his parents. He was diagnosed as having psychological problems, even though he had coped well *before* the school renovations. (Certain chemicals that can directly alter the nervous system and brain can also produce definite changes in behavior, mood, and memory. The stress that some of these teachers and students have endured since September 1992 has been so immense that it could understandably cause adverse secondary emotional effects.)

Six of the teachers were too ill to return to school in 1993. With the help of the teachers' union, some applied for workers' compensation. A few qualified for disability compensation, which was gradually tapered from full, to half, and then to one-quarter payments over a one-year period. Many teachers (and many students' parents) who had health insurance coverage nonetheless could not afford physician visits, diagnostic evaluations, blood tests, or treatments because there was little or no reimbursement. By 1994, three of the six teachers had returned to work, but no one in authority has accepted any responsibility for the health problems of the teachers and students. Nevertheless, for some, their lives and health probably will never be the same.

PARENTS

When their children initially became ill, many of the parents had no idea what to do or where to go for help. They were repeatedly assured by both school officials and local doctors that the problems weren't serious. At the time, there were no readily available avenues for parental communication, and the school appeared extremely reluctant to allow the parents to meet and discuss their common concerns.

Like several of the teachers, some complaining parents said they received anonymous threatening phone calls, warning them to keep quiet and not discuss any aspect of the school situation with anyone. A couple sets of parents reported they were even told that their children would be taken away from them and placed in foster care if the youngsters did not return to school, while others reported they were threatened that if they did not put their sick children back in school, they would be taken to court and fined for truancy. These parents refused to give in, however, because each time their children did return to school, they experienced an immediate flare-up of their illness. Two years later, in spite of a doctor's note, one mother was told to report to the police station. She thought she would be arrested, because her son had missed too many days of school because of sickness. Fortunately, the state health department intervened on her behalf.

The students, of course, had no union to look out for their interests. When the problems initially began, there were no large meetings where parents could compare their children's health problems and discuss their mutual concerns. Many parents remained uninformed about the patterns of illness and the potential seriousness of chemical exposures. Even though some youngsters routinely became sick whenever they went to school, their parents often had no idea, for example, that recurrent headaches, fatigue, or easy crying might be related to a chemical exposure.

After several months, one parent finally conducted an informal survey of parents; it showed that 30 percent of about four hundred students had developed medical symptoms during the month after school started in 1992. Although some parents had sought treatment for their children, few recognized the possible gravity of their problem, or the scope of the problem, for several years. The local newspaper, their sole source of outside information, continually reported statements by school officials that no serious problem existed.

During the period when the building was ''baked out,'' then aired out, the students and teachers were temporarily transferred to different schools. The majority of the ailing children and staff had fewer or no symptoms during that time, but upon returning to their original school building, some of their previous symptoms returned. Many parents did not have insurance that would pay for neurological, psychological, or environmental medical examinations. They had no money for expensive specialists, essential diagnostic blood tests, or special brain-image studies. Some of them could not even afford to buy glass-bottled or filtered water, organic food, and nutritional supplements. In desperation, some sought less expensive alternative forms of medical care, and at times, approaches such as homeopathy and acupuncture were surprisingly helpful.

SCHOOL HEALTH OFFICE PERSONNEL

When some of the sickest children went to the health office, a few were allowed to return home. Nurses or health aides repeatedly reassured the vast majority, however, that they were all right. These children were promptly sent back to their classes and some said they were forbidden to call their parents.

In spite of repeated parental requests, some health personnel refused to notify the students' mothers when their children complained of feeling ill. One nurse was overheard telling a child, "You can make it through the rest of the day." A number of parents wondered who had initiated this policy, and why caring nurses and other health personnel were acting in such an uncharacteristic manner.

PHYSICIANS

In general, local family physicians, as well as some medical specialists, diagnosed the children's illness as a prolonged flu. To be sure, many of the symptoms of a chemical sensitivity, such as headaches, joint pains, fatigue, nausea, dizziness, and weakness, are typical of flu.[9] Other physicians diagnosed these problems as hysteria and referred a few of the students and teachers to a psychiatrist.

As a physician, I was disappointed that some medical specialists refused even to see the ailing students and teachers after hearing details about the situation. One environmental medical specialist openly admitted that he did not want to become involved because he would eventually have to spend many hours collecting documentation related to probable litigation.

Many of the students and teachers were eventually seen by environmental medical specialists (including me or Dr. Patel), who noted that the majority had classic allergies and/or allergic relatives. For the most part, the patients who received the appropriate medical treatment for these conditions improved, but many others could not afford either an initial evaluation or the necessary continued care.

In the ensuing months, although the teachers tended to follow the recommendations for avoiding potentially allergenic items and chemicals better than the students, the children improved more quickly and to a greater degree. However, the teachers in general were sicker than most, but certainly not all, of the students.

THE FINAL OFFICIAL REPORTS—AND THE FOLLOW-UP

The health department and school officials issued reports that, in essence, assured everyone that the situation had been evaluated, the problems had been appropriately addressed, and the school was safe for occupancy. They found no significant toxic chemical levels, and three years later, they had no explanation why certain students and teachers continued to become very ill within minutes after entering the school building.

The medical problems of some of the students and teachers persisted over time. Fortunately, 50 percent (7 out of 14) of the children seen in one doctor's office improved as soon as they were transferred to another school. Another 36 percent (5 out of 14) had to try several different schools before finding one they could tolerate. The other 14 percent (2 out of 14) remained unable to attend their original or any other school; in these youngsters, even minute amounts of innumerable chemicals still cause daily symptoms.

Some of the students and teachers report they continue to have constant or intermittent headaches, nausea, and fatigue. Because some of them remained sensitized, they must stringently limit their exposure to chemicals in foods and water, as well as in the air. This is typical of the "spreading phenomenon," commonly noted in individuals who have been sensitized by a chemical exposure. As I've said, many of these people find that odors in a mall, restaurant, church, public lavatory, movie, or public gathering make them ill. The slightest whiff of chemicals such as perfume, tobacco, freshly dry-cleaned clothing, fingernail polish, scouring powder, disinfectants, deodorizers, or exhaust fumes, can cause a sudden recurrence of some of their original symptoms. For example, in a twenty-month follow-up, one student still developed intense headaches, fatigue, a sharp pain in her left ear, pain in her lower right abdomen, nausea, and shakiness after accidental exposures of these types. From one such exposure, her symptoms can persist for two to ten days!

At that twenty-month point, other seriously ill students and teachers were also unable to tolerate chemical exposures. Only 14 percent (2 out of 14) of these students were still on a home teaching program, but 50 percent (3 out of 6) of teachers remained at home, unable to work or live normally. All of the sickest individuals had to be alert for a sudden recurrence of their illness whenever they ventured outside their homes. They needed to constantly consider what chemicals they might accidentally encounter. Teachers described having to find a full-service station where someone else would fill the gas tank; but even then they were fearful of the health effects from exposure to just a trace of gasoline fumes when they opened the car window to pay for the fuel. At times, just that little bit of smell can trigger an illness that lasts from hours to days.

In general, however, the children and teachers who have received environmental medical care have improved. Some have been treated only or mainly by instructions to avoid as many chemicals as possible. A few children and one teacher unfortunately did not get any type of medical care until 1994; they are certainly not as well at this time as most of those who received earlier treatment and education.

TESTING

A number of tests were conducted on some of these students and teachers, as well as with a piece of carpet from their school. Here is what these evaluations showed:

BLOOD AND ALLERGY TESTS
The majority of the affected individuals who were treated had a number of immunological abnormalities in their blood (see Chapter 13). A few showed evidence of chemicals, and over one-third had antibodies against myelin (the fat covering their nerves) and/or the nuclei of their own cells. Sixty-seven percent (4 out of 6) had signs of nerve conduction abnormalities.

During P/N allergy skin tests (see Chapter 13), most of those tested reacted to dust, molds, pollen, and foods, as well as to common chemicals such as formaldehyde, phenol, glycerine, and hydrocarbons. Single-blinded P/N allergy testing with extracts prepared from the school carpet and/or the school air were positive in 75 percent (8 out of 13) of the students and 60 percent (3 out of 5) of the teachers. These challenge tests reproduced symptoms that were similar or identical to those these individuals had when they entered their renovated school.

BRAIN-IMAGE TESTS
Four students and four teachers underwent brain-image SPECT tests (see Chapter 13). They all showed they had had mild-to-severe brain changes, indicating alterations in normal blood flow and brain function. These changes were of the type caused by exposure to neurotoxic substances. For financial reasons the remaining students and teachers did not have this test performed.

Figures 11.1a to c show the types of changes that were seen in the brain images of one student and one teacher. Both of these individuals continue to have daily symptoms; in the aftermath of the school exposures that began in September 1992, it is highly doubtful that they will ever be the same.

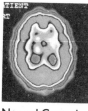 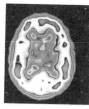 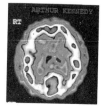

FIGURE 11.1A TO C
SPECT Test Results

Normal Control   Student   Teacher

As you can see, in Figures 11a to c, the brain images of the student and the teacher (on the right) do not look like that of the control (on the left). Their brain structures show a definite variation in color compared with the control. The large white outer areas in the images compared to the control indicate or at least strongly suggest that the blood supply and brain function are not normal. The teacher's image also lacks the smoother outer-edge contour that is typical of the normal control.

CARPET MOUSE TEST

A year-old, eight-by-ten-inch piece of school carpet with no apparent odor was analyzed at Anderson Laboratories (see Resources). During the test, air was blown over this carpet sample into a cage containing four gently restrained mice. They were to breathe this air for a total of four hours over a two-day period. During that time, some of the mice developed facial swelling, breathing problems, skin hemorrhages, eye problems, and paralysis, along with an inability to grasp and turn over in a normal manner. One mouse died after the third hour of exposure. The response of the mice to this carpet sample is shown in the video *Environmentally Sick Schools* (see Resources).

THE DILEMMAS FACED BY HEALTH OFFICIALS

Local, state, and school health officials may face a number of perplexing dilemmas when they investigate potentially sick schools. For example, ASHRAE, EPA, NIOSH, and OSHA all suggest *different "tolerated or safe"* levels of various air pollutants. To further complicate matters, *the recommended guidelines are designed for healthy male adults in workplaces, not for children or pregnant teachers in schools.*

Who should be responsible for setting the standards for children? What should those standards be? Among these agencies, the suggested cut-off levels between "all right" and "a potential problem" can vary from year to year, with a tendency to become more lenient rather than more restrictive as time passes. Sometimes, the "safe" or "acceptable" levels have been raised, possibly for totally nonmedical reasons. If the permissible level of a gas or chemical allowed in indoor air is repeatedly increased, school officials (and health departments) may feel less need to take measures to lower these levels in their buildings, or to be responsible for health problems or other sequelae. The decision whether to take such measures or not is not always based on what is medically best for people, but sometimes also on what is practical and economically prudent.

Sometimes currently acceptable levels of air contaminants are not exceeded, but certain children and teachers continue to become ill. What should health departments do? I believe that this disparity between a supposedly "safe" classroom environment and the persistence of health problems begs for a logical explanation. Perhaps there is something in the air that has not been investigated. Potentially, there can be a vast number of pollutants in the air of a sick building, yet only the obvious or major suspects are routinely investigated unless there is evidence of the presence of other substances. Some water- or fat-soluble airborne chemicals can be particularly difficult to evaluate because they are present in concentrations lower than those routinely detected in the air or in the blood or urine in the human body. Maybe the standard methods of analysis are not capable of detecting low levels of these chemicals, although these can be high enough to cause illness in very sensitive individuals.

Even if the health department's thorough evaluation indicates that no problem exists, realistically there must be a reason why, years later, certain students and teachers become ill within minutes of entering a particular school building. What is present that exceeds their level of tolerance? School officials need to conduct more investigations if individuals continue to become sick. In those situations, logical answers must be found.

The ultimate challenge for a health department is not so much whether a problem exists, but whether the elusive factors causing sudden ill health can be detected and eliminated.

■ GENERAL ADVICE

Many officials show a clear pattern of responses when students and teachers become ill shortly after major school renovations. They may exhibit denial, confusion, anxiety, anger, fear, and other stressful emotions from conflicting observations, recommendations, and conclusions. At times, the effective resolution of school health crises has been delayed by misrepresentation, bias, unsupported claims, and the withholding of information. The various investigators and consultants must cooperate with one another, and officials must help ensure that productive and constructive communication takes place, rather than gossip and rumors. As the level of awareness and knowledge increases among all parties, the potential for future health problems and long-term chronic illness should significantly diminish. The aim of everyone should not be to find fault or blame individuals or systems but to quickly resolve the crisis, by eliminating the root of the immediate health problems, in an effort to prevent recurrences in the future. One critical issue remains, however: Who will pay for the medical care of individuals who desperately need it? More must be done to help sick students and teachers.

The following example, documented in the videotape *Environmentally Sick Schools* (see For Further Reading), illustrates how a school principal helped a teacher, but only after a student also became ill.

HELPING OTHERS BY HELPING ONESELF

Sandra

Sandra had a long history of typical allergies, dating back to early childhood. Her allergies suddenly and significantly flared after she was assigned to a new classroom. She fell ill every year, from October to May, while she was teaching in that particular room. She had congestion, colds, and laryngitis, as well as constant throat, lung, and sinus infections. She started each day with sniffling and excessive mucus. Her chest felt heavy from recurrent coughing. These problems subsided when she was not in school. Later she learned that the teacher who had previously used the same classroom sometimes had had to lie down on the floor behind her desk because of a headache so severe that she was totally incapacitated.

Sandra felt embarrassed because she never felt really well. Her long list of symptoms peaked in May-June 1992, when she became so hoarse that she could barely whisper. She could not speak normally for a full month. Sandra eventually discovered that a combination of dust, molds, an extremely old carpet, smelly lavatory disinfectants, and pollinating grass were more than her body could tolerate.

She improved during the next few months, as she always did during summer vacations. In October, however, she was reassigned to the same room, and her infections returned. She had so many health problems that her school principal joked to others about her "complaint of the week." Her colleagues were skeptical of her endless array of "psychosomatic" symptoms. Her migraines were so excruciatingly painful that she felt her head would explode. Her symptoms at that time included hyperactivity, difficulty breathing, irritability, abdominal gas, full ears, and ringing sounds. In addition, her muscles ached, her feet felt numb, her eyes burned and teared, and her vision was not up to par.

Because she felt worse at school and better at home, she finally concluded the culprit was something in her school building. She went to the new school principal, who listened reluctantly. Not until a student also became very ill did he initiate appropriate action. This student's extreme fatigue and unusual behavior in Sandra's classroom finally convinced him that the teacher's complaints might be valid.

The principal requested that a HVAC firm evaluate factors that might be affecting the teacher and the student. By then Sandra was so ill that she would develop a hoarse voice, flushed face, and severe breathing problems within minutes of entering her classroom each day.

In May 1993, the school opened the ventilation ducts—all but two had been closed for more than ten years. New filters were installed. Odorous chemicals were removed from every classroom, and environmentally safer cleaning agents and disinfectants were used. Air purifiers were placed in Sandra's classroom and the child's homeroom. When it was time to purchase new carpeting, the affected student (but not Sandra) was exposed to several pieces of carpet to see which one appeared to be best tolerated. The chosen carpet was installed in one room, and when the youngster remained well, that carpet was purchased for the entire school.

Sandra further improved after treatment from an environmental medical specialist. She made changes in her home similar to those the school made. She drank pure, glass-bottled spring water and ate more organic foods. She took nutritional supplements to strengthen her immune system and her body's ability to detoxify chemicals. She became more knowledgeable about when and why she was ill, enabling her to avoid some of the more subtle causes of her flare-ups. She presently remains well, unless she is accidentally exposed to certain chemicals, which happens much less frequently now that her classroom, school, and home are environmentally safer.

When Sandra was allergy-tested with an extract made from the school air and the school's original carpet, she developed a hoarse voice and had difficulty breathing in only a minute or two. These were the symptoms that she had had so frequently in her own classroom. She became normal in less than two minutes with a neutralization dose of allergy extract.

When she was tested for toluene, Sandra developed the lower abdominal pain that had perplexed many previous doctors. When she was tested for ethyl alcohol, she reacted as she had when exposed to perfume that contains this chemical. She also was found to be sensitive to dust and molds.

After this testing and treatment, plus the changes in her school, Sandra's subsequent school year was entirely different. She did not develop the discouraging and incapacitating infections that had plagued her for years. Not only was she improved, but others who used her classroom appeared to suffer less illness. Because the school administration had done more than merely listen, Sandra, unlike other EI teachers, did not become a prisoner in her own home wishing to be well enough to return to work. She did not have to subsist on Workers' Compensation or Social Security, and she had no cause to initiate stressful litigation.

This school administration's approach was practical, sensible, appropriate, and farsighted. Its response was cost- and health-effective for both teachers and students. By eliminating the causes of environmental illness—the woefully inadequate ventilation and the adverse chemicals—they have a teacher who feels well enough to work and does not need to be replaced. Certain students feel better, can remain in school, and do not need home teaching. They may also have helped other students and teachers who might have eventually developed symptoms from the woefully inadequate ventilation system and adverse chemical exposures.

This school administration chose very wisely. Denial and cover-up would have only delayed what would have had to be done eventually. A few sensible changes and precautions can defuse a potentially serious medical and legal powder keg, as this teacher's challenging medical history indicated.

The rewards were immense for both students and faculty. Still, Sandra's problems are not entirely solved. She was not compensated for her lost time, her years of illness, her discomfort and worry, or many of her immense medical bills. Although she is able to work, her health will remain labile and brittle for an indefinite period of time. Her symptoms continue to be triggered too easily, too quickly, and too often by minute exposures. For example, a student's stuffed animal that smelled of tobacco smoke, a girl's hair spray, and a whiff of a deodorizer spray have all triggered sudden debilitating flares. Her throat goes into spasm, and her breathing becomes difficult. How will she feel five and ten years from now? We don't know.

The best remedy for exposure to chemicals is avoidance. Improved ventilation and room air purifiers help by reducing dust, molds, pollen, and possibly some chemicals. Dietary changes, better nutrition, glass-bottled filtered water, and allergy extract therapy all lessen allergies and environmental illness.

When treating EI the aim must be to keep the total level of exposures below that which causes illnesses. Each person's tolerance varies, but if the sum of the adverse effects from what you breathe, what you eat, and what you touch is more than you can tolerate, you will be ill; if it is less, you will remain well.

Once you know how easy it is to find helpful answers, you must recognize your obligation to share what you've learned. Many other parents and teachers are floundering as they search for the causes of similar perplexing symptoms. Urge your city and school libraries and health offices to make books and videos available so that everyone's awareness of environmental illness can be raised (see For Further Reading).

Remember, by helping your child's or your own environmental illness, you are also helping every other student or teacher who is exposed to an environmentally sick school building.

NOTES

1. Rowe, Albert, and Albert Rowe, Jr., *Food Allergy* (Springfield, IL: Charles C. Thomas, 1972).

2. N.A. Ashford and C. Miller, *Chemical Exposures: Low Levels and High Stakes* (New York: Van Nostrand Reinhold, 1991).

3. From a letter to parents and colleagues from the office of the superintendent.

4. Ibid.

5. N.S. Green, *Poisoning Our Children: Surviving in a Toxic World* (Chicago, IL: Noble Press, 1991).

6. John Bower, *Healthy House Building: A Design and Construction Guide* (Bloomington, IN: Healthy House Institute, 1993).

7. MSD sheet warning for Burlington Unibond Adhesive.

8. Marion Moses, *Designer Poisons* (San Francisco, CA: Pesticide Education Center, 1995).

9. See Ashford and Miller, *Chemical Exposures*; and Green, *Poisoning Our Children.*

12 Let's Learn from Canada

◼ THE WATERLOO COUNTY BOARD OF EDUCATION, ONTARIO

What can parents and educators accomplish when they work together? Just look at what happened in the Waterloo school district in Ontario, Canada.

The Waterloo increase in awareness began during the early 1980s, when over a period of several years John MacLennan, M.D., Alexander Schauss, Ph.D., Lendon Smith, M.D., Marshall Mandell, M.D., and I presented a series of lectures on school environmental issues to educators and the general public. Those speeches markedly increased the understanding among parents, school psychologists, administrators, and teachers about the possible role of environmental factors in relation to the behavior, learning, and physical well-being of children. As a result, several observant, dedicated school psychologists and concerned parents urged the open-minded and progressive Waterloo school administrators to create a pilot ECO (environmentally controlled opportunity) classroom. Every effort was made to ensure that these rooms provided a safe haven for environmentally ill stuzndents.

This initial effort to create an ECO classroom was so successful that the concept was gradually refined and then expanded to include more schools in the Waterloo area. By 1994, several school districts in Ontario had made significant changes so that their programs evolved into models worthy of emulation by schools around the world (see Table 12.1). Yes, there is still much to be learned and implemented, but the Waterloo area have made tremendous practical and sensible strides to help improve the air quality in their school districts. They have clearly demonstrated the following:

Environmentally cleaner classrooms, which profoundly improve the academic performance, health, and attendance of certain students, can be created in existing school buildings with relatively little additional expenditure.

HOW THE WATERLOO PROGRAM EVOLVED

As the ECO classroom program was introduced in one Waterloo area school district after another, local participation was always encouraged. In some districts, parents shared their knowledge about environmental medicine, providing their own practical input. In addition, "in-service" educational programs were conducted for new teachers, principals, superintendents, maintenance engineers, and purchasing agents. In the process, school employees began to change their own ingrained habits and beliefs, more fully appreciating the role that environmental factors can play in every aspect of student performance and school functioning.

There were a variety of initial goals and concerns among those involved in launching these programs. Astute personnel from the Waterloo County board of education, for example, were looking for alternative or supplementary approaches to help students with behavioral or learning problems. Board members realized that when traditional therapeutic modalities do not resolve the plight of these students, other solutions had to be sought. A number of such students needed home teaching due to school-related illnesses. These children were well at home and at times even on the school bus, but they became increasingly ill because of various exposures that occurred as the school day progressed. They repeatedly required medical attention for health problems, such as asthma, that would develop by the time they arrived at school or during the school day. They were justifiably concerned and worried about how they could receive the education they wanted and needed.

After consulting with individuals knowledgeable about environmentally related engineering and medical issues, the Waterloo school board implemented its pilot program. It began as part of one secondary school's renovation, with the creation of a single ECO classroom. The special classroom proved helpful from both an educational and an economic viewpoint. Particularly it made a difference in the lives of the initial group of eight environmentally ill students who used it. As a result of the pilot program, recommendations for this and successively better-developed ECO classrooms were formulated (see Table 12.1).

How were students chosen for instruction in the first ECO classrooms?

TABLE 12.1

Composite of Changes Implemented for ECO Classrooms in the Waterloo, Guelph, and Halton, Ontario, School Systems

The schools took these steps to implement ECO classrooms:

- They built the classrooms of natural materials, with specially treated walls and ceilings, and sealed concrete floors. They used natural fiber throw rugs, and environmentally safer, nonodorous paint (see Resources). They allowed no regular carpets.
- They furnished the rooms with solid wood furniture whenever possible and applied safe sealers on all plywood furnishings to minimize the "outgassing" of chemicals such as formaldehyde (see Resources).
- They replaced curtains with metal window blinds. If curtains and drapes were used, they were made of natural fiber and were regularly cleaned or tumbled in a dryer.
- They used safer maintenance and decorative materials.
- They undertook renovations at the beginning of school vacations, allowing adequate time for the dissipation of residual chemical odors caused by construction.
- They installed a separate heating/cooling ventilation system with a quality HEPA electronic air-filtering system. High-quality filters were changed four times per year.
- They maintained a positive air pressure within the classrooms so that air did not enter the room when the doors were opened.
- They used natural light as much as possible and installed full-spectrum shielded lighting, which emitted less electromagnetic energy.
- They installed windows that could be opened.
- They used high-quality room air purifiers to remove dust, molds, pollen, and other particles from the air (see Resources). Separate air purifiers were made available to provide a localized pocket of purer air around extremely environmentally ill students.
- They selectively used dehumidifiers and humidifiers.
- They allowed any student to change rooms if specific classrooms caused symptoms.
- They made a portable oxygen tank available for the initial treatment of minor accidental chemical exposures.
- They allowed no plants within the classrooms, reducing the levels of mold contamination.
- They installed bulletin boards made of special nonodorous cork.
- They used magnetic white marker boards with odorless, water-based markers instead of blackboards and chalk (see Resources). The boards were cleaned nightly with safer cleaning materials.
- They restricted the use of odorous art supplies, glues, crayons, duplicate copies, acetone markers, vinyl or plastic binders or containers, and smelly fountain-type pens.
- They provided "pure" nonchlorinated drinking water in glass containers, when it was available.
- They supplied pure organic cotton futons for napping.
- They requested that all students and teachers avoid the use of any scented personal products in the classrooms.
- They were advised to air out all dry-cleaned clothes and not to wear new clothing unless it had been washed—with scented soap or fabric softeners.

■ They were told not to touch pets before coming to school and no pets were allowed in these classrooms.

■ They placed signs on the classroom doors prohibiting the entrance of anyone who smelled of perfume, tobacco, or chemicals.

■ They prohibited highly allergenic substances.

■ They stored boots and coats outside the classrooms to reduce the potential growth of molds.

■ They provided large classroom garbage containers that were to be used only for paper disposal. Lunch waste was immediately removed from the classrooms and placed in an outside, tightly sealed, and frequently emptied container.

■ They swept the floors daily and washed them weekly with safer cleaning and disinfectant products. For dust control, they used dry dust mops (like Saran Material red), which did not need to be sprayed. Separate cloths and dusters were used for each classroom.

■ They cleaned the classrooms with better-tolerated, unscented natural cleaners: Borax, baking soda, vinegar and water, and Bon Ami. The rooms were aired out after cleaning.

■ They provided "clean" taxis or vans to bring selected home-taught students to school. This service was cost-effective, even though a few individual students had to be transported over twenty miles each day.

■ They insisted upon nondiesel and nonsmoking transportation, avoiding bus and auto hydrocarbon exhaust fumes as much as possible.

■ They provided chemically sensitive students with older, used textbooks. When they had to use books that were new and odorous, they spread them open and baked them at 100° F for at least five hours and then aired them out. This procedure diminished ink and paper chemical odors. They used the same procedure to help eliminate the moldy, musty smell in older or improperly stored books.

■ They refrained from spraying with pesticides or cutting grass during school hours. They used safer forms of pesticide control (see Chapter 10).

■ They improved the air quality in the ECO classrooms and throughout the school by restricting all school printing, copying, and lamination equipment to specially ventilated rooms that had automatic closure doors. Photocopies, rather than chemically laden dittos, were used when copies were needed.

■ They had educational programs for students and staff so that everyone became more aware of environmentally related health, behavioral, and learning problems.

■ They provided practical, helpful suggestions to the parents of the children in the ECO classrooms to help them detect food sensitivities and learn how to make their homes more environmentally sound.

■ They instructed school health assistants to become familiar with each student's medical concerns related to foods, odors, contacts, or stinging insect sensitivities. They learned what to do when physical reactions occurred. Refrigerators were available to store needed medications.

■ They gave individualized consideration to alternatives for chemistry and biology classes or labs; preferential seating near natural light; and placement in rooms with non–smoking teachers when youngsters were gradually mainstreamed.

■ They provided a variety of support services for students in the classrooms in both the elementary and secondary school systems. They made provisions for student referrals, assessments for the need for intervention, and individualized modification of each student's program.

■ They regularly monitored and recorded the progress of all students academically, psychologically, and medically. Individualized changes and adaptations were made for each student when indicated.

Their selection was based in part upon attendance records. Most of the students were on home teaching or had a history of repeated congestion, asthma, eczema, headaches, malaise, and/or infections. Their symptoms included sniffling, throat-clearing, wheezing, dark eye circles, red earlobes, red cheeks, or wiggly legs, all occurring at specific times when they were unable to concentrate, behave, and learn in a normal manner. After they were admitted to ECO classrooms, their learning ability and health complaints were carefully monitored, and adjustments were made to maximize their academic performance.

Of course, the most effective way to treat all environmental illness that interferes with learning is to *prevent* it. A questionnaire for preschool children might help parents and school officials or personnel detect which youngsters might be prone to environmentally related learning problems or illness in the future. By identifying the certain characteristic clues— either before or as early as possible after a child begins school—it should be possible to delay or prevent the progression of certain symptoms that could significantly impede a child's future academic career. (An example of a detailed environmental medical history form can be found in Table 3.2.)

HOW EFFECTIVELY DID THE ECO CLASSROOM PREVENT ENVIRONMENTAL ILLNESS?

The first ECO classroom was immensely helpful in improving the health of all the initial students. Within six months, their attendance and academic performance improved dramatically, and their health problems and need for medications diminished significantly. In this school district, for example, the attendance of the typical *well* student had been 88 percent; while among the *environmentally ill* students who went to school, the attendance rose from 64 percent to 84 percent after placement in the ECO classroom. This group of eight students, previously home-taught for about two hours each day, now received traditional, supervised education for a full six hours per day.

In general, all aspects of learning and memory in these children improved. At times, their grades rose to levels that far exceeded anyone's expectations. Their behavior and activity levels also significantly improved because they simply felt better. Their self-esteem increased, in part because they felt happier and more content, and they took pride in themselves and their accomplishments.

Merely breathing cleaner air, avoiding as many chemicals as possible during school hours, and drinking purer water helped these students to a significant degree. This improvement occurred even though few of them were receiving allergy extract treatment or were following special allergy diets (unless such diets had been part of their previous medical care). School officials also accommodated special food restrictions, as well as their need for emergency allergy treatments (for example for asthma or stinging-insect allergy).

At first, some of the students had to be in the ECO classroom all the time, but as their health improved, most were gradually mainstreamed into regular classrooms. Some felt so well that they even were able to obtains part-time jobs.

One of the most significant advantages of this program was that school administrators immediately became aware of any indoor air-quality problem. For example, if students left the ECO room for a regular classroom and suddenly complained of headaches or a rash, school officials were notified at once so the cause could be detected. In a sense, each environmentally ill child served as a "canary in a coal mine." Because of their sensitivities when these youngsters were mainstreamed, they were able to detect any new, potentially upsetting exposures quickly. If a different, supposedly safer cleaning agent, for example, created symptoms, and a cause-and-effect relationship was noted with very little delay. Because of this, the school administrators could take appropriate action before the less sensitive students or staff began to react adversely.

EXPANDING THE CONCEPT

The response to the first ECO classroom was so favorable that school officials soon had to decide whether other sick students would be given the opportunity to learn in that same room. When parents learned of the dramatic improvement in attendance and academic performance in the original students, they naturally wanted their own classically allergic or environmentally sick children to be taught in the ECO classroom. The demand quickly exceeded the availability.

In response to the success of the initial ECO classroom, the Waterloo school board decided to build similar rooms in other schools at different grade levels. By 1995, there were four ECO classrooms in elementary schools and two in high schools, each of them accommodating eight to ten students. Usually, two to four youngsters were assigned full-time in these special classrooms; another four to six students were placed there temporarily for a variety of reasons. For example, if a student's records indicated a recurring decrease in scholastic ability during the pollen or mold seasons, that child might be placed in the ECO classroom at those times of the year. This proved helpful during year-end examinations in the spring, the peak of grass-pollen season, and similarly in September, the peak of the outside mold-spore and weed-pollen seasons.

Other students were placed in ECO classrooms on a short-term basis at the recommendation of the school psychologist or special-education personnel. During this trial period, they could be observed and evaluated to assess whether environmental factors were related to their enigmatic problems. If they were unequivocally better, these children remained in the special ECO classroom. But if they showed no significant improvement, then social, emotional, or other causes for their difficulties were more fully investigated.

In general, this same commonsense approach was implemented in other problematic schools. Waterloo officials found that the application of the ECO concepts sometimes produced fast, sensible solutions due to various adverse exposures that arose in other school buildings or portable classrooms. For example, problem buildings might be temporarily improved by installing air purifiers in select areas, cleaning and replacing filters, repairing water leaks, and eliminating obvious sources of molds and chemicals. At other times, if a building was old, making certain changes was neither practical nor possible.

In addition, school officials incorporated environmental concepts into the design of future school buildings. If funds were not immediately available for those purposes, they constructed the new buildings in such a way that certain desirable but not necessarily essential changes could be implemented easily at some future time.

School officials also decided to use the safest possible materials for all future construction. For example, they now use 100 percent water-based, less odorous latex paint; they clean with less toxic substances; and they decrease bacterial contamination with safer disinfectants (see Resources). (Interestingly, the demands by these schools for less toxic products has prompted the creation of new industries that offer a choice of environmentally safer products.)

Another important aspect of the Waterloo County school district's success was the environmental educational programs that parents and educators created to inform other parents and teachers. These sessions encouraged the parents of children in ECO classrooms to make their homes, particularly their children's bedrooms, more allergy-free and environmentally sound by reducing dust, molds, and chemicals as much as possible. They learned how simple it can be to pinpoint previously unsuspected exposures or food sensitivities. In time, doubting parents, students, and teachers, as well as some cautious, skeptical physicians, became more open to the idea that certain exposures or foods had to be avoided. As these educational programs increased everyone's awareness, adverse exposures were prevented more often and more quickly.

Bear in mind, however, that these students were *not totally symptom-free* in their ECO classrooms; even so, each youngster definitely felt better, and his or her school attendance and academic performance improved. Also, in sharp contrast to their previous experience, most required less or no daily allergy medication.

WHAT DID IT COST?

Ten years ago the initial ECO classroom cost only about $10,000—it was surprisingly cost-effective. (In 1994 the cost was approximately $50,000.) Before the initial ECO classroom became a reality, several students had been taught at home for forty weeks per year at a weekly cost of fifty dollars per student. When these students could stop home teaching, it saved the school district as much as $2,000 per student each school year.

True, the initial cost of making some of the changes inside some of the schools was high. But in time, because of the efficacy of specific modifications related to cleaning, lighting, and ventilation, the changes proved to be both cost- and health-effective. As a result, other school districts subsequently implemented and even expanded upon those changes. For example, in newly constructed schools in one district, the ventilation systems are now computerized; with a simple flick of a switch, the custodians can modify and adjust the air flow, heat, temperature, and humidity in localized areas of several different schools. This advanced technology should improve the scholastic achievements and behavior of *many* students, not only those with obvious environmental illness.

IN THE WATERLOO ECO CLASSROOM

Kathy

Kathy was a teenager who had anxiously waited for three years to be accepted in the Waterloo ECO classroom. She had been unable to attend regular school because, after a typical school bus ride, her throat routinely became tight, she wheezed badly, and she was barely able to see because her eyes became so swollen. These problems made her embarrassed and extremely discouraged.

About once a month Kathy had to be hospitalized because her allergies would suddenly become extremely severe, either at home or at school. One whiff of perfume or tobacco could make her desperately ill in seconds. After she was accepted into the ECO classroom, a "clean" van was assigned to transport her to school, as a result, her eyes were much less swollen, and her need for daily medications decreased markedly. Her incapacitating asthmatic episodes became progressively less evident. In the past, she had missed *two hundred* classes per year; after she moved to the ECO classroom, she missed only fifteen. Her grades, which had averaged below the sixtieth percentile, rose to honors level in some subjects, and she was assigned to an advanced-learning class. In time Kathy became so healthy that she began to socialize and attend outside school functions. She eventually was able to find and retain a job.

There is no doubt that the Waterloo ECO classroom enabled Kathy as she so aptly put it "to receive an education, not a diploma." That simply would not have been possible if her education had been limited to home teaching.

Robert

Six-year-old Robert's mother wrote to the administrators at the Waterloo school to thank them for their ECO classroom. She explained how he was before and after he was assigned to the ECO classroom.

Before he entered school he could write cursive letters. This changed, however, after he began kindergarten. His writing gradually regressed to large irregular printing, with some letters written backward or reversed. In a few months he became moody and progressively more negative. He said that he hated himself and nobody liked him. He often cried because he hated school so much.

Because of the complaints, Robert was seen by an allergist, who found that he was sensitive to many foods, dust, and molds. Later, an environmental medical specialist discovered that Robert was also sensitive to the odor of hydrocarbons (see Chapters 7, 10, and 11). In time, his classroom's carpet was found to be moldy, and his poor behavior in gym was attributed to a ventilation defect that allowed hydrocarbon exhaust fumes from the school's oil heater to blow directly into the gymnasium.

Robert's problems, were finally totally resolved shortly after he was placed in the ECO classroom. His constant winter cough disappeared, and he became calmer, less worried, and much happier. His sleeping improved; he stopped having nightmares and wetting the bed. He became interested in sports, and his coordination improved. He was less irritable and angry with the world and himself, and his depression gradually disappeared. His violin teacher simply commented, "Wow!" and called him "the new improved Robert."

As his schoolwork and concentration improved, Robert felt more positive about school. His ECO teacher called him "an amazing kid." As a result of this improvement, his family's home life also became more peaceful and pleasant. He felt so happy and content that he told his mother, "The days just keep getting better and better."

Unfortunately, the family subsequently moved to a suburb of Chicago, where the same type of special classroom environment wasn't available. Robert's mother checked every school within that district from an environmental viewpoint. Mainly because of his sensitivity to carpets, she could not find a school that he could tolerate. He is, therefore, receiving home teaching again.

■ AN ECO CLASSROOM IN GUELPH, ONTARIO

When two environmentally ill siblings in Guelph did not feel well, learn at a level commensurate with their ability, or behave appropriately in school, their mother eventually determined that the major causes were dust, molds, and chemicals in their school building. This mother singlehandedly recruited a group of other concerned parents and enlisted the cooperation of some visionary school officials. Together they initiated changes that eventually improved their entire school district. Initially, a portable classroom was converted into an environmentally safer room. Later, a room in a school building was converted into an ECO classroom. Both of these classrooms contained a totally separate heating/ventilation/air conditioning (HVAC) system that utilized a heat pump. This system maintained the level of carbon dioxide in the classrooms at a remarkable 400 ppm, which is equivalent to high-quality outdoor air. The lavatory and even the teachers' storage cabinet had a negative air pressure, so that odors from these areas were expelled directly outside through a separate exhaust system. Many other basic concepts (as outlined in Table 12.1) were incorporated in this school district.

ONE GUELPH SCHOOLCHILD

Darryl

Six-year-old Darryl could not attend regular school until appropriate environmental changes were made, initially, in a portable ECO classroom and later in a classroom in his regular school building.

During his initial visit to our center, Darryl was an exceptionally pleasant child. He has a remarkably knowledgeable, caring mother who, slowly but surely, not only resolved his school problems but helped many other similarly affected youngsters. Her ability to take her son's pulse proved to be a key asset.

Let's start at the beginning with Darryl, because his history is classic and typical of so many students who do not feel or learn well because of routine school exposures. If his environmental allergic illness had been diagnosed and treated when it first became apparent, many of his subsequent behavioral and scholastic problems might never have occurred.

Early Preschool History

Like most environmentally ill children, Darryl had many allergic relatives, and he himself had evidence of classic allergies during infancy. He had colic when he was breast-fed, until his mother realized that the problem was the cow's milk *she* drank which passed into her breast milk. In fact, he was congested as an infant until all dairy products were eliminated from his mother's and his own diet.

When Darryl was about eighteen months old, his mother, Mrs. K., mistakenly believed that he had outgrown his milk allergy. As typically happens with many milk-sensitive individuals, within a few months after he resumed ingesting dairy products, *different* symptoms gradually recurred. Dairy products now caused frequent colds, bronchitis, and one ear infection after another. In spite of repeated antibiotics, he was "always" congested or ill.

For years, Darryl also experienced frightening night terrors, sometimes as many as four in one night. Each episode lasted two to three hours. His mother eventually found that the terrors were mainly caused by his routine bedtime milk. Like other well-meaning mothers, Mrs. K. thought warm milk would help him sleep, never realizing that it could cause this type of problem. He did not sleep through the night until he was five years old.

By the time Darryl was age two, whenever his mother said, "Good morning," his usual response was, "No! Get away from me!" He spent his days whining, crying, and complaining. On occasion he would act angry and atypically aggressive. There were times when he was an unusually sweet and lovable Dr. Jekyll; but, then, for no obvious reason, he would suddenly switch to an impossibly nasty Mr. Hyde.

By three years of age, Darryl had already undergone surgery twice to place tubes through his eardrums because fluid repeatedly accumulated in his middle ear. Again, this is typical result of unrecognized and untreated milk- or food-allergy.

If a child's nose is swollen because of allergies, it means that the "doorway" to the middle ear—which is the area between the eardrum and the nose called the eustachian tube—is blocked. When air cannot pass from the nose to the middle ear, fluid fills this area and can cause a temporary or permanent hearing loss. In young children, this blockage is a frequently undetected cause of delayed or poor speech; in other youngsters, the fluid traps germs, so the area becomes a site of repeated infections, which can lead to related ear tube and/or adenoid surgery.

If the cause of Darryl's nose allergies had been recognized and appropriately treated, his eustachian tube might have remained open, and his ear problems probably would have subsided without surgery. His physicians had suggested the removal of his tonsils and adenoids, but proper environmental medical therapy eliminated the need for this surgery.

As a young child, Darryl had periods of truly unacceptable behavior. When he ingested the wrong foods, especially milk or apple juice, or was exposed to molds, pollen, dust, or certain chemicals, he experienced a total change in behavior that perplexed and distressed those around him. But Darryl's perceptive mother remained increasingly vigilant and continually asked herself "why?" What caused her son to suddenly withdraw or crawl under the furniture? Why, at times, did he write in infantile scribbles, stab pencils through his school papers, suddenly seem unable to do simple math, become vulgar, violent, irrational, irritable, self-destructive, depressed, and impossibly negative? Why did he want to hurt others, cling to her, or suddenly act so sad, silly, tired, or withdrawn? Mrs. K. felt impelled to find a logical reason for his outbursts and inappropriate actions.

She faithfully recorded her son's symptoms in relation to everything he ate, the weather, and all environmental exposures (see Chapter 3 for how this is done). When his pulse rate suddenly rose twenty beats above normal, she knew, based on previous experience, that he had eaten, touched, or smelled something to which he was sensitive. She immediately considered the possibilities. Was it something indoors or outdoors? A food or a chemical? Making one connection after another, she found that different exposures caused specific symptoms. As time passed, her detective work became easier, and when she finally figured out the causes of Darryl's problems, she could not believe that she had missed the obvious for so long. No one had ever explained to her that all she needed to do to help her son was to record and analyze her observations.

How Did Darryl's School Situation Change?

Mrs. K. read and studied everything she could about environmental illness, and eventually she came to our center for environmental medical care in Buffalo. She cleaned their home in an environmentally safer way and even did the same at Darryl's school. Fortunately, the principal of the school had allergies, too, and was aware of how this medical problem could affect some students. After she showed him a video in which Darryl's unacceptable behavior was caused by one drop of various allergy extract solutions, the principal implemented her (and our) recommendations about better ways to clean his classroom.

Thereafter, from kindergarten through the second grade, Darryl's school room was routinely cleaned with more environmentally sound substances. She provided the school maintenance supervisor with information as to where these items could be purchased. And was instrumental in replacing the school's chemical cleaners with safer products. She personally washed the classroom curtains with Borax, baking soda, and an unscented detergent. Not surprisingly, when Darryl sat in classrooms where routine chemical cleaners were still used on the desks and surroundings, his work deteriorated. But after these cleaners were also replaced, his performance returned to his grade level and above.

When new textbooks interfered with her son's concentration and caused his pulse to increase to 100 beats per minute (normal for him was about 75), Mrs. K. opened her son's textbooks and baked them in the oven at 100°F for five hours; then she aired them out overnight so that the ink and paper chemicals no longer obviously bothered him. The chemical odor from school marking pens caused Darryl to become extremely irritable, so the blackboard in his room was replaced with a white board and less offending water-based markers.

In the third grade, Darryl's teacher was perplexed because of his sudden inability to learn at that grade level. His IQ was tested at that time. Then about a week after the test, his allergy extract dose for dust was adjusted at our office and we recommended that an air purifier was placed in his classroom. Less than a month later, when the IQ test was repeated, his percentile score in vocabulary rose by nineteen points (an increase of 1.3 grade levels), and his reading score increased seven percentile points. His schoolwork was no longer a problem.

Unfortunately, in 1991, beams that contained formaldehyde were used for roof construction at Darryl's school. In spite of two air purifiers in his classroom and school-air allergy extract treatment, his previous learning and behavioral problems quickly returned. His entire class was subsequently transferred to a six-year-old portable classroom outside the main school building. Because this room contained no carpet and most chemical odors had already "outgassed," he improved dramatically and quickly.[1]

The most frequently missed cause of recurrent ear fluid in infants and young children is an *undetected* sensitivity to milk. To resolve this problem, the consumption of all dairy products must be decreased or stopped, and a calcium nutrient should be supplied. Some children also benefit from treatment with a milk allergy extract so they can drink milk without becoming ill.

THE ECO CLASSROOM IN HALTON, ONTARIO

AN ADVANCED PRACTICAL MODEL

Another Canadian school board—this one in Halton, Ontario—implemented an environmental policy that was even more practical, effective, relatively inexpensive, and worthy of emulation. School officials there incorporated and expanded upon the changes that already seemed to be so effective in the Waterloo and Guelph school districts. In Halton, however, the school board recognized that it was not economically feasible to make all schools in their district environmentally sound, or to scatter the environmentally ill students throughout the entire district. So they implemented various types of environmental precautions in just two schools, calling one a Designated Elementary School and the other a Designated Secondary School. Although both schools were more environmentally sound than normal schools, only the secondary school contained a specially constructed ECO classroom.

This ECO classroom accommodated only about six students—those who were the district's most environmentally sensitive youngsters. The rest of the environmentally ill students were assigned to regular but "improved" classrooms within that same designated school. This school provided parallel teaching in the ECO classroom so that students in that room could be taught the same subjects, at the same time, and in much the same manner as students who were being taught in the regular classrooms. Independent-study correspondence courses and videotaped classes were other available options.

Whenever possible, in both designated schools, major restoration or remodeling was scheduled to start and be completed *as soon as possible after the school year ended*. This allowed the construction odors to dissipate as completely as possible before the next school semester began.

If any child in any secondary school in the Halton district became symptomatic because of an environmental factor, that student had the opportunity to take all classes, on a temporary basis, in the Designated Secondary School or, if necessary, in that school's ECO classroom. Whenever a new exposure caused symptoms, every effort was made to pinpoint and resolve the problem in the child's home school setting. If the mold-spore or pollen count was high, for example, an air purifier would be placed in all of that child's classrooms; alternatively, the student could immediately attend the cleaner ECO classroom. For example, one youngster who was very sensitive to chemicals could not attend the school's science laboratory, so the science material was taught in the ECO classroom. This enabled him to learn without becoming ill.

Also, if an environmental emergency such as a chemical spill or a flooded basement occurred while school was in session, all environmentally ill teachers, as well as parents of students who might become ill from such an exposure, were immediately informed so that they could leave the area and remain home until the emergency situation was corrected.

In addition, in the Secondary Designated School, environmentally ill students had the right to retreat to the ECO classroom at any time. Once a child improved, he or she could either resume classes in the regular classroom in the designated school, or remain in the ECO classroom. Environmentally safe sleeping accommodations were even available in the ECO room. This meant that if an accidental exposure known to cause mild transitory symptoms such as fatigue or a headache occurred, the child did not always have to return home, but could rest in school for a while and then resume classes when the medical symptoms subsided.

THE ROLE OF INTERVENTION TEAMS

If a child in Halton had difficulty in particular areas of the school or at specific times, several teams with varying degrees of expertise on environmental issues were available for immediate consultation.

The Minimum and/or Mild Intervention Teams were the initial contacts. They resolved the simple, obvious problems, quickly spotting and eliminating the cause(s) of students' complaints. For example, they might ask a staff member to refrain from using perfume or tobacco. Or they might change a child's seat within a classroom, place air purifiers in certain classrooms, or suggest the use of safer cleaning materials. In one designated school, when a dust-sensitive child developed symptoms, the team found that some of the radiators and their covers had not been cleaned for years. Thereafter, all the radiators throughout the entire school district were cleaned. The school administrators clearly recognized the many benefits of prevention.

The Moderate Intervention Team was called if the initial teams could not satisfactorily resolve a child's problem. This more experienced group might decide that the student should be transferred to a different classroom, or should be placed in another school better adapted to his or her particular needs.

The Full Intervention Team was an elite group of expert consultants who thoroughly evaluated each challenging situation. If the previous teams had not eliminated or remedied a child's problem, this group might suggest transfer to the designated school that contained the ECO classroom.

Finally, the Extreme Intervention Team would be called in for consultation on all aspects of a student's problems. This usually meant that there were few options left, and home instruction was probably a necessity.

In essence, the aims of the school administrators were both practical and positive. They did not try to make an *entire* school district perfect—just more environmentally sound for everyone. For example, on one occasion they determined that the fumes from tarring a school roof were reentering the school building through its ventilation ducts. They resolved this problem, and then decided how they could prevent similar recurrences. They concluded that future schools should be designed with intake ventilation vents located on the least polluted sides, rather than on the tops of buildings. This would minimize any roof or nearby factory pollution odors from entering the school. The school district's ultimate aim with this approach resulted in faster and more economical resolutions of existing problems, as well as the elimination of potential future sources of health and learning problems.

HOW WELL DID THIS PLAN WORK?

The system implemented in Halton was a remarkable success. Environmentally sensitive students experienced exceptional improvement. In their evaluations, parents and teachers indicated that most of these students unmistakably felt and performed better. For example, one child who had routinely missed school for forty to fifty days each year was absent only seven to eight days per year in the designated school. As his attendance improved, so did his grades.

Officials in the designated schools were justifiably delighted with the program's success. The designated schools had significantly helped many environmentally ill students. *They determined that making these schools more environmentally sound had been less expensive than they anticipated and eventually both cost- and health-effective.* As older school buildings needed environmental improvements or other repairs, recommendations for controlling and reducing potentially adverse environmental exposures were made. These were implemented as extensively as possible if they seemed practical. As new schools were designed and built, these salient environmental concepts were considered for inclusion in their plans.

Because the school officials attempted to increase everyone's awareness of environmental issues, many new problems were recognized early, enhancing the possibility of a quick resolution. Students, teachers, and parents learned to think logically about school-related environmental matters when they arose. As a result, many parents and teachers applied these same environmentally sound principles to their own homes and workplaces. In time, even some of the staunchly skeptical local physicians became avid believers.[2]

■ TWO CARING MOTHERS

I'd like to give special recognition to two resourceful, dynamic Canadian mothers, Karin Cremasco and Heather Holden. They singlehandedly initiated significant efforts to help resolve the problems in their children's school districts. These women, along with a number of dedicated and concerned educational behavioral consultants and school administrators, recognized the link between physical, emotional, and academic difficulties and various chemical exposures. As they shared their knowledge and experience in a nonthreatening, educational, and effective way, their school districts became progressively more informed and desirous of change. They not only investigated the causes of specific difficulties, they helped to determine and personally implement some of the measures needed to remedy the problems. This entire nucleus of parents and progressive educators must be commended for initiating a practical program worthy of universal emulation. The ripple effect from their well-thought-out programs eventually will become more widely accepted and it is hoped that in time, expanded and improved, to help many other children and teachers throughout the world.

HOPE FOR ROBERT IN THE U.S.A.

Fortunately, Gary Oberg, M.D., practices environmental medicine in Crystal Lake, a suburb of Chicago, and as mentioned above, his district plans to build a new environmentally safe eighteen-hundred-student high school by the fall of 1997. With Dr. Oberg's input and expertise, this new high school will be the first in this country whose design and construction will apply the basic principles and practices of environmental medicine discussed in this book. Other schools, such as the Irving school district in Texas, have made significant strides toward making their buildings more environmentally sound. We must hope that in time, more American schools will become as far-sighted as those in Ontario and emulate the progressive accomplishments.

The best answer for perplexing learning, behavioral, and/or health problems is not always more teachers with smaller classes, not more special education, and not more sophisticated expensive drugs, but the willingness to spend the time to find and eliminate the cause of these types of problems.

NOTES

1. The video *Environmentally Sick Schools* shows the type of reactions Darryl had during dust P/N allergy testing (see For Further Reading). It also contains statements from various Ontario educators and staff on the value of ECO classrooms.

2. Information about the Ontario environmental health initiatives is available in the *Environmental Hypersensitivities Resource Document*. If you would like to know more about the progressive Waterloo school system, which is "leading the way," call (519) 570-0300 and ask for your call to be directed to the director of the Waterloo County board of education (ext. 4211); the office of the superintendent of special education (ext. 4233); or the office of physical resources (ext. 4311).

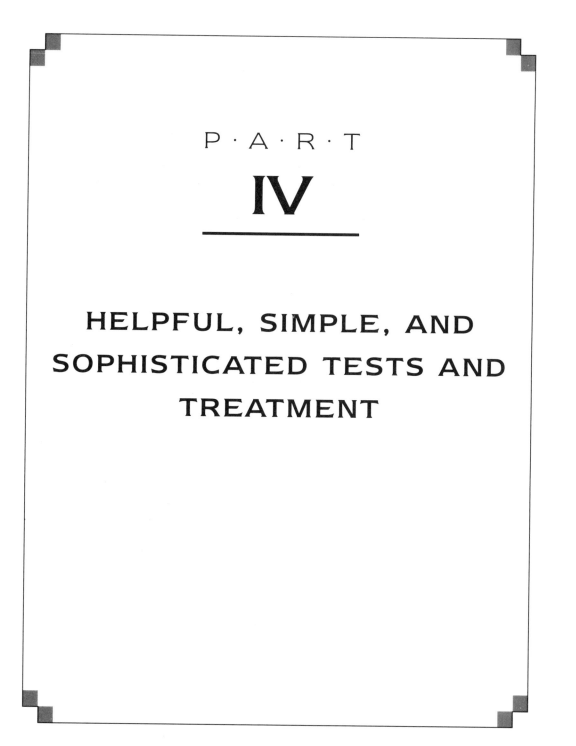

P · A · R · T

IV

HELPFUL, SIMPLE, AND SOPHISTICATED TESTS AND TREATMENT

13 Diagnostic Tests

According to estimates, more than 40 million people now have some form of environmental illness (EI). Many more are unaware that this is their problem, therefore this chapter can be particularly helpful in determining whether your child, or someone else in your family, has unrecognized or unconfirmed EI related to school, home, or work. The diagnostic tests discussed in this chapter will help reveal latent or overt genetic, biological, or immunological weaknesses, which are often related to previous exposures, infections, stresses, or chemical contacts.

How important are these kinds of tests? Just picture the teachers, for example, who are personally distraught over their own environmental illness. Perhaps routine examinations have not indicated any specific abnormality, even though they can no longer perform tasks that they had routinely completed in the past with ease. After a chemical exposure, they become excessively fatigued, and their memory is not normal. They are ashamed to admit that they can no longer think clearly, remember names, or tell time. They are understandably concerned. The information in this chapter will help to confirm that they do have an EI, not an emotional response to some personal stress in their lives.

The lives of too many children and adults have been inexorably changed when the wrong label has been cemented into their medical and scholastic records because doctors and others did not appreciate the role that the environment can play in the functioning of their body.

My aim in this chapter is to show objectively that a person's EI symptoms correlate with certain measurable laboratory changes. A number of these tests will help you sift through the possible causes of your (or your child's) health problems and, at times, provide substantive, definitive answers. They can help differentiate EI from other medical conditions that commonly cause similar symptoms. Conventional medicine, for example, often misses the chemical and food-related causes of an illness. In medicine, it is not enough to find out what is wrong; we must repeatedly ask why it is wrong. For example, we might determine that your fatigue is due to anemia, but why do you have the anemia? The tests in this chapter will help answer this kind of question.

Part of this chapter is rather technical, but it provides you and your physician with important, detailed information that may be needed to explain how to approach certain aspects of environmental illness. Read what is pertinent to you, and don't be intimidated by the technical nature of some of this material (which may actually be particularly helpful to your doctor). The diagnostic evaluation that each child or adult needs must be highly individualized, and the tests indicated for one person may be quite different from those required for another. There is a definite overlap, however, and the tests related to environmental illness will evaluate some combination of the following:

- a typical allergy
- a weakness in the immune system
- a chemical sensitivity
- a nutrient or cellular metabolic deficiency

The tests discussed in this chapter can be performed in a number of laboratories, including those listed in Resources. However, these laboratories represent only a few of the many reliable facilities.

In Table 13.1, you'll find a summary of the major tests that appear to be most helpful in detecting and confirming which *individuals* have an environmental illness. (For a discussion of the most important tests used to determine whether a *building* or its *contents* are environmentally unsound, see Chapter 6.) The aim of the tests described here is to ascertain, for example, if chemicals, dust, molds, or germs are causing the symptoms noted in an individual. Was some chemical or other source of pollution introduced into the person's school or home at the time the symptoms initially developed? Was a specific chemical—possibly implicated on a MSD sheet or detected by a diagnostic laboratory—found in the building? Is that same chemical evident in the blood, urine, or tissues of the sick individual? Were excessive dust, molds, or chemicals also found in the home or school air? Of course, once you pinpoint the EI and then find the source of the illness in a school, you need to urge school officials to remove that cause or lessen the exposure in some way (see Chapters 6, 7, and 12). Similar measures must be taken in homes and workplaces. This may be all that is needed to help some children and adults feel significantly better. The tests discussed in this chapter are an important step in the process of helping you resolve EIs.

For some individuals, you might have to consider the possibility that these tests themselves could pose risks. Thus, you need to weigh the possibility of additional health problems due to continued exposure against the need for proof and documentation of the illness. This choice can create a dilemma for parents, because the health of some affected children is so tenuous that realistically they need to be separated immediately from the cause of their symptoms and, when necessary, to be given appropriate environmental medical care at once (see Chapter 15). If this separation takes place too soon, however, it could interfere with the ability of tests to document the presence of toxic or other offending substances, because certain tests must be conducted within specific time periods after the exposure. On the other hand, if a suspected toxic or harmful exposure is purposely continued so that more objective evidence can be secured, the individual's health may be further jeopardized needlessly.

■ WHO IS A CANDIDATE FOR THESE TESTS?

At least 15 percent of the population of the United States have typical allergies. There is no accurate data on the prevalence of chemical sensitivities, but an estimated 20 to 80 percent of allergic persons have or appear to be prone to developing them as well. Some estimates indicate that up to 80 percent of those who have multiple chemical sensitivities also have food allergies. Any form of stress, infection, and/or emotional upset can precipitate or intensify an EI and/or an allergy.

The human body compensates for chemical exposures to a point, but when an exposure is more than an individual can tolerate, some form of illness will slowly or suddenly become apparent. The precipitating factors that cause obvious illness are often directly related to changes within the person's school, home, or workplace. Remember, such exposures will not affect the health of everyone.

In most patients, the evidence of EI is apparent from the way they look and act. Sometimes the symptoms are easily confused with other complaints associated with more common illnesses—for example, influenza. If fatigue is a prominent complaint, it is common for the EI to be initially confused with infectious mononucleosis.

Possibly your child has already had a detailed physical examination and even a neurological exam but these have failed to reveal abnormalities; this is not unusual when a patient has not had a flare-up of illness at the time of the examination. For example, your youngster may have no evidence of hay fever or asthma except shortly after direct exposure to dust, mold, pollen, or a problem food. He or she may be angelic during the doctor's visit, in spite of a history of frightening emotional outbursts or rages when there is sugar or food coloring in the diet. Heart examinations also can be deceptively normal unless they are performed shortly after the person is exposed to an offending allergenic substance or chemical.

TABLE 13.1

The Most Helpful Diagnostic Tests

Routine Tests (to rule out causes of illness other than EI):

- Complete blood count (CBC)
- Routine blood screening test
- Amino acid assay
- Porphyria blood and urine tests
- Routine urine test
- Nervous system tests

Immune System Testing (to identify allergies and immune weaknesses):

- Total IgE and IgE RAST tests
- Secretory IgA test
- Total IgG and IgG RAST tests
- IgM antibody test
- Delayed, sensitivity tests
- B cell tests
- Tests for T cells and helper/suppressor ratios
- Tal (or CD-26) test for activated T-lymphocytes
- Trimellitic anhydride (TMA) chemical test
- Natural killer cell counts and function tests
- ANA antibody test
- Acetylcholinesterase test
- Autoimmune or autoantibody assay tests
- Interleukin-1 and -2 tests
- Mitogenesis tests
- Lymphocyte transformation tests

Brain-Image Testing (to help determine brain and nervous system malfunctions):

- Nerve conduction tests
- Single photon emission computerized tomography (SPECT)
- Photon emission tomography (PET)
- Electroencephalogram with evoked potentials (qEEG)

Chemical Detection Tests (to identify specific chemicals in humans and air contacts):

- Blood and urine tests
- General volatile screening test
- Hydrocarbon solvent screening test

Advanced Allergy Testing (to verify and/or treat causes of sensitivities):

- Serial end-point titration (SET)
- Provocation/Neutralization (P/N) allergy testing for dust, molds, pollen, foods, and some chemicals
- Enzyme potentiated desensitization (EPD)
- Routine challenge tests
- Controlled challenge tests (in glass booths)
- Air or carpet allergy extract tests

Special Testing

- Carpet analysis for chemicals
- Bioassay tests with mice

Psychological Tests (to help differentiate emotional from physical illness):

- Clinical Analysis Questionnaire (CAQ)
- Profile of Mood States (POMS)
- Minnesota Multiphasic Personality Inventory (MMPI)
- Wechsler Intelligence Scale for Children–Revised (WISC-R)
- Wechsler Adult Intelligence Scale–Revised
- Wechsler Memory Scale–Revised (WMS–R)
- Wide Range Achievement Test (WRAT)
- Harrell-Butler Comprehensive Neuropsychological Screening Test (H–B CNST)
- Clinical Environmental Differential Analysis (CEDA)

To help your doctor in the diagnostic process, consider all possible causes, including school, home, or work exposures. Environmental illness is commonly a mix of many factors, and an attempt must be made to consider, confirm, and document every aspect of your child's problem.

Observe your child's behavior closely. A child who drinks a sweet red beverage and develops red earlobes and a spacey or "demonic" look just before or during a rage rarely responds to anything anyone says or does until that episode has subsided. A change in eye appearance and general demeanor will indicate that the episode is over. (Alkali therapy or the correct P/N allergy extract treatment, discussed later in this chapter and in Chapters 15 and 17, often stops tantrums of this type in less than fifteen minutes.) Certain children have absolutely no recall of what they said or did during their outbursts. Some cannot repress these episodes any more than someone can control a cough, a drippy nose, or a facial twitch. Others definitely can stop or partially control their inappropriate actions, but they need to be highly motivated and encouraged to do so. It is harder to sit still in math class than to quietly watch a favorite television show. Motivation can affect the actions of some children or adults, but unfortunately, not all the time and not completely.

If your child becomes progressively ill or exhibits disruptive behavior more frequently and more intensely from Monday through Friday (school days), it strongly suggests that some school factors need to be considered. Your youngster may simply dislike school, but other subtle yet significant contributory variables can also be at work. The fragrance of a teacher's perfume or the odor of a nearby lavatory disinfectant or pool chemicals

---

WHEN IS AN ENVIRONMENTAL MEDICAL SPECIALIST HELPFUL?

In addition to taking a detailed medical, social, emotional, and occupational history—as well as doing a thorough physical examination—an environmental medical specialist can help identify whether a child has a typical environmental allergy-type illness and/or emotional problem. When these medical problems are frequently intertwined, with primary and secondary psychological aspects, you will also need a psychological consultant to determine exactly which factors are creating symptoms in a child.

Many health professionals, unfortunately, are not aware of certain symptoms commonly due to molds, dust, pollen, or foods. Most would not discern the extent to which a slight exposure to a chemical, for example, could affect the ability of some children to learn, feel well, or behave. If you are suspicious, seek out an environmental medical specialist with expertise in these areas.

can cause extreme fatigue, irritability, and/or constant restlessness in some children. These factors, in turn, can directly cause learning and behavioral problems and, indirectly, a definite dislike of school. In contrast, if children (or teachers) have the same symptoms on weekends and evenings, as well as in school, it is much less likely that the school is the sole cause of a problem. If their symptoms seem worse at home, that is where the problems and answers may lie.

Again, to help diagnose the problem, consider exactly where the behavior is worse. Is it always in one particular room or area? Keep asking why. Combined input from an experienced teacher, school health provider, and school psychologist or counselor may be required to ascertain the cause of school-related symptoms; similarly, a spouse or relative may provide helpful observations at home.

Don't hesitate to obtain professional guidance to help you better understand and learn to respond to your child's unusual behavioral outbursts. Most people accept that the lungs can develop asthma when exposed to dust, molds, and chemicals, but few acknowledge that the brain can react to these same exposures, with changes in mood, actions, or the ability to think clearly.

Your physician will need a detailed list of all the health problems that bother your child. Review your answers to the questionnaire in Chapter 3, and make sure the responses have been honest and without exaggeration or understatement. The key questions to consider are:

- Does your child's medical history indicate an allergy or a propensity to EI? (See Table 3.1.)
- Has your child had a single or long-term chemical exposure in the past?
- How seriously ill is your child?
- Did the illness begin or significantly flare up before, during, or shortly after a minor or major school change or renovation?
- Were chemicals used in the school shortly before your child became ill? (See Chapters 7 and 10.)
- Did your child's school or home have any ventilation or moisture problem prior to or at the time the illness began?
- How many other children are affected?
- Are their health problems similar?
- Are their symptoms typical of those noted after chemical exposures? (See Chapters 10 and 11.)

Answers to these questions will provide clues about which tests might be most informative.

▨ WHAT TESTS ARE MOST IMPORTANT?

The major tests that provide the most information usually include:

- ▨ a thorough examination of the affected body parts. For example, a child with nervous system difficulties needs to be examined by a neurologist; a youngster with hay fever or chronic sinus or ear infections should have an examination by an EI ear, nose, and throat (ENT) or allergy specialist
- ▨ lung, bladder, and muscle studies by other specialists are indicated, if these body areas are involved
- ▨ an immune system profile, especially for T cell function, Ta1, TMA (trimellitic anhydride); and NK cell function tests, as well as various autoantibody tests
- ▨ a toxicology report, to determine the level of certain suspect chemicals in the blood, urine, and/or body fat
- ▨ an analysis to detect chemicals in an offending item such as a carpet, carpet pad, furniture covering, etc.
- ▨ psychological and neuropsychological examinations, to identify the degree and type of memory problems and any emotional aspects of a particular problem
- ▨ brain imaging and brain tomography, to pinpoint brain injury or damage
- ▨ allergy testing for common allergens, especially for air- or carpet-sample extracts made in a suspect school or home
- ▨ bioassay tests, to determine the effects of an exposure to a suspect item upon mice
- ▨ special intestinal and cellular studies to evaluate the adequacy of their function

Knowledgeable physicians can advise you about which tests might be most helpful to confirm a diagnosis of environmental illness in your own child. In some situations, it is a good idea to obtain the opinion of a personal injury lawyer who is knowledgeable about environmental medical injuries and federal and state entitlements, *early in the course of your discussions* (see Chapter 16). Do this not because you intend to sue but because you must know what must be done if your child's or your own problems worsen and you have no alternative. If certain deadlines are not met, you may not be able to initiate a suit at a later date.

▨ ROUTINE TESTS

Let's look closely at each of the routine tests, and the information they can provide. Their main purpose is to rule out possible causes of illness.

THE COMPLETE BLOOD COUNT (CBC)

A total white-blood-cell count and differential can help distinguish a viral from a bacterial infection. This determination is important because chemical exposures typically mimic prolonged viral infections. Chemically sensitive individuals can have a total white-blood-cell count in the range of 2,500 to 4,500, rather than 5,000 or above. Sometimes the CBC indicates an abnormality such as low hemoglobin, which suggest anemia in a fatigued person; or it may detect a markedly elevated white-blood-cell eosinophil count, which suggests allergy, parasites, or a drug reaction.

Exposure to a chemically laden carpet, a defective heating system, or a pesticide can cause definite adverse changes in the blood of some individuals. However, the CBC in certain patients who have chemical sensitivities can be entirely normal. (For an in-depth discussion of various blood abnormalities, see chapter 8 in volume 1 of William Rea's book, *Chemical Sensitivity.*[1])

ROUTINE BLOOD SCREENING TESTS

A routine blood screening test provides a basic overview of the functioning of the liver, lungs, kidneys, muscles, and bones. The results of this test are often normal in environmentally ill people, unless they have another unrelated medical illness. One or two liver function enzymes may be mildly elevated in 40 percent of chemically sensitive patients.[2]

At times, however, distinct abnormalities, such as tics, twitches, or cramps in the facial or body muscles, suggest a magnesium problem, which can be documented with appropriate testing (as discussed in Chapters 14 and 15).[3] Other individuals may have extreme fatigue and swollen lymph nodes or neck glands. This suggests the need for a test to rule out infectious mononucleosis associated with Epstein-Barr syndrome, although a rare child will quickly develop swollen glands from certain foods or exposures. If a patient lives in an area where Lyme disease is a problem, and has a concentric-ringlike skin rash, fatigue, and aches, this illness must be ruled out with a special test.[4] Your doctor will know which special tests need to be ordered.

FOR PATIENTS WITH A BLEEDING TENDENCY

Some young hyperactive children have bruises simply because they have poor depth perception, run too fast, and bump into anything in their way. Others, however, may experience easy bruising, nosebleeds, or vaginal bleeding that is unrelated to any trauma; in some children, these symptoms are due solely to environmental factors.[5] These patients need to be seen by a hematologist.[6] Refer back to the story of Liza in Chapter 2, for example, and you will see that her excessive bleeding perplexed physicians for years. It was eventually found to be related directly to natural gas (hydrocarbon) chemical exposures from furnaces and gas stoves.

AMINO ACID ASSAYS

A number of amino acids are essential for normal brain and body functioning, as well as for the excretion of pollutants and chemicals. Multiple amino acid abnormalities sometimes occur in children who have significant developmental, learning, or behavioral problems. In general, a fasting plasma or twenty-four-hour urine amino acid analysis helps to assess the key metabolic pathways that keep the body performing optimally. These amino acid assays can detect metabolic blocks associated with vitamin and mineral deficiencies.

To utilize the essential amino acids that we ingest, the body needs key nutrients such as various B vitamins, zinc, magnesium, iron, manganese, and molybdenum. Laboratories that do amino acid interpretation and metabolism, such as Bionostics and MetaMetrix (see Resources), can help your personal physician interpret the results of an amino acid assay and explain the need for specific amino acid or nutrient supplements or dietary restrictions to correct an individual deficiency. Nutrient combinations must be balanced and correct. More of a nutrient is not necessarily better; in fact, too much of some nutrients can be harmful. The proportion of various nutrients is critical.[7]

PORPHYRIA TESTS[8]

The symptoms and course of multiple chemical sensitivities (MCS) appear to overlap with the diagnosis of a porphyria disorder in about 50 percent of patients. A porphyrin disorder is an illness that affects mainly females. In some people it can be due to a hereditary enzyme deficiency that affects the production of blood (heme) and other metabolic functions. In others, a wide range of chemicals and toxins, as well as infections and crash dieting, can cause an acquired form of this disease. It may also be caused by antidepressant, antianxiety, and antipsychotic drugs, which unfortunately are commonly used to treat symptoms associated with unsuspected MCS.

A porphyria disorder is present when the liver can't effectively break down red blood cells because of deficient enzymes. This allows toxic porphyrins to be deposited in various body tissues, producing illness particularly in the nervous system and brain. When toxic porphyrins accumulate, they can cause extreme abdominal discomfort and tenderness, leg cramps, muscle weakness and pain, psychiatric symptoms, and a sensitivity to sunlight for select patients. Tiny amounts of previously tolerated odors can also trigger symptoms. Once you know which chemicals cause symptoms, they must be stringently avoided.

Tests to rule out porphyria should be done on all patients who appear to be sensitive to many chemicals. They might also provide answers for some people who appear to have fibromyalgia, silicone breast implant problems, or the Gulf War Syndrome. (Most insurance companies reimburse for these tests without difficulty.)

These special blood-cell tests for the porphyrin enzymes typically show various deficiencies indicating latent or active illness. Elevated twenty-four-hour blood and urine porphyrin levels confirm active disease. With the hereditary form of this illness, these enzymes remain abnormal but stable, while those who have MCS tend to have varying levels directly related to specific chemical exposures.

URINE TESTS

Routine urine tests help to rule out conditions such as diabetes, kidney disease, and dehydration. They should be done first for any child or adult who has urination, bladder, or kidney problems.

Special urine studies for organic acids provide information about how well the cells of the body break down or metabolize proteins, fats, and carbohydrates. These tests can spot errors in B vitamin utilization, neurotransmitters, liver enzymes, and bowel function. (See Resources for laboratories that perform these tests.)

A porphyria urine test can be very important for select patients. One clue suggesting porphyria is that the urine can become dark red in color when it is exposed to sunlight.

NERVOUS SYSTEM TESTS

The following intermittent or constant symptoms suggest that a child or adult may be experiencing undesirable toxic changes in the nervous system, which would indicate the need for a thorough examination by a neurologist. Always notice whether these symptoms are more evident or frequent at school than at home:

- numbness, tingling, or burning of the face, hands, or arms
- persistent headaches, either mild or severe
- problems learning, remembering, or concentrating
- difficulty expressing oneself
- extreme fatigue

- problems walking or moving normally
- unusual sudden behavioral changes or mood swings, such as hyperactivity, aggression, irritability, depression, anger, withdrawal, vulgarity, rages, or panic attacks
- emotional lability or instability, with inexplicable, easy crying or uncontrollable emotional outbursts
- a metallic or unusual taste in the mouth

ROMBERG TEST

The Romberg Test, which you can do at home, is a fast and simple way to help detect possible nervous system damage. First, ask your child to stand on his toes with his feet very close together. Unless he has had a serious back or leg injury, he should be able to stand easily, without swaying or tipping over. Then instruct him to do exactly the same thing, but this time with his eyes shut. If he does that all right, have him do it standing on one foot at a time. Does he fall over in less than ten seconds? Most people will sway a bit but they do not fall over. (Do not have your child try this unless you're ready and able to break the fall if this happens.) If your child *instantly* falls over, the Romberg Test is positive, and he should see a doctor. This simple test can provide a clue that an abnormality is present, especially if chemicals have damaged critical parts of the nervous system or brain.

CURRENT PERCEPTION THRESHOLD (CPT) TESTS

Numbness and tingling of various body parts (face, arms, legs) suggest possible damage to the peripheral nerves. CPT measurements correlate with nervous system problems due to chemical exposures.[9] Physiatrists, who are physicians specializing in this area of medicine, can evaluate these types of symptoms. They can study, for example, the perception of vibration, or measure how long it takes a nerve impulse to travel to the brain and back to a damaged area. If it takes too long, this indicates that something is wrong with the nerve-impulse transmission. These conduction-type tests, unfortunately, are most painful and are not well-tolerated by children and some adults.

■ PSYCHOLOGICAL TESTS

Regardless of age, most children and adults who have EI complain of myriad symptoms. At times, some appear to be unduly upset and to behave most inappropriately. For these individuals, an impartial evaluation of all possible emotional and environmental causes of each complaint is essential.

An emotional evaluation is often more necessary in adults than in young children. Many youngsters appear pleasant and normal until they are tested with a specific allergen; then their unacceptable behavior is suddenly triggered. Even though some children's actions improve significantly after allergy extract treatment, they may need psychological counseling for certain unacceptable response patterns that became a habit before the proper treatment was begun.

Remember that the behavior of a normal child or adult can change with illness, especially if it is chronic and not believed by others. The dilemma, therefore, is to determine whether the person's symptoms are due primarily to a physical condition or partially or totally to a psychological problem. For example, a psychologically upset individual, whether child or adult, may primarily have profound depression, anxiety, and tension, which in turn causes secondary complaints such as headaches and fatigue. In others, the opposite is true: A primary environmental illness may be manifested by a chronic headache and fatigue, which in turn causes secondary depression and anxiety. A mix of physical and emotional problems exists in many patients, so the challenge is to decide which developed first and what is causing the primary difficulty. It is not always easy to tell if the chicken or the egg came first.

There is no doubt that chemicals can temporarily or permanently damage select, as well as generalized, areas of the brain. Such damage can lead to localized specific or nonspecific symptoms of physical and/or emotional illness, which can vary in different age groups. For example, damage to discrete brain areas can affect one or more of the following: a person's mood, level of anxiety, activity, behavior, learning, memory, manner of speech, walking, etc.[10]

PSYCHOLOGICAL COUNSELING

For many who has behavioral and memory problems, psychological counseling can be helpful. However, remember that the EI-related responses of some allergic and/or chemically sensitive people can easily be confused with a purely psychological problem. Professionals who are unfamiliar with EI can fail to recognize the broad spectrum of adverse effects that environmental exposures characteristically have upon multiple areas of the body, including the brain. Physicians commonly attribute such symptoms, particularly in adults, to stress, or else they diagnose it as "somatization," a "functional" illness or a psychiatric problem. Adults, more than children, unfortunately are often told that they suffer solely from an emotional illness, because they simply have "too many" medical symptoms. This is true even when both have the same number and type of medical complaints.

In children, there are some common valid non-EI-related causes for their poor school performance. These youngsters may:

■ prefer to play
■ dislike a teacher who insists that they study
■ be subject to physical or verbal abuse, restraint, or ridicule by peers, teachers, or parents
■ feel stress because of family friction
■ act despondent because they simply never feel well

Of course, there are many other causes for poor school performance, behavioral problems, or ill health. For example, children quickly learn to manipulate their parents and teachers by screaming, becoming negative, or acting inappropriately if they are not given what they want, when they want it. Many parents bend quickly when pressured by "I hate you" or "If you don't let me eat this, I'll kill myself." Behavior modification is obviously essential for such families, and a counselor can help parents implement such a program. Both parents must present a united front and set down hard, fast, fair, and enforceable rules so that their child clearly understands: Do "this," and you will be rewarded; if you do "that," you will be punished. The selection of reward or punishment used for a particular child must be highly individualized. Each child has buttons that can be pushed, depending upon his or her particular likes and dislikes. A reward might be staying up a half hour later at bedtime, while a punishment might be not playing with a favorite video game for one day. Applying rewards and punishments, however, is much more effective and at times is possible only *after* the environmental/allergenic factors have been appropriately identified and addressed.

Note that EI can create *secondary* psychological problems in normal individuals simply because they are not believed and must convince everyone that a morsel of food or a whiff of a passing aroma can cause an illness that may last for hours, days, or weeks. When affected individuals realize the full extent of their injuries and limitations, they are justifiably concerned and upset. How would you feel if you're a teacher who is extremely ill, loses your job, has no money, and is not believed. You would have a right to be depressed and afraid. Or, consider the child who is too tired to play, suddenly can't learn or remember, and must avoid any socialization because of possible reactions to chemicals. It takes time for the denial stage to reluctantly become angry acceptance. This is particularly true when no one will accept responsibility for what has happened, or when you cannot afford to do what you know must be done to help restore your optimum health.

SPECIFIC PSYCHOLOGICAL TESTS

The many possible causes of each symptom must be considered by parents, teachers, counselors, and physicians; for example, a headache or fatigue may be caused by an exposure at school or by a multitude of physical and/ or emotional factors. That's where a battery of tests, which are generally part of a psychological evaluation, can help. Some standard psychological tests check intellectual and personality/behavioral functions, while others assess the ability to move, walk, feel, or touch.

Particularly valuable tests include the Clinical Analysis Questionnaire (CAQ) and the Profile of Mood States (POMS), both of which evaluate normal and abnormal behavior. POMS helps detect anxiety, tension, confusion, fatigue, anger, depression, vigor, and activity. It is included in the core battery of tests that the World Health Organization uses for evaluating the effects of neurotoxins on a person's mood or feelings. It is a simple, fast (ten to fifteen minutes), and convenient way to quickly measure the effects of an environmental exposure, as well as the effectiveness of therapy.

What about the popular Minnesota Multiphasic Personality Inventory (MMPI) test? It is certainly not the answer for those who have an environmental illness, unless the EI has caused or is associated with a significant secondary psychological problem. The MMPI test was originally standardized on psychologically ill adult patients, and this remains its main function. An inexperienced tester using the MMPI can completely miss the detection of EI in older students and teachers and may incorrectly label them as hypochondriacal or neurotic.

The CAQ, POMS, and MMPI tests depend to a degree upon being able to think; an adverse exposure in a chemically sensitive individual can therefore interfere with the interpretation of these tests. It is imperative that psychologists recognize the limitations of each test and be experienced in the vagaries of environmental illness in order to correctly interpret the test data. If a mental health provider does not have this type of expertise, the chances for misinterpretation can be very high. The MMPI is more useful if given in conjunction with the POMS, so that transient emotional aspects of behavior can be more clearly differentiated from those due to neurotoxin exposures.

One study by Lisa Morrow, Ph.D., and her colleagues demonstrated some effective methods to evaluate changes in personality and thought processing in a group of workers who were exposed to organic solvents.[11] A battery of neuropsychological tests strongly suggested that their difficulties in thinking were independent of their reported psychological complaints. The duration and amount of chemical exposure and the changes in their ability to smell odors (cacosmia) pointed to possible neurotoxic changes that interfered with clear thinking. Changes in mood and personality can be the earliest manifestations of neurotoxic brain damage. The neuropsychiatric tests used for such evaluations must be able to detect subclinical or very early levels of impairment. This study demonstrated that, unlike the control or unexposed group, there was evidence of both impaired thinking and psychological stress in the workers who were exposed to chemical solvents.

Other tests to evaluate intelligence or thinking (cognition) include the Wechsler Intelligence Scale for Children–Revised (WISC-R) and the Wechsler Adult Intelligence Scale–Revised (WAIS-R). These tests are divided into verbal and performance scales, with subtests in each scale. They require professional administration, scoring, and interpretation. They measure short- and long- term memory, attention, concentration, speed of mental operations, and language, as well as other factors that tend to lower the IQ and interfere with thinking skills. The score results can vary with toxic exposures.

The Wide Range Achievement Test (WRAT) is another useful measure of intellectual-learning abilities; in particular, it indicates a child's selected academic capabilities or deficiencies in various subjects such as arithmetic, vocabulary, and spelling. For memory assessment, a useful test is the Wechsler Memory Scale–Revised (WMS-R).

NEUROPSYCHOLOGICAL TESTS[12]

Neuropsychological testing is more than helpful; it is absolutely essential to evaluate the role of chemicals in the complaints of older children and adults. It helps differentiate whether certain problems are psychological (functional) or physical (organic or due to a bodily illness).

These tests can detect nervous system damage in individuals who complain of nervousness, anxiety, depression, fatigue, insomnia, confusion, agitation, panic, and learning problems. (This array of symptoms is not surprising in EI patients, since they tend to show localized as well as diffuse changes in the brain and/or nervous system.) The tests can sometimes identify subtle intellectual changes before abnormalities can be detected by brain imaging or other sophisticated electrical brain-function tests. If patients are evaluated using only personality or behavioral tests, their illness can be incorrectly assigned a purely psychological label, when it is actually due to a chemical or an environmentally related physical illness.[13]

Joel Butler, Ph.D., and his colleagues (Ernest Harrell, Ph.D., William Flanagan, Ph.D., and Nancy Didriksen, Ph.D.) have devised two tests to help these evaluations—the Harrell-Butler Comprehensive Neuropsychological Screening Test (H-B CNST) and the Clinical Environmental Differential Analysis (CEDA).[14] Another useful and informative test is the Child Neuropsychological Questionnaire by Melendez. There are also many other helpful tests (Bender-Gestalt, Benton Visual Retention Test, Symbol Digit Modalities Test) and assessment techniques. These tests can help document changes in behavior due to toxic exposures, even when basic psychological and biochemical changes are not fully recognized or understood.[15] (Incidentally, insurance companies, reimburse for most of these tests without difficulty.)

ARE YOU MISSING A CHILD'S CRY FOR HELP?

With psychological testing in mind, the examples below of Annie and Stephen show the extraordinary need for attention, awareness, care, and consideration of the problems of children, particularly during adolescence. Too many teenagers and adults permanently turn in the wrong direction because they have lost all hope. Such children respond well to psychological counseling, but only after their environmental illness is better understood and treated. Only then does it often become clear that they need it. Many children need additional psychological testing and counseling for a variety of reasons. A single factor rarely causes an illness that is so severe or extreme as the behavior described below. But these youngster's histories illustrate how crucial it is for the proper diagnostic tests to be conducted and for appropriate treatment to be prescribed.

SUICIDAL TENDENCIES

Annie

Annie tried to kill herself at 13 years of age. She recalled that she had "never" really felt well for a single day in her entire life. She had headaches that lasted for several hours; they were so severe that her head felt like it would explode. Her abdominal pain was so extreme that she often held her abdomen tightly and rocked back and forth endlessly. She was so tired that she would easily sleep away an entire day or weekend. She could not attend school and she had no friends. In spite of her exceptionally high IQ, she could not read correctly or learn well. Her family did not know what to do or where to go, and they did not have the finances to obtain the type of medical care she obviously needed.

Annie's problems were so distressing that she finally tried to slash her wrists. She thought, no one understood the depth of her despair. The sight of her own blood, fortunately frightened her back to reality, and she survived.

I'll write more about Annie and her disturbing medical problems later in this chapter (under the heading "Learning Disabilities"). She probably would never have been so depressed that she would consider suicide if she had undergone the right tests at an early age, and if her condition had been properly diagnosed and treated.

Stephen

At the age of 15, Stephen took his life. I'm describing this fine youngster here so you, the reader, will be even more conscious of what's happening in your own child's life during the critical and sensitive teenage years. Everyone needs to recognize the early warning signs of a child's despair so that it can be properly treated. Let's examine how Stephen, his family, his friends, his teachers, his home, and his school all unknowingly contributed to his tragedy. What can his story show and teach us? Although it was surely not just his allergies or his environment that caused his tragedy, they certainly played a role and were critical considerations during this crucial time in his life.

As with most allergic children, Stephen had a long medical history dating back to infancy. His mother was unaware of the importance of maintaining a balanced, varied diet during her pregnancy. She did not breastfeed him, so he missed this early natural and necessary boost in immunity. These factors, plus genetics, contributed to his poorly developed immune system. As a result, he developed various allergies early in life. These included milk-related colic in infancy and typical hay fever by early childhood.

Intermittently, Stephen had the classical facial clues associated with allergies. His ears suddenly would become red and hot. He had dark eye bags, creases under his eyes, a puffy-appearing face, and an itchy nose that he rubbed upward so often that he had a typical horizontal nose wrinkle.

During puberty, Stephen felt confused and mixed up, and there was much he did not understand. His father's repeated physical and emotional abuse made his life intolerable (as it already had been for years). Both of his parents were overly busy and had their own unrecognized food and other sensitivities that intermittently made them volatile, moody, and/or emotionally labile. His mother was loving and supportive, but she was pushed to the very brink of her own outer limits by Stephen's father.

During Stephen's teenage years, his father became still more abusive, critical, negative, and picky. His father's belittling remarks whittled away at Stephen's self-esteem until little remained of his sense of who he was or could be.

In adolescence, Stephen gained weight because of his poor diet. He tended to snack and binge on dairy products and baked goods (wheat). He loved pizza and beef jerkies, complete with food additives. Eating was one of the few satisfactions in his life. However, he hated himself for eating because he felt he looked fat. He didn't like his appearance and wanted girls to find him attractive. In reality, any excess weight was barely evident to others.

Then, one fateful spring, in spite of his high IQ (158), Stephen's school grades began to fall. His stress seemed to mount daily because he could not get along with his father, and he did not feel as well as usual because his allergies to tree pollen and molds were causing a flare up of his hay fever. To add to his emotional overload, his family had recently moved to a new house. As his bedroom area was being remodeled, he was exposed to an overload of dust, paint, insulation, construction materials, and carpet chemicals. At that time, he was simply breathing too much of the many allergens (dust, mold, pollen, and chemicals) that bothered him, both at school and at home. He was perplexed because he could not concentrate. He hated school, so he truly could not understand why he was being forced to go.

Stephen became uncharacteristically somber and had withdrawn periods, but no one really noticed them enough to become concerned. No one realized how urgently he needed help. He felt his teachers, parents, friends, and siblings were not there for him.

In desperation, to get the attention, love, and understanding he needed, Stephen killed himself. At the last minute, he desperately tried to reverse his actions, but it was too late.

No single factor could be blamed for Stephen's death, but the possibility of environmentally-related suicide in adolescents and young adults cannot be overemphasized. The stress at this time of life can be so great that irrational thoughts lead to irreversible actions. Watch carefully how your own children look and act at puberty. Try to keep external stressors to a minimum. Take advantage of the proper psychological tests described in this chapter. Feed your youngsters a rotated diet with a wide variety of foods, especially vegetables, in addition to providing the extra nutrients in the form of balanced vitamins needed for the growth and developmental spurt during puberty. A stronger body, less exposure to allergenic factors and chemicals, and more observant relatives, friends, and teachers might have saved Stephen. His mother, Anne Puryear, has written a book entitled *Stephen Lives!* In this book and on an audiotape, she provides valuable uplifting insight to help every parent of a depressed child, as well as every older child or young adult who feels that life is no longer bearable.[16]

A MODERN TRAGIC TWIST—"MOTHERECTOMY"
Could EI Cause a Mistaken Diagnosis of Munchausen-by-Proxy?

A new and frightening trend that is gaining momentum can sometimes lead to misdiagnosed psychiatric conditions like Munchausen-by-Proxy. In this situation the medical complaints of a parent concerning a child are thought to be fabricated to gain medical attention. It may begin with the following scenario: A disruptive and aggressive youngster who does not conform at school or at home is placed on a series of activity-modifying drugs. The drugs do not help. The parents, who are often allergic themselves, at some point realize that the cause of their child's behavior may be a food allergy or a sensitivity to something in his environment. They have their child evaluated and successfully treated by an environmental medical specialist. The parents are relieved because the doctor can pinpoint exactly what triggers their child's unacceptable behavior, sickness, and other responses and they learn ways to do this on their own.

But this is not the end of the story. When children like this one are in school, certain luncheon foods, odors, or other environmental factors may cause them to repeatedly misbehave. In time, some may rebel and refuse to cooperate with the treatment. They may swap lunches at school, eat too much of their craved allergenic foods, or fail to take their allergy injection treatment as often as needed. (Occasionally parents themselves are unable to follow the doctor's recommendations, perhaps due to the lack of insurance reimbursement.)

What sometimes happens next is that the school officials suggest an extensive psychological or psychiatric evaluation. Since this diagnostic investigation requires the child to go to an inpatient facility at that point parents may lose all control over what is done and said to their child.

In this new environment, the child's tolerance level might be elevated or diminished, depending on what he or she is exposed to and how stressful the experience is. Sometimes these children miss their families so much that they are intensely motivated for the first time to prove how well they are in an effort to return home. They may never have tried so hard to control their emotional outbursts. In fact, they may appear normal to anyone but those who are more knowledgeable about EI.

In such facilities, the children are typically exposed—overtly or surreptitiously—to the items suspected of causing reactions. The children may even be told they do not have food allergies and can eat whatever they like. Naturally they are delighted—and sometimes they do so, without having an obvious allergic reaction. The parents are perplexed. One doctor tells them to limit or avoid certain foods; another says that eating a typical American diet is part of normal socialization, and it is unfair and cruel to deny their child favorite foods. In addition, their allergy extract treatment is often stopped as well.

Why would children who were thought to have a food sensitivity no longer react to the problem food? How is this possible? There are a number of logical reasons, other than the absence of a food allergy:

- They may have already received and responded favorably to food allergy extract treatment. (Once you are treated, for example, for a grass-pollen allergy, your reaction to grass pollen decreases or is no longer evident. That's why you were treated. It works similarly for food allergy therapy.)
- They are now eating their problem foods every day. This possibility has been a major missed key to the detection of food allergies for over forty years.[17] (I personally did not recognize food allergies during my first twenty years in practice because I was not aware of this!) It is called food masking. When a food is eaten every day, it is possible to produce a *temporary* disappearance of *obvious* cause and effect reactions in response to the ingestion of allergenic food. When the food is consumed infrequently, once a month or so, it is possible that the food sensitivity is again not *immediately* evident, even though it might be present. By contrast, to detect the specific cause of a food sensitivity, the food should be eaten at the critical five-to-twelve-day interval, so the response is not only clearly evident, but exaggerated (see Chapter 3).
- They are so delighted that they can now eat the foods they crave that it alone motivates them to behave in a way that was not thought possible before.
- They may be experiencing subtle, or even overt, responses to the allergens that are not recognized by institution employees who typically lack a parent's in-depth personal knowledge of the child's responses to various allergenic exposures. Even when the parents are there and point out the symptoms, they are often not believed—which is, of course, very frustrating for the older children as well as the parents. Neuropsychologists can

help to differentiate emotional from environmental illness and environmental medical specialists may become increasingly essential to find valid answers if this most tragic trend persists.

Ironically, once these children return home, they can become worse. At this point the mother, in particular, is sometimes blamed for the child's difficulty. And a diagnosis of Munchausen-by-Proxy is made. In this syndrome, parents are thought to repeatedly make up their child's symptoms in order to get medical attention. The mother might even be accused of child abuse. In certain extreme circumstances, authorities forcibly remove the child from the home and place him or her in a foster home or institution. Sometimes they even tell the family that the child might be placed for adoption. By threatening to remove the other children from the family, authorities can easily keep the mother or parents in line. Even though children in this situation certainly need attention, this drastic approach is unconscionable.

The recurrence of the symptoms at home, of course, is not necessarily the fault of the mother. There is another perfectly logical explanation. It may simply be due to exposure to the same environmental factors that originally caused the youngster's illness. The mother might be feeding her child his or her favorite food or beverage, which was not available at the facility. Their home may be moldy, dusty, or contain certain chemicals or a pet that is contributing to the child's "home" symptoms. The obvious solution is to have an impartial person observe the child in the home *when the mother is not present if she is suspect*. This option, however, is usually not authorized or even considered.

All this is tragically wrong. If a mother protects her youngster by stringently avoiding what makes her child ill, it makes no sense to call it a food obsession or child abuse. Even if the mother is actually contributing to a child's illness, the answer is to treat her along with the child, not to disrupt the family with speculative psychiatry and threats of never seeing each other again. No parents should be faced with the prospect of the loss of their child or children, least of all when there is a medical diagnosis that can be proven. If brain-image testing were more affordable, it would be simple to demonstrate that a child's brain is normal until a certain adverse food or odor exposure occurs (see later in this chapter). A comparison of videotaped responses to blinded challenges with foods or other P/N allergy testing also could easily confirm the effect of various exposures. If a child has already responded well to treatment, however, these contacts would no longer cause symptoms.

There is a tendency in modern-day medicine to blame the individual or family and recommend psychiatric evaluations when a doctor cannot find the answers. This attitude compromises objectivity. An environmental medical specialist should have the opportunity to prove that the mother or father is not inducing their child's symptoms. Someone, however, must provide the money required to obtain this proof. Munchausen-by-Proxy should not even be considered unless the psychiatrist is very knowledgeable about environmental illness or the child is evaluated by an EI specialist (see Resources).

This tragic new twist is reminiscent of the time not too long ago when an accepted treatment for severely asthmatic youngsters was banishment for years to a medical center in Denver. It was called a "parentectomy."[18] When these children were separated from their families, they often improved, but

when they went home, they often became worse. This hardly proves unequivocally that the parents were at fault. Maybe these youngsters had simply been removed from the cause of their allergies—namely, a dusty moldy
house, or the foods, pets, or chemicals that caused their asthma. In those
days, as now, doctors and others frequently did not recognize certain common but elusive causes of problems such as asthma due to foods and chemicals. Munchausen-by-Proxy appears to be a modern "motherectomy." Let us
hope this trendy diagnosis will quickly pass.

■ LEARNING DISABILITIES

If your child has intermittent or daily learning or memory difficulties, he
or she should undergo a comprehensive evaluation that includes a physical
examination by a physician and/or osteopath, as well as various psychological assessments and intelligence tests. Academic strengths and weaknesses, associated performance levels, and the ability to socially interact
must all be evaluated to identify possible causes for learning problems and
to determine appropriate treatment. The IQs of some children have significantly increased after nutritional supplementation and comprehensive environmental allergy treatment[19] (see Chapter 8).

COMMON LEARNING PROBLEMS

Learning problems come in a variety of labels. Dyslexia, for example, was
a favorite term a few years ago. Dyslexia, which merely means difficulty
(dys) reading *(lexia)*, is a mixed bag with many diverse causes. It is so common that about 15 to 20 percent of the middle-class population are
thought to have this problem.[20] Other current "in vogue" learning-
problem labels include LD (learning disabled), MBD (minimal brain dysfunction), and PDD (pervasive developmental disorder), as well as various
cognitive learning disabilities, sensory integration disorders, and "autistic-
like" or "Tourette's Syndrome–like" symptoms.

Learning difficulties may also occur in children with Attention Deficit
Hyperactivity Disorder (ADD or ADHD), a term that unquestionably over-
laps with allergies in children who have the Allergic Tension Fatigue Syndrome (ATFS) (see chapter 1). An ADHD child is not only impulsive, unable
to concentrate, and easily distracted, but also hyperactive. ATFS children
can be tense, nervous, tired, irritable, and sometimes hyperactive. Further-
more, some ADHD and ATFS symptoms overlap with those associated with
Tourette's Syndrome (see Table 1.3). A mix of the symptoms of all three
conditions can occur in the same child, with remissions and flare-ups coin-
ciding with specific exposures or contacts. Also, when allergy and environ-

mental illness are part of the cause of these children's overlapping symptoms, all three conditions tend to improve simultaneously when these sensitivities are treated.[21]

No one knows how often environmental factors or foods are the cause of learning problems. Sometimes the ability to read and see well is directly

---

UNUSUAL VISUAL PROBLEMS

Annie

Thirteen-year-old Annie (whom I wrote about earlier in this chapter) had suffered from incapacitating albeit unrecognized environmental illness for years. She had daily fatigue, headaches, abdominal pain, extreme depression, and chronic infections. At times she would sleep all day, arising only to use the bathroom. Her abdominal pain was so severe that she would rock in a chair for hours holding her abdomen. At times she passed out. She became ill in school and at home as well as in church and stores. On one occasion she was so unhappy with her life that she tried to kill herself. Prior to her visit to our center, she had seen eight different doctors.

About six weeks before Annie's appointment with us, she suddenly developed a new medical problem. For no apparent reason, during a twelve-hour period, her vision became red (probably due to edema in the macula, located in the back of the eyeball). Subsequently, she could read only if the printed matter was upside down. When she looked at one area of the print, the rest blurred or twirled around. The print on the edge of a page tended to disappear. The number 2 looked like a 3, and 6 looked like 9. Letters were mixed up or upside down. L looked like T. Numbers or letters were duplicated, so that if she looked at the numbers 1-4-5, she would see 1-4-4-5.

After the first day of food P/N allergy testing and treatment, her headaches, chronic abdominal pain, and excessive fatigue subsided. The next day, however, when she received an allergy test for a mold, her vision suddenly became much worse, and she could not read anything. Then, when she was given a drop of the right dilution of that same mold extract, her vision suddenly returned, and she could read again but only when the printed material was upside down.

The following day we tested Annie for soy. Much to our surprise, her major visual problems suddenly disappeared when the correct dose of a soy allergy extract was administered. She could clearly differentiate 2 from 3, 6 from 9, and L from T. She could read a book right-side up and upside down. The twirling words and blurred areas were less of a problem. She and her family were jubilant.

It is too soon to know Annie's long-term prognosis, but for several weeks she remained remarkably well. Her complaints, unfortunately, recurred when she returned to school, but after additional P/N allergy retesting, she quickly responded favorably again. Annie's complaints were not due to a "psychological problem" or to being "spoiled." She had a previously unsuspected but treatable environmental illness.

related to environmental exposures. During P/N allergy extract testing, children sometimes do suddenly write backward or upside down (see Chapter 5). Some read or write from right to left rather than from left to right. A few even read better when the print is upside down! It is truly amazing to see these types of difficulties become evident, then subside within ten minutes after exposure to one drop of specific dilutions of an allergy extract.

The abrupt improvement of Annie's serious visual problems with P/N allergy testing suggests the need for much more investigation in this area. How many other children suffer needlessly and cause their teachers and parents to be frustrated, because environmental illness erratically alters their ability to read, write, or learn?

VERY SEVERE LEARNING PROBLEMS

AUTISM[22]

Each child who is labeled autistic or autistic-like must be treated as an individual. The variation in autistic behavior covers a wide spectrum. Most children with this problem have developmental delays, problems with perception, communication, behavior, and attention. Many make poor eye contact and have repetitive patterns of movement (flapping hands, twisting, etc.) and do not respond normally to questions or touch.

There appears to be both an increased awareness and incidence of autism. Many children who have autistic-like characteristics initially appear to be normal, but only until about eighteen months to two years of age. Then they not only stop progressing but often regress in their development. Why do they change? The excessive use of antibiotics, routine immunizations, and possibly increased pollution are three suspect factors that need investigation. Twenty-five books were published in 1994 that question the safety of immunizations; the increasing incidence of autism is, in particular, one aspect that is being considered. In 1992 the television program *20/20* reported about an unusually large number of autistic children whose parents grew up in a particular community. As children, these parents had played on a dump site for plastics and lived downwind from factory pollution in Leominster, Massachusetts. We don't know if that was a factor, but we must wonder why their class reunion revealed so many medical problems such as autism in the offspring of both the males and the females. Was the hormonal development of these youngsters altered in some manner, so that years later, their children were not normal?

Two pregnant women in Maryland, who had headaches and nausea from smelly new carpets and renovated work areas, gave birth to babies who became autistic. Is there a relationship? Isolated cases are difficult to interpret, but there must be some reason why this is happening more often than in the past. We don't have the answers at this time, but obviously we need to find out. Collaborative studies under the direction of Bernard Rimland, Ph.D., are now in progress, which should eventually provide more definitive answers.

Meanwhile, in rare instances, an exceptional autistic child will become *entirely normal* within two weeks after being placed on a diet totally excluding dairy and/or wheat products (see Chapter 5). Because of this remote possibility, such diets should be considered for all autistic youngsters. Studies indicate that autistic-like characteristics in some youngsters can subside to varying degrees after eight to twelve months of other specific dietary treatment, allergy extract therapy, or nutrition regimens. The learning ability and physical limitations of some autistics unquestionably improve dramatically after B_6 or other nutrient or mineral supplementation, and/or intravenous gamma globulin therapy. A number of specialists with differing backgrounds have had varying degrees of success using other approaches. Sometimes autistic youngsters are helped by immunologic, allergic, gastrointestinal, metabolic, neurochemical, nutritional, audiologic, osteopathic craniosacral and specific touch therapy. Appropriate testing and treatment for parasites, chronic localized bacterial infections, lead detoxification, and treatment with certain neurotransmitters have sometimes proven helpful. The bottom line, however, remains, why is autism increasing and how many autistic children can be helped to respond more favorably.

LANDAU KLEFFNER SYNDROME

Normal children between the ages of one and eight years can develop Landau Kleffner Syndrome, which has some characteristics of autism or PDD (Pervasive Developmental Disorder). Either gradually or rapidly, the affected children lose their ability to understand or acknowledge what is said to them, but they retain the ability to express themselves. They tend to be withdrawn, aggressive, hyperactive, stubborn, and prone to repeat phrases. Sleep EEGs, brain waves, and SPECT brain imaging might help in the diagnosis. Early treatment with steroids appears to be helpful.[23]

FRAGILE X SYNDROME

Fragile X Syndrome is a medical condition that must be considered in children who have severe learning problems. It is a genetic illness seen in males and carried by female members of families. These boys tend to have a prominent chin and forehead, a long face, large protuberant ears, poor muscle tone, autistic or strange behavior, altered speech patterns, and enlarged testes (after puberty). They are usually retarded and hyperactive. Fragile X can be diagnosed easily with a simple blood test.

FETAL ALCOHOL SYNDROME

Fetal Alcohol Syndrome occurs in the infants of mothers who drank alcohol during their pregnancy. These infants are often seriously retarded and have multiple malformations, including small eyes, tiny eye slits, abnormal palm creases, heart defects, and tight joints.

■ IMMUNE SYSTEM TESTING

When the adequacy of the body's defense or immune system needs to be checked, certain laboratories (such as Antibody Assay Laboratory and Immunosciences Lab, listed in Resources) can perform these tests. In general, a specialist should be consulted and baseline blood and/or urine specimens should be collected in special tubes supplied by the laboratory. These samples should be taken *as soon as possible* or *at the proper time* in relation to specific offending environmental exposures. If the timing is wrong, certain abnormalities can be easily missed. A temporary tolerance or a waning sensitivity can seriously compromise the interpretation of the test results.

The major tests described below (and listed in Table 13.1) are useful and typically are reimbursed by insurance companies. Although significant deviations from the normal range indicate something is wrong, at times these test results can appear deceptively normal. A lack of evidence of an abnormality in a test result should not be equated to a lack of disease. Maybe the wrong tests were ordered or the timing was incorrect. A knowledgeable physician or biochemist can determine if and when additional tests are needed.

TOTAL IgE AND IgE RAST TESTS

In general, typical allergies such as seasonal hay fever cause an elevated total IgE (immunoglobulin E) level. Similarly, specific IgE RAST (radioallergosorbent-Test) tests are typically elevated in individuals who are allergic to dust, molds, pollen, foods, or pets, but there are exceptions.

Again, even in a patient who has obvious typical allergic symptoms, a test result can erroneously appear normal. For example, an exceptional child may experience repeated learning problems as a result of obvious hay fever during the grass-pollen season every year. Yet the blood test may give a false impression that no such sensitivity exists—showing a normal rather than an elevated total IgE and IgE RAST for grass. Nonetheless, this youngster may respond favorably to routine grass allergy extract treatment.

Another way to show that a child has a grass sensitivity is to add grass antigen to the youngster's basophilic white blood cells to show that histamine is released. This would indicate that a true sensitivity exists, in spite of a falsely negative IgE RAST test. In much the same way, immediately after a classic chemical exposure to formaldehyde, it is very rare to see an IgE elevation. The initial antibody response to a five-day formaldehyde exposure may not be evident for about a week. If the blood sample is taken before that time, the test may not provide proof of an exposure. After the antibody response becomes evident, it lasts for only a couple of weeks. So if a blood sample is taken several weeks *after* an exposure, again it can fail to provide the usual IgE evidence of a past exposure.

Other formaldehyde antibody tests (like IgM, immunoglobulin M) can indicate a previous exposure for about three to four months. Then, after about a year, the formaldehyde exposure will be reflected by an elevated IgG (immunoglobulin G) level. The laboratories that do these studies can help advise you and your physician about which tests to order and when.

In summary, a positive IgE test indicates a probable allergy. If the IgE level is in the normal range, it suggests no allergy, though this interpretation is sometimes misleading and incorrect.

SECRETORY IgA LEVEL TEST

The secretory IgA antibody is present in the mucous membranes, and its level can be measured in saliva. This secretory IgA antibody is the first line of defense to protect the body against germs or allergenic substances that enter the body through the mouth or intestinal wall. Its level is often decreased if a patient has digestive problems, food sensitivities, or yeast problems. Chemical exposures can alter the immune protection in the body so that the secretory IgA level in saliva or mucous membranes is lower than normal.

TOTAL IgG AND IgG RAST TESTS

A normal IgG level in the blood, in general, reflects long-term protection from potentially harmful substances. It is sometimes, but certainly not always, decreased when recurrent infection is a problem.

The results of IgG RAST tests for foods are often elevated in patients who have food sensitivities, especially if they have eczema. Routine P/N food allergy skin tests are usually possible and helpful, when a food **IgG** RAST score is markedly elevated. To ensure safety, however, extreme caution must be taken during allergy testing for a food or any other item that has an inordinately high **IgE** RAST score.

Some reactions to foods can occur immediately after eating; others (such as ear infections, joint pains, colitis, bed-wetting, and canker sores) are not evident for several hours. Delayed sensitivity reactions are therefore difficult for children and their parents to pinpoint on their own, and thus testing of the IgG$_4$ subclass has been increasingly used as an indicator of these delayed reactions. But even though these tests are most useful in detecting "hidden" food reactions, they too can appear falsely normal. For example, if a child stops eating a problem food for a few weeks, the IgG$_4$ level can appear to be entirely normal, even though the child actually has a sensitivity. If a person uses cortisone or other steroids, the IgG$_4$ production can be suppressed so the test result can be deceptively normal.

Other circumstances can raise IgG$_4$ levels. For example, repeated exposure to food antigens can alter the intestinal wall so the gut becomes leaky and foods pass through the allergically damaged tissues. The spaces between the cells in the intestines can be so open that undigested food particles and larger molecules that are normally blocked can directly enter the circulation, this can cause problems in the immune system, such as an increased IgG$_4$ production. When these immunoglobulins unite with food particles, they form immune complexes that can cause a wide range of symptoms affecting multiple body areas.

TESTS FOR IgM ANTIBODY LEVELS

The level of this antibody in the blood is often the first to increase after a harmful exposure, and it can remain increased for a year or so afterward. In time, however, this antibody will decrease as it is usually replaced by an IgG form of protection.

TESTS FOR B CELLS

The white blood cell lymphocytes called B cells make protective antibodies. Abnormal increases or decreases in this type of cell in the blood are important, but they are possibly less meaningful than the white blood cell level of T lymphocyte cells. Overzealous B cells can increase the IgE-type antibodies associated with typical allergic-type responses. This abnormality is often genetic and found in allergic families. However, if certain types of B cells become stimulated, the less readily recognized (but equally prevalent) forms of allergic reactions (see Table 3.1) can occur and make excessive IgG, not IgE, antibodies. This latter type of antibody response can be caused by chemicals, infection, or stress.

TESTS FOR T CELLS AND HELPER/SUPPRESSOR RATIOS

T cells, the commanders that regulate the immune system, must function well in order to tell the B cells exactly when and how much to help the body. T cells may be deficient in allergic individuals, or in those whose immune system needs protein or nutrients or when immunity has been compromised by infection, toxins, cancer, chemicals, or stress. When the T cells are not functioning correctly, the B cells have lost their leader. When that happens, the B cells can get out of hand and they can overproduce either IgE or IgG-type antibodies. A significant increase or decrease in either the T or B cell population is abnormal and indicates illness.

The T-helper cells (CD4) signal the B cells when the body needs more antibody production. The T-suppressor cells (CD8) tell the B cells that they have done their job and that no more antibodies are needed. Individuals with a chemical sensitivity often have an abnormal level of T-suppressor (CD8) and/or T-helper (CD4) lymphocytes, with a corresponding abnormal change in the helper/suppressor (H/S) lymphocyte ratio. For example, the T-suppressor cells can be increased after an individual has experienced an organophosphate pesticide exposure, but they tend to be lower than normal in a person with allergies. The H/S ratio can appear to be too high, too low, or even normal, depending on a patient's exposure.

T-helper cells also produce lymphokines, which are cells that enable the lymphocytes to communicate with one another. Lymphokines increase in number when there is a need for an enhanced immune response.

Nutrient deficiencies can adversely affect various components of your immunity. A decrease in the total T cell lymphocytes, for example, can be associated with an impaired cellular response associated with a zinc deficiency.

Ta1 TEST FOR ACTIVATED LYMPHOCYTES[24]

The Ta1 or CD26 test is **the most informative** test that checks the level of activated white blood cells (lymphocytes). It is a so-called "nonspecific" indicator and tends to become elevated in sensitive patients who have had even a minimal exposure to a foreign substance, chemical pollutant, or toxin.[25] This level can increase within one to two days after a chemical exposure in symptomatic patients, and it tends to remain elevated for three to four months.

NATURAL KILLER CELL COUNT AND FUNCTION TESTS

Natural killer cells (NK) normally protect against viruses, bacteria, and cancer. An NK cell *count* does not necessarily reflect NK cell *function*, which is the essence or crux of a critical evaluation. The NK *function* test is a nonspecific test, but it initially shows a decrease in a patient who has chronic fatigue secondary to a chemical exposure. The results of this same test, however, are more apt to be normal if a patient has other symptoms caused by chemicals. Vitamin C enhances NK cell function, so challenge tests with this nutrient can be used to monitor damage to NK cells (see Resources).

ANA ANTIBODY TEST

About 20 percent of chemically sensitive patients have ANA (antinuclear antibodies). When chemicals damage cell nuclei, nucleic acids are released, and antibodies are formed against them. Systemic lupus erythematosus, viral pneumonia, and silicone breast implants can also cause a rise in ANA antibodies.

ACETYLCHOLINESTERASE TEST[26]

Certain blood tests can help detect whether a chemical exposure has reversibly or irreversibly impaired the functioning of the cholinesterase enzyme. Cholinesterase is normally produced in the area where a nerve impulse must jump from one cell to another to carry messages swiftly throughout the nervous system. If the cholinesterase level is low and the enzyme is not functioning properly, the nervous system goes awry. This can cause a variety of symptoms such as muscle weakness, pains, or cramps, tiny pupils, blurred vision, headache, nausea, twitches, drooling, heart irregularities, and even convulsions can occur. If these symptoms arise, be suspicious of an organophosphate or carbamate pesticide exposure, especially if atropine is mentioned as an antidote on the label of a suspect substance.

For the acetylcholinesterase test itself, the serum or plasma blood level must be drawn within seventy-two hours of the exposure. The red-blood-cell level will remain low for about sixty days after a chronic toxic exposure. This test, however, is not accurate in patients who use oral contraceptives.

AUTOIMMUNE OR AUTOANTIBODY ASSAY TESTS[27]

As mentioned earlier, humans normally form antibodies to protect against foreign substances that enter the body. Chemical exposures, however, can damage normal tissues so that the body becomes confused and no longer recognizes these tissues as its own. When this happens, the immune system can form *auto*antibodies (*auto* means "self") that can attack its own tissues, especially in patients who have a history of a significant chemical exposure.

These individuals should be tested for various autoimmune or autoantibody-type illnesses. Your physician can order these autoantibody tests (from Antibody Assay Laboratory and Immunosciences Lab, for example, listed in Resources). Although the development of autoantibodies does not necessarily indicate an autoimmune disease, it is evidence that an abnormal body response has occurred.

Here is what often happens: When an individual is exposed to a chemical, there is a response in the body. Reactive breakdown products cause antibodies to form, which can potentially cause tissue damage. Some people form autoantibodies against the nuclei of cells and various stomach, intestine, thyroid, liver, muscle, and/or nervous system tissues.[28] As soon as the exposure ends, the antibody production stops and its level gradually falls back into the normal range. But by then, some injury may have already occurred. For example, formation of antimyelin antibodies indicates that there has been damage to the protective covering of the nerves; this damage can lead to significant alterations in nervous system function. Similarly, these antibodies can damage the fat normally found in the walls of each cell in the body.

Antibodies to various body tissues develop in individuals who have been exposed to organic solvent chemicals (such as the halogenated hydrocarbons, tetrachloroethylene, formaldehyde, or chloroform), organophosphate pesticides (such as chlorpyrifos, called Dursban, or diazinon, called Spectracide) used in buildings and for agriculture. In addition, aerial crop spraying near populated areas with chlorinated pesticides such as heptachlor, chlordane, or hexachlorocyclohexane (found in lindane) can cause tissue autoantibodies to develop.[29] (Lindane is a powerful pesticide found in preparations commonly used to treat head lice. When a product containing lindane is used improperly, some youngsters can become seriously ill.)[30]

Because the types of exposures mentioned in the previous paragraph can alter nerve impulse transmission, they can possibly increase the time needed for protective impulses to reach the brain. Not only do some patients with memory or thinking problems, headaches, and/or unusual behavior have abnormal antibodies, but they have altered brain scan images as well. Comparative before-and-after studies by Dr. William Rea and his colleagues have shown that in some patients, abnormal autoantibody levels and brain scans will reverse and become more normal after appropriate detoxification and comprehensive environmental medical care.[31]

OTHER TESTS

A cell called the macrophage can increase the production of protective substances called lymphokine interleukins after pesticide exposures in people with chemical sensitivities. Interleukin-1 stimulates T-helper cells to make interleukin-2, which boosts immune functioning. This test is useful but expensive and not really critical in the treatment of most patients.

Mitogenesis, an aspect of cell division, may also be impaired after a chemical exposure.[32] If it is impaired in genetic cells, it can cause abnormalities in newborns; hence a test for these changes may be appropriate for certain patients.

▪ CHEMICAL DETECTION TESTS

A number of tests can be conducted to determine if there is too much of a particular chemical in the blood or urine. The major laboratory tests that detect the chemicals associated with environmental exposures in schools are discussed below. If you have questions about which specific tests are necessary, call a laboratory and explain which product exposure might have caused certain symptoms. AccuChem, Antibody Assay Laboratory, and Immunosciences Lab (see Resources) are just three of the capable labs that have the necessary expertise to advise you or your physician about or concerning which tests might be most helpful, and the best time to collect the samples.

BLOOD AND URINE TESTS

Blood and urine tests can determine if your child has elevated levels of a specific chemical caused by an exposure to that chemical at the time he or she became ill. For example, if wall paneling, inexpensive wooden cabinets, and new carpeting were installed in a school building just before a number of students or staff members became ill, elevated results from a blood or urine formic acid test would indicate that an excessive exposure to formaldehyde had occurred. These tests, however, are valuable only if they are performed at the correct time after an exposure, and if the sensitivity of the lab test is adequate to detect the levels of the chemical in question. In other words, the tests are not 100 percent accurate. At certain times, they might be unable to detect a harmful chemical in your body, even though it is making you ill.

TEST FOR TRIMELLITIC ANHYDRIDES (TMA)

This key test indirectly measures the level of major volatile (gaseous) organic compounds, such as benzene, styrene, toluene, phenol, or 4–PC (phenylcyclohexene) in the blood. In response to these chemicals, patients with increased TMA antibodies would tend to have specifically elevated IgG, IgM, and/or IgE antibodies. For example, these levels remain elevated for up to three or four months after an illness due to an exposure to certain carpet chemicals, carpet glue, roof insulation, or printing shop fumes. If the person avoids subsequent exposures, these levels should drop, so follow–up blood studies should be conducted.

After exposure to toluene and xylene, moreover, a urine organic acid analysis may find that the compounds methylhippurate and hippurate are elevated. This technique is a standard way to assess a massive exposure to these common solvents. A negative result with this test, however, does not exclude the possibility of an exposure, since there is a marked variation in sensitivity among different individuals. For example, a minimal exposure might cause a chemically sensitized person to become extremely ill, even though the urine organic levels are within the usual normal range.

GENERAL VOLATILE SCREENING TEST

The volatile (gaseous) aromatic chlorinated organic compounds are found in synthetic products such as carpets. In simple terms, this test measures the level of certain volatile organic compounds (VOCs) in the blood and/or the urine (see Chapter 10 and Appendix for more details).

HYDROCARBON SOLVENT SCREENING TEST

This blood test can detect whether someone has been exposed to an excessive level of hydrocarbons. A hydrocarbon is a substance derived from organic material—something that is or once was alive. Anything that originally came from coal, oil, or gas is a hydrocarbon. People are exposed to hydrocarbons predominantly by inhaling vapors and fumes (such as bus or auto exhaust, and vapors from gas stoves, gas or oil furnaces, and gasoline). Hydrocarbons also can be absorbed through the skin (chlorine during showers), or through the intestines after ingesting nonorganic grocery store foods or beverages that often contain traces of pesticides and chemicals. Hydrocarbons, in fact, are routinely found in thousands of consumer products and are used in innumerable industrial processes. Individuals who are bothered by hydrocarbons have a heightened sensitivity that enables them to quickly detect furnace or stove gas leaks, and they tend to become ill particularly when they put gasoline in their car, go to church, or shop in malls.

■ ALLERGY TESTING

We have seen throughout this book, allergy extract testing is used to determine whether the symptoms a patient is experiencing are caused by sensitization to an allergenic substance. These "newer" allergy testing methods are used today by more than three thousand ear, nose, and throat (ENT) and environmental medical specialists, who have found some combination of them to be effective and helpful for the past thirty-five years.[33]

SERIAL END-POINT TITRATION

One new diagnostic method used by environmental medical specialists to find the best dose of allergy extract to use for treatment is called serial end-point titration (SET). It is used primarily to find the initial treatment dose of extract for inhaled substances such as dust, mold, and pollen. Several such allergenic items are tested in different concentrations at the same time. From the response of the skin at the test site, the starting treatment dose of allergy extract is found.

PROVOCATION/NEUTRALIZATION ALLERGY TESTING

The form of allergy testing called provocation/neutralization (P/N) is a precise but exceedingly time-consuming method that has proven helpful because it can pinpoint the specific cause of certain health problems. Using this method, it is possible to reproduce the exact symptoms that an individual is experiencing in school or at home. Carlson Lee, M.D., discovered P/N testing in 1959, and Joseph Miller, M.D., of Mobile, Alabama, taught the technique to many of the physicians who presently practice environmental medicine.[34] This test should be conducted in relatively environmentally safe and allergy-free office. However, in rare cases, an individual is so sensitive to certain foods or exposures that such testing is possible only in an environmental medical hospital (see Resources).

PROVOCATION

A provocation skin test can provoke or suddenly reproduce a patient's typical medical complaints. Provocation tests are typically performed single-blindedly, which means that only the nurse (and not the patient, parents, or doctor) knows exactly what is being tested at a particular time.

A single drop of progressively weaker dilutions of stock allergy extracts (1:5, 1:25, and so on) is injected into the outer layers of the skin every ten minutes. The skin test site where each drop is injected is carefully watched for any significant change. If a sensitivity exists, symptoms are often produced by the stronger concentrations of allergy extract. This is why it is called the provocation dose.

During the testing period, patients should be observed constantly for changes in how they appear, feel, act, behave, breathe, and write. Any symptoms should be roughly gauged on a scale of one to four, making it possible to tell if they are becoming more or less ill or affected as the testing procedure progresses. In addition, some environmental medicinal specialists check the pulse and blood pressure of select patients, between each skin test. If asthma or breathing is a problem, it can be monitored with a simple Peak Flow Meter breathing test (see Resources) before and after each dilution of allergy extract is administered. In addition, more thorough lung function studies, called spirometry, can be conducted at the beginning and end of each skin testing session.

If a child has an allergy, for example, to a mold, one drop of a relatively strong concentration of a mold allergy extract injected into the outer layer of the skin can suddenly and unequivocally cause a significant increase in the size of that skin test site within ten minutes. For instance, if an injected substance causes a skin wheal that is 5×5 mm and it increases in less than 10 minutes to 7×7 mm or more, this suggests an allergy to that substance. Other symptoms, such as congestion, red ears, wiggly legs, asthma, headaches, leg aches, abdominal pain, and/or hyperactivity may also suddenly become apparent during that same period of time. During this period the child's writing may become illegible, his pulse may increase, and there maybe a decreased ability to breathe, as measured by a decline in the Peak Flow Meter reading. Using these combined clues, environmental medicine specialists can usually find one dosage and dilution of allergy extract that *provokes* the patient's typical symptoms, and another that relieves or *neutralizes* many of them.

NEUTRALIZATION
Neutralization is the part of the provocation/neutralization testing procedure that gives the patient treatment. It uses the dose and dilution of allergy extract that stops the symptoms that were produced during provocation. Once the neutralization dose is found, it can be used to prevent an allergic reaction if given *prior to* an offending exposure to that test item. It can also help relieve symptoms if administered *after* an allergic reaction has begun. This treatment dose often diminishes or stops symptoms in less than ten minutes. In time it also can significantly or completely diminish the need for drug therapy.

In general, once the patient is given the provocation dose, then fivefold weaker dilutions of the allergy extract are administered every seven to ten minutes. When the correct neutralization dose, is injected, the skin test area will again look normal. In addition, as the patient's pulse decreases and his breathing improves or returns to normal, he will suddenly feel, look, act, and write normally again.

The exact doses and dilutions of each test item—for example, mold, milk, dust, or pollen allergy extracts—can be combined. This combination of extracts can then be used to prevent, decrease, or eliminate future symptoms caused by everyday contact with these substances. The drops of allergy extract can be administered either under the tongue (sublingually) or by injection. Although most physicians in the United States are unaware of the efficacy of sublingual allergy treatment, it has been used for more than thirty years.[35] A recent Belgian study found that twenty-nine patients with nasal allergic symptoms had significantly fewer problems after receiving low doses of grass allergen sublingually.[36] Many studies conducted in several other countries, indicate this form of therapy is helpful (see For Further Reading).

SOME PRACTICAL EXAMPLES

How does P/N allergy extract testing and treatment help in real-life exposures in schools? Commonly, some children will have problems writing and will complain of headaches in a dusty, moldy classroom. When they undergo P/N testing, it is possible to provoke writing changes during the dust allergy skin test and a headache with the mold test. Then, if the correct neutralization dilutions of dust and mold allergy extract are given before school, both reactions should be prevented. If a child is already experiencing an allergic reaction, it frequently can be eliminated in less than ten minutes, as soon as the correct neutralization dose is received.

The video *Environmentally Sick Schools* demonstrates these types of responses, showing how a teacher's voice became hoarse, and how she developed breathing difficulties within seconds after a skin test with a drop of a weak allergy extract made from her school's carpet. Then, within seconds after receiving one drop of the correct weaker dose of that same allergy extract, her symptoms subsided. This P/N allergy test, therefore, reproduced, and then promptly eliminated the reaction that occurred every day shortly after she entered her carpeted classroom (see the description of Sandra in Chapter 11).

A similar response, unfortunately, can now occur whenever this teacher inhales the slightest bit of perfume or enters a lavatory where there is a deodorizer because she has become sensitized not only to carpet chemicals, but to anything that also contains ethyl alcohol. With that P/N allergy test, it was possible to determine exactly what caused her to react. Because ethyl alcohol is present in deodorizers, disinfectants, and perfumes, as well as in some synthetic carpets, it was clearly the common denominator. This procedure helped explain why many of her distressing and misunderstood symptoms eventually occurred in places other than her classroom.

Similarly, if your child has food sensitivities, these reactions can be prevented if the correct food allergy extract is given before eating, either at school or at home. If symptoms have already begun to develop after eating a particular food, the reaction can be relieved quickly with the right food allergy extract. But the extract must be made from the right food. Suppose a sweet red cherry beverage causes your child to become hyperactive in a few minutes. Is the cause the red dye, the sugar, or the flavoring? Environmental medical specialists would test each item separately and determine if a drop of a sugar, the cherry flavor or the dye allergy extract precipitates the hyperactivity. Once the culprit was found, future disruptions could be controlled by having your child either avoid the offending food item and/ or by using that specific neutralizing dose of allergy extract before (to prevent) or after (to treat) such an exposure. The latter, therefore, may make it possible for your child to drink or eat most offending food items, in moderation, without difficulty.

MY INITIAL SKEPTICISM ABOUT P/N ALLERGY TESTING

I was extremely skeptical when I first heard about P/N allergy testing. I had practiced traditional pediatric allergy medicine for eighteen years and had been told that P/N techniques were unreliable. However, when I tried to disprove the effectiveness of P/N testing, I was astounded to find that it was indeed possible to repeatedly reproduce or precipitate, and then quickly eliminate, specific medical complaints. Even now, I am surprised, at times amazed, that such a wide range of medical symptoms, as well as changes in writing and drawing, can be caused by a single tiny drop of properly diluted standard allergy extract. This certainly does not happen with each P/N allergy skin test or with every patient, but dramatic responses definitely can be produced and quickly eliminated in many patients. This has occurred in centers throughout the United States and been documented by the thousands of videos taken at our own office.

It is certainly not an universal panacea, but it surely quickly and effectively identifies and relieves many previously elusive causes of certain children's chronic health or learning problems. I was more and more perplexed, however, because I did not understand how our bodies can so quickly identify a drop of the "wrong" dilution as harmful and capable of causing illness. Even more challenging was why did one drop of some fivefold weaker dilution of a substance prevent and/or quickly relieve symptoms that had been caused by a stronger solution of the same item? Why did the "right" dilution (in the range of 1:1,000 to 1:100,000) enable a child to eat a food to which he or she was clearly sensitive, or allow increased exposure to dust, pollen, molds, foods or even some chemicals with fewer or no symptoms?

Theories abound which attempt to explain the efficacy of P/N testing, including those proposed by Hartmut Heine, Ph.D., in his book *Matrix and Matrix Regulation*, but we really do not know exactly how and why the procedure is so helpful.[37] This lack of a valid scientific explanation is one reason for the skepticism, especially on the part of those who have neither observed, tried, nor learned these methods. The absence of an adequate explanation, however, in no way indicates that P/N allergy testing and treatment do not help. It merely demonstrates that the human body remains much more complicated, amazing, and magnificent than present-day physicians can explain, understand, or appreciate.

For a more detailed, critical, and fair evaluation of this procedure, see Chapter 17.

P/N TESTING CONFIRMS THE CAUSE OF A STRESSFUL FOOD REACTION

Jacob

Jacob was eight years old when we first saw him in our office. His mother was desperate and described being badly bruised and bitten by him during his recurrent episodes of "mother battering." This violent behavior was not unusual for him and included frequent attacks on his younger brother and sister as well. He also sometimes stabbed his school-mates with pencils and sharp rocks when he suddenly became uncontrollable in school.

On one occasion, shortly after Jacob had just begun his allergy treatment, he refused to dress for school and kicked his brother after eating breakfast. When he finally arrived at school, his teacher immediately noticed that he was even more uncooperative than usual. He was totally negative and refused to comply with the simplest request. In addition, he had that "look" that his teacher (and mother) had learned to recognize as a sign of impending trouble.

It did not take long, before Jacob's teacher became exasperated and sent him to the principal's office. Once there, he promptly grabbed a pile of papers from the top of the principal's desk, ripped them in half, and tossed them into the air. Then with one dramatic sweep of his arm across the desk, he quickly propelled everything else within reach to the floor. The principal called for four security guards, who were able to restrain Jacob, but not without a struggle. They advised taking him to a hospital because they thought it was unsafe for his mother to drive alone with him in her car. Because his mother did not know at that time what had caused this reaction, she gave Jacob his neutralization treatment dose for histamine under his tongue. He promptly spit it out. Within fifteen minutes, after he finally accepted this extract, he became normal, pleasant, quiet, and calm. His mother had no difficulty taking him home, and his behavior and activity were exemplary the rest of that day.

Why did the histamine neutralization dose help? When allergic reactions like Jacob's occur, histamine is usually released. If the correct treatment dilution of histamine is available, it can be used as a nonspecific "turn-off." Similar to aspirin, which nonspecifically relieves headaches, the correct treatment dilution of histamine will frequently relieve a wide variety of allergic symptoms in a few minutes, because this is one of the major offending substances released during allergic reactions.

Sometimes seeing is believing, and this is one of many examples cited in this book that was included in the videotape *Environmentally Sick Schools.*

Later, we asked his mother what was unusual about that day when he had become exceptionally uncontrollable. She told us the prime suspect were strawberries he had eaten at breakfast. We then precipitated an episode of extreme hostility and intolerable behavior, like the one that had occurred at school, by placing a single drop of strawberry allergy extract in his arm. During this episode, in spite of our attempts to intervene, he proceeded to cover his mother's arms with bite marks. His face looked almost as if he were possessed. He glared at his mother, and jabbed at her with his fist, striking her in the eye. As she held her eye and quietly wept, he emphatically and defiantly said, "Good!" He cried at times, but his major activity during this episode was aggression directed at his mother. Fifteen minutes after he received the correct neutralization or "turn-off" dose of strawberry allergy extract, he again became a normal, pleasant, and cooperative youngster. There was no further need for outside restraint.

One must wonder how many other "Jacobs," in school and elsewhere, are misunderstood because they have allergic reactions in areas of the body where most people do not realize they can occur. The brain, bladder, muscles, joints, and blood vessels can react in much the same manner that the lungs react in asthmatics or the nose in those who have hay fever.

Not every individual or test provokes such a dramatic response, but P/N allergy testing certainly helps to detect, pinpoint, and treat the specific cause of perplexing and challenging health problems. A sublingual dose or an injection of the neutralization allergy extract can be safely administered by either parents or older children to relieve or prevent symptoms. It is extremely unfortunate and unfair that many children and adults are deprived of this most effective form of treatment because certain insurance companies refuse to reimburse for P/N allergy testing or treatment (see Chapter 17).

ENZYME POTENTIATED DESENSITIZATION

A new form of allergy extract therapy called enzyme potentiated desensitization (EPD) has been studied and used since 1966. Preliminary blinded studies have confirmed its efficacy, and larger-scale investigations are presently under way for a more comprehensive evaluation.[38]

EPD therapy uses injections of very weak homeopathic dilutions of allergenic substances, combined with an enzyme called beta-glucuronidase. These injections appear to help as many as 80 to 90 percent of treated patients. The treatment method has its pros and cons, but it is promising because patients need only six or fewer injections each year. For some conditions—such as seasonal hay fever or a simple dust allergy—only one to three annual injections are eventually required. In time, the need for injections can further diminish, so that several years can actually elapse between doses. Some patients can eventually stop this treatment because they are so well.

EPD seems to be particularly helpful for people who have food sensitivities. Sometimes, after a year or so of therapy, multiple food allergies are dramatically relieved. Typically, once patients have responded favorably, they can eat many previously symptom-producing foods without concern or other treatment, except for strict dietary and other restrictions near the time of each booster injection.

There is a down side, however, to EPD. Many potentially allergenic foods, drugs, and other items must be strictly avoided for several days before and after each injection. Also, P/N allergy treatment must be discontinued for two weeks before EPD treatment can be started, and if patients aren't helped by treatment, they cannot start or resume P/N therapy for six months. Fortunately it may be possible to use a histamine P/N treatment dose during this period.

Patient responses to EPD can vary considerably. Although some individuals improve quickly, others need one to three years before EPD begins to relieve their typical allergies or chemical sensitivities. During that period symptomatic drug therapy is typically required. Also, keep in mind that EPD does not help everyone, and some patients temporarily worsen during the course of this treatment. Although EPD is still considered experimental, it appears to be a most promising form of allergy treatment for some children and adults.

ROUTINE CHALLENGE TESTING

The purposeful exposure of people to foods or to chemicals such as phenol, glycerin, formaldehyde, or hydrocarbons, can show whether these common offending substances cause symptoms. This testing sometimes can be done at home or more scientifically in a doctor's office—in a single-blinded manner with appropriate controls. The response to eating a food or smelling some chemical can be documented on a videotape. With this approach, sensitive individuals will often experience the exact symptoms that occur when they eat an offending food or are exposed to a chemical. For examples of chemical challenges conducted in our center, see the discussion of Tom below, and of Ryan in Chapter 1. The actual responses of many more children to challenge testing appear in the video *Environmentally Sick Schools* (see Resources).

We usually test patients only for those chemicals that they cannot routinely avoid. The test exposure is often minuscule by comparison to what they normally encounter on a daily basis.

LEARNING PROBLEMS DUE TO FOODS AND CHEMICALS

Tom

Tom was a 12-year-old boy whose parents and brothers were all allergic. His story is typical of many children. He was so hyperactive as an infant that his crib had to be nailed to the floor. He had difficulty going to sleep. His bed-wetting continued until his mother stopped his bedtime citrus drinks. He coughed excessively and had temper tantrums—until he began food allergy treatment in 1988 after undergoing challenge and P/N allergy testing.

At that time Tom's parents became aware that his learning problems were in part related to foods. So severely did his food cravings affect him that he would set his alarm clock to eat pizza in the middle of the night. After his parents restricted his diet, his grades improved markedly. At one point, however, Tom again began to eat routine school lunches and swap snacks with his classmates. Once again, his grades promptly slipped to C's. His teachers recognized the problem and urged his mother to insist that Tom resume his restricted diet. When he did, his grades improved again.

Further allergy testing confirmed that part of Tom's learning problems were related to offending school chemical exposures. After Tom began home schooling he had no difficulty finishing his work. He could complete his assignments easily at home, earn higher grades, and sit still without difficulty while this was not possible when he was in school. He was obviously better in his more controlled, allergy-free home environment, providing his diet continued to be closely supervised.

Then, in the late summer of 1992, Tom returned to his recently remodeled school. Within five days, he had developed eye circles and bags under his eyes, a bandlike throbbing headache and a burning throat. These sensations lasted all day and did not subside until one to two hours after he left the building. He was typically sickest by Friday afternoon and felt the best by Sunday evening. He seemed worse when the weather was colder and the school windows were closed. At these times he also exhibited poor judgment and manifested behavioral problems, such as complaining, crying, confusion, forgetfulness, tantrums, and irritability.

When he attended school, his mother noted that Tom's (and his brothers') clothing smelled of mop oil. (One brother repeatedly had facial tics or twitches in reaction to this odor.) The oil contained petroleum distillates (hydrocarbons), N amyl acetate, propylene glycol, and nonionic surfactants. Only seconds after taking one whiff of this oil, Tom developed his usual headache and burning throat. As is typical of many chemical sensitivities, oxygen completely relieved his discomfort within ten minutes. Tom's reactions to the mop oil were videotaped, in order to document his response to this exposure.

Then other chemical odors began to bother Tom. He felt ill whenever the school bus engines idled nearby; the ventilation intake for his school drew these fumes directly into the building. This odor made him feel "bouncy" and sick. Whenever he smelled perfume, he tried to pull his shirt over his face to protect himself. When a laundry room in his school was being remodeled, his symptoms recurred because of the many chemicals being used during this process. He became irritable and obnoxious and cried with a headache from the fumes associated with lawn mowing. He had similar symptoms when he was exposed to phenolic cleaning agents (Lysol), lavatory deodorizers, and odorous marking pens.

Although Tom had food sensitivities, as well as problems with dust and molds, chemicals proved to be his largest and most challenging problem. It was impractical for Tom's parents to buy an air purifier for each of his classrooms; home teaching has therefore became a necessity for him.

What was the response of school officials to Tom's problems and to the video demonstrating his response to the mop oil? The school continues to use the oil, and it also permits the buses to continue to idle where fumes can enter the school's ventilation system. The maintenance workers still routinely exterminate with pesticides each month, whether they are needed or not.

CONTROLLED CHALLENGE TESTING

Controlled challenge testing can be conducted in specially ventilated rooms that resemble glass telephone booths.[39] These cubicles contain elaborate exhaust systems and devices to deliver minute, specifically measured amounts of individual chemicals into the booth's air. A patient sits and breathes the altered air. Sometimes a patient is exposed to such a small amount of a chemical that it cannot be identified or smelled. Even such a minuscule amount of a problem chemical can often exactly reproduce the symptoms that a person has in response to an unavoidable everyday exposure.

AIR EXTRACT TESTS

If the indoor air is causing an environmental illness in your child, it is possible to prepare an allergy extract of the school air. You must obtain authoritative, written permission, however, to take a sample of indoor air from a school or workplace. Once you have obtained written permission from school officials, you can have an allergy extract made from the air in the specific areas of a school building that appear to adversely affect your child. (Read Chapter 3 to find the problem areas of a school.) At times, this sample can also be used for treatment, allowing your child to remain in that school.

Environmental medical specialists can advise you how you can use such samples to document your suspicions.

An air-extract machine is used to prepare school, work, or home air allergy extracts (see Resources). It operates much like an aerated fish tank, bubbling the air sample through a small bottle of saline, a salt solution, for about eight hours. This solution is subsequently filtered and checked for sterility to create an allergy extract, which is then used for testing, either under the tongue or in the skin.

P/N allergy testing can sometimes demonstrate exactly which health or learning problems are related to the water soluble contaminants found in the sample. This testing should be blinded to reduce bias. Also, you should videotape the changes that occur in your child during each test to document the response. Again, as your child is tested, watch the skin test site and carefully observe your youngster (as previously described in this chapter). Once a causal relationship is confirmed, appropriate comprehensive treatment (as detailed in Chapter 15) should begin. Your child must avoid proven offending items, such as chemicals, as much as possible if such exposures cause serious illness.

Sometimes treatment with an air extract will enable a child to continue to attend a school that has caused mild to moderate symptoms. Such an extract would contain an exceedingly tiny amount of the dust, molds, and chemicals that were present in the school air at the time the sample was prepared.

CARPET CHEMICAL ANALYSIS

Similarly, you can make an allergy extract from a carpet. If you cannot obtain permission from the school to make a carpet sample, perhaps you can purchase or test an "identical" sample of carpet. (Be aware that there can be variations in the exact contents of different lines and even of single specific run during carpet production.) You can also prepare allergy extracts from a variety of other suspect items, such as chemically-treated paper, a newspaper, a plastic water container, or tooth braces, by soaking them in a small amount of normal saline. Such extracts prepared from ordinary items can be used to clearly demonstrate a cause-and-effect relationship. Contact an environmental medical physician to find out exactly how to prepare this type of extract and how to test for such a sensitivity (see Resources).

You can send a piece of carpet to a laboratory to find out more about the chemicals it contains (see Resources). Your ultimate aim is to ascertain if a chemical in a suspect substance is also present in the blood or urine of your sick child. Normal blood should not contain any chemicals, and certainly no elevated levels of those which are toxic. Remember, only some of the offending components in carpets are listed on MSD sheets.[40] The most toxic may not appear on these information sheets because they are erroneously called "inert" (see Chapter 10).

You can obtain an extensive and relatively inexpensive analysis of a number of gaseous chemicals found in carpets, as well as in foods and in indoor or outside air.[41] One indoor air environmental evaluation team can come into a suspect building and perform an on-the-spot gas-chromatography, mass-spectrometry test, which can provide accurate and meaningful information. Other labs can provide similar information in one to three weeks using other methods of detection (see Chapter 6). These chemical studies can be much more helpful than an evaluation by a regulatory agency, which usually preannounces the date of its inspection and thus allows officials time to improve the ventilation and purge any suspect chemicals. You might want to video the activities prior to health department visits. Such pre-inspection cleanups can result in health department reports that are relatively benign, even though large numbers of individuals in a building continue to become ill when they enter the building. Independent unannounced inspections can be much more informative.

BIOASSAY TESTS

Once you obtain a sample of school carpet or some other potentially offending substance, it is possible to prove whether it is safe for mice by purposely exposing them to its vapors in an impartial scientific laboratory.

If exposed mice quickly become significantly ill, we have to wonder how safe that substance is for human beings.[42]

Anderson Laboratories (see Resources) uses such bioassays to examine samples of carpet and tile, as well as adhesives, glues, and paper, mattresses, synthetic clothing, and baby products. Hundreds of carpets, varying in size and age, have been studied at the Anderson facility.

The testing procedure begins by placing the suspect item in a sealed glass chamber. The temperature, humidity, and airflow are carefully monitored as pure air is blown over the carpet, directly into another glass chamber, where four gently restrained mice breathe it for a total of four hours. They are exposed on two consecutive days, for two one-hour periods each day. After each hour of exposure, the mice are examined. Their appearance, coordination, breathing, behavior, and alertness are noted. They are examined for physical changes and tested for their ability to grasp an object, for example, or to right themselves when placed upside down.

Exposure to some substances produce no ill effects in the mice. Others, however, cause them to act and behave abnormally. They may develop mild to severe congestion, breathing or coordination problems. A few gasp to breathe and turn blue with severe respiratory distress. Some have lung, eye, or skin hemorrhages or facial swelling. They may develop obvious changes in their nervous system, with loss of balance, twitching, abnormal reflexes, and paralysis. A few die, sometimes after only fifteen minutes of exposure to a chemical odor or a sample of school air. Pathological studies show muscle and kidney damage.

Yves Alarie, Ph.D., a research scientist and professor from the department of environmental and occupational health at the University of Pittsburgh, developed this bioassay test used by Anderson and several other laboratories. His results clearly confirm that carpet chemicals can cause illness in mice. He has stated, "At low exposure concentrations of chemicals as emitted by carpets, I have never observed [such] severe neurotoxic effects or deaths in mice as I observed with certain carpets."[43]

It is most perplexing that the Maryland State Department of Education recently stated that conclusions should not be drawn from the reported test results on mice.[44] Why not? Does someone have some vested interests? Are the stakes too high to inform the public? Is there something we don't know or that someone does not want us to know?

Interestingly, the Environmental Protection Agency (EPA) was able to duplicate Anderson Laboratories' results while using the Anderson facility; *but after it significantly altered the testing procedure (testing wet carpet sam-*

ples, for example, instead of dry ones), the agency was no longer able to consistently replicate those findings at its own laboratory.

If your child has allergies or chemical sensitivities, you may want to ask your school to run a bioassay on a sample of new synthetic carpet *before* it is installed throughout the school (or your home or workplace). If a suspect carpet already has been installed, a large piece (two feet square) should be examined as soon as possible, because the "outgassing" chemicals are most evident initially. Even so, pieces of carpet as small as seven inches square and others more than ten years old, without an obvious odor, have adversely and profoundly affected some mice. The most critical factor is the chemical content of the carpet, not its age or size.

We obviously need more extensive, large-scale scientific evaluations of the health risks associated with carpets. But for now, it certainly appears that some carpets do cause serious illness in some mice and possibly in humans. Until we know more, I believe it is prudent not to install carpets in schools or homes unless the type that is going to be purchased—along with any adhesive or pad used for installation—are thoroughly prescreened for safety.

Bioassay testing is of little value unless it is conducted in *a totally impartial and highly scientific laboratory*, such as Anderson Laboratories. Obviously the same laboratory that provides safety labels for the carpet industry should not also be paid to evaluate the safety of the same carpets. This would create a potentially serious and significant conflict of interest. The fox should certainly not be the one to decide the design of the henhouse.

■ BRAIN-IMAGE TESTING

An estimated nine million people are exposed to neurotoxins at work.[45] We have no idea how many people have been affected by such exposures at school, at home, or at work. Because of this, more must be done to recognize and more fully understand the types of illnesses that chemical exposures can and cannot cause.

In the past researchers found it difficult to prove that a nerve-damaging chemical was the cause of someone's headache, fatigue, loss of memory, confusion, agitation, or unacceptable behavior. Today, however, brain-image tests can determine if such nervous system symptoms are related to chemical exposures. These tests can prove that certain responses do not have a purely psychological origin. For example, in one study by Thomas Callender, M.D., and his colleagues, thirty-three workers became ill after a chemical exposure. The researchers discovered that seven percent had an abnormal CT (computerized tomography) scan, eight percent an abnormal EEG (electroencephalogram), 29 percent an abnormal MRI (magnetic resonance imaging), and 94 percent an abnormal SPECT (single photon emission computerized tomography) test.[46]

A CT scan shows gross anatomical changes, such as atrophy or tumors, while the MRI is better for soft tissue changes. These tests are readily available and relatively inexpensive compared with some of the newer techniques, such as SPECT. The newer, more advanced brain-image techniques, however, provide details about brain circulation and function that explain some of the distressing changes in activity, behavior, and memory that are present after certain chemical exposures in both children and adults.

PET (PHOTON EMISSION TOMOGRAPHY)

PET tests provide a way to compare the effects of various chemicals and to document exactly which area of the brain is adversely affected by different chemicals among individuals. During these PET tests, radioactive substances are injected into a patient to evaluate brain function. Dr. Callender has stated that PET tests are more flexible and more easily quantified than SPECT tests (which is described more fully below).[47] Both SPECT and PET tests provide a dynamic global picture of the localized blood flow and brain function changes that can occur during and after a chemical exposure. But while the PET image can provide insight, for example, into how glucose or other radioactive-tagged substances are *metabolized* in the brain, the SPECT test shows how these same substances are *distributed* in the brain.

SPECT (SINGLE PHOTON EMISSION COMPUTERIZED TOMOGRAPHY)

SPECT is a sophisticated way to study the brain. This brain-image test has been used and refined for more than twenty years and it provides a three-dimensional snapshot of the brain (see Resources). The initial SPECT pictures show the blood flow in the brain, and fifteen minutes later, they indicate brain function. Preliminary carefully controlled studies indicate that this technique can accurately and safely demonstrate important brain changes in children and adults.[48] However, this test can be deceptively negative unless it is conducted by a specialist specifically trained in this complex nucleus-medicine technique.

The findings of a SPECT test can explain some environmentally caused headaches, fatigue, numbness, tingling, behavioral problems, confusion, and memory difficulties. For example, if your child has balance problems (as determined by a Romberg Test discussed earlier in this chapter), difficulties recalling recent events, lack of concentration, an intermittent inability to speak or move, and/or confusion, it is possible for a SPECT test to show the significant brain-image changes that are causing these complaints. If your youngster has ADHD, the SPECT evaluation can show an increased blood flow to the frontal cortex.[49]

With this technology, the brains of students age five and older have been shown to have undergone typical brain-image pattern changes after certain toxic and low-level chemical exposures. Environmentally ill children characteristically have changes in both brain blood flow and in brain function, due to scattered localized and generalized lesions within as well as on the surface of the brain. (These changes are similar to those seen in patients who have had known chemical or pesticide exposures—like Gulf War soldiers, glue-sniffing youngsters, or woman with leaky silicone breast implants.)

One SPECT study found significant brain abnormalities in thirty-five of forty individuals with multiple chemical sensitivities, and in three of three silicone breast implant patients. However, none of fifteen healthy controls, nor any of thirty depressed patients, exhibited these brain changes. This finding suggests that the latter group's depression was unrelated to environmental illness.[50]

A number of chemically sensitive patients have demonstrated significantly worse SPECT scans following brief controlled exposures to low concentrations of such common chemicals as toluene and acetone.[51] Studies by Dr. Gunnar Heuser and his colleagues have demonstrated a normal or slightly abnormal baseline SPECT test on one day; then, after these patients were exposed to an adverse chemical the next day, a repeat test showed significant brain-image alterations.[52]

A SPECT test can help distinguish among problems such as depression, schizophrenia, strokes, and brain infections. Patients with multiple chemical sensitivities, as well as cocaine addicts and alcoholics, have characteristic brain-image patterns that help explain how these affected individuals think, act, and behave. Levels of chemical exposures, so subtle that they are not detected by smell, can still produce obvious changes in brain images. Sometimes the characteristic areas in brain tissue are so damaged that they show "cortical holes" (craters on the brain surface) or large round areas of obvious abnormalities scattered throughout the brain.[53]

The brain images of individuals who have abnormal SPECT tests can improve, at times merely by avoiding the factors that caused these changes. Most people need detoxification of some kind before their brain-related symptoms and their brain images will improve. Because of the cost of this test, follow-up studies are not routinely performed.

ELECTROENCEPHALOGRAM (EEG)

When doctors conduct traditional EEGs, they visually evaluated them for abnormal areas, such as spike waves suggesting seizure activity. This type of examination, however, reveals no convincing changes in chemically sensitive patients. Newer computerized methods are now available, which assess neurological function and perform brain topography or brain mapping. The quantitative electroencephalogram (qEEG) can detect a brain response caused by a minute chemical exposure.[54] It can greatly enhances the interpretation and detection of obvious, as well as the more subtle, forms of brain damage.

This test can also be adapted to more objectively and precisely measure various electrical brain signals using evoked potentials (EVP). Auditory or visual stimuli, for example, create or evoke potentials (brain signals) that cause changes in the brain tissues, which can be interpreted because of various modifications in certain peaks. One variation of the test is called the P300 evoked response, referring to a peak response noted at 300 milliseconds after certain forms of auditory stimulation.

Many doctors remain skeptical that a child or an adult can have a dramatic reaction or become seriously ill within seconds after a single whiff of a perfume or aerosol. These brain-image tests, however, show that the brain can respond in less than a second to certain exposures. They demonstrate objectively and sequentially what happens after someone smells an odor that alters the ability to think, speak, walk, act, or behave appropriately.[55]

By the use of qEEGs with evoked potentials, it is possible to show:

■ why temporary memory loss, drowsiness, or an inability to move and communicate suddenly occurs when a sensitized individual smells a damaging chemical
■ why odors cause brain fog or an inability to think clearly, at times when alpha and delta bursts of electrical activity dull the normal brain function. (Using thyrotropin-releasing hormone, or TRH, the duration of a brain fog episode can be diminished from weeks to a couple of hours.)
■ why an electrical impulse from a stimulus to the eye can cause a ringing sensation in the ears[56]
■ subtle responses to chemicals at levels below those that can be detected by smell

Olfactory or odor evoked potential tests using newer electrical and magnetic encephalographic techniques have been performed for years in Germany.[57] Their studies provide objective documentation that brain changes can occur within 100 milliseconds after an odor, such as perfume, enters the olfactory nerve or the nose and throat mucosa. SPECT and PET tests reveal "immediate" changes, but they cannot record brain responses this rapidly.

A major deterrent to the use of brain imaging with evoked potentials is cost. Even though this testing correlates a patient's symptoms with what happens inside the brain, few can afford the cost of having the test performed. This type of test can cost as much as $5,000.

As these radiological techniques become more refined (and hopefully less expensive), labeling physical problems as "psychological" will decrease because their true medical causes will be better understood. Documentation of certain more subtle types of brain malfunction certainly is now possible.[58] These tests are going to add a new dimension to our full appreciation of the overwhelming chemical threat in our society. The public and particularly politicians must realize that there is no safe level for many everyday chemicals, and that the brains of humans and animals can be at risk.

Dr. Jaumann, a German research physician, has stated, "There is more and more proof that there is no safe level of many chemicals and toxic substances. The delicacy and complexity of our nervous system and the brain, and the information transported by molecules and neurohormones, makes our nervous system and brain most vulnerable to changes in the chemical environment.

"Many doctors are not aware of this upcoming challenge. Intensive education is needed as many neurotoxic diseases are 'mislabeled' today. Public health care has to understand that only prevention of pollution will pay."

NOTES

1. William Rea, *Chemical Sensitivity* vol. I and II, (Chelsea, MI: Lewis Publishers, 1991–1995).
2. Ibid., vol. 3, p. 1,465, regarding chemical sensitivity.
3. See Sherry Rogers, *Wellness Against All Odds* (Syracuse, NY: Prestige Publishing, 1994) and *Depression Cured at Last* (Syracuse, NY: Prestige Publishing, 1996).
4. Kenneth Bock, M.D., Pinnacle Place, Suite no. 210, 10 McKowan Road, Albany, NY 12203, tel. (518) 435-0082, fax (518) 435-0086.
5. See G. Heuser, A. Vodjani, and S. Heuser, "Diagnostic Markers in Chemical Sensitivity," in *Multiple Chemical Sensitivities: Addendum to Biologic Markers in Immunotoxicology* (Washington, DC: National Academy Press, 1992), pp. 117–38.
6. See Rea, *Chemical Sensitivity*, vol. I.
7. Billie Sahley, *The Natural Way to Control Hyperactivity with Amino Acids and Nutrient Therapy*, 2d ed. (1994); *Breaking Your Addiction Habit* (1990); and *The Anxiety Epidemic*, 2d ed. (1995); all pub-

lished by Pain and Stress Clinic (see Resources). These books provide practical, easily understood information about key amino acids and nutrients, what they do, and why they help.

8. Gordon P. Baker, "Porphyria and MCS Overlap Symptoms," *Our Toxic Times* (a publication of the Chemical Injury Information Network), vol. 5 (August 1994), p. 3; and Grace Ziem, *NYCAP News* (Summer 1995). To order a protocol or fact sheet on chemical sensitivities and disorders of porphyrin metabolism, contact MCS Referral and Resources, 2326 Pickwick Road, Baltimore, MD 21207. Also contact Mayo Labs (1-800-826-5561).

9. Editorial by G. Heuser, "Diagnostic Markers in Clinical Immunotoxicology and Neurotoxicology," *Journal of Occupational Medicine and Toxicology*, vol. 1, no. 4 (1992), p. 88.

10. See Sahley, *Natural Way; Addiction Habit; Anxiety Epidemic.*

11. Lisa A. Morrow et al., "A Distinct Pattern of Personality Disturbance Following Exposure to Mixtures of Organic Solvents," *Journal of Occupational Medicine*, vol. 31, no. 9 (1989), pp. 743–46; and Lisa A. Morrow et al., "Alterations in Cognitive and Psychological Functioning after Organic Solvent Exposure," *Journal of Occupational Medicine*, vol. 32, no. 5 (1990), pp. 444–50.

12. Bonnye L. Matthews, *Chemical Sensitivity* (Jefferson, NC: McFarland & Co., 1992).

13. See K.H. Kilburn, R.H. Warsaw, and M.G. Shields, "Neurobehavioral Dysfunction in Firemen Exposed to Polychlorinated Biphenyls (PCBs): Possible Improvement After Detoxification," *Archives of Environmental Health*, vol. 44 (Nov/Dec 1989), pp. 345–50. For articles about evoked potentials and chemical injury, contact EARN (see Resources). See also Muriel Lezak, *Neuropsychological Assessment*, 2d ed. (New York: Oxford University Press, 1983).

14. For more information on these tests, write Joel Butler, Ph.D., and Susan Franks, Ph.D. (see Resources).

15. See Lisa Morrow, "A Distinct Pattern."

16. Anne Puryear, *Stephen Lives!* (New York: Simon & Schuster, 1996).

17. Herbert Rinkel, Theron Randolph, and Michael Zeller, *Food Allergy* (Springfield, IL: Charles C. Thomas, 1951).

18. M.M. Peshkin, in H.A. Abramson, ed., *Somatic and Psychiatric Treatment of Asthma* (Baltimore: Williams and Wilkins Co., 1951), p. 202.

19. S.J. Schoenthaler, W.E. Doraz, and J.A. Wakefield, "The Impact of a Low Food Additive and Sucrose Diet on Academic Performance in 803 NYC Public Schools," *International Journal of Biosocial Research*, vol. 8, no. 2 (1986), pp. 185–203; S.J. Schoenthaler, D. Benton, and G. Roberts, "Effect of Vitamin and Mineral Supplementation on Intelligence, a Sample of Schoolchildren," *Lancet*, vol. 664 (1988), pp. 140–43.

20. Harold Levinson, *Dyslexia, A Solution to the Riddle* (New York: Springer-Verlag, 1980); and D.J. Rapp, *Is This Your Child?* (New York: William Morrow & Co., 1991), chapter 16.

21. Rapp, *Is This Your Child?*

22. Karl-L. Reichelt, Jonny Ekrem, and Helge Scott, "Gluten, Milk Proteins and Autism: Dietary Intervention Effects on Behavior and Peptide Secretion," *Journal of Applied Nutrition*, vol. 42, no. 1 (1990), pp. 1–11; Harris L. Coulter, M.D., *Vaccination, Social Violence, and Criminality: The Medical Assault on the American Brain* (Berkeley, CA: North Atlantic Books, 1990); C. Kotsanis, M.D., 1600 West College Street, Grapevine, TX 76051, tel. (817) 481-6342; Autism Research Institute, 4182 Adams Avenue, San Diego, CA 92116, tel. (619) 281-7165; Bernard Rimland, Ph.D., "Controversies in the Treatment of Autistic Children: Vitamin and Drug Therapy," *Journal of Child Neurology*, vol. 3 (1988), pp. 568–72; B. Rimland et al., "The Effect of High Doses of B_6 on Autistic Children: A Double-Blind Crossover Study," *American Journal of Psychiatry* (Apr. 1978), pp. 472–75; Bernard Rimland, *Autism Research Review*, vol. 9, no. 3 (1995), p. 3; and Temple Grandin, Ph.D., *Thinking in Pictures* (New York: Doubleday Books, 1995).

23. See the various works by Bernard Rimland in note 22.

24. A. Broughton, J. Thrasher, "Antibodies and Altered Cell Mediated Immunity in Formaldehyde Exposed Humans." *Comments Toxicology*, vol. 2, no. 3 (1988), pp. 155–174.

25. Ta1 tests are done at the Antibody Assay Laboratory (see Resources).

26. Tinsley Harrison, *Principles of Internal Medicine*, 12th ed. (New York: McGraw-Hill, 1991).

27. G. Heuser, "Diagnostic Markers."

28. Kilburn, Warsaw, and Shields, "Neurobehavioral Dysfunction."

29. EPA, *The Recognition and Management of Pesticide Poisonings*, pub. no. EPA-540-9-88-001, 4th ed. (see Resources).

30. Marion Moses, *Designer Poisons* (San Francisco: Pesticide Education Center, 1995).

31. W.J. Rea and G. Ross, "Food and Chemicals as Incitants," *Nurse Practitioner*, vol. 14, no. 9 (1989), pp. 17–40.

32. G. Heuser, "Diagnostic Markers."

33. Doris J. Rapp, "Environmental Medicine: An Expanded Approach to Allergy," *Buffalo Physician* (Feb. 1986), pp. 16–24; and David L.J. Freed, "Part I. The Provocation-Neutralization Technique. Part II. Can We Diagnose Allergies, Do We Know What We Are Doing, Does It Matter?" in *Food Intolerance*, John Dobbing, ed. (London: Bailliere Tindall, 1987), pp. 151–84.

34. Joseph B. Miller, *Relief At Last* (Springfield, IL: Charles C. Thomas, 1987).

35. D.L. Morris, "Use of Sublingual Antigen in Diagnosis and Treatment of Food Allergy," *Annals of Allergy*, vol. 27 (1969), pp. 289–94. (More sublingual studies are listed in the Appendix.)

36. A. Sabbah, S. Hassoun, J. Le Sellinet, C. André, and H. Sicard, "A Double-Blind, Placebo-controlled Trial by the Sublingual Route of Immunotherapy with a Standardized Grass Pollen Extract," *Allergy*, vol. 49 (1994), pp. 309–13.

37. Edited by Hartmut Heine, Ph.D., *Matrix and Matrix Regulation* (Brussels: A. Pischinger and Haug International, 1995), English edition 1991.

38. J. Egger, A. Stolla, and L.M. McEwen, "Controlled Trial of Hyposensitization in Children with Food-induced Hyperkinetic Syndrome," *Lancet*, vol. 339 (May 9, 1992), pp. 1150–53; P. Fell and J. Brostoff, "A Single Dose Desensitization for Summer Hay Fever," *European Journal of Clinical Pharmacology*, vol. 38 (1990), pp. 77–79; "Preliminary Studies with Enzyme Potentiated Desensitization in Canine Atopic Dermatitis," *Environmental Medicine*, vol. 8 (1991), pp. 140–41; W.A. Shrader and L.M. McEwen, "Enzyme Potentiated Desensitization: A 16-Month Trial of Therapy with 134 Patients," *Environmental Medicine*, vol. 9, nos. 3–4, pp. 128–38.

39. For more information on challenge booths and air chemical testing, contact the American Environmental Health Center (see Resources).

40. Moses, *Designer Poisons*.

41. The Citizens Environmental Laboratory in Massachusetts will examine extracted chemicals from carpets and screen for substances such as 4-PC. Reed and Associates Laboratory in Kentucky (see Resources), will help determine which chemicals "outgas" and can be extracted from carpets. This type of information can be most helpful, both medically and legally, if the same chemicals are also found in a person's blood.

42. The video *Environmentally Sick Schools* shows what can happen to mice during such testing of a year-old piece of school carpet (see Resources).

43. Affidavit of Yves Alarie, Ph.D., department of environmental and occupational health, Graduate School of Public Health, University of Pittsburgh. See also Y. Alarie and J. E. Luo, "Sensory Irritation by Airborne Chemicals: A Basis to Establish Acceptable Levels of Exposure," *Toxicology of the Nasal Passages*, ed. C.S. Barrow (Washington, DC: Hemisphere Publishing Co., 1986), pp. 91–100; Y. Alarie, "Sensory Irritation by Airborne Chemicals," *CRC Critical Reviews in Toxicology*, vol. 2 (1973), pp. 299–363; Rosalind C. Anderson, "Toxic Emissions from Carpets," *Journal of Nutritional & Environmental Medicine*, vol. 5 (1995), pp. 375–86.

44. Maryland State Department of Education, Division of Business Services, Technical Bulletin, "Carpets and Indoor Air Quality in Schools" (Oct. 1993).

45. *Organic Solvent Neurotoxicity*, NIOSH Current Intelligence Bulletin no. 48 (1987), DHHS publication no. 87-104.

46. Thomas J. Callender et al., "Evaluation of Chronic Neurological Sequelae After Acute Pesticide Exposure Using SPECT Brain Scans," *Journal of Toxicology and Environmental Health*, vol. 41 (1994), pp. 275–84; and Thomas J. Callender et al., "Three-Dimensional Brain Metabolic Imaging in Patients with Toxic Encephalopathy," *Environmental Research*, vol. 60 (1993), pp. 295–319.

47. Thomas J. Callender, personal communication, Jan. 20, 1995.

48. T.R. Simon et al., "Abnormalities in Scintigraphic Examinations of the Brains of Desert Storm/Desert Shield Veterans," presented at the twelfth annual international symposium on Man and

His Environment in Health and Disease, Dallas, TX, 1994; Heuser, Vodjani, and Heuser, "Diagnostic Markers in Chemical Sensitivity"; Heuser, "Diagnostic Markers in Clinical Immunotoxicology."

49. Gunnar Heuser, personal communication (1994).

50. *Human Ecologist*, no. 64 (1994), p. 18.

51. Ibid.

52. See Heuser, Vodjani, and Heuser, "Diagnostic Markers in Chemical Sensitivity," and Heuser, "Diagnostic Markers in Chemical Immunotoxicology."

53. See Simon et al., "Abnormalities in Scintigraphic Examinations."

54. See Morrow, "A Distinct Pattern," and Morrow, "Alterations in Cognitive and Psychological Functioning."

55. Ibid; *Human Ecologist*; A.S. Aslanov and G.I. Lvretskaya, "Effect of TRH on the Central Nervous System," translated from *Problemy Endokvinologii*, vol. 33, no. 4 (1987), pp. 51–55; and J.G. Bajorek, R.J. Lee, and P. Lomax, "Neuropeptides: Anticonvulsant and Convulsant Mechanisms in Epileptic Model Systems and in Humans," *Advances in Neurology*, vol. 44 (1986), pp. 489–500.

56. Ibid.; and M. Miyata, "Development of Myopia Following Chronic Organophosphate Pesticide Intoxication: An Epidemiological and Experimental Study," in W.H. Merigan and B. Weiss, ed., *Neurotoxicity of the Visual System* (New York: Raven Press, 1980).

57. By researchers such as G. Kobal, T. Hummel, and M. Jaumann. See M.P. Jaumann, W. Eckrich, and G. Schwinger, "Early Detection of Neurotoxic Effects of Organo-Halogen Compounds by Auditory Evoked Potentials (AEP)," *Organo-Halogen Compounds*, vol. 7, no. 2 (1980); G. Kobal, "Process for Measuring Sensory Qualities and Apparatus Therefore," U.S. Patent no. 4,681,121 (1987).

58. Matthews, *Chemical Sensitivity*.

14 Tests for Special Problems

To make and confirm an accurate diagnosis for some common medical problems frequently seen in environmentally sensitive patients, your doctor should consider certain specific tests beyond those more general tests described in Chapter 13. These tests should be considered in individuals with specific types of health problems of the type discussed in this chapter.

In diagnosing and treating these complaints, sometimes the expertise of other specialists (as indicated in Table 14.1) is needed to help evaluate specific body areas. You may need a specialist in pediatrics, internal medicine, environmental medicine, and/or occupational medicine in addition to the doctor you already are using. True, many of these specialists are not fully aware of the role of the environment in their specialty, but nevertheless they will surely be more knowledgeable than the average doctor in their specific area of expertise. At times, they can find or explain something that is totally unrelated to environmental medicine.

A point that you and your doctors must appreciate is that when a product label states "no known health hazards" this in no way means that the bodies and brains of individuals cannot be seriously and, at times, permanently damaged. You must raise your guard and become more cautious in managing conditions like those described in this chapter. The best place to start is with the tests cited below, followed by the most appropriate treatments (some of which are mentioned here as well).

■ YEAST OR CANDIDA INFECTION

A child or adult with a possible candida (yeast or monilia) overgrowth often have a white-coated tongue, itchy genitals, smelly hair and feet, a bloated abdomen, and a red rectal area as listed in Table 14.2. For each of the listed complaints, there are other possible causes, but if several of them are present, and there is a history of an excessive need for antibiotics, or the use of

---

TABLE 14.1

Specialists Sometimes Needed for Environmental Illness Evaluations

Cardiologist: heart, circulatory system problems

Endocrinologist: thyroid, hypoglycemic, menstrual-related symptoms

Gastroenterologist: intestinal disorders

Hematologist: bleeding symptoms

Neurologist: nervous system, brain-related symptoms

Neuropsychologist: emotional, behavioral, or mood disorders

Ophthalmologist: visual problems

Osteopath and/or Chiropractor: bone, joint, or movement discomfort

Otolaryngologist: ear, nose, or throat problems

Psychologist: learning, mood, attitude, or behavioral difficulties

Physiatrist: muscle or nerve problems

Pulmonologist: breathing or lung symptoms

Rheumatologist: joint pain or swelling

Toxicologist: identifies poisons or toxins

Urologist: bladder and kidney complaints

---

birth control pills or cortisone (steroids), a candida overgrowth should be considered. Most people with this condition have the typical history as well as more than one of the classical symptoms in Table 14.2.

The symptoms of a yeast problem typically smolder in some minor form for long periods, and then flare up each time an antibiotic is used to treat an infection. In addition, regular P/N yeast allergy skin testing will typically reproduce some of the many symptoms associated with this sensitivity. For example, one drop of a yeast extract in a skin test can cause a chronic, unexplained rash to suddenly become itchy or red. This might be the first clue pointing to yeast and a possible way to eliminate the rash. If considerations like these point to candida, a trial of yeast treatment is certainly indicated.

This diagnosis, however, is not always suspected, easy to prove, or even believed by many doctors. Because yeast is so commonly found in

---

TABLE 14.2

Common Symptoms of Yeast Overgrowth

■ white-coated tongue
■ red ring around the anus
■ bloated abdomen
■ persistent hair or foot odor
■ itchy genital area causing touching
■ recurrent or constant body rash
■ sudden vaginal discharge after eating sweets

everyone's body, it is normal to have yeast in the bowel and the vagina, as well as some yeast antibodies in the blood. As a result, doctors disagree about the value of candida antibody tests and the newer tests for candida IgG immune complexes. Sometimes a comprehensive digestive and parasite stool examination provides the needed answers for more complex yeast-related illness.

The best proof of a candida infection is a satisfactory response to appropriate yeast therapy in a patient who has the typical history of a yeast overgrowth (as discussed in Chapter 15). At times this therapy will quickly eliminate symptoms that have not been relieved by previous treatments. Dr. William G. Crook's informative books have greatly increased public awareness of this common medical condition, and as a result many children and adults have been helped after years of discomfort, distress, and misdiagnosis.[1]

■ INTESTINAL PROBLEMS

Intestinal problems often clear up after the use of a rotation diet, food allergy extract therapy, and candida treatment. Sometimes this is even true for various forms of colitis or Crohn's disease. However, if symptoms per-

---

TESTING FOR INTESTINAL PROBLEMS

The intestines protect us by preventing the wrong substances from entering our bodies. If the intestines are leaky or too permeable, undigested food particles and/or germs can directly enter the circulatory system. This can make us more prone to develop food allergies, and it can affect our immune systems.

To check the intestines for this type of problem, your physician can arrange for the following test: You (or your child) will be instructed to swallow two forms of sugar, one called lactulose and the other called mannitol.[2] (Lactulose has nothing to do with lactose, which is milk sugar.) A urine sample is subsequently collected and analyzed, which may provide the answer to the problem. Normally mannitol is absorbed well and easily passes from the intestines into the blood, so eventually a large amount should be present in the urine. In contrast, lactulose is absorbed poorly, very little of it will pass into your blood, so most would leave your body in your bowel movements. This means that only a small amount should be detected in your urine. However, if *both* are well-absorbed, then too much of both will be found in the urine, which indicates you have a leaky gut. By contrast, if *neither* is absorbed, very little of either will be found in the urine. This would suggest a malabsorption problem. Once you understand the basic problem, specific appropriate therapy can be immensely helpful. Check with your doctor or the lab that conducts this test for more information (see Resources).

sist in adults or children, and they cannot move their bowels easily each day with formed and odorless stools, then certain tests are indicated. These tests usually include a thorough stool examination to look for digestive abnormalities, or for evidence of malabsorption and/or parasites (see Resources). Some patients may be helped by digestive enzymes, drinking more water, and sometimes an acid to adjust the stomach pH.

Whenever bowel problems persist, consult a gastrointestinal specialist. Many bodily processes depend upon proper bowel functioning, and initial minor complaints should be considered early warnings. They should not be ignored, because they might lead to more serious health problems. At least some bowel problems today are due to overuse of antibiotics. These drugs can disrupt the normal balance of intestinal organisms, so that there are not enough lactobacilli and too many yeast or candida in the intestines. This imbalance in part, can be due to the excessive use of chemicals in foods and beverages.

■ ASTHMA AND OTHER LUNG PROBLEMS

Breathing or lung function tests include the simple Peak Flow Meter (PFM) test, as well as the more precise spirometry or pulmonary lung tests. They should be conducted on anyone over five years of age who has recurrent coughing, asthma, irritable airway disease, shortness of breath, or difficulty breathing. These breathing tests can be immensely helpful in pinpointing the cause of pulmonary (lung) complaints, such as difficulty breathing air *out of the lungs*, which typifies asthma, and difficulty breathing air *into the lungs*, which in children is more apt to be due to an infection. A comparison of baseline PFM readings, before and after an exposure, can often give you and your doctor the clues needed to find the cause of your respiratory problems (see Chapter 5).

The key to long-term relief from an allergic cough or asthma attack is not a better drug that temporarily relieves it, but finding out why you cough and wheeze. If you can eliminate the cause, you might be so well you may not need asthma medication.

If a breathing problem becomes severe, consult an environmental medical specialist, allergist, or pulmonologist (lung specialist) for a thorough evaluation. Depending on your own (or your child's) history, the doctor's evaluation will include specific tests for lung diseases such as tuberculosis, coccidioidomycosis, and aspergillosis. Whenever chest symptoms persist for several weeks, additional tests must be done to determine the cause.

A word of caution: If you or your child have breathing difficulties and have ever turned blue or choked badly while eating, tell your physician. Special X-ray techniques can help demonstrate if certain foreign substances have entered the lung. If undetected and untreated, this type of condition could cause a lifetime of breathing problems.

Environmental medical specialists can be particularly helpful for children or adults who have one infection after another. Various bacterial and influenza vaccines and nutrients, along with comprehensive allergy treatments, can be surprisingly effective for some.

■ HYPOGLYCEMIA

Hypoglycemia, or low blood sugar, appears to be inordinately common in environmentally ill allergic children (and their parents). In a nutshell, hypoglycemia means that the brain is screaming for help; it needs glucose (or sugar). If hypoglycemia is suspected, your doctor should obtain a fasting blood sugar and/or do a five-hour (not three-hour) glucose tolerance test.

Here is some basic information about hypoglycemia.

SIGNS OF HYPOGLYCEMIA[3]

Hypoglycemia can cause some children to repeatedly develop to feel unwell, tired or to have change in attitude and behavior, *particularly just before it is time to eat.* Each youngster, however, reacts in a highly individualized manner. Common physical symptoms include headaches, drowsiness, whining, shaking, irritability, anger, aggressiveness, and hyperactivity. Some children typically develop such severe hunger that they cannot wait for a school snack or food to be placed on their plates. They characteristically *demand*, not *request*, food, and some, when the blood sugar is low, will fight or kick other children or any nearby adult. This illness obviously can interfere with a child's ability to learn.

If hypoglycemic children also have a food sensitivity, they will develop symptoms before they eat because of their low blood sugar, and after they eat because of their food allergy. This can lead to much confusion, at school and at home, unless both are recognized and treated. Symptoms from both of these tend to diminish after appropriate, comprehensive environmental medical care.

Hypoglycemic symptoms tend to occur on a daily basis, including weekends, particularly between 10:00 and 11:30 A.M. and between 2:00 and 4:00 P.M. Some hypoglycemic children routinely awaken in a nasty mood and start their day by greeting their mothers with unkind remarks, such as "I hate you!" because they have not eaten for several hours. In these youngsters the treatment can be as easy as providing food at the bedside so children can eat as soon as they awaken.[4] Another solution is to feed your youngster a nut butter (like peanut or almond) at bedtime (providing he is not allergic to it). Nuts contain enough fat that they help to prevent a significant drop in blood sugar during the night.

Even though the symptoms of hypoglycemia are easy to recognize and to stop, the diagnosis is sometimes difficult to *prove*. Simply by feeding a child a tablespoon of a nonsweet food, it is possible to relieve a low blood sugar level within a few minutes. The challenge, however, is to confirm the diagnosis. As I mentioned earlier, if you suspect you or your child has this problem, ask your doctor to obtain a fasting blood sugar level, which should range between 60 to 105 milligrams per deciliter (mg/dL); the body carefully regulates the blood sugar to stay within this limited normal range. If the blood sugar level is too *high*, however, as it is in diabetes, it can affect the brain so much that a person can lose consciousness. By contrast, if it is too *low*, the brain can respond vigorously, causing symptoms such as headache, hunger, fatigue, shaking, and irritability. If a random fasting or a spur-of-the-moment blood sugar test is normal in your child, but you remain suspicious that hypoglycemia is a problem, be sure to ask your doctor for a *five*-hour glucose tolerance test. Do not accept a three-hour test because symptoms typically appear during the third to fifth hour of such a test, rather than in the first three hours.

Ironically, at times, feeding food to the child can immediately relieve a child's symptoms, *even though the blood sugar level at that time appears normal.* There are a number of possible explanations, but we really do not know exactly why this happens. Perhaps some bodies adjust so quickly that a blood sample cannot be obtained before the body has already responded by releasing enough sugar to correct the hypoglycemia. If possible, check the blood sugar level *immediately*, as soon as symptoms are evident. In this way you can usually obtain a blood sugar test result that clearly indicates a subnormal blood sugar level.

THE EFFECTS OF HYPOGLYCEMIA[5]

By definition, hypoglycemia means that the blood sugar level drops below 60 mg/dL. Very simply, the reason is that sometimes the pancreas produces too much insulin, which lowers the blood sugar below this critical level. When this occurs, a signal is sent to the liver to immediately release some of its stored sugar into the bloodstream. This process is similar to your car engine sputtering until you give it more gas. The combination of the right amount of insulin from the pancreas and the right amount of glucose (sugar) from the liver are key factors that help keep the blood sugar level within the normal range. The adrenal and pituitary glands are also part of the team that plays a role in keeping the blood sugar level normal. However, outside influences such as stress and allergic reactions can definitely alter this delicate balance.

If any part of the elaborate system of blood sugar control malfunctions, the body quickly tries to reestablish equilibrium. Each of us has a body full of wonderful checks and balances, which assist one another so the body functions optimally and keeps us feeling well. But at times, when glucose and insulin are not kept within their specified ranges, such as during a hypoglycemic episode, the body quickly becomes ill.

Drs. William Philpott and Dwight Kalita have observed that eating certain foods can alter the function of the pancreas, so the blood sugar level quickly changes.[6] This confirmed observation should provide fresh insight into the complexities of diabetes. In some diabetics, exposure to a common allergenic substance can significantly affect their disease. For example, one youngster's dose of insulin repeatedly decreased after P/N allergy retests for his mold allergy. We must ask why mold exposures appeared to alter the normal functioning of this child's pancreas. How many other diabetics have found certain aspects of their disease particularly puzzling because they are unaware of such possible relationships? The blood sugar level in a mold-sensitive person may routinely be too high or too low on rainy days, which may necessitate an alteration in the usual dose of insulin. Similarly, dust, mites, or a certain food or chemical may alter the dose. Appropriate allergy treatment should be helpful for such individuals. For this reason, the "Big Five" described in Chapter 3 should include a blood sugar test in diabetics in whom unexplained fluctuations in the need for insulin are a recurrent problem, as well as in individuals known to be prediabetic.

MANAGING HYPOGLYCEMIA WITH DIET

Remember that the human body can be smarter than present-day medical pundits. Even if we don't understand why eating a little food temporarily relieves hypoglycemia symptoms, it works, so why not do it? If it helps and does not hurt in any way, feed your child frequent small snacks. A proper breakfast and one or two appropriate midmorning and afternoon snacks will help considerably to reduce hypoglycemic episodes during school hours. Some children learn better at home than at school simply because at home it is easier to eat whenever they are hungry.

Also, consider giving your child certain natural nutritional supplements that appear to help hypoglycemia. These include glutamine, amino-tate (see Resources), chromium, and a neurotransmitter powder called balanced neurotransmitter complex (BNC) with GABA (gamma–amino butyric acid). In addition, drinking more water (not other fluids) can be helpful.[7]

ONE WAY TO PREVENT OR RELIEVE A HYPOGLYCEMIC EPISODE[8]

Surprisingly, the best treatment to prevent or relieve hypoglycemia is not to eat candy, fruits, or fruit juices but to eat some protein, vegetable, or fat every hour or two. Hypoglycemia can be relieved by eating a tablespoon of nuts, carrots, celery sticks, a hard–boiled egg, a chicken drumstick, or a pork chop. *Remember, no one should ever eat any food known to cause an alarming allergic reaction.* If you or your child cannot eat nuts or eggs, for example, do not try to control hypoglycemia with these foods.

A CHILD WITH FOOD ALLERGY *AND* HYPOGLYCEMIA

John

A 12-year-old youngster named John was seen in our office because of his extreme mood swings and irrational behavioral outbursts. He was depressed and repeatedly said that he did not want to live anymore. He tended to act spacey, break things, punch holes in walls, become vulgar, and swear. During his outbursts he developed red earlobes and wiggly legs, which is typical of youngsters who have allergies affecting the brain. These episodes occurred several times a week, at times lasting up to thirty minutes.

John's recurrent behavioral problems could erupt at any time. For example, if someone in a mall passed by and glanced at him in a manner he disliked, his facial expression immediately became violent and angry. He did not become physical, but his sudden and severely fierce appearance frightened even his parents. In one incident, when he had "that look," he picked up a knife and stabbed his favorite football. He repeatedly gave his parents other strong indications that he was under too much stress.

John's attitude and actions caused many difficulties for him. In spite of his normal intelligence, his grades were F's. He had the characteristics of ADHD or Attention Deficit Hyperactivity Disorder (see Chapter 2). In hopes of managing his behavior, he had been placed on Ritalin about two months before we saw him. This drug, however, made him act so wild, emotional, weepy, and enraged that it had to be discontinued within a week.

Finally, John tried a food-allergy diet and improved dramatically in less than seven days. During the second week of the diet, his mother found that sugar, cocoa, and citrus were definitely contributing to his hyperactive outbursts.

How Is John's History Typical of Allergy?

Like the parents of many environmentally ill youngsters, John's parents had allergies. John's own symptoms dated all the way back to infancy. He was not cuddly as an infant but had to be "walked and bounced." He spit up, drooled, and perspired so much that his mother had to change his formula and his clothing repeatedly. He had recurrent ear infections before he was a year old.

At the age of two and again at six, John had tubes placed through his eardrums. By the time he was four, his adenoids had been removed. Because of repeated antibiotics he had a white-coated tongue, suggesting an overgrowth of yeast. He also had "growing pains," which are typical in milk-sensitive children.

By the age of five, John experienced seasonal tree-pollen allergy with stuffiness, nose rubbing, and recurrent nosebleeds. By ten he had developed eye allergies with redness, eye circles, and puffy eyebags. These symptoms are all typical of allergic children.

How Is John's History Typical of Hypoglycemia?

Other symptoms, however, strongly suggested that John also had hypoglycemia. On some mornings he was so groggy that it would take him almost forty-five minutes to wake up. It was a real struggle for him to begin his day. He tended to fall asleep in class. He repeatedly became angry and lost control *before* meals, although this sometimes also happened *after* he ate. When he was being allergy-tested in our center, his blood sugar was only 50 mg/dL—a level definitely below the normal range—just before he left for lunch. At that time he looked as if he would fall asleep. He acted tired and irritable, had wiggly legs, and was angry. He improved as soon as he ate, however, which again is typical of hypoglycemia.

Overall, John's combination of symptoms—occurring before he ate due to hypoglycemia, and after he ate if he consumed foods to which he was allergic—explained many of his perplexing, irrational outbursts. Not surprisingly, John appeared to be on an emotional roller coaster. His allergy testing indicated he had multiple sensitivities to foods, as well as to molds, pollen, and dust. His improvement while he was on the diet we recommended (see Chapter 3) suggested that he would respond favorably to appropriate allergy treatment, providing his diet and nutrition were adjusted (as indicated on Table 14.3) to help prevent and/or control his hypoglycemic episodes.

Within eleven weeks of environmental allergy treatment was begun, John's overall health and demeanor were dramatically better. In school, his grades improved by ten points, and his parents believed that on the whole, John was 80 percent better. He no longer had to be placed in the room with the "bad" kids.

TABLE 14.3

Nutrients Suggested for Hypoglycemics

Amino Acid Nutrients	Typical Dosage
500 mg. L-glutamine	Children usually take half a capsule 30 minutes before meals. The contents of an open capsule are placed under the tongue for 5 minutes or until dissolved. The mouth is filled with water and it is swallowed.
700 mg. aminotate (a combination of amino acids that convert to glucose)	Children 12 years and older take 5 to 7 capsules each day: 2 in the morning, 2 in the afternoon, and 1 at bedtime. A six-year-old child might take 3 capsules per day. It helps in 15 minutes or less.
Chromium	The daily dose is 200 mcg. for children 5 to 12 and 400 mcg. for children over 13.
Balanced neurotransmitter complex (BNC) with GABA	The usual dosage for children is $1/2$ to 1 tsp. twice a day. It is tasteless and water-soluble. It may help in minutes.

■ HAY FEVER

If your child has hay fever, your doctor should evaluate his nose and throat tissues for typical allergies, or for infection of the tonsils, adenoids, or sinuses. If nose complaints are allergic, microscopic nose mucus smear examinations usually show an increase in a type of white blood cell called eosinophils. If there is evidence of too many white blood cells called neutrophils, as well as bacteria, this is characteristic of an infection. If the problem is a combination of allergies and infection, both excessive eosinophils and neutrophils are seen.

SPECIAL EVALUATION OF NOSE TISSUES

Quite often physicians (or parents) can merely glance in the nose and determine whether an individual has an allergy, infection, or both. An otolaryngologist (an ear, nose, and throat specialist) might also use a technique called fiberoptic rhinolaryngoscopy, which is simply a more thorough way to examine these tissues. Here is what they're looking for:

■ With allergies, the tissues inside the nose tend to be swollen, and whitish or bluish in color. They are often covered with watery mucus if the nose is drippy, or they appear swollen if stuffiness is the major complaint.

■ If there is an infection, these same nasal regions become red, inflamed, and covered with gray, green, or yellow mucus.

■ Chemically irritated tissues mimic the signs of infection.

■ Shrunken, atrophied tissue can indicate the overuse of nose spray, while a cobblestone appearance can indicate chronic irritation.

Look in your child's nose with a flashlight. If the normal pink color has changed, try to determine why.

■ FLUID BEHIND THE EARDRUMS

Serous otitis is a condition in which fluid accumulates in the middle ear, the space between the eardrum and the nose. This can develop each time your child's nose tissues swell because of a food, dust, mold, or chemical sensitivity. It commonly causes a hearing loss, feelings of fullness in the ears, and problems when toddlers are trying to learn how to talk. If germs are trapped in the fluid, the youngster will have repeated ear infections.

For the ears to function properly, there must be air on both sides of the eardrum. But if the natural doorway or opening between the nose and eardrum is blocked by allergic or infected swollen nose tissue, fluid accumulates.

One early clue strongly suggesting a milk allergy at any age is a past history of one ear infection after another during infancy. To test for such an allergy, stop a child's intake of all forms of milk and dairy products for a week.[9] A dairy-free diet, with calcium supplementation, can entirely resolve some chronic ear problems in infants and older children. Also, avoid tobacco smoke and gas heat, because these factors contribute to some recurrent ear problems.

To temporarily relieve fluid accumulation, your doctor might recommend placing a tiny tube through the eardrum. This, however doesn't resolve the basic problem, which is the blockage at the nasal end of the tube. If this swelling can be eliminated by treating the allergies, then other common therapies—one course of antibiotics after another, prophylactic antibiotics, removal of the adenoids, and/or placing tubes through the eardrums—may not be needed.[10] Once those allergies are treated, the tendency for repeated infections decreases, and there is less need for antibiotics. When the infections are gone, the adenoids often shrink. (They also normally decrease in size after about the age of ten years.) The end result is that ear problems disappear.

To repeat, if you and your doctor do not recognize and appropriately treat the *cause* of chronic ear fluid buildup, particularly in babies, some of them will not hear properly. This deficiency can lead to secondary speech and learning problems, yeast overgrowth due to antibodies and repeated and unnecessary ear, adenoid, and/or sinus surgery. To make matters worse, the latter entails exposure to an anesthetic, another powerful chemical. Although a loss of brain function after anesthetics is not noticed in most individuals, surgery can definitely permanently diminish the memory in senior citizens.

One other note about surgery: It can relieve recurrent infections caused by a deviated septum, a condition in which the divider between the two parts of the nose is not centered. If a deviated septum impedes the proper drainage of mucus on one side of the nose, sinus surgery might be required. Fortunately, the treatment of routine allergies alone will often improve the drainage to such a degree that an operation is unnecessary. Also, physical manipulation and structural adjustments by an osteopath, along with environmental allergy therapy, can be more helpful in relieving recurrent otitis than either treatment used alone.

■ HEART AND PULSE PROBLEMS[11]

Cardiac function tests are necessary, primarily in adults, if hypertension or significant pulse or heart irregularities are present. Surprisingly, most cardiologists seldom consider environmental causes for these symptoms. However, if the cause can be found and eliminated, drug therapy for symptoms such as high blood pressure, angina, and heartbeat irregularities might be reduced or eliminated.

Older children and adults—as well as the parents of young children—may recognize that their heart is not beating in a uniform, steady manner. Sometimes the beat suddenly becomes too rapid, irregular, or too slow. If it does, a key question is: What did that person smell, eat, or touch?

Although many environmental factors and foods affect the circulatory system, it appears to be particularly sensitive to chemicals. A single whiff of lavatory deodorant, perfume, tobacco, gasoline, natural gas, or outside factory pollution can precipitate immediate cardiac or blood vessel changes. Sometimes chemical exposures can even cause repeated blood clots, particularly in the legs or blood vessels of the heart or brain. In some individuals, an allergenic craved food eaten during the evening meal routinely causes delayed heart complaints, such as a frighteningly rapid heartbeat (tachycardia) in the middle of the night.

During routine cursory heart examinations, your physician can easily miss changes due to such intermittent exposures, but with a bit of thought and some record-keeping, you can sometimes alert your doctor to a problem. Your physician can help document any heartbeat irregularities with a twenty-four-hour Holter monitoring device, so you can pinpoint the exact time they occurred.

When you or your child are at rest, a pulse increase of twenty or more beats or an abnormal change in heartbeat rhythm can constitute an alarm signal. Most people have a normal pulse between 65 and 85. When you are at rest and the pulse routinely goes over 95, you should ask yourself: What did I eat, touch, or smell? Was the cause something inside or outside, a food or a chemical? Again, if you can determine the cause of such changes and eliminate your exposure to offending substances, you may eventually feel so well that your physician can decrease or stop your cardiac medications. Don't decrease or stop them on your own, however, as it could be dangerous. Merely note any possible cause-and-effect relationships and discuss them with your doctor.

■ BLADDER PROBLEMS

Routine urine tests can be helpful in detecting certain bladder, kidney, or other problems, but in general they are of little help in detecting an environmental medical problem. Because the body excretes offending substances in the urine, however, it is possible that the urine sediment or mucus will show eosinophilic white blood cells. If these cells are present, they certainly suggest a possible allergy in individuals who have bladder complaints. Remember, your urine collects and concentrates what your body must excrete, so it often contains the very substances to which you are sensitive. In some individuals the bladder reacts with pain or spasms because these offending substances contact the bladder wall. In other words, youngsters and adults can have bladder contractions from an exposure in much the same way as an asthmatic's lungs go into spasm from contact with offending foods or chemicals.

A food sensitivity can certainly contribute to a child's daytime or nighttime bed-wetting problems. For example, a sensitivity to milk, fruit juice (especially apple, pineapple, orange, and grape) or any other food can be a common undiagnosed cause of:

■ bed-wetting
■ daytime accidents in school
■ a frequent or urgent need to urinate in the daytime
■ a painful urge to urinate but inability to do so

Following a simple allergy diet by excluding all suspect food items for one week or liquids other than water (see Chapter 3), sometimes entirely eliminates these problems in children. If these youngsters then ingest each single suspect beverage or food item on a separate day during the next week or so, it is often easy to pinpoint exactly which one is causing some medical problem.

If a change in diet only partially helps a child's daytime or nighttime wetting difficulty, or if there is no obvious evidence of an allergy at all, consult a pediatric urologist. Sometimes an allergy is only part of the problem. For example, if avoiding apple juice reduces the incidence of bed-wetting from seven times a week to twice a week, apple is only one factor contributing to this condition. A pediatric urologist should check for an anatomical abnormality that needs correction. Sometimes minor surgery *plus* an allergy diet and/or allergy extract treatment can totally eliminate a child's excessive need to urinate.

Surprisingly, molds, dust, pollen, and chemicals can cause some children and adults to urinate too quickly and too often. Major school problems can result unless these allergenic substances are reduced or removed. Some youngsters will need to receive mold and/or dust allergy extract therapy. Children can't learn well if they get sudden, frequent urges to urinate whenever they are in a dusty classroom or whenever a rainy day causes mold problems. Parents and teachers should become aware of such clues.

When children tend to wet their pants during the daytime, most parents believe they are simply too busy playing to bother to urinate. The majority of children, however, want to keep playing but *do not* wet their pants. Once again, keep asking why is your child different?

Essential fatty-acid deficiencies can also cause an increased thirst and need to urinate. Supplements with fatty acids sometimes help such patients (as well as some who have hyperactivity), often within a few weeks.[12] Diabetes can cause similar urinary complaints, but it is easy to spot with a urine dip-stick test.[13] If you are suspicious, check with your family doctor.

In rare cases, a child or adult will have blood in the urine, but only during the mold or pollen allergy season. Again, look for a pattern. Is the blood evident each year at the time when a certain type of pollen is in the air, or when molds are a major problem because of rain or dampness? On occasion, bladder pain associated with cystitis (a urinary tract infection) can be caused or aggravated by environmental or allergic factors.[14]

■ STRUCTURAL OR SPINAL PROBLEMS

Some individuals have neck or spinal injuries related to some trauma at birth or later in life. These people routinely tend to tip their head or body to one particular side while sitting or walking. If the spine is not properly aligned, however, the blood, lymph, and nerve supply to and from the brain will not be normal. This can cause a variety of subtle-to-serious health problems that will not improve without appropriate osteopathic or chiropractic diagnosis and adjustment. For example, if your child's skull became severely deformed during birth, perhaps it was damaged in some manner from the forceps or suction so that it does not feel perfectly smooth child craniosacral manipulation might be beneficial. However, only adept and knowledgeable doctors should attempt these types of adjustments, particularly in infants and young children. If you or your doctor suspects a structural problem, such therapy should be implemented prior to other forms of treatment. Sometimes this will help when other more traditional treatments have failed.

Why would a child experience sudden recurrent headaches? They can be due to sporadic muscle spasms that force the neck and spine out of alignment. If a muscle spasm is caused by eating chocolate (which it sometimes is), a cervical adjustment may help, *but only if your youngster stops eating chocolate.* The neck adjustment must be accompanied either by a diet that sharply limits or excludes chocolate and/or by treatment with an allergy extract for chocolate. Of course, other foods or exposures can cause a similar response leading to chronic headaches. Tight or painful joints and peculiar ways of walking or even talking can be caused by foods, chemicals, or typical allergenic exposures. Keep asking why. The elusive answers can be one thought away. Specific nutrients and homeopathics also can help relieve various types of muscle spasm. Dr. F. Batmanghelidj claims that a markedly increased water intake is also beneficial.[15]

■ SERIOUS VISUAL PROBLEMS

Most visual problems are unrelated to environmental exposures. When children complain of eye pain or irritation, they may simply need to wear glasses. If these eye complaints, however, suddenly appear after major school renovation or construction, there certainly may be an association. The most common eye problems that are due mainly, but not exclusively, to chemicals include burning or pain in, around, or behind the eye, blurred vision, an exquisite sensitivity to light, and sometimes double vision.

What tests should be conducted? The histories of a number of children in this book indicate that certain eye changes are reversible during P/N allergy testing. On occasion, a child will read upside down, as Annie did (see Chapter 13); her vision dramatically improved after mold and soy allergy testing and treatment. Others are like Wallace (in Chapter 10), who developed multiple temporary visual problems each time his school's carpets were cleaned. We must wonder how many other children have transient or permanent reading problems owing to unrecognized environmental factors.

Some environmentally ill people become perplexed after a proper eye examination when they realize their new prescription glasses do not correct their poor eyesight. Some need to have their eye exam in a medical office that does not smell of chemicals, dust or molds or their evaluation will be inaccurate. They may need to breathe oxygen during an eye examination so their glass prescription will be correct.

IRIS CORDER

Some very observant mothers or teachers can tell when certain children are reacting to a chemical or allergenic substance because the pupils of their eyes routinely change in size. An instrument called an Iris Corder can measure and provide specific data and analysis concerning such eye changes. Unfortunately, this instrument is not yet commercially available.

Ongoing studies using this instrument are presently being conducted by a team of Japanese ophthalmologists under the direction of Dr. Satoshi Ishikawa at the Environmental Health Center in Dallas, Texas.[16] They have documented that minute exposures to chemicals can interfere with sympathetic or parasympathetic nerve pathways and cause pupil and other significant eye changes. (Specific portions of the eye can also definitely undergo detectable changes during provocation/neutralization allergy testing or after minute exposures to chemicals.)[17]

■ NUTRITIONAL DEFICIENCIES[18]

At the cellular level the body requires many critical nutrients. Environmental medical specialists believe that vitamins, minerals, trace metals, essential fatty acids, and amino acids must be available if a person is to feel really well.[19] If these nutrients are present in the correct amounts, the total body feels and functions better. If one or more is lacking or excessive or the proportion of one to another however, is not correct there will be a progression of subtle to obvious medical symptoms.

While it is true that measuring the blood level of a particular vitamin, mineral, or other nutrient does not accurately reflect its level in the cells or tissues (where it is really needed), an abnormal blood level of that nutrient—accompanied by health problems corresponding to that type of nutrient deficiency or excess—certainly indicates a possible connection.[20] The initial signs of a vitamin deficiency, however, are always subtle. For example, if you have a slight need for more vitamin C, your gums may bleed when you brush your teeth. There is evidence of a shortage long before someone develops scurvy.

Unfortunately, most medical schools do not give a high priority to the clinical significance of cellular nutrition. To educate yourself (and your doctor) about nutrition, *for example*, read the excellent books written for the general reader by Drs. Majid Ali, Jonathan Wright, Alan Gaby, Billie

Sahley and Sherry Rogers (see For Further Reading). Various audiotape series for physicians from HealthComm International are also most valuable and informative (see Resources).

A trace metal examination for red-blood-cell magnesium, plasma zinc, and serum copper can be particularly informative to detect abnormal levels in both children and adults (see Resources for laboratories).[21] Magnesium and zinc are required for so many metabolic cellular body processes that these deficiencies must be detected and treated if the human body is to function optimally.

MAGNESIUM

As with other nutrients, the level of magnesium in the blood *serum* may not necessarily give a valid indication of how much magnesium is in the cells. For this reason, testing for a person's *red-blood*-cell magnesium level can sometimes be more informative. However, the best test to request from your doctor for is a *magnesium loading test* because it most accurately reflects how much magnesium the cells actually need.[22]

To conduct this test, a doctor will give your child a known amount of magnesium, and then measure the amount excreted in the urine. If most of it is excreted, your youngster has no magnesium deficiency. If only a little or none is found in the urine, your child's cells needed this essential nutrient so much that little was left over to be excreted. This is very important information if your child appears to have symptoms of magnesium deficiency. Common symptoms can include muscle cramps, spasms, tics and/or twitches, heart spasms or irregularities, cold hands and feet, blood pressure problems, a poor appetite, headaches, visual problems, weakness, numbness, dizziness, anxiety, confusion, and hyperactivity.

As with everything in our bodies, both too little or too much can create health problems. Thus, too much magnesium can cause symptoms such as a dry mouth, flushing, a slow heartbeat, muscle weakness, nausea, and thirst. Of course, the same symptoms can be a signal of many other health problems, and thus a magnesium deficiency or excess is not the only possible diagnosis. Unfortunately it is certainly a critical one that is often not even considered by many health providers.

ZINC

Children who have inadequate zinc levels may not learn well, and the growth of their body, genitals, and brain can be impaired. In adults, a zinc deficiency can cause brittle nails, apathy, poor wound healing, lethargy, and impotence. It also often causes white specks on the fingernails or stretch marks on the skin. This tends to be particularly evident at puberty, when youngsters normally have a growth spurt. Affected children and adults often crave highly seasoned foods and tend to put ketchup or salsa on everything because of a decreased sense of taste. In addition to checking for these signs, your doctor can conduct tests to measure plasma zinc levels in the blood.

COPPER

If your child has a copper deficiency, look for hair loss, anemia, depression, skin problems, fatigue, and weakness. However, if the copper level is too *high*, watch for irritability, joint or muscle pain, nervousness, diarrhea, depression, or a metallic taste in the mouth. Your child must be careful to avoid a high copper level, because it can lower the vitamin C level and weaken the body's defense systems for example, in relation to infection. Also, the zinc and copper levels must be in balance; if one is too high, the other goes down.

Note: The copper level in the blood can appear to be falsely high during an infection. So rather than reflecting excess copper in the tissues, the test actually indicates a mobilization of copper to fight the infection. Thus, in spite of this temporary elevation, a relative deficiency can actually be present. The opposite is true of iron; a blood level of iron can be falsely low during an infection, even though iron stores within the body are adequate. To avoid these types of misinterpretation, whenever possible have blood nutrient samples taken when there is no infection.

LEAD AND OTHER METALS

Lead is found in solder on pipes, in older paint, and until recently, in gasoline. An elevated lead level detected in the blood or hair, or a positive screening free erythrocyte protoporphyrin (FEP) test, sometimes explains why certain children are hyperactive, behave inappropriately, and can't learn. The results of a FEP test can be misleading if a patient is zinc-deficient or anemic. Therefore, discuss any abnormalities in these tests with your child's physician.

A hair analysis and a blood test are actually excellent screening tests for toxic metals (see Resources for laboratories). Elevated lead levels in the hair indicate a definite abnormality. Once a lead problem is documented, you must find and eliminate the source. Chelation therapy (in which metals are drawn out of the tissues and into the blood so they can be excreted) is one way to treat this problem.

Other metals that can cause illness:

■ Aluminum appears to be a possible factor in Alzheimer's disease. Be cautious about exposure in cooking pots, coffee makers, motor exhaust,

antacids, food additives, underarm deodorants, and beverage cans. It is also used as a flocculant in your tap water, combining or aggregating particles so they precipitate, thus making the water clear rather than cloudy.
■ Cadmium is present in tobacco smoke, automobile exhaust, and plating factory fumes.
■ Arsenic is found in seafood, wood preservatives, and plating factory fumes.
■ Mercury is present in dental fillings, seafood, and scientific instruments. Studies in humans and animals have repeatedly confirmed the many medical problems that can occur when the mercury in dental amalgams leaks into the body.[23] In some adults, mercury fillings must be *cautiously* removed or the procedure can make them feel worse.

VITAMINS[24]

To help detect whether a lack of nutrients is contributing to your environmental illness, various laboratories (see Resources) can conduct vitamin evaluations in your child. These tests may find, for example, that vitamin levels in white blood cells, especially pyridoxal-5-phosphate levels, are low. This is common in chemically sensitive individuals. As for the B vitamins, many are coenzymes that are necessary to break down or properly utilize what we eat. In general, any excess of vitamins B_1 (thiamine), B_2 (riboflavin), B_3 (niacin or niacinamide), and B_6 (pyridoxine), as well as C, is excreted in the urine, so they are *usually* considered to be quite safe. One exception is an extremely high dose of B_6, which can be toxic to the nervous system.

Excessive levels of the fat-soluble vitamins A, D, E, and K definitely can cause illness. The recommended vitamin A dosage, for example, should not be exceeded unless it is monitored by your doctor. Vitamin A is available in a potent droplet form that can be toxic if not taken **exactly as prescribed**. This vitamin can cause liver disease, as well as birth defects in infants, if taken in excess during pregnancy. So remember: More is not always better. Vitamin levels must be in the proper range and balanced.

Vitamin C helps our bodies in multiple ways and detoxification is part of its role;[25] if your child takes too much of this water-soluble vitamin, however, it typically causes abdominal discomfort, diarrhea, and/or canker sores in the mouth. Some physicians believe that the more expensive ester form of vitamin C is best because it is available to the body twenty minutes after ingestion and can help for about twenty-four hours. Ester C, unlike vitamin C, typically does not cause diarrhea or gastrointestinal upsets because it has a neutral pH of 7. This vitamin is particularly helpful to take during stressful travel because it reduces the tendency to develop infection.

■ BIOCHEMICAL AND METABOLIC ABNORMALITIES

Many qualified laboratories can perform nutrient tests that can indicate specific deficiencies or intestinal, metabolic, or biochemical abnormalities. (See MetaMetrix, Doctor's Data, SmithKline Beecham, and SpectraCell in Resources.) Specific tests can evaluate the liver's ability to adequately detoxify chemicals after a toxic exposure. Your doctor can order these tests and assist you in interpreting the results. (The physicians listed in Resources can be most helpful in determining which tests are most appropriate for you or your child.)

In general, a twenty-four-hour urine amino acid study will reveal how well the cells of your body are carrying out their metabolic processing. Other helpful tests include those evaluating organic acids, trace minerals in whole blood, red or white cells, functional vitamin levels, and enzymatic deficiencies. These tests are often required in chronically ill or developmentally delayed patients to provide further information about their body's ability to metabolize and detoxify at a cellular level. In other words, they can tell you whether your child's body has the nutrients it needs to function properly, and whether it can eliminate unwanted circulating or stored toxic substances. If each cell in the body is well and happy and have what is needed, the body in turn should be functionally optimally.

Amazingly, insurance coverage is sometimes denied for these tests, even though they can accurately reflect bodily function. It is perplexing that an insurance company would deny such reimbursement, particularly since this type of knowledge could certainly promote long-term wellness, reducing not only chronic illness but also the need for repeated insurance reimbursement.

■ DETOXIFICATION

Tests called depollution or detoxification enzyme panels can help pinpoint which nutrient or enzymatic deficiencies or inadequacies may be preventing the cells of your body from functioning optimally (see Antibody Assay Laboratory, Immunosciences Lab, and Great Smokies Diagnostic Laboratory in Resources). For the human body to feel well, it must be able to break down or convert certain chemicals or foreign substances into less toxic forms that can either be used or excreted. Unwanted substances normally are eliminated through the urine, bile, bowel movements, expired air, perspiration, saliva, and/or skin oils (sebum). The liver is the body's main detoxifying organ. It plays a major role in eliminating chemicals, drugs, poorly digested food particles, and other irritants that have oozed into the circulation from leaky or improperly functioning intestines. Bile from the liver eliminates chemicals through the intestines. Other water-soluble chemicals are routinely excreted in the urine. The liver, intestines, and kidneys must work well and in unison to withstand the daily onslaught we all face in today's heavily polluted world.

If the human body has been exposed to such an overload of toxic chemicals that it can't efficiently eliminate them, they tend to be stored in fatty tissues. When these harmful chemicals are allowed to remain there, these areas literally become toxic dump sites that can eventually cause a variety of illnesses.

There are a number of ways to enhance the excretion of toxins. Adequate amounts of substances such as glutathione, zinc, magnesium, B complex, vitamin C, selenium, taurine, and superoxide dismutase can help to prevent this toxic buildup and thus protect us. Dozens of other nutrients—including CoEnzyme Q10, glutathione, and taurine—assist the liver in excreting chemicals. Certain therapeutic programs place more emphasis on one or more of these nutrients, but in essence, seriously ill children and adults need many of the suggestions outlined in Table 15.4. Unfortunately, what determines the care a sick child or adult receives is too often not what is needed but what the family can afford.

Ideally, your doctor should test your child's blood, urine, and stool before, and again several weeks after, a detoxification nutritional program. This would help to objectively provide evidence of improvement. The results of these tests can indicate if a diet, for example, has created a better balance of the normal intestinal organisms and allowed fewer chemicals to be absorbed into the blood. (Initially, the levels of chemicals in the fat decrease as they enter the blood so they can be excreted. Once the chemicals are eliminated from the body, their levels in the blood, fat, and urine usually decline, along with the symptoms.) In some youngsters, these tests have shown that after detoxification the level of foreign chemicals in the urine drops by as much as one-third; at the same time, the imbalance in the intestinal flora is corrected. In addition, there is evidence of increases in IQ after the Hubbard detoxification method is used.[26]

The following information about available tests is rather technical, but you might ask your physician if some of these newer functional challenge laboratory studies would be helpful in understanding and relieving your child's health problems after a toxic exposure. They provide warning clues of liver malfunction long before the routine liver tests would indicate that something is wrong. These tests identify the competence of a person's biochemistry and the detoxification pathways. Detailed information and tapes about these tests are available from HealthComm International (see Resources).

1. The lactulose and mannitol test (discussed earlier in this chapter) determines if the intestinal mucosal barrier is intact. Is it doing its job? Does it let the right substances get into the circulation? Does it exclude and excrete those that are undesirable?
2. The caffeine challenge test, using sodium benzoate, which checks Phase I of detoxification.
3. A test using acetaminophen evaluates a number of pathways used by the liver during Phase II conjugation and detoxification process.
4. The salicylate challenge test checks for oxygen free radicals. They can be either helpful or harmful, depending upon how many you produce. Antioxidant therapy helps if these free radicals pose a problem.
5. A variety of urinary nitrate, sulfate, or sulfite-to-creatinine tests check different aspects of the immune system, glutathione reserves in the liver, and the activity of different key enzymes.

These tests enable physicians to specifically tailor a child's (or adult's) nutritional requirements to the unique weaknesses he or she manifests. You need to know the extent of your youngster's reserves. Can the body handle additional life stresses in the form of pollution, or is it already in overload? These types of tests represent the cutting edge of medicine and are discussed in more detail in Chapter 15.

■ SOME UNPROVEN ALTERNATIVES

If your child has gone through a lengthy, expensive, and at times traumatic series of tests, without turning up any conclusive evidence of where the problems lie, you may decide to pursue still other options. There are some easier ways to test and treat various forms of illness effectively, *even though these methods are certainly not scientifically proven, understood, or accepted.* If you decide to try them, be aware that some illnesses worsen or become irreversible when appropriate regular therapy is delayed. On the positive side however, even though these methods are not proven to the satisfaction of the medical establishment, they often help and do not hurt. They even sometimes spell success when all the traditionally accepted methods have failed.

Some chiropractors, in particular, are using newer rapid approaches that seem to be particularly helpful.[27] These approaches include various forms of muscle testing, acupuncture meridian stimulation, chiropractic adjustments, nutritional supplements, and "body modification and balancing." These techniques do not use any needles and are not painful. Two such promising methods are Total Body Modification (TBM) and Neuro-Emotional Training (NET) (see Resources). Some of the patients described in this book, such as Darryl in Chapter 13, *have been helped to such a degree by these approaches that they no longer require a special ECO classroom, diet, or allergy extract therapy. These methods, therefore, urgently need more study and critical evaluation.*

Similarly, some environmentally ill individuals have definitely been helped by homeopathy,[28] naturopathy, herbal, and Edgar Cayce remedies (see Resources). These approaches can be particularly useful for the treatment of infections in persons who cannot tolerate antibiotics or most other drugs. Some of these forms of treatment have been used successfully for centuries. Such modalities including blue-green algae and pycnogenol, certainly need more investigation and critical study, but scholarly physicians and scientists must be less closed-minded when these methods prove safe, effective, less traumatic, and less expensive.

Do not err by equating benefit to in-depth understanding. The body can recognize what helps, even when today's academic medical physicians cannot presently explain why. As long as an alternative therapy does no harm and the patient feels better, it must be given serious consideration, especially when the usual forms of therapy have not proven beneficial.

There are also a number of machines that in strange ways appear to detect and diagnose illnesses and provide a guide for treatment. These machines are variously called Vega, Enterro, Dermatron, and Computron. They are used, for example, in the offices of some physicians to find the "approximate" correct allergy extract doses. Then routine P/N testing is used to pinpoint or verify the *exact* treatment dilution and dose. Once again, if they help, save time, and do not hurt, why not encourage their use? If these methods decrease the number of needle-type allergy skin tests that a youngster or adult needs, are they not most worthwhile? Studies are needed and some are in progress to evaluate the efficacy of these machines as credible diagnostic tools.

Lastly, some investigators examine fresh and dried blood samples with exceptionally precise electron microscopes and claim to be able to diagnose various illnesses from their observations (see Resources). This method is not that different from examining and counting the white blood cells to help differentiate a probable viral infection from one that is bacterial. Perhaps a blood smear can provide more diagnostic information than mainstream medicine presently recognizes or appreciates. We need to evaluate these methods and use them *if* they provide diagnostic and/or therapeutic clues.

All these options should be more available, especially when traditional medical therapies fail to help. Remember, much that we presently do in medicine was not fully understood for many years but was used solely because it helped. Aspirin is the classic example. It would never have been approved to relieve pain if today's restrictions on the release of drugs had been applied years ago. However, not understanding the mechanism of action of aspirin or other therapeutic modalities does not negate its value. If scientists are given enough money and time, they can usually discover why something is beneficial, but the lag time between obvious help and documented proof can exceed twenty years. That's how it was with the ideas of Dr. Ignaz Semmelweis, who advocated washing contaminated hands to prevent childbirth fever; and those of the nurse Sister Kenny, who suggested that exercise could help to decrease the long-term paralysis associated with polio. The sick children of today cannot wait for a lifetime to get answers—they have a limited window of time in which to receive an education. The bottom line is that if it is safe and effective, why should it not be used.

In time, of course, scientists must thoroughly research and document the veracity of unusual claims and methodologies. Although I have personally observed (but not used) these "different" methods, I strongly believe that we must investigate each one to either confirm or refute its value.

■ SOME FINAL THOUGHTS

If we always do everything exactly as it has been done in the past, there will never be any progress in medicine. We must continually search for faster, easier, safer, more effective, and more inexpensive methods to prevent and relieve sickness, including the environmental illnesses discussed in this book. We must combine the beneficial aspects of proven Eastern and Western methods of healing in the practice of modern medicine.

Present-day physicians concentrate almost exclusively on the physical aspects of medicine and drug therapy. When indicated, or if they are perplexed, they investigate the emotional aspects of illness. But they have neglected another important category—the spiritual aspects—which truly need much more consideration. Illness is not due to one isolated malfunction in a single obviously sick body part; instead, it is a warning that something is wrong in the total being. We must try to determine why an illness is in the left leg, for example, and not the right ear. Why does a child's body suddenly seem to completely malfunction? We must look at patients in their entirety. Mind, body, and spirit are interrelated, and hopefully the physicians of tomorrow will consider each of these elements when they try to relieve the pain and anguish of those who cross their paths in a quest for better health. If this book helps to create an educational medical center in Phoenix, this will be a fundamental principle used in a most comprehensive approach to treat patients.

NOTES

1. William G. Crook, *The Yeast Connection* (Jackson, TN: Professional Books, 1989), and *The Yeast Connection and the Woman* (Jackson, TN: Professional Books, 1995).

2. HealthComm International, 5800 Southview Drive, Gig Harbor, WA 98335, tel. (206) 851-3943.

3. Carlton Fredericks, *New Low Blood Sugar and You* (New York: Perigee Books, 1985); and William Philpott and Dwight Kalita, *Brain Allergies: The Psychonutrient Connection* (1980); and the same authors' *Victory Over Diabetes* (1983). Both books are published by Keats Publishing, 27 Pine Street, New Canaan, CT 06840.

4. Fredericks, *New Low Blood Sugar*.

5. Billie Sahley, *The Anxiety Epidemic* (San Antonio: Pain and Stress Clinic, 1994).

6. Philpott and Kalita, *Brain Allergies* and *Victory over Diabetes*.

7. F. Batmanghelidj, *Your Body's Many Cries for Water* (Falls Church, VA: Global Health Solutions, 1995).

8. See Sahley, *The Anxiety Epidemic*, and Fredericks, *New Low Blood Sugar*.

9. Doris J. Rapp, *Is This Your Child?* (New York: William Morrow & Co., 1991), chapter 27.

10. Michael A. Schmidt, *Childhood Ear Infections* (Berkeley, CA: North Atlantic Books, 1990); and Michael A. Schmidt et al., *Beyond Antibiotics* (Berkeley, CA: North Atlantic Books, 1994).

11. William J. Rea, M.D., "Environmentally Triggered Small Vessels Vasculitis," *Annals of Allergy*, vol. 38 (1976), p. 245; William J. Rea, "Recurrent Environmentally Triggered Thrombophlebitis," *Annals of Allergy*, vol. 47 (1981), pp. 338–44; William J. Rea and O.D. Brown, "Mechanisms of Environmentally Vascular Triggering," *Clinical Ecology*, vol. 3 (1985), pp. 122–27; William J. Rea and C.W. Suits, "Cardiovascular Disease Triggered by Foods and Chemicals," in *Food Allergy: New Perspectives*, ed. John Gerrard (Springfield, IL: Charles C. Thomas, 1980); William J. Rea et al., "Environmentally Triggered Large-Vessel Vasculitis," *Annals of Allergy*, vol. 38 (1977), pp. 245–51; Gerald Ross and W.J. Rea, "Environmentally Triggered Hypertension, Part II; Environmental Health Center—Dallas Treatment Experience," presented at the eighth annual international symposium on Man and His Environment in Health and Disease, Dallas, TX, Feb. 22–25, 1980; Joseph Harkavy, *Vascular Allergy and Its Systemic Manifestations* (Washington, DC: Butterworth, 1963).

12. L. Galland and D.D. Buchman, *Superimmunity for Kids* (New York: Dell Publishing, 1988).

13. Philpott and Kalita, *Brain Allergies*.

14. Patrick Kingsley, *Conquering Cystitis* (London: Ebury Press, 1987).

15. Billie Sahley, *The Anxiety Epidemic* (San Antonio: Pain and Stress Clinic, 1994); and F. Batmanghelidj, *Your Body's Many Cries for Water* (Falls Church, VA: Global Health Solutions, 1995).

16. Satoshi Ishikawa et al., "Evaluations of the Autonomic Nervous System Response by Pupillographical Study in the Chemically Sensitive Patient," *Clinical Ecology*, vol. 7, no. 2, (1990).

17. W. Rea et al., "Confirmation of Chemical Sensitivity By Means of Double Blind Inhalant Challenge of Toxic Volatile Chemicals," *Clinical Ecology*, vol. 6, no. 4 (1989), p. 113.

18. Majid Ali, *The Butterfly and Life Span Nutrition* (Denville, NJ: Life Span Press, 1992); and Majid Ali, *RDA: Rats, Drugs and Assumptions* (Denville, NJ: Life Span Press, 1995). The publisher's address is Life Span Press, 95 East Main Street, Denville, NJ 07834. See also Frank Murray, *The Big Family Guide to All Minerals* (New Canaan, CT: Keats Publishing, 1995). The publisher's address is Keats Publishing, 27 Pine Street, Box 876, New Canaan, CT 06840.

19. Sahley, *The Anxiety Epidemic*.

20. Murray, *Big Family Guide*.

21. The Carl Pfeiffer Treatment Center does these tests (see Resources). See also Jonathan Wright, *Dr. Wright's Guide to Healing with Nutrition* (New Canaan, CT: Keats Publishing, 1991); and the audiotape series from HealthComm International (see Resources).

22. Sherry Rogers, *Wellness Against All Odds* (Syracuse, NY: Prestige Publishing, 1994).

23. Joyal Taylor, *The Complete Guide to Mercury Toxicity from Dental Fillings* (San Diego, CA: Scripps Publishing, 1988); Jukka T. Salonen et al., "Intake of Mercury from Fish, Lipid Peroxidatin, and the Risk of Myocardial Infarction and Coronary, Cardiovascular, and Aneurysm Death in Eastern

Finnish Men,'' *Circulation*, vol. 91, no. 3 (1995), pp. 645–55; Murry J. Mitchell, and J.R. Butler, ''Neuropsychological Dysfunctioning Associated with the Dental Office Environment,'' *International Journal of Biosocial Research*, vol. 10, (1988), pp. 45–68.

24. Lendon H. Smith, *How to Raise a Healthy Child* (New York: M. Evans and Co., 1996).

25. Linus Pauling, *How to Live Longer and Feel Better* (New York: Avon Books, 1986).

26. R. Michael Wisner et al., *Treatment of Children with the Detoxification Method Developed by Hubbard* (San Diego: Proceedings of the American Public Health Association National Conference, 1995); David W. Schnare et al., ''Body Burden Reduction of PCBs, PBBs and Chlorinated Pesticides in Human Subjects,'' *Ambio*, vol. 13, no. 5–6 (1984), pp. 378–80; Kaye H. Kilburn et al., ''Neurobehavioral Dysfunction in Firemen Exposed to Polychlorinated Biphenyls (PCBs): Possible Improvement after Detoxification,'' *Archives of Environmental Health*, vol. 44, no. 6 (1989), pp. 345–50; David E. Root et al., ''Excretion of a Lipophilic Toxicant Through the Sebaceous Glands: A Case Report,'' *Journal of Toxicology: Cutaneous and Ocular Toxicology*, vol. 6, no. 1 (1987), pp. 13–17; Ziga Tretjak et al., ''PCB Reduction and Clinical Improvement by Detoxification: An Unexploited Approach?'' *Human and Experimental Toxicology*, vol. 9, (1990), pp. 235–44; ''Is Detoxification a Solution to Occupational Health Hazards?'' *National Safety News* (May 1994).

27. Dean Black, *Inner Wisdom* (Springville, UT: Tapestry Press, 1990); John Diamond, *Your Body Doesn't Lie* (New York: Warner Books, 1983).

28. On homeopathy, see J. Benveniste et al., ''Human Basophil Degranulation Triggered by Very Dilute Antiserum against IgE,'' *Nature*, vol. 333, (1988), pp. 816–18; ''Various Rebuttals,'' *Nature*, (1988), pp. 285–91.

15 Treatments for Environmental Illness

The best place to start is to find a doctor with expertise in illnesses like yours (or your child's). That means looking for an environmental medical (EM) physician who is experienced in treating environmentally related health problems. Many EM doctors are board certified in one to three medical specialties (see Resources). As in any specialty, however, they have varying degrees and levels of expertise. If possible, find a doctor who is familiar with your specific problem. For example, if your child has a stuffy nose and ear problems, an ear, nose, and throat allergy specialist may be best for you. (Many ENT allergy physicians, in particular, are knowledgeable about this type of medicine because of the far-sighted teachings of Dr. Herbert Rinkel in the 1950s.[1]) If your child has extreme fatigue and typical allergies, find a pediatric environmental specialist; adults should seek an internist or EI specialist.

The doctor you select should be able to advise you concerning exactly what you and your child personally need to do. This advice will depend on your youngster's age, the degree and duration of the illness, and the nature and amount of chemicals or other substances to which your child has been exposed. Whether the problem lies with a student or teacher who feels unwell in a school building, or a family member who becomes sick at home, the answer is sometimes gratifyingly easy. Many times, merely making a few minor changes inside a sick building is all that is needed. However, people with the most severe EI will find the solutions more challenging. If they don't or can't make dietary adjustments or drastic changes in their lifestyle, they may be faced with a prolonged period of feeling unwell. Fortunately few are this ill, although their numbers are growing even among the children.

To complicate matters, after some individuals have been significantly sensitized to chemicals, it can be difficult for them to find *any* school or home that will not cause similar symptoms. Some severely ill people become prisoners in their own homes because eventually their sensitivity to minute amounts of any chemical—even perfume and tobacco—incapacitates them to an extraordinary degree. If this happens, the advice of a specialist in environmental medicine is essential. These physicians have the special expertise to recognize and treat chemical sensitivities.

In addition to finding a doctor, you need to equip yourself with as much information as possible. This chapter will help you to do that. It will discuss comprehensive environmental medical treatment, which typically requires allergy therapy. Dust, mold, pollen, pet and food allergies, chemical sensitivities, nutritional deficiencies, yeast overgrowth, and, at times, parasites and hormonal imbalances may all need to be treated in the total therapeutic program. (Problems related to lead, radon, asbestos, and electromagnetic exposures were discussed in Chapter 9.) Sometimes each aspect must be addressed. If symptoms are extreme, psychological counseling is essential as well.

In general, younger children respond more quickly and easily to treatment than adults. But *all* environmentally ill individuals must learn to help themselves. EI is typically not a simple medical problem that can be eliminated by a few weeks of drug therapy. Parents, older children, and teachers must read and study about their illness. There are many books, audiotapes, and videotapes to help in that process (see For Further Reading).

You do not have to read this entire chapter. Just scan the various parts and read in depth only the portions related to you or your child. If some aspect seems pertinent, ask your physician to look at it and decide if what's written might be applicable and possibly helpful for you.

As I've mentioned in many parts of this book, the lack of insurance reimbursement prevents many individuals from continuing to receive proper environmental medical care even when it proves helpful. In everyday life the cost of treatment is a real issue; therefore, whenever possible, the information provided in this chapter has been divided into:

- what's fast, easy, and inexpensive
- what's better but more expensive
- what's best but expensive

Armed with this knowledge, you can make some personal strides to help your child or yourself feel better. No one knows your youngster's medical history as well as you and your own physician, so obtain professional advice before you make any changes in your own or your child's health care.

HOW CAN YOU DETERMINE THE SEVERITY OF YOUR CHILD'S ILLNESS?

Your child's prognosis improves if his or her symptoms either lessen or disappear within a few days after eliminating an allergenic or chemical exposure. In other words, after your youngster leaves school each afternoon, does he or she feel better? Does your child feel healthier on weekends? If you can honestly say yes, your youngster should improve if the exposure to the offending substance ends. Try to change the environment of your child's school sufficiently that he or she no longer becomes ill there. Similarly, change your home if this is where your youngster seems sicker. (Another option is to transfer your child to another school or move your family into a different house with a healthier environment.)

For most of the rest of this chapter, I'll discuss ten major treatment options that may prove helpful to you or your child. They are:

- avoidance
- allergy diets
- allergy extract treatment
- improved overall nutrition
- psychological counseling and family support
- detoxification
- nondietary aids to help excrete toxins
- treatments for yeast problems
- treatments for parasites
- hormone treatment
- alternative less proven methods of treatment

Let's look at each one of these therapeutic modalities in detail.

■ AVOIDANCE

FAST, EASY, INEXPENSIVE

The most cost-effective, fastest, and easiest way to feel better is simply to avoid as many chemicals and allergenic substances as is sensibly possible. Many children (and adults) who are allergic to common substances such as dust, molds, pollen, foods, and pets are also sensitive to chemicals. For youngsters to regain their health and remain well, parents must strive to find and eliminate as many of these potential causes as possible. A combination of the following steps is relatively inexpensive and effective for many children:

■ Take the measures outlined in Chapter 6 to diminish exposure to dust, molds, pollen, pets, and chemicals. For example, improve the ventilation, install new and better duct filters, open windows, and clean with safer products (see Resources).

■ Have your child keep a charcoal face mask handy at all times to help absorb odors when he or she has no choice but to breathe pollution. Sew a pocket into a hanky so your youngster can use it without feeling self-conscious. Keep one handy in your own pocket, purse, and car as well (see Resources, under PARF).

■ Remember, even after your child feels well, you must remain cautious. Any massive chemical exposure in the future could cause a devastating recalcitrant recurrence of the original symptoms (see the story of Jerry in Chapter 7).

■ If a single food such as bananas, cinnamon, etc. causes allergies, eliminate it totally from your diet.

■ As much as possible, have your child wear clothing made of 100 percent natural fibers, such as cotton, silk, wool, or ramie. Avoid polyester and all synthetic "no iron" fabrics because they often contain formaldehyde. Use 100 percent natural fabrics for everything from blankets, sheets, and furniture coverings to cotton diapers.

■ Wash all new clothing with baking soda or vinegar before wearing. Thoroughly air out all freshly dry-cleaned clothes before hanging them in the bedroom closet.

■ Ask your school officials to stop the formaldehyde emissions coming from pressed wood, plywood furniture, and paneling by using a safer sealing substance (see Resources).

Our schools cannot be expected to control every possible environmental exposure, but they must at least begin to improve the air quality inside school buildings. This alone would greatly enhance the health and well-being of many students and teachers. In time, the quality of school lunches will also have to be addressed.

BETTER BUT MORE EXPENSIVE

Place an air purifier in your child's major classrooms at school and in the bedroom and family room at home. Environmentally ill youngsters don't need to study, live, or work in total pristine purity, but they must not be exposed to a level of offending substances that is higher than their bodies can tolerate. If air purifiers decrease the total daily exposure to below the critical tolerance level, symptoms should develop less readily. (See Chapter

EMERGENCIES HAPPEN:
Responding to Illness from Chemical Exposure

When a chemical exposure occurs, here is how to minimize the problems associated with it:

- If possible or practical, your child should quickly get away from the odor, and breathe in the direction of cleaner air. Have him leave any area that suddenly makes him ill, and he should avoid returning if the odor persists. He can hold his breath in obviously polluted areas and distance himself quickly from avoidable chemical exposures. Many become ill from school buses, crowded parking lots, and lavatories that smell of chemicals.
- Have your child breathe oxygen, which diminishes his symptoms. If no oxygen is available, take your child to the nearest emergency room.

If breathing a chemical cannot be avoided, ask your physician for a prescription for a portable refillable tank of oxygen. The oxygen should be inhaled at a rate of four liters per minute for several ten-minute intervals throughout the day. Use a ceramic (not plastic) mask connected via special, less-allergenic Tygon tubing (see Resources) to the oxygen tank. A small tank can be kept at school, in your car, and at home and/or the workplace for treating accidental exposures.

- Sometimes vitamin C, taken in amounts just below those that cause adverse symptoms, can be beneficial. The initial dosage is generally small (500 mg.) and is gradually increased to tolerance in a few days. As much as 3,000 mg or more per day can be helpful for adults after an acute exposure (or for an infection). Take a smaller dosage on a daily basis for maintenance.[2] Your body will tell you if you are consuming too much vitamin C because it will cause an intestinal upset or canker sores in the mouth. If you are in doubt, ask your doctor how much you should take. For children, consult a doctor for the appropriate dosage.
- Antioxidant nutrients can be purchased in supplement form at health food stores to help prevent oxidation. The release of single, unpaired electrons or oxygen free radicals, which can be harmful to the body. Antioxidant preparations typically include vitamins A, B_2, C, and E, pyridoxal-5-phosphate, selenium, L-glutathione, and taurine. The latter two help excrete toxic chemicals in the urine and bowel movement.[3] Your child may particularly need antioxidants before, during, and after art, biology, or chemistry class, or spending time in a polluted school bus. These matters will be discussed in more detail later in this chapter.
- A drop or two of heparin under the tongue appears to help prevent some reactions to chemical odors. Ask your doctor for a prescription for your child to use prior to obvious odorous classes, such as art, biology, or chemistry. It is also helpful when shopping in malls, or in other polluted areas.

6 for more about ventilation and air quality.) If you can lower your child's exposures at home as much as possible, then he or she can tolerate more in school without a recurrence of symptoms. The opposite is also true: the more you're able to reduce school exposures, there will be fewer problems with exposures at home.

■ ALLERGY DIETS

If avoiding a single suspect food does not resolve a food allergy, this type of problem typically can be helped by a variety of diets.[4] The major exception is the foods that cause a life-threatening response. They must be avoided in all forms, at all times. You must also be aware that approximately 80 percent of chemically sensitive people are sensitive to foods, or the chemicals such as pesticides found on or in them. These people improve providing they eat only organic foods. When dietary avoidance or restriction is not practical or possible, food allergy extract therapy is a realistic option.

FAST, EASY, INEXPENSIVE

- A simple seven-day Multiple Food Elimination Diet can be very helpful (see Chapter 5).[5] Many children and adults improve dramatically during the first three to seven days. It is a diagnostic diet, however, not a treatment diet. It helps pinpoint which food causes each specific health problem.
- Alkali products are frequently useful to relieve food sensitivities; they can also quickly decrease or stop some symptoms from chemical exposures. Use commercial products such as Alka Aid, Trisalts (available in health food stores), or Alka-Seltzer Antacid Formula (in drugstores). (See Chapters 3 and 8 for more details.)
- If possible, grow your own vegetables and fruits *without herbicides and pesticides*.[6] This method is very cost-effective. Remember, the Food and Drug Administration found 108 different pesticides on twenty-two fruits and vegetables.[7]
- Read every label of every food or beverage your child ingests. Detect hidden problem foods or additives and avoid them. Don't allow your youngster to eat anything stored or served in plastic or Styrofoam.
- Urge your youngster to be exceedingly careful in the school cafeteria and any restaurant. Talk to the cook if your child's food reactions can be life-threatening and you are concerned about the content of something on the menu. No one wants a serious allergic emergency in his or her place of business.

BETTER BUT MORE EXPENSIVE

■ Drink and cook with only purer filtered or glass-bottled water. (To check for a school or home tap water sensitivity, see Chapters 5 and 8.)

■ Organic or less chemically contaminated foods and beverages are much preferred. They are more nutritious but less readily available and usually much costlier.[8]

■ A Rotation Diet of regular or, preferably, organic foods is one way to detect and treat food allergies.[9] This diet (discussed in Chapter 3 and below) often makes it possible for children to eat a wide range of slightly-to-moderately allergenic foods without becoming ill. It allows limited amounts of tolerated problem foods, *provided they are eaten no more often than every four days.*[10] Over time, even a moderately allergenic food sometimes can be tolerated if the initial amount is very tiny. The challenge is to start with such a small amount of a food that it will not cause symptoms (check with your doctor to decide how small is small). Then at four-day intervals, the amount ingested can be doubled until a normal-sized portion is eaten. If symptoms occur during this buildup, you must back down and then increase the amount your child ingests more slowly. You will need the help of a number of books or an EM specialist and experienced nutritionist/dietitian to try this diet. (Also see Chapter 3.)

BEST BUT EXPENSIVE

The Rotation Diet is helpful, but it can take months before problem foods can be consumed in normal amounts—unless the diet is combined with relatively expensive allergy extract therapy. For example, if your child receives allergy extract treatment for dairy (milk) or wheat, a normal portion usually can be ingested (at four-day intervals) either immediately or a couple of weeks or months after treatment. By contrast, if you gradually increase the amount of a food your youngster eats at four-day intervals, but don't give food allergy extract therapy, it may require many months or even a year or more before a normal-sized portion of dairy, baked goods, or other problem food is well-tolerated.

Fortunately, allergy extract treatment for most food sensitivities has been available and in use for over thirty-five years.[11] This therapy unquestionably has helped many children and adults tolerate previously offending foods. However, when foods obviously interfere with a child's ability to think or behave appropriately, they should be avoided during school hours *unless* allergy extract therapy prevents these symptoms. Regrettably, similar to myself during the first twenty years of my practice, many well-trained, board-certified allergists have not personally tried or even observed this form of therapy. We were never taught about these methods during our training and most doctors have not read the abundant number of articles showing its efficacy (see For Further Reading). As a result, many well-trained physicians simply do not believe that such treatment is possible.

■ ALLERGY EXTRACT TREATMENT

If avoidance and/or allergy diets do not quickly and adequately relieve environmental illness, treatment with extracts for typical allergenic substances, including foods, is often helpful. This type of allergy extract therapy raises a child's or adult's tolerance to an offending item so that exposure causes less or no difficulty.

For example, before your youngster receives allergy extract treatment, a pollen count of 50 may cause episodes of asthma when dairy products are ingested. But after pollen and milk allergy extract treatment, asthma may not be experienced even when the pollen count is 100. At that time dairy products can be ingested every four days. Allergy extract therapy gives your youngster a "larger barrel" or increased tolerance. It often enables children to eat foods or to be exposed to items that previously bothered them with less or no difficulty. It also tends to diminish or eliminate the need for drug treatment.

ARE YOU CONFUSED ABOUT ALLERGY TREATMENT?

As mentioned before, the majority of doctors may be unfamiliar with or most skeptical of some types of allergy therapies. That leaves many patients confused, because one group of specialists says one thing, while another group, who appears to be equally well-trained, says the opposite.[12] How can you decide who is right? Who do you believe when well-written medical articles reach opposite conclusions? One suggestion is to see what and who effectively helps your child's medical problems.

If your youngster is always sick and always using medications, and no one really knows *specifically* what causes the illness, maybe it's time to try another way. If you notice that something repeatedly causes your child to feel differently or unwell, but your physician maintains that this is not possible, maybe you need to provide more proof to your doctor—or find a physician who is more familiar with other causes for these types of problems. Unfortunately many doctors continue to believe that food allergies rarely occur, or that the only treatment is total avoidance of all obvious offending foods.

Look for a specialist who says, "I treat food sensitivities all the time and recognize chemical sensitivities in many patients." Seek out a doctor who knows that dust, mold, pollen, foods, and chemicals can affect not

TABLE 15.1

Comparison of Allergy Testing and Treatment Methods

Typical Method	Provocation/Neutralization Method
Used for testing:	
Uses stock allergy extract with phenol preservative for testing.	Uses the same allergy extract, but many avoid the phenol preservative.
Tests with weak, less precise, and less reliable scratch skin tests or with 1:10 dilutions of allergy extract placed on or into skin (intradermally).	Tests with more precise 1:5 dilutions, placed either intradermally or sublingually.
Tests with weak-to-strong concentrations of various allergy extracts (1:10,000 to 1:10).	Tests with strong-to-weak concentrations (1:100 to 1:100,000 or weaker).
Tests many items at one time on the back or arm, and observes *only* the skin test site.	Tests one item at a time, not telling the patient which is being tested. Before and after each test, the skin test site is observed and, in addition, the symptoms, pulse, breathing, writing, behavior, and appearance may be monitored.
Can rarely pinpoint which item causes a specific symptom.	Can often pinpoint the exact cause of each symptom.
Very fast and easy testing method—takes about 15 minutes.	Extremely time-consuming testing method—takes hours or several days.
Used as treatment:	
Takes months to improve.	Often helps in minutes, hours, or days.
Symptomatic drug therapy is routinely needed.	Fewer, less, or no drugs are needed.
Administered by injection.	Administered by injection or sublingually (unless insurance won't pay).
Administered only in doctor's office.	Can be safely administered at home.
Many visits are needed for ''buildup'' injections.	No ''buildup'' injections are needed (set therapy requires buildup injections).
Administered according to a standard schedule, with the same desired ''arbitrary'' top dose for all patients.	An optimum **individualized** dose is found for *each* item. Requires no buildup booster doses.
Rarely requires retests.	Requires retests whenever effectiveness of therapy diminishes.
Virtually no danger.	Virtually no danger.
Less precise and sensitive—often misses some food and/or chemical sensitivities.	Detects missed food and chemical sensitivities.
Can give a false impression that there is no allergy when there is (especially with scratch or prick tests).	Can give a false impression that an allergy is present when it is not.

only how individuals feel, but how they behave and/or learn. Find a physician who has no doubt that yeast and candida are common problems and that sometimes chronic fatigue is caused by environmental exposures. The answer for some patients is a physician who is both knowledgeable and experienced in environmental medicine (see Resources). These doctors often provide meaningful answers, *particularly if you are tired of giving your child daily medications to control symptoms and are willing to make an effort to help find and eliminate the cause of the illness.*

Treatment for environmental illness is often effective, especially P/N allergy treatment. For complete details about P/N allergy testing as a diagnostic method, see Chapter 13. Because there is a difference of opinion among physicians about this form of therapy, let's look more closely at the pros and cons of this treatment (see Table 15.1).

PROS OF P/N ALLERGY EXTRACT TREATMENT

■ Once P/N testing helps identify *why* your child is ill—pinpointing specific causes of an allergy—then avoidance and/or allergy extract therapy can be used to prevent, eliminate, or treat flare-ups of illness. (However, if you only want a drug that will quickly but temporarily make your child feel better, *this is not the treatment for you.*)

■ Some patients actually feel better within minutes after treatment has begun. For many others, it can take several days. For a few very challenging individuals, it can take many months or they may be helped very little or not at all.

■ The need for medications is often reduced or eliminated.

■ After a child's nose and chest allergies respond to therapy, his or her tendency to develop secondary infections decreases. That translates into using fewer antibiotics, which means less overgrowth of yeast and fewer bowel disturbances. Quite often, this eliminates the need for repeated ear, nose, throat, and/or sinus surgery.

■ You can safely self-administer P/N allergy extracts by injection, or treat children sublingually under the tongue, reducing the need for costly doctor visits.

■ Although P/N treatment is initially expensive, in time it is usually both cost- and health-effective. As time passes, there should be fewer drug bills, doctor visits, specialist consultations, surgeries, and/or hospitalizations. It is truly not unusual for patients to feel better for the first time in many years.

CONS OF P/N TREATMENT

■ P/N testing is most time-consuming. Many patients need tests for histamine, dust, molds, pollen, pets, yeast, some major foods, and possibly chemicals, such as phenol, formaldehyde, glycerine, hydrocarbons, tobacco or chlorine. Testing for each item can require from twenty minutes to an hour or longer, so it typically requires several days to complete the initial evaluation.

■ You and/or your child must help monitor the effect of each test dose. Thus this form of therapy definitely requires direct and continued patient/parent involvement.

■ P/N treatment doses often change with time, so retesting is often required at intervals of one to three (or more) months, at first and in time, possibly once or twice every year or two. (The retests are much less time-consuming and therefore less expensive than the initial tests.)

■ Another form of treatment called EPD was discussed in Chapter 13. It appears to be most helpful for some patients.

The American people need to be able to choose their physicians, as well as the type of medical care they receive. Unfortunately and surprisingly, managed care organizations (like HMOs) and similar health-provider groups often have little expertise, knowledge, or interest in environmental medicine. Thus, some patients have to make a difficult choice. They must decide whether they want a limited choice of non-environmental physicians who will provide less expensive medical care and repeated drug therapy; or the right to choose their doctor and the type of medicine they believe will be helpful. Initially environmental medical care entails increased medical costs, but potentially it is possible to restore the health of some to many individuals while decreasing the need for drugs.

■ IMPROVED OVERALL NUTRITION

After you have implemented the treatment options for avoidance, allergy diets, and allergy extract treatment, then a relatively easy and inexpensive nutritional program is essential. Be sure that any nutritional therapy diet you undertake is approved by a physician (and dietitian) who is knowledgeable about your youngster's personal health needs and who understands nutritional and environmental medicine.

On a long-term basis, your child requires improved nutrition, supplied by a better diet and supplements. This is an essential aspect of comprehensive environmental medical therapy and a critical part of his or her recov-

---

HOW EFFECTIVE ARE AVOIDANCE, DIET, AND ALLERGY THERAPY COMBINED?

In 1992 a two-part study by British environmental specialists D.J. Maberly and H.M. Anthony documented that a combination of avoidance, diet, and allergy treatment can help dramatically.[13]

Here's how the study was conducted: Asthmatic patients were admitted to an environmentally sound, allergy-free clinic for three weeks. Each patient's ability to breathe was repeatedly monitored using a Peak Flow Meter. During the test period, patients drank pure water while they fasted for five days, Then were given challenge meals of single foods. By deliberately exposing the patients to different single foods, the effects of each could be evaluated. In addition, the patients received P/N testing for foods and serial endpoint titration (SET) treatment for dust, molds, pollen, and chemicals (see Chapter 13).[14]

By the sixth day, most of the patients were symptom-free or needed less medication. By the third week, the reduction in their medication was statistically significant. (For the scientifically minded, the P-value was <0.0005!) Six months after discharge, thirteen out of nineteen patients (68 percent) were significantly better and five others (26 percent) were well or almost well. Similar results in the United States have been reported by Dr. William Rea and colleagues and by W.P. King and colleagues.[15]

---

ery. This nutritional regime usually includes a combination of vitamins, trace metals, minerals, essential fatty acids, amino acids, digestive enzymes, and other substances that enhance the metabolism and excretion of body toxins. These also aid the digestion, absorption, assimilation, and the metabolism of what we eat. They help convert what we ingest into various hormones, neurotransmitters, and other substances that our bodies need to function optimally.[16]

Nutritional supplements do more than strengthen the immune system and reduce susceptibility to infections and allergies.[17] They are needed to help combat everyday wear and tear of the body, as well as to maintain, repair, and enhance the body's ability to excrete chemicals. Two types of toxins can cause internal confusion or mayhem in our bodies.

■ *Exotoxins*, such as pesticides, enter our lungs from the air we breathe, from the foods and beverages we ingest, and via direct skin contact. Once inside, they circulate throughout the body through the blood vessels. Some damage specific vulnerable areas such as the brain, the nervous system, and the immune system. Certain pesticides, for example, can mimic the natural female hormone estrogen and disrupt normal sexual function, particularly in males[18] (see Chapter 18). There are even substances that are *not* harmful when they enter the body, but surprisingly they can be transformed into something injurious once they are inside.

▪ *Endotoxins* are substances that are naturally formed within our own bodies from intestinal bacteria. At times, they too can be harmful.

CHOOSING NUTRIENTS CAREFULLY

When selecting nutritional supplements, look for relatively inexpensive, hypoallergenic forms that don't tend to cause adverse reactions.[19] For infants and small children, special liquid or chewable vitamins are available and rarely cause difficulty because they are free of corn, sugar, dyes, artificial flavors, and preservatives.[20] Some vitamins can be swallowed, crushed, or blended with food or juice. If vitamins have caused problems for your youngster in the past, secure the help of a knowledgeable physician to determine which forms your child might tolerate better. (A few nutrition specialists and consultants are listed in Resources.)

HOW TO DETERMINE IF YOU CAN TOLERATE A NUTRIENT SUPPLEMENT

Even nutrients labeled hypoallergenic may not be problem-free. Some chemically sensitive or allergic individuals are unable to tolerate components commonly found in certain nutrients. Some even become ill from the mere odor of the yeast in B vitamins, but fortunately this is true for only the most sensitive patients. Some can tolerate vitamin C derived from sago palm, carrot, or potato, but not the usual corn-based form. Many extremely environmentally ill individuals find that they cannot tolerate or that they poorly absorb oral nutrients. For some, preservative-free intravenous vitamin therapy is the only form of nutrients that they can take.[21]

Many companies now sell nutrients with low allergenicity, and while most of them should be safe, *each person is different.* The bottom line is how you or your child responds to a particular product. Even if your physician suggests a particular nutrient, double-check it with the simple screening test outlined in Chapter 5. If vitamins have been a concern in the past, talk with your doctor *before* you do this test. Most can do the "Big Five" by placing the nutrient on or under the tongue for about three to four minutes. Then remove it from the mouth and wait to see if there is any indication of a problem within the next hour. If your youngster remains well, and the "Big Five" does not change, that nutrient *probably* will be tolerated without difficulty.

Dr. Lendon Smith believes that you should not take vitamins if their odor is offensive to you.[22] Once again, use common sense. If a vitamin makes you or your child feel worse in some way, stop taking it until you can discuss it with your doctor.

DO YOU NEED CERTAIN NUTRIENTS?

Ideally, you would check your need for a nutrient by determining the blood level for each vitamin, mineral, and trace metal. Unfortunately we do not presently have the expertise to determine the nutrient status *inside* our body cells, even though this method would be much more informative. If each body cell has the nutrients it needs, the body should feel and function better. Fortunately, at the present time there is a trend among some doctors to learn more about nutrition.

Particularly, if growth or nutrition is a problem with your child, you should try to consult with a physician who has special knowledge of nutritional biochemistry (see Resources). Realistically, however, blood vitamin studies are not always practical and it can be difficult to find a doctor who has had advanced nutritional training. In addition, insurance companies are reluctant to pay the cost of blood vitamin evaluations. Nevertheless, the difference between the correct amount and an excessive amount of nutrients, and the relationships among certain nutrients, can be critical. It is best if both you and your doctor are knowledgeable as possible in this area. Even so, much more emphasis is needed in this area.

Some doctors may still try to convince you that the ordinary American diet supplies all the nutrients your child needs, or that the RDA (Recommended Daily Allowance) listing for vitamins is adequate for optimum health. A wealth of scientific evidence, however, documents that larger amounts of nutrients are required to compensate for the increased pollution in our world. Truly, nutritious foods cannot be grown on soil that is depleted or contaminated. In addition, we contribute to our own poor nutrition by eating "refined" foods. These foods have been stripped of their inherent nutrients but are then called "enriched" because a mere token of these nutrients has been replaced. Yes, skeptics joke that taking nutritional supplements is simply a way to make expensive urine; however, many sick patients excrete *no* nutrients in their urine because they are so deficient in the very substances that are essential for optimal health.

RELATIVELY INEXPENSIVE NUTRITIONAL SUPPLEMENTS

Many excellent hypoallergenic vitamins are available (see Resources). The following are some examples of those recommended in our center.

For Infants

■ Floradix Liquid Multivitamin can be given to infants, and it appears to be hypoallergenic. The dose for infants is $1/4$ to $1/2$ teaspoon per day. It does contain wheat germ, so those sensitive to wheat might have to avoid this. Check with your doctor and do the "Big 5."

For Toddlers

■ Kid's Companion Cherry-Flavored Chewable Multiple Mineral/Vitamin with Iron can be given to children two to six years of age in a two-tablet-a-day dose. Children over six can take four tablets a day.

■ Schiff's Children's Chewable Vitamins with Minerals (No Sucrose) are low in allergenicity. Children under four can be given one tablet daily; those over four can take two tablets.

For Children Under Twelve

■ Vital Life Multi-Vitamin Complex capsules can be taken in the morning. They can be swallowed, or opened and mixed with juice. The daily dose is one capsule.

■ The Vital Life Multi-Vitamin Complex, mentioned above, can be used with the Multi-Mineral Complex, which is taken at night for better absorption. The daily dose is two capsules. Hyperactive children take only one at bedtime.

For Adults

■ Maximum by Vitaline is a relatively inexpensive vitamin with low allergenicity. The dose is six per day for adults and children over twelve. This preparation is high in all the water-soluble B vitamins and vitamin C, so the body will take what it needs and excrete the rest. It also contains the recommended doses of the fat-soluble vitamins (A, D, and E), as well as many needed trace metals and minerals. These vitamins can be obtained from health food stores or direct-mail suppliers (see Resources).

Maximum daily doses of vitamins are listed in Table 15.2.

To see if a supplement is water-soluble, merely place it in water. Does it dissolve readily? If it does not, it may be intact when it leaves your body. An undigested vitamin tablet in your child's bowel movement is of little use.[23] If this type of problem is evident, your youngster may benefit from digestive- and intestinal-enhancing supplements to improve the absorption of nutrients. A natural herbal digestive enzyme and acidifying substance such as Floradix Bitters may be helpful for some environmentally ill patients.[24] Sometimes a thorough stool examination is most helpful in detecting why nutrients are not being utilized properly (see Resources).

ESSENTIAL FATTY ACID SUPPLEMENTATION

Essential fatty acids (EFAs) are polyunsaturated oils that are divided into two major groups or families, called omega-3 and omega-6. The EFAs

TABLE 15.2

Maximum Daily Doses for Adults

Vitamin A* (10,00 IU is beta-carotene)		Iron	20 mg.
	15,000 IU		
Vitamin D_3	400 IU	Copper	2 mg.
Vitamin E	400 IU	Manganese	20 mg.
Vitamin C (ascorbic acid)	1,200 mg.	Iodine (kelp)	150 mcg.
Vitamin B_1 (thiamine)	100 mg.	Chromium	200 mcg.
Vitamin B_2 (riboflavin)	50 mg.	Selenium	200 mcg.
Vitamin B_3 (niacin and niacinamide)	190 mg.	Molybdenum	50 mcg.
Vitamin B_6 (pyridoxine)	100 mg.	Vanadium	25 mcg.
Vitamin B_{12}	100 mcg.	Silicon	2.4 mg.
Pantothenic acid	400 mg.	Liver concentrate (sod)	100 mg.
Folic acid	800 mcg.	L-lysine	600 mg.
Biotin	300 mcg.	Choline bitartrate	200 mg.
Calcium	500 mg.	Inositol	100 mg.
Magnesium	500 mg.	PABA	50 mg.
Potassium	99 mg.	Citrus bioflavonoids	100 mg.
Zinc	30 mg.		

*This level of vitamin A can cause birth defects if it is derived solely from vitamin A and not beta-carotene. The latter is considered safe. See Melvin R. Werbach, *Nutritional Influences on Illness*, 2d ed. (New Canaan, CT: Keats Publishing, 1990), p. 638.

lower cholesterol, help prevent heart disease, and keep cell membranes flexible. They help the liver, bile, and intestines to excrete chemicals into the bowel movement. They are especially important in the biochemistry of prostaglandins, which are hormonelike messengers that play a key role in immune and sexual functioning. They help prevent inflammation and modify allergic reactions.

In general, choose only virgin cold-pressed or nonchemically contaminated (without hexane or bleach) or nonhydrogenated oils. Be careful to use only fresh oils that are not rancid. Taste the oil. It's easy to tell it's not right. High levels of EFAs are found in beans (soy, navy, and kidney), nuts, seeds, and fish—foods that are often scarce in the typical American diet.

EFA supplements are discussed in detail in Dr. Leo Galland's excellent *Superimmunity for Kids* and in *Essential Fatty Acids in Health and Disease* by Edward M. Siguel, M.D., Ph.D.[25]

Guidelines for EFA Supplementation

Here are important points to keep in mind when choosing EFA supplements:

■ Human beings need a proper balance of *both* omega-3 and omega-6 forms of EFA.

■ Read the labels of supplements before you purchase them. Capsules contain different amounts of various forms of omega-3 and -6. Omega-3 refers to the *alpha linolenic acid series*, which are converted into EPA (eicosapentaenoic acid) and finally into DHA (docosahexaenoic acid). But you also need the omega-6 family, containing the *linoleic acid series*, which must be converted into GLA (gamma linolenic acid) for the body to use it. Various nutrients and enzymes are necessary to make these conversions.

■ Children under four years of age should not try to swallow capsules because they can choke on them.

■ Do not take too much of either form of Omega without medical supervision. An excessive amount can lead to inflammatory and nervous system disorders, among other problems. One way to check for imbalances is to request a red-blood-cell membrane or plasma phospholipid analysis (see laboratories listed in Resources). If this is not possible, be sure to ask your physician to check with a nutrient specialist.

■ Be sure to check with your doctor about the initial dose and then every three months thereafter—or even sooner if there is a problem.

Alternative Sources of EFA

■ The easiest way to obtain both omega-3 and omega-6 EFA is to drizzle one tablespoon of flaxseed oil once or twice daily over the food of children three to twelve years old; or to give one to two tablespoons of flaxseed oil to adults. (Flaxseed oil contains 56 percent omega-3, while whole canola, corn, and walnut oil contain 12 percent, and soy oil only about 6 percent.) However, if you or your child is allergic to buckwheat or linseed, you cannot use flaxseed oil in any form. For children who can't swallow oils, rub them directly onto the skin, where they will be absorbed. Keep in mind that flaxseed oil can stain clothing and bedding.

■ Fortified Flaxseed Flakes are another form of EFA. They can be sprinkled over food or cereal. These flakes are predominantly omega-3, with some omega-6. The dosage for children over six years and for adults is two to three tablespoons per day. If diarrhea occurs, decrease the dosage. Remember that solid forms of flaxseed provide much less omega-3 and -6 than do the liquid forms; one tablespoon of flaxseed oil equals approximately three tablespoons of flaxseed flakes.

■ Marine or fish oils are another source of omega-3, although some people should show caution when taking them. These fish oils could cause grave problems for anyone who is allergic to fish. They are often contaminated with pesticides.

CLUES OF AN EFA DEFICIENCY

The following suggests possible EFA deficiency:

- bumpy skin on the upper outer arms
- dry skin that lacks a luster
- excessive thirst and perspiration
- dry, hard ear wax
- brittle soft fingernails that split easily
- dry hair and dandruff
- hyperactivity
- allergies, particularly eczema

If a child or adult takes flaxseed oil for a month or two, but continues to have some of the above problems, their body may not be able to utilize EFAs properly. This can result in a deficiency with a continued need for EFA.

Such clues may indicate that the flaxseed oil is not being changed into a form that the body needs. This can occur when other nutrients—especially vitamins E, B₆, A and C, plus zinc, magnesium, copper, and selenium—are lacking in the body. Check with a nutrition expert.

WHAT ABOUT PRIMROSE OIL?

Your child can also obtain EFAs through the GLA (gamma linolenic acid) derived from omega-6 in primrose oil. The dosage of the active ingredients varies from capsule to capsule and from company to company, so check with your physician about the correct dose.

The usual dosages are listed in Table 15.3. (Efamol is one good brand.)

If your child cannot swallow the primrose oil capsule, make a hole in the capsule with a pin and squeeze out the contents onto a slice of bread, and have the youngster eat it. If that's a problem, rub the oil into the child's scalp at bedtime.

TABLE 15.3

Gamma Linolenic Acid Omega-6 Requirements
(by age)

Age	Dose GLA
Up to 1 year	40 mg.
1 to 2 years	80 mg.
3 to 5 years	120 mg.
6 to 9 years	160 mg.
10 to 12 years	200 mg.
13 years and older	240 mg.

Even larger amounts of GLA as a source of omega-6 can be found in black currant seed oil and borage oil capsules. Lesser amounts are present in one to two tablespoons of safflower oil.

AMINO ACID SUPPLEMENTATION

The intake of specific amino acids can be helpful in overcoming blocks in the metabolic pathways within the body. This form of therapy is sometimes particularly beneficial for children who have significant learning or developmental delay problems. Youngsters on vegetarian diets may also lack certain essential amino acids, especially if their diet is not appropriately supervised and monitored.

Before you begin supplementation, your physician should obtain a complete blood and/or urine amino acid analysis (see Resources for laboratories).This amino acid testing can also help pinpoint specific vitamin and mineral deficiencies.

When supplementation is necessary, about six capsules or six grams per day of Amino Acid #5 from Klaire Laboratory, for example, will help provide the necessary amounts of the essential amino acids (see Resources). Another amino acid mix, called balanced neurotransmitter complex with GABA, is available for both children and adults (see Resources). Because it is readily absorbed, many parents put this powder in their child's lunch drink. This amino acid mix appears to help some children think and remember better.

Brain Link is an amino acid complex powder that is soluble in juice. It is recommended to enhance brain function in children and adults. It contains glutamine which has helped for ADD and ADHD. GABA which is anti-anxiety, glycine which lowers anxiety, hyperactivity and aggression and reduces constant sugar craving, taurine to reduce excessive movements and tyrosine which helps depression.

WHAT ABOUT ANTIOXIDANTS?

When choosing nutrients for yourself or your child, you need to consider the role that antioxidants may play. A few of these nutrients were mentioned earlier in this chapter, but here is some more specific information about them.

The antioxidant nutrients include the beta–carotene form of vitamin A, vitamins C and E, selenium, coenzyme Q, a number of minerals and trace metals, pycnogenol, and bioflavonoids. They are found in fruits and vegetables, and in various commercial antioxidant supplements.

Antioxidants help to control or neutralize the excessive number of electrons or free radicals that can be so damaging to the human body.[26] They stop the production of free radicals and scavenge those that are running around in the body. For example, they help combat the billion or so free radicals that are produced in a person's lungs and that spread throughout the body after someone takes a single puff on a cigarette.

EXACTLY HOW ARE FREE RADICALS FORMED?[27]
When oxygen combines with fat or protein to make energy, it is called oxidation. This is the process that occurs when food spoils, fire burns, iron rusts, or humans fight infection.

During oxidation, free radicals are produced. In essence, they are incomplete single electrons. If an electron is not paired, it is unstable, so it steals another electron from one that is paired. This is what happens during oxidation. Although this produces energy, which is good, the process also has the bad effect of creating a chain of new unpaired electrons capable of damaging others. Even when single electrons manage to become paired, their structure is altered so they can be damaged in form and function.

WHAT'S GOOD ABOUT FREE RADICALS?
Free radicals normally form to create energy in living cells. We all know that bacteria, viruses, fungi, and parasites can make us ill; to help protect the body from these invaders, free radicals are produced from oxygen, and their energy can help combat germs. Not only do they help when we have infections, but they increase when we are stressed from physical exercise or exposed to pollution such as cigarette smoke or barbecued meat. Free radicals also play a role in the functioning of our hormones, and they act as chemical messengers to send information from one body part to another.

DOES NUTRITION HELP INCREASE IQ?

Both Stephen Schoenthaler, Ph.D., from California, and David Benton, M.D., from England have published studies indicating that appropriate nutrients can increase the IQ of some students by as much as 30 points.[28] The behavior and activity levels definitely improved in children studied by Dr. Schoenthaler.

Some children who received environmental medical care unquestionably have a dramatic increase in IQ. (See Marsha in Chapter 8.) In some children, this increase may be due, in part, to nutritional supplements, an increased tolerance for a wider variety of foods, and an overall feeling of well-being that helps their concentration.

WHAT'S BAD ABOUT FREE RADICALS?

For our bodies to function well, everything must be in balance. This is certainly true in relation to free radical production. Unless the production of free radicals is controlled, they can damage normal healthy tissues. If there are too many of them, they definitely *cause* illness. They can damage the integrity of cell walls, hurt the mitochondria in our cells (which generate energy), interfere with enzyme and hormone functioning, and attack our DNA (or genetic material). This damage can cause cataracts, atherosclerosis, heart disease, arthritis, cancer, genetic problems, wrinkles, or premature aging.

Certain forms of free radicals are particularly worrisome:

■ A particular type of reactive free radical called a singlet oxygen arises from exposure to ozone, ultraviolet light, and radiation.

■ Another particularly damaging type of free radical is called superoxide. It is destroyed by an enzyme called superoxide dismutase.

■ A third type of free radical is the hydroxyl radical, which is formed from hydrogen peroxide. It is destroyed by the enzymes catalase and glutathione peroxidase, which converts hydrogen peroxide into water. The enzymes that can destroy these free radicals need zinc, copper, manganese, magnesium, selenium, and iron, which are found in most antioxidant nutrients.

So, in our precisely created human body, everything should be in the correct ratio. We need some free radicals to protect us, but if this type of response is excessive, it damages more than it helps. Internal defenses help to rescue our bodies from too many free radicals, but this process can be enhanced by taking antioxidant supplements and eating fresh organic fruits and green and yellow vegetables which supply these types of nutrients. Antioxidants are particularly necessary at this time because of the enormous compensation which is needed for our bodies to adjust to the immense amount of pollution in today's world.

OTHER SUPPLEMENTS

When selecting supplements, you'll find other types that may be beneficial as well. Individuals with environmental allergies or chemical sensitivities (or their parents) **should check with their doctor about the following**. Many of them are available from the sources for nutritional supplements listed in Resources.

■ Reduced L–Glutathione—two 75 mg. capsules per day for children; three capsules per day for adults. Sherry Rogers, M.D., states, "For every molecule of a chemical that you detoxify, you forever throw away a molecule of glutathione."[29] To detoxify the many unwanted and harmful chemicals that enter our bodies every day, we need daily glutathione.

■ Taurine—250 to 500 mg. capsules; 250 to 500 mg. per day for children; 250 to 750 mg. per day for adults.

■ Coenzyme Q-10—10 mg. daily for children who weigh up to 100 pounds; 30 mg. for anyone over 100 pounds. Some patients require much larger doses.

■ Cal-Mag Zinc or Cal-Mag Aspartate—The dose for children six years of age is one capsule nightly; for those over 100 pounds, two capsules nightly; for those over 125 pounds, three capsules nightly. The adult dosage is one to four capsules daily, preferably at bedtime. If the dose of magnesium is too high, it can cause diarrhea.

■ Chemically ill children and adults often need digestive enzymes to help break down food particles for proper absorption and utilization. Many varieties are available, so check with your doctor before deciding which ones to take. InFla-zyme Forte is a dietary supplement that contains enzymes, zinc, and other digestive adjuncts. Similase or Ness Digestive Enzymes are available for those who want a totally vegetable-derived product (see Resources).

■ Stomach acidity can be altered by infections, chemicals, or age. Supplements that appear to gently enhance and restore normal stomach acidity include Gastric Protocol #4 and Floradix Liquid for Infants. These are two brands that provide natural herbs.

■ Pycnogenol is an antioxidant bioflavonoid herbal nutrient derived from the bark of maritime pine trees. Since about 1960 some European physicians have used pycnogenol to decrease inflammatory swelling and to control hay fever, in place of antihistamines.[30]

■ Various forms of *blue-green algae* are grown wild and harvested from natural fresh water lakes (Lake Klamath Blue-Green Algae) or in syn-

---

WILL INSURANCE PAY FOR VITAMINS OR VITAMIN MONITORING?

Insurance companies and big business presently dictate how medicine is practiced in this country by arbitrarily limiting or denying reimbursement to both patients and physicians for certain tests and/or forms of therapy. Insurance firms are reluctant to pay for nutrient laboratory tests (see Chapter 17 for a discussion of the possible reasons). When payment is denied, patients with environmental sensitivities have few options. Due to these reimbursement problems, most individuals take vitamins without any monitoring. Many struggle on their own with difficult choices and are forced to accept the type of medical care they can afford, rather than what helps or what they know they need.

thetically engineered food ponds (chlorella and spirulina). It is available in powder, capsule, and pressed tablet forms. Repeated anecdotal observations by parents, as well as scientific studies, indicate that it can be helpful, particularly for nervous and immune system deficiencies.[31]

■ PSYCHOLOGICAL COUNSELING AND FAMILY SUPPORT

When children and adults are sick, other people may not believe they are really ill.

In fact, few families, colleagues, principals, administrators, or school health personnel fully understand the dreadful scope of environmental illness. Too often those seriously afflicted with this problem encounter a paucity of compassion, understanding, sympathy, patience, and help in their desperate, lonely lives. The brain and nervous system can be directly damaged by chemicals; therefore, some who are ill can have periods when they simply cannot think clearly or act appropriately. Yet those who are unaware of EI tend to interpret their actions as entirely psychological or emotional in nature.

As a result, these sick individuals as children or adults, are reprimanded, ridiculed, punished, and criticized much too often. The sensitive self-images of children in particular often are crushed to such a degree that some are desperately depressed. Both teachers and parents feel helpless and, at times, guilty, even though they have good reason to be upset. Sometimes they simply don't know where to turn.

Affected children and adults need psychological counseling, but it is most effective *after* they have received environmental medical care. The correct diagnosis often requires a counselor or psychologist who is knowledgeable about environmental medicine and knows how to differentiate an emotional problem from neurological brain changes due to chemicals and/or allergenic substances such as foods, molds or pollen (see Chapter 13).

For those who have a severe form of EI, the resulting limitations upon their lifestyle can justifiably cause secondary psychological problems. Adults and youngsters who are afflicted have a right to ask, "Why me?" Many adolescents are already typically stressed and distressed during the process of becoming young adults, but the load can become overwhelming when it is combined with the unrecognized allergies, scholastic problems, loneliness, and strained interpersonal relations. Some teenagers truly cannot understand why they look or feel unwell, act inappropriately, lose total control, or have difficulty learning. A few, even at the tender age of five years old, are so overwhelmed that they express a desire to die. In *Stephen Lives!* Anne Puryear gives more insight about one allergic, severely depressed teenager (discussed in Chapter 13); his total burden simply became too great.[32]

A ROLE FOR TEACHERS AND PARENTS

When a child or adult has a chemical or environmental sensitivity, it is often possible to tell at a glance that something is not right. Teachers and parents, in fact, can often find meaningful answers just by observing these affected youngsters. Teachers can sometimes uncover answers when everyone else has failed to do so, because of their experience in watching normal children. Teachers see each student for a prolonged period of time every day. They can compare each child with the many others they have taught over the years.

HOW ARE MANY TREATED?

The use of one antidepressant drug after another (Paxil, Haldol, Ativan, nortriptyline, bethanechol chloride, and Prozac) is certainly not the best answer if a child's or adult's depression is due to environmental factors. Nor is shock convulsion therapy, despite the recent upsurge in its use in children as young as two years old.[33] We need repeated SPECT brain-image tests to show that electroconvulsive therapy does not permanently alter the brains of youngsters who receive it.

Ask the psychiatrists who use such measures if they have investigated the less traumatic and effective methods used by environmental medical physicians. They might not be applicable and possibly helpful for some of their patients. For example, P/N allergy testing and treatment certainly needs more serious consideration as a possible answer for some of the growing number of allergic youngsters who have depression.

For pro and con information on this subject, contact the American Psychiatric Association at (202) 682-6000 and the National Empowerment Center at (800) 769-3728. Once again, insurance coverage is rarely denied for drugs and/or repeated shock therapy, but it can be rejected for detecting and testing environmental allergies. If such treatment is proven to be safer and definitely helpful for some, we must ask why it is not covered by insurance.

■ DETOXIFICATION

As discussed earlier, exotoxins enter the body through the nose, lungs, mouth, skin and/or hair; meanwhile, various endotoxins are normally produced inside the body. Detoxification is a natural process that helps rid the body of toxic substances, such as the vast array of foreign chemicals (xenobiotics) to which we're exposed every day. However, the vast majority of chemically sensitive individuals are ill because they are unable to detoxify properly. Your physician can determine your ability to detoxify by ordering special blood immunotoxicology tests (for laboratories, see Resources).

> The key for many to feel better and regain their health on a long-term basis is more than avoidance of exposure to foreign chemicals. The water- and fat-soluble foreign chemicals stored in the body must be excreted, through the process called detoxification.

The stomach, intestines, bowels, liver, kidney, heart, adrenals, and thyroid must all function well to effectively control what enters or remains within the body. Also, as you'll read later, certain dietary adjustments can facilitate the detoxification process. One comprehensive and practical book, *Staying Healthy with Nutrition* by Elson Haas,[34] provides a detailed discussion of detoxification diets, as well as many other aspects of nutrition. Other exceptionally informative books that describe how to eat, what to eat, and why, include *The Canary and Chronic Fatigue*, and *RDA: Rats, Drugs, and Assumptions*, both by Majid Ali, M.D. Your physician will find the audiotape series on nutrition from HealthComm International particularly practical and informative (see For Further Reading).

THE ROLE OF YOUR INTESTINES IN DETOXIFICATION

When you properly digest food, your body breaks down large food particles into little ones to enhance their absorption and decrease the risk of allergies. A healthy intestine is a key to this process. An intact intestinal barrier keeps the wrong or harmful substances that you ingest out of the rest of your body. If it is functioning optimally, it allows only the right substances to enter the bloodstream. The intestinal wall helps filter out or eliminate harmful germs or chemicals in your gut.

However, this process does not always work to perfection. Repeated or prolonged courses of antibiotics and a poor diet can markedly alter normal intestinal function and flora, causing a loss of the needed lactobacilli and other "good" bacteria, and an overgrowth of yeast and other "bad" bacteria. If your intestine does not have the right type and balance of organisms, it can become leaky, or you may develop a nutritionally related illness or a weakened immune system.

How can you tell if you are experiencing abnormal digestion? Some clues include bad breath, recurrent diarrhea, chronic constipation (often due to dairy products), soft or poorly formed bowel movements, bloating, rectal gas, belching, belly noises, strong body odors, and excessive stool mucus. The stool should not routinely float or look clay-colored, black, bloody, or be covered with mucus. If these problems are noted frequently, check with a nutritionist and your doctor.[35]

If a urine and/or blood analysis from a laboratory (see Resources) indicates an elevated level of foreign chemicals, it is possible that a cleansing diet or preparation is indicated. Stool samples can be examined at a laboratory (such as the Great Smokies Medical Laboratory) to check for digestive inadequacies and to ascertain if yeast, parasites, or abnormal types or amounts of bacteria are causing additional problems.

LIVER DETOXIFICATION

The major detoxification organ in the body is the liver. It helps eliminate what the body does not want or need. If the intestines are "leaky," then the chemicals and undigested molecules that get inside the body can go to the liver and may overwhelm its capacity to detoxify them. Toxins that commonly cause problems come from alcohol, tobacco, perfumes, the fat in red meat, grilled meats, fumes from car exhaust, and the chemicals in cleaning agents, carpets and paints. Sometimes even ordinary prescribed medicines can be toxic to the liver. When these toxins are not properly eliminated, they tend to be stored in the fatty tissues of the brain, nervous system, and various body organs such as breast tissue.

There are two phases of liver detoxification, and although Phases I and II overlap, both must function correctly for you or your child to feel really well. If the detoxification paths are blocked or are out of sync with each other, then health problems can develop, including intestinal difficulties, muscle aches, headaches, irritability, fatigue, confusion, memory loss, facial flushing, and even a feeling of drunkenness that is unrelated to drinking alcohol.

HOW TO CHECK PHASE I
If you or your doctor are concerned about whether detoxification problems exist or not, ask about tests to determine specifically how well your liver functions. While routine liver blood tests can detect some late evidence of pathological function, most environmental medical specialists use special earlier detection tests to help assess the ability of the liver to do its job: Can it properly detoxify and excrete particularly noxious substances?

For example, your doctor can use a test to spot-check how well your liver can eliminate a simple foreign substance. In this test, you simply drink a specified amount of caffeinated coffee. Then a measurement will be taken of how well and how fast it takes for 50 percent of the caffeine in the coffee to be excreted in your saliva. If it takes a half hour, your liver is functioning well; but if it takes longer, your liver is not up to par.

This test evaluates Phase I of liver detoxification, or the ability of what's called the cytochrome P450 enzyme system to "deactivate" toxic substances so they are less harmful. If your liver is functioning too slowly or is deficient in this phase, you need your physician's advice about ways to improve it.

HOW TO CHECK PHASE II
The second phase of liver detoxification is called conjugation. Something must attach, conjugate, or combine with a toxic chemical so it can be excreted from the body. The body has a number of choices for conjugation and each affords a possible pathway for elimination. When certain conjugation pathways are blocked, the body hopefully can use alternative ones. The aim, however, is to keep as many of these pathways functioning as well as possible so there will be no unnecessary buildup of toxins within the body.

It is also easy to spot-check another possible pathway, this time by drinking sodium benzoate. If this so-called glucuronidation conjugation pathway is working properly, a breakdown product called hippuric acid will be excreted in the urine within a specified period of time. If Phase II is not functioning properly, however, you may need to take a number of nutrients to enhance the pathway. In addition, hope that your remaining conjugation paths are optimally effective.

TWENTY-FIRST-CENTURY DETOXIFICATION
Jeffrey Bland, Ph.D., his associates, and other researchers have recently devised another comprehensive test to evaluate the Phase I and II liver detoxification pathways.[36] This test uses what is called an acetaminophen challenge. In essence, it extends the value of the sodium benzoate test so that several additional critical pathways of liver detoxification are all evaluated at one time. It checks not only the Phase II glucuronidation conjugation pathway but the alternative paths related to glutathione, sulfonation, and acetylation.

So in addition to requesting the caffeine challenge test used in Phase I testing, you might ask your physician to check into the other functional challenge tests that are suggested by Dr. Bland's group. These tests identify the competence of the biochemistry and the detoxification pathways in various body systems:

■ The lactulose and mannitol test (described in Chapter 15) checks the intestinal mucosal barrier. You should know if it is intact and doing its job.
■ The salicylate challenge test checks for oxygen free radicals that can be harmful, as well as the Phase II glucuronidation pathway.
■ A number of urinary nitrate, sulfate, or sulfite-to-creatinine tests check

different aspects of the immune system, the glutathione reserves in the liver, and the activity of different enzymes.

These various precisely devised tests enable physicians to specifically tailor a patient's nutritional treatment to his or her unique weaknesses. To make the best treatment decisions, doctors need to know how large a person's reserves are. Can the individual's body handle additional life stresses, or is it already on overload? Dr. Bland's group is definitely on the cutting edge of the medicine of tomorrow.

DIETARY DETOXIFICATION AND OTHER METHODS

EASY AND INEXPENSIVE

There are a number of diets designed to cleanse the body of toxic substances and chemicals.[37] In addition to copious amounts of pure glass-bottled water, they should include plenty of organic, less pesticide-contaminated fruits and vegetables. Certain grains, nuts, legumes, and beans are usually allowed, while white flour or baked goods, white sugar, fatty or fried foods, coffee, tea, alcohol, and tobacco are not. Some physicians also suggest consuming cleansing herbs such as garlic, silymarin, cayenne pepper, red clover, and echinacea. Remember, your physician should be consulted before you attempt to detoxify with these substances.

Nature's Pure Body thirty- to ninety-day program is a relatively inexpensive herbal method to cleanse and detoxify. If you feel as well on the days you don't take the herbal tablets, as you do on the days when you take them, you probably do not need to continue the program. One of its preparations, called the Colon Formula, helps excrete chemicals. Another is called the Whole Body Formula. The aim with these preparations is to slowly and gradually cleanse and purify the body naturally. If you move too quickly, symptoms can temporarily reappear. Be sure to ingest adequate pure water, not juice, with these products.[38] (See Chapter 5 for a cursory screening test to check out these tablets if your doctor says you can start this program.)

Another practical resource for detoxification information is Dr. Haas's book, *Staying Healthy with Nutrition*, which describes a low-calorie, low-sugar, low-fat, nonchemical diet with unrefined foods that are easily handled and eliminated by the intestine.[39] This diet helps food exit the bowel faster, which helps prevent the reabsorption of bowel waste back into the body.

A number of other diets may also be used to cleanse the body. Those discussed in ayurvedic (traditional Indian) medical books use various beans, rice, and spices to help rid the body of wastes in turn.[40] In general, however, these and most other detoxification diets have not been scientifically evaluated for use in children; therefore, you need the approval of your personal physician, who must monitor your child's growth and nutritional status if you attempt one of these approaches. Similarly, teachers and other exposed adults also need constant medical supervision if they want to try various diets or preparations, particularly if they have chronic fatigue.[41] Everyone is different, and each person's treatment must be individualized. You can enhance any detoxification program by following the suggestions in Table 15.4.

TABLE 15.4

Basic Ways to Enhance Detoxification

▪ Eat organic foods and drink glass-bottled or filtered water to minimize chemicals entering the body.
▪ Avoid prolonged showers or baths in chlorinated water.
▪ Take specific nutritional supplements orally and/or intravenously.
▪ Replace the glutathione, taurine, and vitamin C that are normally depleted during detoxification.
▪ Chew your food more slowly and thoroughly.
▪ If needed, take digestive enzymes.

BETTER BUT MORE EXPENSIVE

Jeffrey Bland, Ph.D., and his team of nutritional experts have developed a series of complete but relatively expensive formulations for detoxification. They are available in carefully prepared, tasty nutritional beverages. These programs use a variety of "Ultra" products, such as Ultraclear and Ultra-sustain, which significantly help to cleanse the body of toxic water- and fat-soluble substances. These nutrient-powder preparations should be mixed with water or natural juice and ingested over a period of weeks or possibly months to replace or supplement a regular diet, as suggested by your physician. (Test each product as suggested in Chapter 5 to be certain that your child has no sensitivity to any component.) An UltraKid preparation has recently been developed specifically for children.

For adults, a questionnaire can help you compare how you feel before and after you use these preparations. Check with your physician, or contact Dr. Bland's HealthComm International (see Resources) to find a nearby specialist knowledgeable in the use of Dr. Bland's cleansing and maintenance preparations.

NONDIETARY DETOXIFICATION METHODS

Here are some details about a few basic inexpensive, nondietary ways to help eliminate chemicals from the body.

WATER[42]

Drinking plenty of water is important—but it has to be the right kind of water. An adequate intake of *pure* water will help eliminate chemicals via bowel movements, urine, saliva, and skin. Water increases urination and decreases constipation by softening the bowel movements. Adults need to drink at least eight large glasses of glass-bottled pure spring or filtered water per day. If you can't afford bottled water or a filter, at least boil your water for five minutes to remove some of its chemicals. Remember, any liquids stored in plastic will contain plastic; if they are stored in styrene, they can contaminate the body with styrene. Both of these substances are undesirable inside the body. (See Chapter 8 for more information about the critical role that water plays in our lives.)

BOWEL CARE[43]

Regular and thorough bowel elimination is essential so that chemicals that enter the intestines can be excreted as quickly as possible. To aid in excretion, you (and your child) should eat a diet high in pesticide-free (organic) vegetables and fiber.

Your bowels should move easily every day. Constipation is analogous to your bowel movement being stuck in a leaky garbage can. The waste material and toxins in the hard stool can reenter your circulation and further contaminate your body.

Dr. Majid Ali's books for the public, and his courses for physicians, stress the "seed, feed, and occasionally weed" principle of using natural products to restore normal bowel function.[44] Many environmentally ill children and adults have cold hands, which Dr. Ali believes indicates poor blood circulation, not just in the extremities, but in the intestines as well. Intestines that are functioning properly, however, will help keep noxious substances out of the circulation, discourage parasites, enhance immunity, and digest foods more fully. This in turn will decrease the tendency to develop allergies. As you've already read, the intestines must contain the correct balance of organisms if they are to do its job well. If you have recurrent intestinal complaints, this is a strong signal that something is not right.

The answer to bowel symptoms is not simply to take an antacid or yeast treatment but to resolve the cause of the problems. Laxatives and antacids are a quick fix that allows the cause to remain and provides an opportunity for a minor symptom to insidiously progress into a major illness.

What approaches make more sense? Charcoal supplements are one possibility. Charcoal enhances the excretion of chemicals, impedes noxious substances from reentering the circulation, and decreases the odor of the bowel movements. It can also help lessen abdominal symptoms that may occur during detoxification.

The proper dose of charcoal varies with age, so again, check with a doctor who is knowledgeable. Do not use charcoal supplements for prolonged periods, however, because charcoal can deplete the body of needed vitamins and minerals. Also, take care that a specific charcoal allergy is not present and does not develop (see Chapter 5).

In adults, organic coffee enemas are well recognized as an aid in liver detoxification. They appear to be helpful even in people with a sensitivity to coffee. This form of therapy has been used for over one hundred years and is presently part of the cleansing Gerson and Kelley diets, which appear to help some individuals who have cancer or arthritis. For more details, see Dr. Sherry Rogers's most informative *Wellness Against All Odds.*[45]

EXERCISE
Physical activity contracts your muscles, shaking up and moving the chemicals stored in your fat. To get the greatest detoxifying benefits from exercise, do it when it is warm or until you feel warm, because perspiration helps to eliminate chemicals.

Talk to your doctor about the best type and intensity of exercise for you. Good choices are often running in place for twenty to thirty minutes, or using a stationary bicycle, rowing machine, or treadmill. If you run outdoors, select a chemically clean area, not a congested street.

OTHER NONDIETARY DETOXIFICATION AIDS
There are some additional alternatives to help you or your child excrete toxins and aid digestion. The following substances may help you cope better with chemical exposures—but be sure to check with your doctor before using them:

- *Silymarin* is a most helpful detoxification adjunct. It works by raising the glutathione level by 30 percent.[46]
- The liver transports fat-soluble chemicals into the bile. When bile enters the intestines, a drug called *cholestyramine* (or Questran) can absorb or hold on to these chemicals so they can be eliminated in the bowel movement and not be reabsorbed into the blood. Check with your doctor about cholestyramine, which is available only by prescription, in a powdered or a suspension form from Bristol-Myers Squibb. You should be aware that this product contains food dyes, artificial flavors, sucrose, aspartame, and citric acid, any of which could cause illness in certain sensitive individuals.
- *Psyllium husks* bind chemicals and provide bulk to the stool. They are the basis for the "regularity" medicines used by older adults.
- *Chlorophyll* soothes and heals the intestines. It also helps to stimulate detoxification and decrease body and breath odors.

■ Muscle aches and headaches sometimes can be lessened by using an *al-kali* such as Trisalts or Alka Aid (see "General Supplies" in Resources), plus a large amount of filtered or glass-bottled spring water, vitamin C, and magnesium.

■ *Organic germanium*, found in some health food stores, may be helpful if it is taken during the aura phase, just before a migraine begins. It also can reduce severe muscle aches.

HOMEOPATHIC REMEDIES[47]

Homeopathic physicians practice a system of medicine that treats illness with a minute dose of the substance that has caused the illness. In the nineteenth century, homeopathic medicine was prescribed extensively throughout the world. It continues to be available throughout Europe, but its use declined in the late 1920s in the United States. Now its acceptance is again on the rise because informed mothers are finding that it can be helpful, particularly in treating some children and adults who cannot tolerate antibiotics.[48]

A number of remedies promote "drainage" or relief of congestion in various organs. Some were developed to cleanse various organs or to assist in the elimination of unwanted by-products and toxins through the body's normal channels, such as the liver, kidneys, lymphatics, lung, skin, and blood. Specific inexpensive mixtures and individual preparations are available for dental toxins, heavy metals, chemicals and drugs, insecticides or pesticides, perfumes, vaccines, and industrial pollution (see Resources).

Homeopathic preparations are considered to be very safe. Even when homeopathic treatments do not help, they rarely hurt. *The exception is when they delay the use of more appropriate treatment—for example, surgery for appendicitis or antibiotics for a stiff neck that can be an early warning sign of meningitis.*

Resources are available if you want to discuss natural detoxification methods with a trained homeopathic physician, obtain homeopathic kits or read articles or books for the public or physicians about homeopathy and herbal treatments for children or adults (see Resources).

HERBAL REMEDIES

Books for the general public suggest a variety of herbs for natural detoxification.[49] You should find a trained naturopathic physician if you want to try this form of therapy. Contact the American Association of Naturopath Physicians (see Resources).

EXPENSIVE BUT COMPREHENSIVE DETOXIFICATION PROGRAMS

DEPURATION

Depuration is a process that combines sauna or heat therapy with the detoxification methods that have already been discussed. This is a more thorough method to help cleanse and purify the body. Its aim is to enhance perspiration with dry sauna heat so that chemicals and stored drugs can be excreted through the skin. Unfortunately, only a few facilities with medical supervision presently offer depuration, although some adults can learn what to do at a medical facility, and then continue certain aspects of this therapy at home.

A comprehensive detoxification program such as depuration requires several weeks of daily therapy. Each person's program must be individualized by a physician to be certain that the offending substances are released safely and slowly. For this reason doctors conduct laboratory studies to monitor several key body functions, particularly during the initial phases of this process.

WHAT ABOUT CONTINUED USE OF HOME SAUNAS?

A number of companies make saunas for personal home use (see Resources). In general, these well-aerated saunas are heated to temperatures of 140° to 160° F (or 62° to 68°C) and then they are used for gradually increasing periods of time. (Most sports health saunas, in contrast, have a temperature of 180°F.) Nevertheless, children should undergo sauna therapy only in well supervised units under a physician's personal care. Adults, too, must be advised by a knowledgeable physician before self therapy with sauna treatment.

All sauna salons must be well-ventilated and have dry heat chambers. They are usually made of special poplar wood, glass, aluminum, and/or ceramic tile. The better, more elaborate and costly saunas are made of glass and ceramic tile. Care must be taken so the ceramic tile has been installed with decontaminated grout. The electrically heated units should be cleaned with natural soap and hydrogen peroxide.

DETOXIFICATION CENTERS

You or your child can be cared for in special centers, where treatments are available to help move the toxins stored in the fat into the circulation for excretion. This type of care is very expensive, but it is essential for seriously chemically sensitized (or radiation exposed) children or adults (see Resources). Detoxification treatment must be modified according to what is needed, available, and affordable. Less ill individuals can be seen in special outpatient units that offer three-to-four-week comprehensive detoxifica-tion programs. If someone is very young, weak, debilitated, and ill, detoxi-fication is safest if carried out very slowly and cautiously, preferably in a hospital-based unit supervised by experienced environmental physicians. (Components of this care, however, are not recommended for persons who have severe kidney disease.)

The typical pattern of care consists of some combination of sauna heat, cooling down, fluids, nutrients, massage, and exercise, which can last up to several hours each day for several weeks. More specifically, a two-to-six-week detoxification or depuration program combines aerobic exercise, carefully controlled and gradually increased doses of short-acting vitamin B_3 (niacin/nicotinic acid), and monitoring and replacement of water, other nutrients, and electrolytes such as potassium. An increased fluid intake helps excrete chemicals through the urine. Reabsorption of the toxin or chemically laden bile after it enters the intestines can be retarded by the use of cold-pressed, nonrancid, polyunsaturated oils and increased fiber in the diet. These substances will help to increase the excretion of chemicals in the bowel movement.

Dry sauna heat in the range of 120° to 180°F or 60° to 80°C enhances the orderly excretion of chemicals, particularly through the perspiration and oil (sebum) of the skin.

BALANCING BENEFITS AND ADVERSE EFFECTS
Several keys can help prevent the adverse reactions sometimes noted during detoxification. These include constant monitoring and individualized incre-ments of fast-acting niacin that help release the toxins slowly from the fat. (Slow-released high-dose niacin can cause liver damage.)

Detoxification benefits, however, can be enormous. In one medical re-port researchers showed that 155 patients with elevated levels of pesticides in their fat experienced decreased levels after this form of treatment.[50] Other articles discuss not only the many health and cost benefits but evi-dence of improved memory or increased IQ (see note 28 in this chapter).

Studies have associated decreases in xenobiotic (pesticide) storage in the body with *measurable* improvement in nerve, muscle, and immune function.[51] This treatment process can remove specific chemicals, such as formaldehyde, that tends to cause chest pain, muscle aches, and headaches, or the solvent chemicals such as toluene or benzene (used for cleaning printing presses) that can cause memory and learning problems.

After a detoxification procedure is begun, the chemical levels in fat tis-sue tend to decrease slowly, over a period of months. The level of this de-crease roughly correlates with a patient's degree of improvement. Chemicals are not excreted all at one time, but are released in a sequential pattern, one layer at a time.[52]

INFRARED RADIATION DETOXIFICATION

A German pediatrician, Dr. Thomas Meyn, in Neuharlingersiel has effectively and safely used infrared radiation for detoxification. Adults and children, as young as one to two years of age, have been treated in a chamber located in a special "clean" room.

These youngsters are treated in the following manner: The children are suspended in a net in the chamber, while their bodies are heated from below to a temperature of 38.5°C, using short-wave, water-filtered, infrared radiation. This heat increases the body temperature gradually so that chemicals are safely released into the blood and through the skin within an hour. The children are given five or six treatments, approximately once a week.

Once the body and skin temperatures have reached the desired levels, the treatment session is finished. The children must drink fluids and receive proper nutrients before and after the process.[53] They must also be monitored carefully so they do not develop a fever from dehydration. The released chemicals can be measured using spectroscopy. Various chemicals and the carbon dioxide levels can be monitored every three minutes during this procedure, so it is possible to demonstrate, for example, exactly when a chemical, for example, benzene, is being excreted from the body. In addition, the blood levels of certain chemicals, such as the chlorinated hydrocarbons, will show definite decreases between the first and the last treatment session.

A TWENTIETH-CENTURY CHALLENGE: HOW DO WE DETOXIFY INFANTS?

At the present time the health of more and more and younger and younger infants is not up to par. These babies cry and scream hour after hour. Some cannot even tolerate breast milk. The problem is much more than allergic parents. When they were in the uterus, via their mothers, some of these babies were exposed to toxic chemicals at home or work, in schools or factories. After birth, they may be so sensitive that they cannot be held in the arms of parents who wear polyester (which contains formaldehyde). Some cannot be placed on a bedspread that has been laundered with a fabric softener.

How can we detoxify these babies? The majority of detox centers will not treat children under three years of age, although the Environmental Health Center in Dallas does care for infants (see Resources). Must they remain ill for several years when they can be helped? Is there a way to safely give nutrients such as niacin to babies? Should they perspire in a sauna, or would a hot bath using pure water be better? Should they be helped to exercise? How much of which cold-pressed oil can they tolerate?

P/N allergy testing can definitely relieve the allergic component of the illnesses of these youngsters; but this will solve only part of the problem. Too few physicians and nurses know how to properly or safely do P/N allergy testing on infants (see Resources). In time let us hope that we shall be more knowledgeable about how to help them.

■ YEAST TREATMENTS

Although many physicians have discounted or continued not to recognize or treat yeast or candida illness seriously, its existence simply cannot be denied. Many medical publications explain yeast-related illnesses dating back to 1974. In addition, many books on this subject, such as those written by Dr. William G. Crook, are available.[54] For the clues that suggest a yeast problem, see Chapter 14.

Yeast treatment usually consists of several major steps:

1. All sugar, white flour, and highly yeasty foods such as bread are eliminated from the diet. Mushrooms and fermented foods such as vinegar, alcohol, and soy, also cause yeast-sensitive people to have a flare-up. Some adults require a strict yeast-free diet, which can be very challenging, especially if combined with the four-day Rotation Diet. Children tend to grow poorly if both diets are attempted at the same time, so a nutritionist and a doctor must closely monitor your youngster's health and growth while following an abridged or relaxed, highly individualized version or combination of these diets.[55]

2. The normal balance of organisms in the intestines must be reestablished. Milk-free lactobacillus, such as Vitalplex, which combines lactobacillus acidophilus and bifidus with streptococcus faecium, is thought to be most helpful in helping to restore the normal intestinal flora and aiding in the control of diarrhea and excessive gas (see Resources). Another product, called Bio-Bifidus Complex, is a blend of lactobacillus bifidus and lactobacillus acidophilus. New products also contain fructoligosaccharides (FOS) that enhance the growth of the "good" bacteria.

3. The yeast overgrowth found in and on various parts of the body must be controlled. Think of a yeast problem as a lawn with too many weeds. You must not only "reseed the lawn" (your intestines) with lactobacillus, you also must "eliminate the weeds" by using a candida- or yeast-controlling substance. Your doctor may prescribe Mycostatin powder, Nystatin tablets, or Mycocidin capsules, or stronger preparations such as expensive Diflucan or Sporanox tablets. Your doctor should routinely conduct liver function studies when the latter two preparations are used. P/N allergy extract treatment for candida and baker's and brewer's yeast are also helpful. Natural preparations such as garlic, Pau

d'Arco tea, certain herbs (such as goldenseal), and digestive enzymes all appear to help improve intestinal yeast problems.

Remember, after your child's nose and chest allergies are appropriately treated, the tendency to develop infections in these areas, as well as in the middle ear and sinuses, will decrease. This improvement will reduce the need for antibiotics, which in turn will decrease the chances of yeast overgrowth. This will certainly enable your child to feel better in school and at home.

■ TREATMENTS FOR PARASITES[56]

Parasites are relatively common, but they are frequently missed in the routine medical care of both children and adults. If doctors fail to recognize the need for parasite treatment, the rest of their recommended therapy for chemical sensitivities and/or allergies may be much less effective. If your child responds poorly to an initial program of environmental medical care, a thorough stool examination is needed. Test results will indicate if appropriate traditional and/or homeopathic anti-parasite forms of therapy is indicated.

■ HORMONE TREATMENT

Many environmentally ill older girls and women have a multiple hormonal imbalance. For example:

■ They tend to have cold hands and feet, pallor, thin hair, fatigue, memory loss, edema, sudden unexplained weight gains (several pounds a weekend), and other subtle-to-obvious clues of hypothyroidism. Doctors can miss the diagnosis of this problem because routine thyroid tests can be deceptively normal. In Europe, twenty-four-hour urine thyroid studies and morning basal temperatures are often most helpful in the detection of this problem.[57] Broda Barnes, M.D., has suggested that *normal* morning basal temperatures should be higher than 97.8°F. If yours is frequently below this level, check with a doctor who is familiar with Barnes's studies.[58]

■ They frequently have some form of adrenal malfunction, or patterns indicating that their adrenals cannot handle stress well. (A chemical overload is a major stress.) Some affected women crave salt.

■ They often have intestinal problems along with an array of PMS-related (Premenstrual Syndrome) and other menstrual complaints. Charles R. Mabray, M.D., in Victoria, Texas, is knowledgeable about this complicated hormonal interplay, and has helped many women with these types of complaints (see Resources).

■ They tend to crave sugar or chocolate, are overweight, and may be hypoglycemic due to pancreatic and cellular dysfunction.

■ They may have mitral valve prolapse (a heart valve irregularity). We don't know exactly why this is so frequently evident in environmentally ill adult females.

IF ALL ELSE FAILS, WHAT ABOUT DRUGS?

There is no doubt that drugs are helpful and necessary at times, even though they can cause undesirable side effects and/or merely mask symptoms. Some drug-treated (or related) illnesses, however, will recur, persist, and become progressively worse unless a doctor spends the time to find and eliminate the basic cause.

Consider nightly hay fever, for example. It can be caused by sleeping on a feather pillow. When symptoms occur, you have several choices. You can take an antihistamine before bed, receive allergy injection treatments for feathers for years, or replace your pillow with a cotton towel in a cotton pillow case. If you choose to depend solely on drugs for therapy, your allergically swollen nose tissues could become infected; polyp swellings can form inside the nose; and you might need repeated antibiotics, yeast therapy, hospitalizations, and/or surgeries.

Once you eliminate the cause of a problem or allergy, you must go one step further. You need to determine why you are prone to it. Ask why your immune system is weak, and find out how it can be strengthened. A better diet and judicious nutrient supplements can be a critical missing link. Spend more time thinking about where, when, and why you become ill. Sometimes the resolution of such challenges is amazingly simple.

■ A MORE DETAILED BIOCHEMICAL EXPLANATION

What biochemistry underlies the information in this chapter?

Your body may use up certain essential nutrients in its effort to eliminate the excessive daily load of chemicals to which you are exposed. Without these nutrients, necessary and proper body processing can't take place. For instance, let's say you eat lots of sugar, which will cause your body to use up its reserves of magnesium so you become magnesium deficient. This mineral is needed for about three hundred necessary metabolic body processes. The lack of this one critical nutritional substance can affect the functioning of the entire body.

THE STORAGE OF CHEMICALS

When chemicals can't be excreted, the body tends to store them in the obvious fatty areas such as the breast tissue, as well as in the much less evident fat in every cell wall and in the sheaths or myelin that cover our nerves. (Some studies indicate that the breast fat of women with cancer may contain four times more pesticides than the breast tissue of women without this disease.)[59] Up to three hundred chemicals have been found in human fatty tissue, so we truly do have toxic dump sites scattered throughout our bodies. (Studies have shown that human breast milk contains the chemicals that a mother has taken into her body. Some human milk has such a high pesticide level that it would be declared unacceptable for consumption if it were cow's milk.)

Sometimes the body neither excretes nor stores certain chemicals; rather, it incorporates them into the tissues themselves, which can damage cells. Cadmium from automobile exhaust, for example, can become part of the kidney tissue, which in turn can lead to high blood pressure. Mercury from dental fillings and eating certain fish can sometimes cause nonspecific but serious problems such as exhaustion and extreme irritability.[60]

Our bodies do their best, but sometimes as certain chemicals are detoxified, even more potentially harmful substances are produced. This process is called biotransformation. This means the structure of a chemical is altered, so it forms a new substance that can be more, not less, toxic than the original one. This new substance definitely can harm body cells and tissues. If, for example, genetic material is damaged by certain harmful breakdown products, the injured genes in an unborn baby can cause congenital deformities. If the immune system or other body systems, are damaged, this can cause an individual to develop serious incapacitating illnesses later in life.

The simplest way to explain how the body detoxifies chemicals is to imagine that A must be converted to B, B to C, and then C to D. D is what the body really needs. However, if there is a block so B can't go on to C, then the body will have too much B and not enough C and D. Doctors can conduct expensive tests to find the blocks in the degradation or breakdown of chemicals. (These tests assess amino acids, organic acids, vitamins, and nutrient levels in the blood and urine.) From the location of the block, and with the knowledge of what is needed to move from one step to the next, it is sometimes easy to correct a deficiency. In fact, some medical and learning problems can be eliminated merely by supplying certain essential substances needed for the normal stepwise conversion of A through D.

GETTING TO THE CAUSE

The rest of what happens is better explained in Dr. Sherry Rogers's excellent, informative books.[61] She discusses, simply and humorously, why the body needs all of the nutrients previously mentioned to correct metabolic problems caused by chemical exposures, and shows exactly how these can interfere with normal cell functioning and cause ill health.

Nevertheless, because some chemical effects may not become evident for many years, the cause-and-effect relationships of certain exposures can be easily missed. Benzene in gasoline, organophosphates in pesticides, phenol in aerosol disinfectants, formaldehyde in paneling, tetrachloroethylene in dry-cleaned clothing or synthetic carpets, toluene in paints or plastics, and/or mercury fillings in teeth may not be suspected as the culprits causing an illness until years after the exposure.

The patients of nutritionally oriented physicians are truly fortunate because these doctors now have the knowledge to better recognize the basic causes of many illnesses that were previously not recognized or understood. No panacea will treat everything or everybody, but many children and adults can be helped to feel truly well on a permanent basis after the body is supplied with the nutrients that are required to function optimally.

ONE CHILD'S REPEATED FIGHT WITH CHEMICALS

Carl

Twelve-year-old Carl's story illustrates many of the recurrent problems that can face an environmentally ill person. As you read his story, consider how often he not only needed the causes of his illness to be detected but also required detoxification. He demonstrates the need for the types of therapeutic modalities discussed in this chapter.

Carl had typical allergies, which he was able to handle without much difficulty until he was accidentally and unknowingly exposed to furnace exhaust fumes. Eventually this exposure caused him to develop an exquisite sensitivity to progressively more and more chemicals. Subsequent accidental pollutant exposures, both at home and at school, escalated his illness to a frightening level. These exposures caused a dramatic downward spiral in both his emotional and his physical health, which eventually led to very challenging medical, learning, and behavioral difficulties. He was able to attend school, but a single whiff of perfume could cause a total loss of control. At that time he could and would hurt himself or others. Few understood why he suddenly acted in such an unacceptable and inappropriate manner.

Some Background on Carl

Carl has many allergic relatives, and by the time he was five months old, his history strongly suggested that he also personally had allergies causing his repeated ear infections. He had classical hay fever and asthma by the age of three.

In 1992, when he was eight years old, Carl's parents were perplexed. He could no longer even sit through a meal. Why had he suddenly developed serious behavioral problems and depression? At times he even acted suicidal, especially on rainy days. In addition to headaches and leg aches, he experienced extreme hunger, blackouts, and frequent crying spells when he did not eat on time. This pattern suggested that he had hypoglycemia (low blood sugar), which was confirmed at a later date.

A Major Exposure to Gas Fumes

In May 1992 Carl's parents realized for the first time that harmful exhaust fumes had leaked from their home furnace, exposing the family. These fumes definitely caused Carl to become ill.

Doctors and his parents learned more about the causes of his unacceptable behavior when he tried the Multiple Food Elimination Diet, which excludes highly allergenic foods (see Chapter 5). His mother said that he improved by 95 percent in six days. He became "the nicest and most delightful child" she had ever seen, and his leg aches subsided. During the second part of the diet, she found that sugar, eggs, and preservatives bothered him, and that milk and dairy products contributed to his temper tantrums.

The diet helped so much that even though Carl's typical hay fever allergies were present during the summer of 1992, he no longer had depression, leg aches, or sudden, terrifying mood swings.

Carl's Response to P/N Allergy Testing

Carl was seen in our center in July 1992. During P/N allergy testing, he acted perfectly normal most of the time, but the following behaviors were noted: Certain dilutions of mold extract made him exceedingly tired; others caused him to become hyperactive and aggressive. At one point, he playfully pulled his mother's nose and called her names, and shortly thereafter he banged his head on the floor. During this reaction his ears and cheeks became a brilliant red. His mother finally understood why he repeatedly became aggressive, depressed, and nasty on damp, moldy days. Sometimes his depression was so intense and severe on those days that he said he hated life and wanted to die; on one occasion he even tried to jump off a balcony.

During allergy testing for tree pollen, Carl hit his mother and became exceedingly nasty. While undergoing yeast testing, he called his father names. During a test for natural gas, he became mean, uncooperative, withdrawn, and so depressed that he hit his own face. During a phenol allergy test, he developed red cheeks, became uncooperative, started to kick and hit, yawned, would not talk, and became withdrawn.

Later, after Carl saw a videotape of his response to these allergy tests, he looked surprised. He sincerely could not recall behaving this way.

Other Tests

Blood studies showed that Carl had formed antibodies against his own nervous system and against formaldehyde. This phenomenon can usually be seen in persons who have been exposed to exhaust fumes from furnaces.

His brain-image SPECT test showed alterations both in the blood flow and in the functioning of specific portions of his brain. These alterations could be attributed to neurotoxic damage from chemical exposures.

Carl's Treatment

After he received comprehensive environmental care, which included avoiding chemicals, improving his diet, receiving nutritional supplements, psychological guidance, living in an environmentally safer home, and receiving allergy extract therapy, Carl responded well. He and his family learned to recognize, understand, and control many of his adverse responses to typical allergenic substances, foods, and chemicals. Both he and his family found that in spite of diligently avoiding all chemicals each day proved to be challenge. Every unavoidable exposure became a potential source of immense distress and concern.

A Second Major Gas Leak

In November 1992, shortly after the family turned on the furnace for the winter, Carl's actions and behavior changed again. His pulse, which was normally 80, increased to 110 whenever he was at home. His parents recognized that this indicated a problem with their home's indoor air. They found a gas leak and determined that their furnace again needed repair. Once the leak was corrected, his behavioral outbursts, depression, episodes of meanness, and other problems quickly improved. His pulse returned to 80 when he was inside his home.

However, the exposure to this second major leak had tipped his balance. Carl developed the dreaded "spreading phenomenon." His sensitivity became so intense that even the slightest odor of a chemical caused him to act mean and/or exhausted. He could not stay awake in church, and upon arousal, he would become extremely nasty. The smell of burning wood caused him to complain of nausea and a burning throat, and he would quickly be overcome with violent urges. He could no longer attend his regular school. After November, the slightest chemical exposure could precipitate an uncontrollable episode of rage. Carl's life became increasingly restricted. He could no longer swim in a chlorinated pool. Once, when he and his family stayed in a motel that contained a new, smelly synthetic carpet, he became so violent that he picked up the mattress and threw it at his mother. Another time, the odor of pesticides caused him such excruciating head pain that he fell to the floor.

Carl's mother needed to be warned before lawn spray trucks were scheduled to come into their neighborhood. At these times, if Carl did not stay indoors with the windows tightly closed, he could become violent. The odor of fabric softeners or scented products also caused him to become violent, and to spit, scream, and swear. When upset, he could tear his room to pieces. On one occasion, he became so out of control, cranky, irritable, and hostile that he threatened to hit his mother with a baseball bat.

When these episodes finally subsided, Carl would fall into a deep sleep or become almost unconscious. When he finally awakened, he could not walk or speak for five or ten minutes, and his body was totally limp. Then, just as suddenly, he would become normal again.

Surprisingly, during P/N allergy testing, this pattern of responses was repeatedly noted. Carl's parents were justified in their increasing concern about his angry outbursts and difficult behavior.

Problems at School

Carl became worse again as soon as he returned to school after the Christmas holiday in January 1993. This time he manifested extreme depression and again made suicidal statements. He told his counselor, "I think I am going to die." Scented substances in his classroom caused him to become oblivious to what was going on in class. At times he would fall asleep so suddenly that his teacher heard the thump of his head hitting his desk. On one occasion the odor from a fire entering the intake ventilation ducts caused him to suddenly change completely and to act in a most inappropriate manner.

Chemicals such as perfume had not caused Carl to experience symptoms of this intensity, or such anger or depression, in the past. But now, within minutes after an exposure to a disinfectant containing phenol, his eyes became framed by black circles. This change in his face helped confirm that a chemical was bothering him. Later the same day, after he smelled a neighbor's perfume and some lawn spray, he attacked his brother with such vengeance that two adults could not hold him down. When the rage stopped, he simply fell asleep.

On another occasion, a new carpet and pressed wood furniture in Carl's school were thought to be the cause of his elevated blood level of formaldehyde. His teachers also complained that they did not feel well. Later on his school discovered a gas leak a short distance from his classroom, his grades had begun to slip, his vision was blurred, his joints ached, and he had become totally exhausted during school hours. This added exposure surely could be one more reason why he was inordinately tired or misbehaved at school.

In February 1993 Carl finally switched to a more spartan parochial school that allowed no perfume or hairspray. His parents asked the school officials to discourage the use of chemicals for cleaning and maintenance, and with this kind of full cooperation, his condition improved. Whenever he returned to his former school, however, his original symptoms recurred within fifteen minutes.

And Yet Another Major Exposure to Furnace Fumes

In March 1993 Carl and his family again began to experience headaches, aching joints, blurred vision, and flulike symptoms. Even the family's dog and turtle became ill. Once again Carl's pulse increased, but only when he was at home. It decreased back to normal when he went outside. This observation strongly suggested again that something inside the house was bothering him.

This time the problem was traced to a large hole in the furnace heat exchanger. After the furnace was replaced, everyone gradually improved. Carl's bouts of depression decreased, but his serious behavioral changes after exposure to chemical odors persisted.

How Is Carl Today?

The smell of perfume continues to cause Carl to develop a spaced-out, squinty look to his eyes, as well as tension, extreme anger, and hostility. His brother develops asthma, and his father becomes "testy" from the same odor. (Chemical or environmental illness rarely affects just one person; it is usually a family problem.)

Carl can no longer attend church, shop in malls, or stay at the homes of friends. The slightest odor can cause a violent rage or outburst of hitting, biting, kicking, and foul language. During these episodes he may threaten to seriously hurt others. Fortunately, these outbursts are now better controlled with allergy extract therapy, nutrients, an alkali, and certain homeopathic remedies.

Carl received comprehensive environmental allergy treatment and homeopathic care. He now must eat and drink only organic foods; regular grocery store foods contain so many pesticides that eating them causes his behavior to change quickly.

Carl has recently shown great improvement, particularly after his family moved to a more environmentally sound house. His grades are excellent except when there is a chemical exposure in school. At those times his family and teachers understand what causes his episodes and know how to treat them. If his pulse increases over 100 and he suddenly develops dark eye circles and/or red earlobes and acts inappropriately, they quickly detect which chemical has started the chain reaction and attempt to immediately prevent the situation from getting out of hand. If he takes an alkali or his allergy extract without delay, he can usually abort his uncontrollable behavior and he returns to normal within about ten minutes.

Even so, Carl's chemical sensitivities have made his daily life demanding and difficult. We can only wonder where and how he might be today if the many causes of his behavioral outbursts had been found sooner. If the repeated accumulation of chemicals in his body had been significantly reduced through detoxification, would he not have had much less difficulty? How and why do so many substances bother him? How can he be protected in our increasingly polluted world? What's the long-term prognosis for him? Will he eventually hurt himself, or someone else, badly?

We don't know the answers, but one thing is certain: Without appropriate environmental and homeopathic care, Carl would certainly not be as well as he is at present. With proper but expensive detoxification, he probably could and would be better. Once again, the bottom line in relation to a child's health and education, present and future, can be, amazingly, insurance coverage. Will his family be reimbursed for what is needed to restore his health, or will insurers limit his future by denying him medical care that might be helpful but costly?

On a long-term basis, an insurance company can lower its costs and surely improve Carl's health by permitting him to have the best and most appropriate comprehensive treatment available. He desperately needs help now, because as he becomes older it becomes increasingly difficult to constantly and carefully control his environment. Detoxification should make his future less demanding and challenging. Unfortunately, this is an unrealistic option at present, ironically due to a large degree to medical reimbursement limitations.

NOTES

1. Herbert J. Rinkel et al., *Food Allergy* (Springfield, IL: Charles C. Thomas, 1951).
2. Leo Galland, *Superimmunity for Kids* (New York: Dell Publishing, 1989); Majid Ali, *The Canary and Chronic Fatigue* (Denville, NJ: Life Span Press, 1994); and Majid Ali, *RDA: Rats, Drugs and Assump-*

tions (Denville, NJ: Life Span Press, 1995); Billie Sahley, *The Natural Way to Control Hyperactivity with Amino Acids and Nutrient Therapy*, 2d ed. (San Antonio, TX: Pain and Stress Clinic, 1994); Lendon Smith, *Feed Your Body Right* (New York: M. Evans and Co., 1995); J. Bland and A. Bralley, ''Nutritional Upregulation of Hepatic Detoxification Enzymes,'' *Journal of Applied Nutrition*, vol. 44, nos. 3 and 4 (1992); J. Bland et al., ''A Preliminary Outcome Study of a Medical Food-Supplemented Detoxification Program in the Management of Chronic Health Problems,'' *Alternative Therapies in Health and Medicine* (Nov. 1995); Edward Siguel, *Essential Fatty Acids in Health and Disease* (Brookline, MA: Nutrek Press, 1994); and Udo Erasums, *Fats and Oils* (Burnaby, B.C.: Alive Books, 1986).

3. Ali, *Canary*; and Ali, *RDA*.
4. William Rea, *Chemical Sensitivity*, vol. 2 (Chelsea, MI: Lewis Publishers, 1991–1996), p. 619.
5. Doris J. Rapp, *Is This Your Child?* (New York: William Morrow & Co., 1991); Doris J. Rapp, *The Impossible Child* (Buffalo, NY: Practical Allergy Research Foundation, 1989).
6. Howard Garrett, *Organic Manual* (Fort Worth, TX: Summit Group, 1993).
7. L. Mott and K. Snyder, *Pesticide Alert: A Guide to Pesticides in Fruits and Vegetables* (San Francisco, CA: Sierra Club Books, 1987); and Regenstein, *Cleaning Up America*.
8. Bob Smith, ''Organic Foods vs. Supermarket Foods: Element Levels,'' *Journal of Applied Nutrition*, vol. 45, no. 1 (1993), pp. 35–39.
9. Rapp, *Is This Your Child?*
10. For more details, see Donna Powell, *Why Five?* (Cobra Limited, 1989); and Natalie Golas and Frances G. Golbitz, *If It's Chicken, It Must Be Tuesday* (New Canaan, CT: Keats Publishing, 1981).
11. R.N. Podell, ''Intracutaneous and Sublingual Provocation and Neutralization,'' *Clinical Ecology*, vol. 2, no. 1 (Fall 1983), pp. 13–20.
12. Doris J. Rapp, ''Environmental Medicine: An Expanded Approach to Allergy,'' *Buffalo Physician* (Feb. 1986), pp. 16–24.
13. D.J. Maberly and H.M. Anthony, ''Asthma Management in a 'Clean Environment': 1. The Effect of Challenge with Foods and Chemicals on the Peak Flow Rate,'' *Journal of Nutritional Medicine*, vol. 3 (1992), pp. 215–30; ''Asthma Management in a 'Clean Environment': 2. Progress and Outcome in a Cohort of Patients,'' *Journal of Nutritional Medicine*, vol. 3 (1992), pp. 231–48.
14. Joseph Miller, *Relief at Last* (Springfield, IL: Charles C. Thomas, 1987).
15. William J. Rea et al., ''Elimination of Oral Food Challenge Reaction by Injection of Food Extracts,'' *Archives of Otolaryngology*, vol. 110 (Apr. 1984), pp. 248–52; and W.P. King et al., ''Provocation-Neutralization: A Two-Part Study. Part I. The Intracutaneous Provocative Food Test: A Multi-center Comparison Study,'' *Otolaryngology—Head and Neck Surgery*, vol. 99, no. 3 (Sept. 1988), pp. 263–71; ''Provocation-Neutralization: A Two-Part Study. Part II. Subcutaneous Neutralization Therapy: A Multi-center Study,'' *Otolaryngology—Head and Neck Surgery*, vol. 99, no. 3 (Sept. 1988), pp. 272–77.
16. Jonathan Wright, *Dr. Wright's Guide to Healing with Nutrition* (New Canaan, CT: Keats Publishing, 1991); Ali, *Canary*; Ali, *RDA*; and Sahley, *Hyperactivity*.
17. Galland, *Superimmunity*; and M.A. Schmidt et al., *Beyond Antibiotics* (Berkeley, CA: North Atlantic Books, 1994).
18. As reported on *Eye to Eye With Connie Chung*, CBS, Jul. 28, 1994.
19. See Ali, *RDA*; and Sahley, *Hyperactivity*.
20. Ibid.
21. See Ali, *RDA*.
22. See Smith, *Feed Your Body Right*.
23. Smith, *Feed Your Kids Right*.
24. See Ali, *RDA*; and Sahley, *Hyperactivity*.
25. See Galland, *Superimmunity*; Siguel, *Essential Fatty Acids*; and Erasums, *Fats and Oils*.
26. Regenstein, *Cleaning Up America*.
27. David Lin, *Free Radicals and Disease Prevention* (New Canaan, CT: Keats Publishing, 1993); Jean Barilla, ed., *The Nutrition Superbook*, vol. 1, *The Antioxidants* (New Canaan, CT: Keats Publishing, 1995); Borek Carmia, *Maximize Your Health-Span with Antioxidants* (New Canaan, CT: Keats Publishing, 1995).
28. Stephen Schoenthaler, *Improve Your Child's IQ and Behavior* (London: BBC Books, 1991); S.J.

Schoenthaler, W.E. Doraz, and J.A. Wakefield, "The Impact of a Low Food Additive and Sucrose Diet on Academic Performance in 803 NYC Public Schools," *International Journal of Biosocial Research*, vol. 8, no. 2 (1986), pp. 185–95; and S.J. Schoenthaler, D. Benton, and G. Roberts, "The Effect of Vitamin and Mineral Supplementation on Intelligence, the Sample of School Children," *Lancet*, vol. 664 (1988), pp. 140–43.

29. Rogers, *Wellness Against All Odds.*

30. Richard A. Passwater, and Chithan Kandaswami, *Pycnogenol: The Super Protector Nutrient* (New Canaan, CT: Keats Publishing, 1994).

31. For more information on blue-green algae, see D. John Apsley, *The Genesis Effect* (Northport, AL: Genesis Communications, 1996). Lake Klamath Blue-Green Algae is available from Cell Tech (see Resources).

32. Anne Puryear, *Stephen Lives!* (New York: Simon & Schuster, 1996).

33. Dennis Cauchon, "More Children Undergo Shock Therapy," *USA TODAY*, Dec. 7, 1995.

34. Elson Haas, *Staying Healthy with Nutrition* (Berkeley, CA: Celestial Arts, 1995).

35. See Ali, *RDA.*

36. Bland and Bralley, "Nutritional Upregulation"; and Bland, "Preliminary Outcome Study."

37. See Ali, *RDA.*

38. F. Batmanghelidj, *Your Body's Many Cries for Water* (Falls Church, VA: Global Health Solutions, 1995).

39. Haas, *Staying Healthy.*

40. David Frawley, *Ayurvedic Healing: A Comprehensive Guide* (Salt Lake City, UT: Passage Press, 1989).

41. Ali, *Chronic Fatigue.*

42. Batmanghelidj, *Your Body's Many Cries.*

43. Ali, *RDA*; Haas, *Staying Healthy*; Bland and Bralley, "Nutritional Upregulation"; Bland, "Preliminary Outcome Study."

44. Ali, *RDA.*

45. Rogers, *Wellness.*

46. Michael T. Werbach and N.D. Murray, *Botanical Influences on Illness* (Tarzana, CA: Third Line Press, 1994), p. 30.

47. For information about homeopathy, see Trevor Smith, *Homeopathic Medicine* (Rochester, VT: Healing Arts Press, 1989). See also Lyle Morgan, *Homeopathy and Your Child* (Rochester, VT: Healing Arts Press, 1992); Sheila Harrison, *Help Your Child With Homeopathy* (Garden City Park, NY: Avery Publishing Group, 1989); Paul Callanan, *Family Homeopathy* (New Canaan, CT: Keats Publishing, 1995).

48. See Schmidt, *Beyond Antibiotics.*

49. Steven Horne, *The ABC Herbal* (Winona Lake, IN: Wendell W. Whitman Co., 1994); and Daniel B. Mowery, *Herbal Tonic Therapies* (New Canaan, CT: Keats Publishing, 1993).

50. Z. Tretjak, M. Shields, and S. Beckmann, "PCB Reduction and Clinical Improvement by Detoxification: An Unexploited Approach?" *Human and Experimental Toxicology*, vol. 9 (1990), pp. 235–44.

51. D.W. Schnare et al., "Evaluation of a Detoxification Treatment for Fat Stored Xenobiotics," *Medical Hypotheses*, vol. 9 (1982), pp. 265–82. See also Moses, *Designer Poisons.*

52. Tretjak, Shields, and Beckmann, "PCB Reduction."

53. Thomas Meyn, presentation on "The Use of Infrared: A Hyperthermy in Detoxification in Neuharlingersiel, Germany," at the tenth international symposium for environmental medicine, Bad Emstal, Germany, Sept. 1995.

54. For information on yeast illness, contact International Health Foundation (see Resources). See also William G. Crook, *The Yeast Connection and the Woman* (Jackson, TN: Professional Books, 1995). See also C. Orian Truss, *The Missing Diagnosis* (Birmingham, AL: C. Orian Truss, 1983).

55. J. Krohn, F.A. Taylor, and E.M. Larson, *The Whole Way to Allergy Relief and Prevention* (Port Roberts, WA: Hartley and Marks, 1991).

56. Ibid.; Ali, *RDA.*

57. Personal communications from Jacques Hertoghe, M.D., and Thierry Hertoghe, M.D., Antwerp, Belgium.

58. Broda O. Barnes and Charlotte W. Barnes, *Hope for Hypoglycemia* (Fort Collins, CO: Robinson Press, 1978), p. 29. Call the Barnes Foundation for more information at (203) 261-2101.

59. F. Falck, Jr., et al., "Pesticides and Polychlorinated Biphenyl Residues in Human Breast Lipids and Their Relation to Breast Cancer," *Archives of Environmental Health*, vol. 47 (1992), pp. 143–46; N. Kreiger et al., "Breast Cancer and Serum Organochlorines: A Prospective Study Among White, Black, and Asian Women," *Journal of the National Cancer Institute*, vol. 80, no. 8 (1994), pp. 589–99; P.J. Lewis, "Risk Factors for Breast Cancer. Pollutants and Pesticides May Be Important," letter, *British Medical Journal*, vol. 309 (Dec. 17, 1994), p. 1662; comment: *British Medical Journal*, vol. 310 (Mar. 4, 1995), p. 598; and H. Mussalo-Rayganaam et al., "Occurrence of Betahexachlorocyclohexane in Breast Cancer Patients," *Cancer*, vol. 66 (1991), pp. 2124–48.

60. Ibid.

61. S.J. Rogers, *Tired or Toxic?* (Syracuse, NY: Prestige, 1990); and Rogers, *Wellness Against All Odds* (Syracuse, NY: Prestige, 1994).

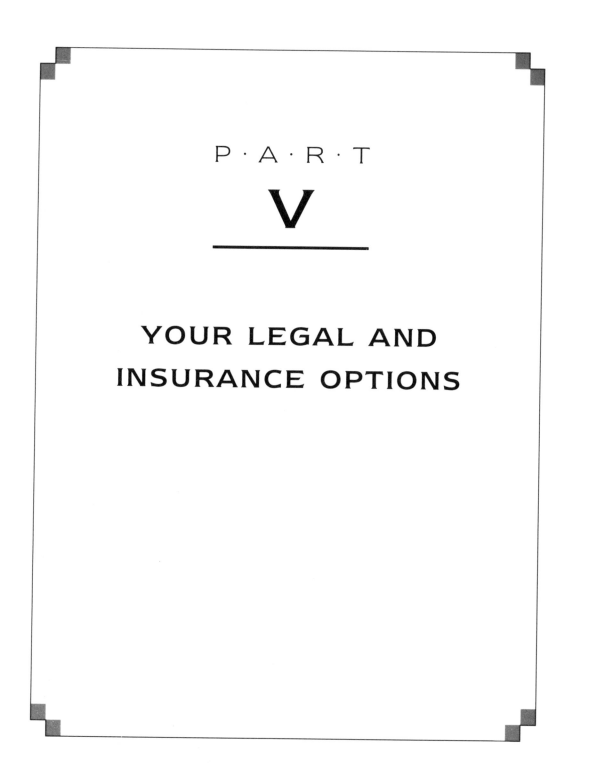

P · A · R · T

V

YOUR LEGAL AND
INSURANCE OPTIONS

16 When You Need Legal Help Because No One Is Listening

If you or your child is obviously ill because of a recent school exposure, there is much that you can do. Your actions will be determined by the intensity of the symptoms and the school administration's attitude.

First, you should advance through the chain of command, starting with the school nurse or health personnel, followed by the principal, the school superintendent, and finally the local and state boards of education. If necessary, contact the commissioner of education and health officials in your state. Determine which agencies, organizations, and individuals can encourage your school to cooperate fully. Many have information that will help the school do what is right, without recourse to personal threats. *Keep a detailed written record of your inquiries and each person's response* if possible. Your aim is to remedy the situation without legal intervention. You need not blaze a new trail through unknown territory. Several Canadian mothers and their progressive Ontario school districts have clearly shown cost-effective ways to successfully and amicably resolve many environmental health issues, as discussed in Chapter 12.

You will encounter no lack of disbelievers, and the burden of proof sometimes will rest solely upon you to prove you have an environmentally-related illness. Skeptics who are not knowledgeable about chemical sensitivities and the true scope of allergies will assume that any sudden illness in a school is primarily an infection or some emotional or psychological problem. If no one believes you or your child feel unwell, it is entirely normal for you to develop realistic fears about the future. These fears, in turn, can certainly cause *secondary* psychological problems. Over time unresolved health issues can become more and more complex and challenging. The bottom line often rests with one simple question: **Initially, did you or your child suddenly become ill after an environmental change in a school?**

■ HOW TO KEEP RECORDS AND OBTAIN DOCUMENTATION

You must record in detail exactly what you believe happened that created the unhealthy school situation. Start a notebook, and keep it updated and in order. Record and date every environmental exposure in a sequential manner. Make a rough drawing of the building and the areas that affect you, your child and others. Pinpoint potential sources of difficulty. If you can, videotape your own or your child's visible responses to school exposures. Videotapes and/or photographs of dust, mold, ductwork, dirty filters, basement leakage, bus pollution, pesticide use, and other environmental problems can also be helpful.

Keep an organized paper trail of all your letters and responses in a notebook. Phone calls are of less value because you may forget exactly what was said—unless you can obtain consent to tape pertinent conversations at the time of your discussions. *Keep written, dated copies of what is said and done.* To be able to provide the right information to concerned parties, you must be organized. No one else can or will do it for you. If you neglect to record your documentation, for whatever reason, you may lose much more than your insurance coverage.

You cannot legally take samples of various school items such as a piece of carpet or even a sample of school air without authorized written permission.[1] Check with your lawyer about using samples found in outside trash cans. Alternatively, try to purchase exactly the same brand or type of product. If possible, keep samples of potentially harmful items (like cleaning solutions or adhesives) well marked, labeled, and dated. Store the samples in glass jars, in a safe place in your home. You may need them in the future.

■ STATE AND FEDERAL AGENCIES

A number of governmental agencies enforce regulations pertaining to environmental health issues. You need to know which agencies at the local, county, state, and federal level can be helpful. Make your local reference librarian your friend—he or she can provide a wealth of information. Always obtain information from organizations in your locality, such as the local bar association, before attempting to enter the maze of state and/or federal bureaucracy.

Check the government agency listings in your telephone directory. More federal agencies that may be helpful are listed in Resources. Call your various local, state, and federal agencies at mid-week—never early Monday morning or near closing time. Briefly explain your concerns. Some contacts will prove more helpful than others. Since laws vary from state to state, individual investigation is required. For example, some local social service agencies will provide benefits but only if certain eligibility requirements are met. You must learn what stipulations assist or restrict the needs of your child. Some states, such as New Jersey, provide informative booklets. Write your state board of education.

■ IMPORTANT FEDERAL LAWS

Two important laws may provide you with great help.

1. The Rehabilitation Act of 1973 (Section 504) states, "No otherwise qualified individual with handicaps in the United States . . . shall solely, by reason of his handicap, be excluded from participation in, or denied the benefits of, or be subjected to discrimination under any program or activity receiving federal financial assistance." This law has been interpreted to mean that schools receiving federal funds must provide each qualified "handicapped" individual with an appropriate free education. A handicap is defined basically as "any physical or mental impairment which affects one or more body systems or substantially limits one or more major life activities, such as breathing." Environmental illness can certainly cause such handicaps and therefore should meet the eligibility requirements for aid. An increasing number of parents are receiving specific individual help for their children under this law.

This law also requires that schools follow prescribed procedures to safeguard parents' rights. Schools must implement fair measures appropriate to each child's needs. Schools and parents must act as equal partners in planning and decision-making.[2] Because instituting the changes required for one child can affect the rest of a school, many children may be helped every time one environmentally ill student is helped.

2. The Americans with Disabilities Act (ADA), passed in 1990, can help students who no longer have access to an education and teachers who have been denied employment and workplace accommodation.[3] In essence, ADA states that at the expense of the school district, federally subsidized schools must do what is "readily achievable" to accommodate access to their school facilities. This includes persons with handicapping conditions.

■ Title I prohibits employers who have more than fifteen employees from discriminating against the disabled.

■ Title II prohibits discrimination in relation to providing public services.

■ Title III prohibits private entities from discriminating in the provision of public services.[4]

In reference to schools, both Titles II and III have been interpreted to mean that students, faculty, and other occupants cannot be denied education or employment because of an illness or chemical sensitivity that has developed due to an offending factor in a school environment.

The Department of Justice enforces Titles II and III of the ADA (and Title I for government workplaces). The office of the attorney general specifically refers to environmental illness or Multiple Chemical Sensitivities (MCS), which may be considered a disability if it substantially limits one or more major life activities.[5] The *ADA Handbook* describes environmental illness as a "sensitivity to environmental elements." Although it declines to state categorically that these types of allergies or sensitivities are disabilities, it specifically asserts the following: "Sometimes respiratory or neurological functioning is so severely affected that an individual will satisfy the requirements to be classified as disabled under the regulations. Such an individual would be entitled to all the protections afforded by the Act."[6]

On the basis of this statute, individuals can request less polluted accommodations that do not cause serious illness. People suffering from MCS have had some success using ADA. In Texas environmentally ill people have forced a county government to decrease the use of pesticides in public buildings because MCS patients could not use a building. Recently in one case the general counsel for the Department of Housing and Urban Development made a determination that pesticides used in a condominium and by a lawn service could constitute discrimination against a resident on the basis of MCS.[7]

A number of appellate court decisions have supported MCS disability.[8] The following story is just one example of what a number of parents have accomplished.[9]

Alexandra, Joseph, and Jared, all children with environmental illness and MCS, are now able to attend elementary school in Baltimore, Maryland, because of the following accommodations:

■ None of the children should be exposed to colored chalk, felt pens (except Crayola water-based), paints, mimeographed copies, carbonless copy paper, cleansers or disinfectants (including Pine Sol, Lysol, bleach, green soap), Play-Doh, rubber cement, model glue (Elmer's glue is allowed), pesticides or fertilizers, perfumes, scented stickers or candy "rewards," or any oil-based or acrylic-based products.

■ The children's parents are to be notified in advance of any painting or floor stripping and waxing, and they are to be told immediately if any child in the class has head lice. (A common therapy for head lice is an organochloride pesticide, lindane, which can cause serious illness if it is not used correctly or if it is used to treat someone who is very sensitive to it.[10] For more information, see Chapters 10 and 15.) Spraying with insecticides has been discontinued, and teachers are asked to wear no perfume, cologne, or other scented personal-care products.

■ The children have been placed in classrooms with the best ventilation, and the vents are cleaned twice a year.

- New books are to be aired out and, when necessary, sent home for "baking" (see Chapter 6).
- Food service personnel prepare only organic food to which the children are not allergic and that contains no artificial colorings, flavorings, or preservatives.

In New York State, a few schools have implemented similar changes in relation to MCS because of the federal Rehabilitation Act of 1973. In addition, a teacher with MCS should check into state vocational rehabilitation programs.

While it is unrealistic to demand totally uncontaminated classrooms at this time, designating cleaner, less-polluted Canadian-type ECO classrooms is not unreasonable (see Chapter 12). School districts can and should provide cleaner, safer classrooms and buildings and offer a variety of home educational programs.

HOW TO FILE COMPLAINTS

Title I

Complaints about violations of Title I (employment) by units of state and local government or by private employers should be filed with:

> Equal Employment Opportunity Commission
> Program Development and Technical Assistance Division
> Office of Program Operations
> 1801 L Street, N.W., Room 9405
> Washington, DC 20507

Title II

Complaints about violations of Title II (public services) by units of state and local government should be filed with:

> Civil Rights Division, Coordination and Review Section
> Department of Justice
> P.O. Box 66118
> Washington, DC 20035-6118

Title III

Complaints about violations of Title III (public services) by public accommodations and commercial facilities should be filed with:

> Civil Rights Division, Public Access Section
> Department of Justice
> P.O. Box 66738
> Washington, DC 20035-6738

Home teaching has distinct disadvantages. The academic and social development of a child can be seriously restricted. The estimated two hours per day of supervised instruction that home-schooled children receive over a three-year period is equivalent to only one year of school education. Moreover, most parents lack the necessary training to be educators. Even though they are willing and capable in many ways, they should not be forced to become educators.

For more information on ADA and other laws, contact the organizations listed in Resources. For copies of settlement agreements and legal documents, write to the Freedom of Information/Privacy Act Branch (see Resources) or to MCS Referral and Resources (see Resources).

■ HOW YOUR PHYSICIAN CAN HELP

Before any educational authorities or governmental parties will listen to you, you must be able to provide documentation from your physician that you are significantly ill or incapacitated. It helps if you have selected a board-certified physician who has in-depth knowledge of environmental illness and who keeps precise records. Has your chosen physician had specific training in environmental and/or occupational medicine? Does he or she believe in the existence of MCS?

Be sure your physician has a copy of all your past and present medical records. Send all available information from each previously consulted physician and specialist, and all laboratory findings, including X-ray reports if these are requested. *Be sure to keep copies of all medical records and X-ray reports yourself.* Sometimes records are lost and cannot be replaced.

SOMEONE ELSE SELECTS A PHYSICIAN FOR YOU

An insurance company may request an "independent" medical examination in an effort to ascertain whether you are truly ill. It is best if such an evaluation is conducted in the home of another MCS patient or in a place that can reasonably comply with your environmental limitations. It can be a challenge for these doctors to be truly independent, since they are being paid by the insurance company. Some of these physicians appear to be rewarded in proportion to the number of people they claim are not ill. The conclusion that such a doctor reaches in one hour may weigh equally in court with that of a doctor who has seen you for many years. The Freedom of Information Act can force the insurance company to turn over such doctors' reports, except when they belong to the federal government. In that situation your rights are limited.[11]

■ SELECTING A LAWYER[12]

You may very well find yourself in need of a lawyer, especially where personal injury, Workers' Compensation, and insurance problems are concerned. Finding the appropriate lawyer can be as challenging as finding the right physician. Interview a prospective lawyer prior to hiring and evaluate his or her capabilities. Ask for references from past EI patients: Were their cases won or lost? Will the lawyer or a paralegal handle your case? Will you pay double for both? Will the lawyer meet with you in an environmentally safe place and be careful not to wear offending scented preparations? Is he or she willing to accommodate an MCS patient? Will he or she return your calls?

If you cannot find a local lawyer to represent you on a contingency basis (meaning that you do not pay unless your lawyer wins), contact your local (county) bar association. They will provide information concerning which attorneys handle your type of case in a particular area. If that referral is not satisfactory, the next best choice is the state bar association. There are many state and federal "litigation groups" that focus on specific types of products or substances (asbestos, breast implants, and lead, among others). Although these groups are not directly connected to state bar associations, a bar association can provide you with the phone numbers of various litigation groups. More sources of referrals are listed in Resources.

Sometimes an attorney is willing to pay for certain aspects of medical and bioassay evaluations (see Chapters 10 and 13). If so, it suggests that the lawyer feels confident of winning.

■ TYPICAL STUDENT PROBLEMS THAT REQUIRE ASSISTANCE

If your child is in any of the following rather common situations, you may need help to find an individualized solution.

■ *The school refuses to transfer your child to another room or school, in spite of a medical request from a qualified physician.*
From a medical perspective, do not continue to expose your child if you and your physician believe it can be harmful. Remove your child from the offending school as soon as possible, and consider your options: home teaching, a private school, transportation to another school district, or moving your family to a different school district. Ask your doctor to contact the principal or superintendent on your behalf. If the school's problem is identified and corrected, returning your child there is certainly possible, providing that your child feels entirely well in that environment.

■ *Your child continues to become ill shortly after entering the school building, even though local, county, and state health departments have reported that minor inadequacies have been corrected.*

Your child may represent the "canary in the coal mine." Ask for a transfer to another school, or for home teaching. Most schools, however, will do little if the health department cannot confirm a significant problem. The reports do not necessarily mean that no problem exists. Rather, it is possible that the cause is elusive and challenging to identify. Impartial, on-the-spot evaluations for chemicals inside and outside a building should be available soon. (see Resources).

■ *The health department detects some problems, but the school appears not to have made all the appropriate changes needed to prevent your child's school-related symptoms from arising again.*

Once again, consider home teaching or a transfer to another school. Call the state commissioner of education. Ask if the state can force further changes within a possible sick school building.

■ *You have requested home teaching for your child at the state's expense, but months pass without any action.*

Ask your child's school principal for a form requesting immediate home teaching. Keep records of all written requests to school officials. If the school is nonpublic, request an evaluation for special education. If your request is ignored or delayed, check with your district superintendent or your local or state board of education. Parents in some states may be entitled to the assistance of an attorney.

In New York State a disabled child who reaches the age of three is entitled to an appropriate public education within an adequate, least restrictive environment that meets his or her needs. Children are entitled to a complete physical and psychological evaluation. The committee on special education classifies disabled children. Some allergic or chemically sensitive children are classified as "learning disabled" or as "other health impaired." Additional meetings with appropriate agencies can be scheduled if required.

If you believe there is an injustice, file a claim under the 1973 Rehabilitation Act with the U.S. Department of Education, Office of Civil Rights. (Claims also can be filed with the Justice Department and with ADA officials. See Resources at the end of this book.) Ask for the address and phone number of the regional office for your school. You must file a complaint directly to your regional office within 180 days of the alleged discriminatory action. If the action is ongoing, you may file a complaint at any time. This department will act as investigator, mediator, and enforcement agency. They routinely resolve complaints, from start to finish, without attorneys.

■ *You are told that your child must return to a school that you know causes illness each time he or she enters the building.*
At times it can be seriously harmful to reexpose someone to the original source of an illness. Whether short or prolonged, the exposure can be the straw that breaks their health. Check with your environmental medical physician before you comply. Some parents have been threatened with truancy violations, fines, and placement of their children in foster care. Teachers have been intimidated in various ways and threatened with charges of insubordination if they speak out.

■ *You can't find a lawyer to help you, and you have no money.*
File for "pauper" status if you can, and find a knowledgeable advocate or ombudsman who will help you *pro bono.* Call the local or state bar association referral service. If none is listed in the phone book, call Legal Aid. Your aim is to find a lawyer who will represent you at no cost except for a small initial fee to pay for incidentals, such as copies of salient materials, or one who will represent you on a contingency fee basis. A contingency fee means that the lawyer is paid a certain percentage of the final settlement. If the case is lost, the lawyer is not paid. Unfortunately, many attorneys will not handle cases involving MCS on contingency, in part because they lack in-depth knowledge of the illness and also because of the mood disturbances and the intense desperation that is sometimes associated with this illness.

■ *A lawyer states that he will represent you, but after an initial flurry of interest, he does little.*
This situation is unlikely, but if it should happen, discharge the lawyer and request that all records be sent to your new attorney. If you paid a retainer fee, ask for a detailed record of exactly how the money was spent, and ask in writing for a refund of the balance.

■ *You disagree with the school about your child's placement in a special class.*
It sometimes happens that a bright child with a learning disability caused by environmental illness is placed in a classroom with severely retarded or behaviorally disruptive youngsters. This placement can lead to a loss of interest in school, to mimicking undesirable behavior, or to reasonable fear. Sometimes after EI children respond favorably to appropriate medical care, their school will unjustifiably refuse to transfer them back into a regular classroom. Ask for a temporary trial period within the desired classroom. If your child is truly better, this may resolve such a problem.

■ *You receive anonymous, threatening phone calls.*
Contact the phone company. It is now easy to trace such calls.

■ WHAT SPECIFICALLY CAN TEACHERS DO?

Teachers can apply for ADA, Social Security Disability Insurance, and/or Workers' Compensation if they are disabled by a chemical or other environmental exposure while at work.[13] If applicable, teachers can also contact their union lawyer and apply to their state health insurance for payment of their medical care. However, the statistics are not encouraging. Approximately 50 percent of EI patients receive no benefits at all; about 20 percent collect some form of Social Security disability, and 16 percent secure state (not federal) workers' compensation.

SOCIAL SECURITY DISABILITY INSURANCE

Teachers may be eligible for Social Security disability through the Social Security Administration, an independent federal agency. (For your local office, check your phone directory under "United States Government.") This agency on a case-by-case basis, recognizes chemical sensitivities due to environmental exposures and disabilities not related to exertion. Social Security Disability Insurance (SSDI) is provided to everyone who has "an inability to engage in work" by reason of "severe physical or mental impairment." It must be "medically determinable and expected to last at least 12 months or result in death." The Federal SSDI determines nonmedical disability; the state DDS (Disability Determination Service, as in New York State) decides about the medical requirements.

You can apply for benefits if you have worked long enough and within the designated time period to be eligible. SSDI assistance then requires a waiting period of six months, and your disability must be present for at least a year before you are eligible to apply.[14] The agencies will evaluate your claim on a case-by-case basis. If you feel well enough to work but cannot work in your school because of unavoidable environmental factors, a disability exists, so you may qualify for benefits. There are many income and resource limitations that deter application for this form of aid, but you can check by calling (800) 772-1213. (For children or adults who have never worked, there is the federal program called Supplemental Security Income, or SSI.)

The payment you receive will be affected by other benefits you may receive. Regular reviews are necessary to ascertain if you continue to require aid. You can appeal a negative decision. This type of aid has been only minimally obtainable in school-related complaints from teachers. Local social service and public assistance agencies may help you as well; call them to find out what restrictions they have in relation to age and eligibility and what you must do to obtain help.

If your efforts fail, contact your congressperson, who has a staff whose job is to assist constituents that meet the government requirements to obtain social security or other federal benefits. This must be done, however, before the matter goes before an administrative law judge.

WORKERS' COMPENSATION

Teachers can receive help through Workers' Compensation providing they can show a clear causal relationship between an environmental exposure in their workplace and their illness or disability. It is part of a federal, state, or self-insured program. Workers' Compensation benefits are nontaxable and are *supposed* to cover medical expenses. (In contrast, disability retirement is taxable, and part of the medical expenses must be paid by the recipient.)

Workers' Compensation rules differ from state to state, but in general, an adult who has had a work-related accident, injury, or disease is eligible for compensation for lost pay and medical expenses. You cannot be forced to work if you are clearly ill from a work-related exposure. Some states have a stipulation limiting remuneration in relation to preexisting illnesses.

To obtain Workers' Compensation, you must prove that you can no longer work due to a work-related medical impairment, which also can include a flare-up of a preexisting condition. The burden of proof is the responsibility of the disabled worker. You must provide expensive, extensive, time-consuming medical proof. Unfortunately, rejection is possible even when you have given adequate proof. Address appeals to your teachers' union or your attorney.

A complicated system requires you to undergo stressful hearings at varying intervals to determine the degree of limitation and your eligibility for compensation. You do not have to prove a permanent disability, but you must provide evidence that you have a temporary/chronic or partial/total disability. Armed with such evidence, your teachers' union or HUD can urge your school to make changes—for example, repair a building, improve ventilation systems, change duct filters, buy air cleaners, and/or accommodate your schedule. If Workers' Compensation is not helpful, contact your teachers' union for assistance. *Time can be critical because environmental illness is more apt to be reversible when treated as early as possible.*

TIPS ABOUT CLAIM FORMS

Have your attorney review your claim forms, for either Social Security Disability or Workers' Compensation, before you submit them, because the exact wording can be crucial to the outcome. It is best to itemize each complaint as a diagnosis, such as asthma, cephalalgia (headache), myalgia (muscle aches), porphyria disorder, vertigo, and toxic encephalopathy. Such diagnoses are more widely understood than is MCS, even though MCS typically includes many of these problems.

Similarly, you should file claims for lost wages and medical expenses by the accepted diagnoses of ICD-9 codes, not for environmental illness. The exception is if the health problem is job-related. A job-related environmental *injury* results if, for example, a worker has an incapacitating accident while installing a carpet. In contrast, a teacher who becomes ill from a new school carpet has an environmental occupational *illness* that developed after an accidental exposure. The distinction and final decision about the label (illness versus injury) is not always clear, and at times it is of little importance.

In some states a teacher cannot personally sue a school district, but you can sue a manufacturer or an installer who did not use the proper materials or methods. Regardless of who is to blame and who should pay, your expertise and talent should not be lost because your classroom is environmentally unsafe. You must be able to work, and your students must be able to participate normally in school activities. You can enhance cooperation among other teachers, students, and parents if you can provide them with any information you have about environmental illness and cost considerations. However, some MCS teachers are so ill that they have neither the energy nor the will to pursue their rights. If they lack the support of family or friends, their stress can be incredibly distressing and totally incapacitating.

TYPICAL TEACHER PROBLEMS THAT REQUIRE ASSISTANCE

■ *Your application for Social Security Disability Insurance benefits is rejected.* In general, Social Security appears to be denied for patients with MCS. Consult with your lawyer. James Ross's *Social Security Benefits: How to Get Them! How to Keep Them!* is a helpful source of information.[15] Other sources of help are listed in Resources.

■ *Your Workers' Compensation application is considered to be inadequate or is rejected.*
Even if a Workers' Compensation claim is paid initially, the amount can dwindle after each hearing or review. You may be too ill to resume work, and you may have inadequate resources for medical care and/or basic living expenses during this period. Discuss your concerns with your union representative, if you have one. If you are initially paid and your claim is later rejected, you must repay the money you received.

■ *You have little money and are so ill that you want to apply for disability. To prove that your health is impaired, however, you are told that you need special medical or psychological examinations, which you cannot afford.* Neuropsychological examinations and other tests (see Chapter 13) are highly desirable, but they are costly and are not readily available in many communities. Necessary blood tests and brain-image tests are also very expensive. To secure money to pay for them, try a local church or other "help" group. You can contact the feature editor of your local newspaper, or discuss your problems on a local radio or public television show.

■ *You are denied transfer to another school and must continue to work in the building that causes your illness.*
This is unlikely but it can happen. Your answer is Workers' Compensation which originally was a liberal system and basically pro-employee. In recent years, however, this approach is less evident. If you can provide any valid evidence that your work environment is medically harmful, a Workers' Compensation judge will not force you to return to it. The unemployment benefits system is also rather liberal in this regard: If you are forced to quit your job because of a harmful (or hostile) environment, you are entitled to collect unemployment benefits. If, like most teachers, you belong to a union, it should be your first contact. The ADA requires "reasonable accommodation" for a known limitation, unless it would impose a hardship on the employer.

If necessary, your lawyer can seek an injunction in state court stating that it can be dangerous to your health to return to work. You must provide proof that you have suffered irreparable harm, not simply lost wages. If there is a visible change in your health upon exposure in the building, make a videotape of yourself before and after an exposure. The challenge is to prove that you actually have a headache, muscle aches, nausea, or intermittent blurred vision. Sometimes it is difficult to verify an illness, even when one truly exists. Documentation is possible, but it cannot be done easily or inexpensively. Both an environmental medical specialist and neuropsychologist should be able to help you. (see Chapter 13).

■ *Inordinate delays occur while various agencies contact other agencies for initial reviews by your union or other representative.*
If this happens, complain to those involved and keep written records.

■ WHAT SHOULD YOUR SCHOOL DO?

Environmental illness associated with school buildings is an old problem, with it has a relatively new twist. Dust and molds have been around for a long time, but the combination of increasingly poor ventilation, tighter building construction, better insulation, and the more extensive use of potentially harmful chemicals have greatly increased the health risks and number of learning problems. Those who advise schools about their liabilities related to health issues often do not fully appreciate these factors. This is one reason why many school officials will not accept the fact that changing the school environment will enable some children and teachers to safely attend school. They do not understand that one's health and ability to learn can be affected by such routine exposures. For some, school attendance is impossible unless changes are made in certain classrooms or school buildings. All school occupants, including secretaries and maintenance personnel, are also potentially at risk.

A health department or HVAC evaluation may fail to identify all the causes of school-related illness (see Chapter 11). In addition, some school officials, who are fully aware of the factors causing illness refuse to make the necessary changes. A school's obligations also include provision of services, such as the administration of prescribed medications. It should modify its policies to meet the needs of individual students and teachers who are acutely or chronically unwell (see Chapter 12).

You need to know what your school system should, will, and will not do in relation to school-related illness. All children have the right to participate in the programs and activities that their educational system offers. Some states appear to be interested in providing environmentally healthy schools. They state that: "Children, including those with chronic health conditions, deserve the opportunity to develop to their fullest potential through the benefits of education and health care."[16] However, individual parents who ask for practical help are not always provided with it.

Unless each state's education department accepts the responsibility to issue mandates and enforce legislation rather than advance recommendations, guidelines, and suggestions, the health of present and future generations will remain in jeopardy.

> The ultimate aim in schools must be to restore the health and well-being of children so they can learn and of teachers so they can teach.

■ MEDIATION AND ARBITRATION

Mediation may be a way to encourage a school to remedy an unhealthy condition.

Serious questions about what is fair and right can arise in relation to environmental health issues. If those who are responsible for correcting a problem deny their obligations, litigation can result that makes everyone a loser. It is better to resolve challenging issues by eliminating the cause, making some adjustments, bending old rules and/or creating new rules. For example, a school may ultimately have to choose between paying many thousands of dollars for appropriate medical care and legal fees, or paying a few thousand dollars for room air purifiers.

For either mediation or arbitration to work, everyone must agree to discuss the issues. A neutral professional can sometimes help each side see the opposing point of view (for sources of mediators, see Resources). As early as possible, this attitude should be part of any discussion to avoid the kind of emotional confrontation that can easily escalate to a major conflict. A trained, impartial mediator will consider the needs of the students and teachers, while remaining sympathetic and realistic about the constraints of the school district officials. Although theoretically mediation and arbitration sound like sensible approaches, realistically it is unlikely that most school officials would agree. For additional information, check with your local library, civil organizations, and university or community college.[17]

The litigation process can take a tremendous emotional, physical, and financial toll on everyone concerned. If a school exposure seriously incapacitates a few individuals, it can also affect others unless changes are made. It is extremely important to appreciate the total effect of what you choose to do, or not do, on everyone else concerned. Your choice may affect the well-being of many others.

If litigation appears imminent, know what is needed to correct the problem before taking legal action. Stay open to negotiating a settlement even after filing a suit. At times, your initiation of legal action may serve to convince your opponents that they need to take your claim seriously.

The following account illustrates what can and does unfortunately happen to some teachers. I have deliberately left in the details so that you can appreciate the scope of this devastating illness. As you read her story, know that almost five years later, Mary still has not received any payment from the school that caused her illness.

ONE TEACHER'S PROBLEMS AFTER CHEMICAL EXPOSURE

Mary

Thirty-five-year-old Mary was teaching preschoolers at a college community day care center. She felt well until the fall of 1989, when her school building was renovated and remodeled to make it more energy-efficient. Carpets and linoleum were installed; rooms were drywalled and repainted; ceilings were dropped; new rooms were created within existing ones; and the parking lot was expanded and asphalted. The odors of plastic from materials that had melted in a dishwasher and tobacco from the teachers' lounge and outdoor designated smoking areas also permeated certain school areas. In addition, the building housed a poorly ventilated print shop. Ever since these changes were instituted, Mary has never really looked or felt well.

Shortly after the renovations began, Mary would sneeze, cough, and gasp for air as soon as she entered the building each day. Her health problems became progressively worse, so that within a few months she was so tired, she could hardly stay awake in the afternoon. As time passed, she complained of frequent headaches, laryngitis, an inability to read print, loss of short-term memory, a total lack of energy, moodiness, irritability, agitation, clumsiness, and problems carrying on ordinary conversation or making eye contact. She had cold hands and feet, nosebleeds, skin rashes, burping, numbness and tingling all over, chest pains, palpitations, dry crusty eyes, earaches, heart palpitations, a lack of perspiration, bone and joint aches, weakness, muscle cramps, recurrent flulike illnesses, and intense food cravings. This vast array of symptoms is unfortunately typical of many chemically sensitive individuals, but too many physicians and psychologists, erroneously believe it's an emotional problem. Her symptoms were less evident when she was away from the school, and she routinely felt better by Sunday night and during vacations.

Until about December 1990, she was able to participate in her usual outside activities. But by then she had become so incapacitated that she could barely cope with her daily personal needs. She was so sensitive to all exposures that her social interactions were significantly impaired. The "spreading phenomenon" completely changed her life, leaving her unable to go into areas that smelled of any chemical. Her illness had progressed from the Sick Building Syndrome to Multiple Chemical Sensitivities.

As so frequently happens, those who were not sensitive to chemicals doubted the veracity of Mary's complaints because they personally did not notice or become ill from faint odors that bothered her. The reality is that environmental illness, which can affect both the body and brain, is often not believed by employers, union officials, loved ones, relatives, and friends. This ignorance results in numerous misunderstandings. Schools routinely contain a smorgasbord of chemical odors and allergenic substances that are perceived only by those unfortunate children and adults who happen to be sensitive or allergic to them, as well as by those who have weakened immune systems.

The officials in Mary's school had virtually no appreciation of her illness. She reports they responded to her complaints with numerous confrontational, belittling, and stressful reprimands and insisted she return to work in spite of her doctor's advice. She felt intimidated and humiliated. Ultimately she was fired for "neglect of duty" and "insubordination."

The incident that precipitated her firing was a doctor's appointment that she had mistakenly scheduled during school hours. Her illness could easily have caused confusion because chemicals can alter brain function. At the time of this incident, there were a myriad of chemical exposures within her school.

According to Mary, she received letters from school officials that "misrepresented and distorted" facts and made unsubstantiated claims and only recourse to legal maneuvers allowed her to ultimately change her firing to a "resignation based on health reasons." The COBRA law enabled her to continue receiving medical insurance coverage. Her school tried unsuccessfully to deny her long-term disability benefits.

Mary says efforts were also made by the school officials to impede her attempts to obtain specific factual information about the air quality in the school. She eventually learned about OSHA's "right-to-know" Standard 1910.20, which states that she had the right to see the Material Safety Data (MSD) sheet for any toxic substance that the school had used. OSHA's investigation showed that the building's carbon dioxide and radon levels were elevated. Eventually the administration did remove the print shop from the building.

Accomplishing the above was far from simple for Mary because she felt very ill and had little energy. Her financial resources were rapidly depleting, and she had little support or understanding from anyone. She received what she felt were humiliating phone calls from the in-house union representatives, who should have shown compassion and helped her. Her teachers' union showed as little comprehension of her problem as the school. People with EI can sometimes become unduly upset, abrasive, negative, moody, irritable, and even volatile. Unfortunately, affected adults receive much less understanding than affected children, even when chemical exposures are recognized as the cause of their illness.

Mary eventually found an environmentally trained physician who implemented a comprehensive medical program that helped relieve many of her symptoms. The program consisted of chemical avoidance, a rotated organic diet, a more allergy-free and environmentally safer home, and allergy injection therapy after P/N testing. In addition, she received various forms of nutrient therapy.

Over a period of four years, Mary improved significantly but certainly not completely. Her coordination, hearing, and vision are better. Her blood pressure, pulse, and heart irregularities have decreased. She has fewer muscle aches, spasms, and infections. Her faintness, dizziness, hair loss, headaches, intestinal complaints, food cravings, and weakness are less frequent and less obvious. She has less daytime drowsiness, irritability, skin itching, and tingling.

In spite of her strict adherence to her medical program, however, exposure to the slightest amount of an odor—be it perfume or a cleaning solution—quickly produces confusion and problems concentrating and even conversing. She mixes up numbers, letters, and/or words, and acts disoriented in relation to time and space. She experiences memory loss, fatigue, muscle stiffness, skin rashes, and mood and behavioral changes. Surprisingly, her symptoms can return with the same intensity they originally had in 1989. These flare-ups, however, are usually short-lived if she quickly distances herself from the offending contact. For several days after such a flare-up, she must be exceedingly careful, because her tolerance level has stabilized at a lower plateau than usual. Her symptoms seem to lie just below the surface and are much too easy to trigger.

She is justifiably distressed that four years after her initial EI diagnosis, the slightest odor continues to wreak havoc in a life that was once productive, helpful, and rewarding. She has to struggle each day to keep her life on course. The constant challenge to prevent a recurrence of her incapacitating symptoms is like walking on eggshells. Her awareness of what causes her to become ill has become most acute and accurate. This helps, but she is justifiably concerned that her illness may never end.

P/N allergy testing provoked several different distressing responses typical of the type she noted in school. Even when she was totally unaware of what was being tested, one drop of allergy extract could quickly cause reactions. Like flipping a light switch, in seconds, she would vacillate from one extremely uncomfortable emotion to another. Some reactions, she said, felt like a fog gradually settling over her body, in the slow change that has been called brain fog. When that feeling finally subsided, she felt uplifted and much improved. Another common feeling she described as a short-circuiting of the brain and reception interference. She seemed unable to clear her thought channels and developed inner turmoil that made her want to crawl into a dark corner and cringe. At that time, she was unable to communicate with anybody about anything. She simply could not think. She felt as if she could "barely hang on." Her brain circuitry was jumbled, and her thoughts disconnected. Fortunately, she felt, looked, and acted in a more normal manner within a few minutes of receiving the right dilution of her allergy extract.

Her laboratory tests clearly demonstrated that her immune system was not up to par. She had antibodies against the fat (myelin) that covers the nerves, and against other body tissues. Other blood tests indicated immune changes of the type noted after exposure to chemicals. The SPECT test in Illustration 16.1 clearly demonstrates alterations in her brain image. These changes appear to be typical of adults or children who have had toxic exposures affecting their brain or nervous system.

ILLUSTRATION 16.1
MARY'S BRAIN-IMAGE SPECT TEST

Control Test	*Mary's Test*
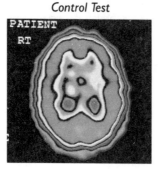	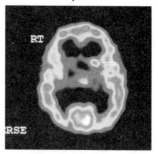

During the past four years, Mary's Workers' Compensation board hearings have been nonproductive and unrewarding. The board's refusal to pay has resulted in a series of hearings at two-to-four-month intervals and ongoing testimonies that have yet to culminate in a decision. Eventually a judge's decision will be reached, but it could take another six months, and it will likely precipitate another delaying series of reviews and appeals. It took her two years to become eligible for Social Security Disability benefits, but these have continued.

Throughout her ordeal, Mary's concern has not been limited to herself. Many children were similarly exposed at the time of the renovation. At one point she attempted to raise the awareness of her students' parents by informing them of the possible deleterious effects of the exposures. Many neither appreciated her warnings nor wanted any insight, even after children had developed some health, emotional, or memory problems at the time of the construction. Some parents who were employed by the college feared reprisals if they "caused any waves." During Mary's Workers' Compensation hearings, however, one parent did discuss her son's Dr. Jekyll/Mr. Hyde behavioral and mood changes, nosebleeds, difficulty in concentrating, and problems with eye contact. These symptoms had begun at the time of the school renovation. This child improved after receiving comprehensive environmental medical therapy.

At one time Mary reported to OSHA that nine out of ten teachers and other employees who were exposed to the remodeling pollution had developed symptoms. Some had flare-ups of previously quiescent allergies. Others developed flulike symptoms that they did not recognize as responses to a chemical exposure. One employee had several miscarriages, and another had an infant with birth defects. (No one knows if these were related to the school exposures.)

As happened to Mary, the lives of many children and teachers can irrevocably go into a downward spiral if they do not receive appropriate medical care. Too few will understand the cause of their problems. Those who were ill but eventually feel better well may not realize the full extent of their present and future risk. For an indefinite period they will be prone to develop their original health problems after any minute allergenic or environmental chemical exposure. This is exactly what happened to many of the children and teachers discussed in this book. Once they are sensitized, they must do everything cautiously and in moderation, and every potentially harmful exposure must be anticipated and prevented. One error may mean extreme precautions will again have to be implemented perhaps for months, before the threshold of tolerance will increase again.

Mary's story clearly reveals the unique problems facing chemically sensitive teachers. Their illness can be misinterpreted as noncompliance rather than an inability to comply; as a lack of cooperation, rather than an attempt to protect against further injurious exposures; and as a lackadaisical lazy attitude, instead of legitimate fatigue. The future well-being, careers, promotions and responsibilities of some teachers can be undermined by a single significant adverse exposure and a school administrator's lack of comprehension and understanding of environmental illness.

If justice is to prevail when no one is listening, you must take action. Obtain the names and addresses of your governor and local, state, and/or federal representatives from the League of Women Voters or the local board of elections. Write to them. If you do not feel uncomfortable, consider discussing the issues on radio or public television talk shows. Much more is at stake than the health of a single individual. The future of our present and future generations depends upon our no longer tolerating the senseless pollution of our environment and our universe.

NOTES

1. Bonnye L. Matthews, *Chemical Sensitivity* (Jefferson, NC: McFarland & Co., 1992).

2. According to Ellie Goldberg, M.Ed., an educational rights specialist, 79 Elmore Street, Newton, MA 02159. (Send a self-addressed stamped envelope for more information.)

3. Human Ecology Action League, *Multiple Chemical Sensitivities and the Americans with Disabilities Act: A Guide to Accommodation* (see Resources); see also *Human Ecologist*, no. 68 (Winter 1995).

4. Alice Kaswan, "The Americans With Disabilities Act As a Weapon Against Indoor Pollution," *Environmental Law in New York*, vol. 4, no. 7 (July 1993), p. 107.

5. MCS Referral and Resources, *Recognition of Multiple Chemical Sensitivities* (Mar. 13, 1995).

6. Ibid., and Human Ecology Action League, *Multiple Chemical Sensitivities.*

7. *Human Ecologist* (Spring 1995), p. 23; see Resources for address.

8. For more information, contact the National Center for Environmental Health Strategies (see Resources). See also Deborah Dubin, "Accommodating Environmental Illness/Multiple Chemical Sensitivity," *Disability Law Reporter Services*, vol. 3, no. 9, (Englewood Cliffs, NJ: Prentice Hall Law and Business, 1991, p. 8).

9. Susan Molloy, "Access in the Works," *New Reactor* (Nov./Dec. 1993).

10. Marion Moses, *Designer Poisons* (San Francisco, CA: Pesticide Education Center, 1995).

11. See Matthews, *Chemical Sensitivity.*

12. Ibid.; see also Charles B. Inlander and Eugene I. Pavalon, *Your Medical Rights* (Boston: Little, Brown, 1990).

13. James W. Ross, *Social Security Disability Benefits: How to Get Them! How to Keep Them!* (Slippery Rock, PA: Ross Publishing Co., 1984).

14. *Human Ecologist.*

15. Ross, *Social Security Disability.*

16. Quoted from the American Academy of Pediatrics (Oct. 1990). Write for a copy of "A Parent's Guide to Special Education for Children 5–21: Your Child's Right to an Education in NY State," from the New York State Department of Education, Office for Special Education Services, Albany, NY 12234, or contact the equivalent office in your own state's department of education.

17. Popular books that promote mutually beneficial outcomes include Roger Fisher and William Ury's *Getting to Yes: Negotiating Agreement Without Giving In* (New York: Viking Penguin, 1983); and William Ury's *Getting Past No: Negotiating Your Wars from Confrontation to Cooperation* (New York: Bantam, 1993). Also consider Thomas Crowley's *Settle It Out of Court: How to Resolve Business and Personal Disputes Using Mediation, Arbitration, and Negotiation* (New York: John Wiley, 1994).

17 Insurance Considerations

Who will pay for medical care arising from school-related environmental illness? This is a key question. All too often, everyone effectively dodges this essential responsibility.

Your school's liability insurance, Workers' Compensation insurance, and your own insurance should be considered as possible sources of compensation for your environmental medical care expenses.

Various insurers can have marked differences in approach and attitude. Examine the written and implied limitations of your own personal and your school's insurance policies. What will the company not reimburse, and why? Schools have limited umbrella policies that cover accidental injuries—for example, related to a child who falls and is hurt on a school playground. Coverage for environmental illness, however, can be another issue.

If your school's or your own insurance policy specifically states that environmental medical care is not covered, or if the policy has a "pollution exclusion" clause, you should be concerned. This clause will obviously diminish the school's fiscal responsibility for chemical problems occurring on its property. There is considerable dispute in legal terms as to what constitutes "pollution." In general, if there is any chance of interpreting a child's medical situation in favor of the insurance company, the company will deny coverage.

The rules can change in the middle of an insurance dispute, so it helps to know exactly what your original policy states. Read the fine print. If you need a copy, you can call the insurance company for one, but make your request in writing, so there is a record. If you can't interpret the insurance policy, check with a contract lawyer.

A ONE-YEAR-OLD INFANT

Ashford

In the case of the infant Ashford, an inordinate delay in providing a copy of his insurance policy proved to be the key for his parents' reimbursement. This one-year-old had constant wheezing, repeated infections, and frequent hospitalizations. His first year's medical expenses totaled $35,000. The insurance company paid all these charges even though the baby did not improve.

Within days after Ashford received environmental medical care, he was so well that steroids were discontinued and other daily medications were rarely needed. However, his insurance company refused to pay for this care because certain required permission procedures had not been followed prior to his emergency consultation. His parents finally received reimbursement, but not because the child was helped. Rather, they were paid solely because their employer had not provided them with a copy of their insurance contract within a specified period of time!

While some insurance companies partially or fully honor their obligation to reimburse patients and/or physicians for treatment of legitimate illness, others fail to do so. Some use excuses that are weak and arbitrary (yet legal and quasi-justifiable) to refuse payment. So you must file all claims in *exactly* the correct manner, or a rejection can be valid. If you have been denied reimbursement, read your health insurance policy carefully. Pay close attention to any ways in which you can appeal any negative decisions.

It is totally unfair that when some individuals finally locate a physician who can successfully treat them, they must discontinue this care because their insurance company denies coverage. Is it possible that powerful special-interest medical groups, who lose money because of competition for the same patients, can negatively influence the decisions of insurance companies?

■ TYPES OF MEDICAL INSURANCE

Before discussing insurance any further, you must understand certain general aspects of present-day medical insurance. There are two major types of insurance in the United States today. The frills vary, but the nuts and bolts are much the same.

TRADITIONAL INSURANCE

The traditional type of insurance does not require your physician to be a member of any plan or to accept assignments. You are able to choose your doctor, and all medical decisions about your care are made by this physician alone. The result is simple. You pay your insurance premiums, your insurance company reimburses you, and you pay your doctor. The insurance company will probably pay you if the doctor's charges are reasonable. This type of insurance is much costlier than the newer kind. In addition, if the insurance company fails to reimburse you, you can take more legal action, at least theoretically, if, for some reason, you are prohibited from selecting your physician and choosing the type of medical care you want.

MANAGED CARE

In the newer form of medical insurance called managed care, you typically pay less and you have relatively unlimited, inexpensive access to a highly specified form of medical care. You must select your physician from a list of your plan's members, and he or she, in turn, usually must accept the agreed set policies and fees for specified allowed services under the managed group plan. In this system the physician's fees are typically lower than traditional fees. In addition, physicians are restricted, even monitored, as to what they can and cannot do. They are told when, why, and to which specialists they can refer you, which drugs they can or cannot order, and how often and how long each medication can be given.

Because of the time and cost, an in-depth study of your complicated medical history and records, however necessary, may be totally unrealistic. In practice, this means that symptomatic drug therapy is usually the first line of treatment. The drugs prescribed by HMOs (health maintenance organizations) are often sharply limited to the less expensive "generic" medications. Costly diagnostic tests and referrals for extensive consultations are often discouraged or inordinately delayed. Because HMO-like facilities are primarily in the *business* of medicine, their major emphasis is unquestionably cost containment. For most patients, managed care is certainly helpful, but for those who require special attention and more time, it can fail to provide the needed treatment. If you are unhappy with your care, be aware that an appeal or review process is available to you.

Some HMOs have a "gatekeeper" policy, which means that the physicians who participate in the plan are strictly regulated. If a doctor does not follow the rules exactly, he or she can be dropped. Physicians who do exactly as they are told and as big business dictates are rewarded. To reduce costs, certain managed care groups collect an "incentive to comply" pot of money that is split among the member doctors, *after business expenses*, at the end of each year. This system makes it possible for the HMO, not the doctor, to make the final decisions relating to each patient's medical care.

■ TAKING LEGAL ACTION WITH TRADITIONAL INSURANCE

In essence, traditional insurance gives you some choices. If your insurance company refuses to pay for treatment of an environmental illness you should first request a complete copy of the insurance contract between you and your employer or between you and your insurance company. If the company will deny coverage for certain routine diagnostic measures and treatment, the policy must state explicitly that certain procedures are not covered. Unless exclusions are specifically spelled out in the policy, the legal obligation tends to fall on the insurance company to cover the legitimate costs of diagnosis and treatment. Check the policy for time restrictions concerning when action can be taken.

If your contract has no specific exclusion, the legal obligation to pay for such costs can fall upon your insurance company. If the company fails to pay, you can take them to small claims court to demand that your health care expenses be covered. Call your local court system to find out where court hearings are held and what maximum claim is allowed in small claims court. (In some states the total bill can't be over three thousand dollars, for example. Your local court can tell you the maximum amount for your area.) You do not need a lawyer to file in small claims court, but you may need your physician to appear as an expert medical witness.

Make sure that you have exhausted all administrative remedies before you pursue the legal route. Case law shows that it is possible for a patient to successfully sue an insurance company for legitimate health care reasons. A growing number of patients have been successful in doing so. For information on how to take action in small claims court and the results of such actions, see Resources.

Since insurance is contractual, any legitimate claim essentially involves a breach of contract. For better or worse, the written policy is controlling. If your particular medical problem is specifically not excluded in the policy, as we have seen, the courts will generally construe this "ambiguity" in your favor. However, insurance law has become a subspecialty in the practice of law. There are many gray areas regarding insurance issues and related laws and regulations. It is often possible to obtain a "declaratory judgment" that states that an entire course of treatment or type of claim is covered, past, present, and future. If a case is complicated and involves a significant amount of money or a protracted course of treatment, contact an attorney who is knowledgeable in insurance law (see Resources).

In some states insurance companies are allowed to "bump" claims up from small claims court to a civil court. This step can intimidate a patient because civil courts require lawyers, juries, and so on. If this happens to you, you can go to the judge in your local civil court and ask for a bench trial. This means that the judge will be both judge and jury and will decide on the merits of a case. Here again, you do not need a lawyer to represent you if your treating physician will agree to be an expert medical witness. Some insurance companies will not challenge this legal maneuver and may even back down. On your own, you must have the fortitude to press on if you know you are right. With the participation of your attending physician, you may ultimately win.

In general, the courts have upheld the principle that medical necessity is determined by the treating physician, not by an insurance company. Contract law is complicated, but doubts, ambiguities, or uncertainties arising from the language in a policy may sometimes be resolved in your favor.

> The purpose of health insurance companies should be to pay honest claims, not to decide what kind of medicine individuals can receive.

■ THE SCHOOL'S RESPONSIBILITY

All school districts carry insurance to compensate for injuries that arise on school grounds. Depending upon the rules in your district, a school principal, superintendent, school board, or state education department may be culpable for an injury. Ask your attorney to check with the school's lawyer. Perhaps the school will obviate the need for litigation by asking its insurance representative for reimbursement.

State education and health departments have general guidelines and suggestions to investigate the indoor air quality in schools but without mandates or laws, they lack the authority to take meaningful action. It appears that when their suggestions or guidelines have not been followed, they are not forced to pay for illnesses created by school exposures.

It is not always easy to determine when and how seriously a health department should be concerned if one or a few students become ill. From a medical viewpoint, someone must decide if the health problem is non-school-related or partially school-related. A single student or teacher who warns that something is awry may possibly help defuse a potentially serious situation, as Canadian schools have repeatedly demonstrated (see

Chapter 12). Realistically, however, schools and health departments tend to discount complaints when only one or a few individuals claim environmental illness. (The validity of an illness is more readily accepted if a member of a school official's family is that single exception.)

The onus of responsibility may actually be borne by:

■ The individuals who brought harmful chemicals into the school or who installed products incorrectly. They and/or the manufacturer may be culpable for their actions, the selection of merchandise, or the workmanship. They typically claim they only did what they were told.

■ The school principals, supervisors, and school district administrators. They may say that their decisions were approved by the school board.

■ The school board members. They sometimes have insurance to help protect them in relation to their decisions.

A realistic concern is that the key players—that is, the principal, superintendent, and the board members—will no longer hold the same position years from now, when the litigation takes place. Because it can take many years for the long-term health effects of an exposure to become fully evident and because the litigation process is so lengthy, action cannot be taken when children and teachers have become ill.

The bottom line in much of today's society is economics, and responsibility for school health or indoor air quality problems often lie with those who have a vested or monetary interest. From a purely financial outlook, if a sick teacher is able to resume work or a child is no longer ill, the insurance company saves money. What logical explanation can there be for their lack of sincere interest? All too often, appropriate medical care is delayed and/or denied because no one wants to accept the responsibility for school-related health problems. Someone must face these issues squarely, so that the health and brains of the present and future generations are protected.

The keys to recovery for environmentally ill students and teachers are:

• prompt, appropriate, and thorough care from a physician who knows environmental medicine
• immediate antidotal treatment for toxic exposures
• baseline comprehensive diagnostic tests and treatment
• appropriate follow-up monitoring of both the patient and the school building.

■ YOUR INSURANCE COMPANY'S RESPONSIBILITY

Insurance reimbursement issues are critical for people with environmental illness because appropriate treatment usually requires physicians with special expertise. Some injured individuals absolutely require a most comprehensive, and at times costly, diagnostic and treatment program, or they will not improve. Instead, they will continue to become ill because of unavoidable slight exposures to innumerable chemicals.

If your insurance company does not pay your claim for environmental medical care, contact the company, either by phone or by mail, and explain your concerns. Document or tape-record all discussions and statements (with permission, if required in your state) so that you can more accurately remember the details. In general, to learn what must be done to have your claim paid, you will have to advance through the insurance company's hierarchy to find a supervisor. Comply completely with their rules, but repeatedly emphasize what is cost-effective. Further a model for a basic letter to an insurance company is outlined on Table 17.1.

Everyone theoretically wins if the underlying causes of a health problem are found and eliminated. The result should be a decreased need for drugs, along with any associated side effects. Acute flare-ups of illness reuiring costly emergency room or office visits, specialist consultations, surgeries, and hospitalizations should diminish. If the causes are not found and eliminated, some patients will unquestionably be left with permanent medical illness.

A TWENTIETH-CENTURY ENIGMA

Why do most major health insurers not pay for environmental medical care, when it can improve the health of the insured and save the insurance company money?

HOW CAN YOU SUPPORT YOUR CASE?

After you read your policy carefully, go through any appeal procedures that it suggests. If you are unsure about your rights or possible remedies, contact a lawyer.[1]

The following questions may be asked during an appeal (or in arbitration, mediation, or trial discussions) relative to an insurance denial:[2]

■ *Was the insurance company's decision-making process fair?* Did an experienced physician, nurse, or other medical professional specifically make

---

TABLE 17.1

Suggestions for Insurance Company Letter

Dear [name of insurance company]:

1. List your general health problems.
2. Compare:
   a. the present cost and number of doctor visits, drugs, and other expenses with those you incurred during the previous two or so years.
   b. the number of consultations, emergency room treatments, and hospitalizations, before and after EI treatment.
3. Generalize how well you have responded to your present EM treatment compared with previous forms of treatment.
4. List how many doctors—including specialists, such as allergists, neurologists, psychiatrists, psychologists, and counselors—you saw prior to your consultation with an EM physician, and what they charged. How long were you on their treatment? How many doctors and how much treatment do you need now? What are your present costs?
5. If questions arise regarding your choice of therapy, offer to show a videotape of significant reactions to allergy extract testing. Videotape yourself or your child before and after school. Show obvious differences in appearance, breathing, behavior, and writing. Label everything with dates and exact times. Check with your lawyer before submitting about this documentation.
6. Enclose the list of studies that have documented the efficacy of the type of therapy your child received (see the allergy testing studies listed in For Further Reading).

---

the decision not to pay? What is the name, or names, of the decision-maker(s)? It is extremely important to obtain a copy of all documents upon which the company based its decision to deny your claim. Insurance carriers will strenuously resist revealing all pertinent information, but ultimately they are obligated to do so. If they call in an "independent medical expert" to review your claim and/or examine you, you are also entitled to a copy of that report. At times, it is difficult to determine whether such individuals are truly "expert" or truly "independent." Attorneys who practice in the personal injury field know from experience whether the conclusions made by an "independent" examiner routinely tend to be biased or not.

▪ *Were the insurance decision-makers truly familiar with the environmental medical technique?* For example, one insurance company's physician admitted that nurses, not physicians, decide who will and will not be reimbursed. It was only nurses, not physicians, who read and critiqued the double-blinded studies on the efficacy of environmental medical procedures that a patient had submitted with her claim.

▪ *Were the decision-makers familiar with* all *the pertinent medical literature?* Did they properly evaluate favorable as well as unfavorable studies of environmental medical procedures? For example, did they read the Davidoff-Fogarty article on MCS and preexisting psychological illness?[3] Did they consider the key articles comparing the efficacy of environmental medical methods? (see "Studies of Allergy Testing" in For Further Reading).

■ *Were the studies that were used to deny payment current and of a high caliber? Or was the rejection based on position papers and editorials?* Position papers are merely opinions, often prepared by competing specialty physician groups. They are not scientific studies. They can contain biased, deceptive, incomplete, and incorrect information about critical issues. If you find that the company based its denial upon published studies that were unfavorable to environmental medicine, try to find out who paid, directly or indirectly, for the research. Studies paid for by the sugar or food industry, for example, tend to conclude that sugar does not cause hyperactivity.

■ *Did an outside medical "expert" render an opinion?* Was that "expert" qualified in terms of training and clinical experience? An allergist is not an environmental medical specialist unless he or she is also trained or board certified in environmental medicine. Inquire if the "expert" had ever observed, been trained in, or tried P/N allergy testing.

■ *Was the "expert" impartial?* Did that individual have a direct or indirect economic interest in the denial of your claim?

■ *Was the denial sensible?* The medical director of a local division of a large insurance company confided to the author that P/N allergy treatment simply takes "too much time." And therefore is too costly. Could this be a significant reason to deny claims for this type of medical care? While this argument may make economic sense to insurance companies in the short run, it makes no sense in terms of patients' long-term health.

■ *Did the insurer act within a reasonable amount of time?* Sometimes an insurance company will repeatedly flood a patient and/or physician with paperwork. The forms are completed and returned, but the insurance company claims it never received them. Such delaying tactics usually precede a reimbursement denial. Don't allow your insurance company to catch you in this web. Send all forms by certified mail, with return receipt requested.

Environmentally ill individuals need immediate medical care because unnecessary delays can seriously impair or impede their degree of recovery. Insurance companies that deny timely appropriate medical care should be held responsible. Delaying tactics unquestionably can increase their own expenses because some insured patients ultimately become more seriously ill and incapacitated as a result of these maneuvers.

■ INSURANCE COMPANIES' RELUCTANCE TO PAY FOR ENVIRONMENTAL MEDICAL CARE

One reason that insurance companies tend to refuse to pay claims for MCS treatment and other environmental medical care is that their advisers do not recognize MCS and/or EI.

MULTIPLE CHEMICAL SENSITIVITIES

Environmental medical physicians who routinely see MCS in their patients find it difficult to believe that others do not recognize it as an obvious illness.[4] Yet many medical professionals are unaware, uninformed, or misinformed about MCS, or they are so closed-minded they simply refuse to consider the possibility.[5] They often discount the complaints of MCS sufferers because of what they were taught (or not taught) in medical school. Medical students learn, for example, that a multiplicity of symptoms, particularly in a female patient, typically indicates a psychological illness; a 1994 review article clearly refuted this common misconception.[6] Having many symptoms is the norm for children as well as adults with MCS.

The medical literature began to discuss chemical sensitivities as long ago as the 1880s. Since then, innumerable scientific articles and books for physicians as well as the general public, have been published concerning this problem both here and abroad. Recently the Americans with Disabilities Act, along with several government agencies, have acknowledged MCS to be a medical illness under certain circumstances.[7] Fortunately, an expanding number of physicians, in America as well as abroad, are accepting MCS as a diagnosis. As a result, vast numbers of individuals have finally recognized the source of their illness and received successful treatment.

> The crux of MCS is not whether a person was exposed to chemical is present at an "accepted, tolerated" level, but whether that particular individual can tolerate that level of that chemical. What makes some individuals ill, will not necessarily affect others.

The amount of a chemical that causes a reaction in chemically sensitive people usually is considerably less than the amount recognized as unsafe.[8] A major reason for a discrepancy is that nonchemically sensitive individuals neither smell nor become ill from exceedingly low levels. In contrast, chemically sensitized people not only perceive but quickly become genuinely ill from exceedingly minute amounts of an ever-growing number of chemicals. Moreover, the amount of a chemical that causes symptoms varies not only from individual to individual, but in different periods of an individual's life, the amount of exposure needed to cause symptoms can change.

Most doctors are unaware that many objective tests can show physiological abnormalities in MCS patients. An authority on MCS, Grace Ziem, M.D., has stated, "Laboratory abnormalities have been demonstrated in so many parameters in chemically sensitive patients that the physician's difficulty now is to select the best tests, that is those which are more sensitive, specific, and best correlate with the clinical status and prognosis. There is no difficulty demonstrating abnormalities unless one does not conduct tests on specific organ systems shown to be abnormal in MCS patients."[9]

Some insurance companies discount MCS as well as the tests used to document it. This attitude is most difficult to understand, when the following procedures can show damage to the nervous or immune system:

■ a physical examination
■ neuropsychological testing
■ brain imaging or tomography
■ certain immune function blood studies
■ blinded P/N allergy testing
■ blinded chemical testing in a glass chamber
■ various tests for organ damage
■ tests for toxicological damage
■ initial and follow-up pesticide screening tests
■ properly conducted bioassay tests on mice

This negative attitude seems particularly illogical since a large number of patients who remained ill after undergoing more traditional, expensive, and drug-oriented treatments obviously have regained their health after receiving environmental medical care.[10]

Ironically, some individuals who have problems with carpets have lost their legal battles because they have been told they do not have a chemical sensitivity. When they try to obtain medical insurance, however, it is denied because they have a chemical sensitivity. This no-win unjustifiable situation has caused many frustrated environmentally ill people to suffer for years with progressively deteriorating health and dwindling, meager finances.[11]

In *Toxic Carpet III* Glenn Beebe recounts real-life health insurance MCS battles. He explains the common pitfalls and cautions that you must understand them if you hope to win when your illness is related to a toxic carpet exposure.[12]

In spite of the inordinate lag time, both the traditional medical establishment and the insurance companies are beginning to listen—but only because the public is demanding that they do so. The preponderance of evidence appears to have almost reached a critical mass. Changes in attitude, despite heavily vested economic interests, are becoming apparent.

One of the first indications that someone is listening is the availability of a new type of medical insurance. A number of alternative health care plans are being offered to subscribers throughout the United States. Their members are allowed to see "any licensed physicians acting within the scope of their license to treat any illness or injury or to provide preventive services." That is, they can see physicians who use acupuncture, homeopathy, naturopathy, chiropractic, traditional Chinese medicine, or Indian ayurvedic medicine. Some of these plans pay for a limited amount of homeopathic and herbal remedies per year but refuse to pay for vitamins. Most require a one-year waiting period before they will cover preexisting conditions.[13] Americans certainly deserve not only a choice of medical care but a choice of physicians.

ENVIRONMENTAL MEDICINE

Approximately 3,500 physicians, both in the United States and abroad, now practice various aspects of environmental medicine. Many are board certified in two or more medical specialties. The vast majority (2,500) are ear, nose, and throat specialists. A few progressive medical osteopathic schools now offer lectures about EM in their curriculum.

The American Medical Association (AMA) has approved the training courses in environmental medicine for continuing medical education credits. They have an approved curriculum, including both written and oral examinations.

Because the basic concepts of environmental medicine are being atztacked, you should have a complete understanding of them in your dealings with your insurance company. With this knowledge you can provide lucid, logical counterexplanations when necessary.[14]

It is difficult to understand why there is any disagreement over environmental medicine. It can provide many answers because it impacts on so many other medical specialties since dust, molds, pollen, foods, and chemicals can potentially adversely affect any part of the human body. Many times in the past, drug therapy was the only answer because the cause was so elusive. In contrast, EM physicians stress educating patients to detect and eliminate the cause of their illness, as well as to make dietary changes, take nutritional supplements, and use allergy extract therapy. This approach markedly decreases the need for symptomatic drug treatment. It enables people to feel well, sometimes for the first time in years.

WHY ARE ENVIRONMENTAL MEDICAL INSURANCE CLAIMS REJECTED?
Sometimes insurance companies deny claims for environmental medical treatment because too few studies have been published in peer-reviewed journals that support this form of therapy. Such published studies are desirable because they are admissible in courts of law. Medical journals, however, can be selectively edited and biased. Advertisements from drug companies pay the bulk of expenses for the production of medical journals. The medical scientists who decide which articles to accept or reject are often the same ones who do research for pharmaceutical companies. If you were an editor or reviewer for a medical journal, routinely paid to evaluate drug therapy, would you be more inclined to publish an article about the effectiveness of a drug that you or a friend had studied, or one explaining the effectiveness of a short, simple diet?

At various levels, such conflicts of interest seriously impede the publication and dissemination of environmental medical research. (The author once received a letter from the editor of a prominent allergy journal rejecting a single-case report of an extremely ill child who had rapidly improved with a short diet and P/N allergy treatment. Among other things, the editor wrote that one reviewer was so upset with the article that he said, "I feel so strongly about it that if [the journal] publishes it, I would give careful consideration to resigning from the editorial board." The article was eventually published in the *Medical Journal of Australia*.)

In *Newsweek* for September 14, 1992, an article discussed censorship in scientific publications. It gave examples of obvious bias and suppression, including medical journal reviewers who purposely repress information because they are "uneasy about informing people" about a problem. For example, papers linking fluorescent light to leukemia, linking bladder and rectal cancer to chlorine in drinking water, and linking bone cancer in rats to fluoride were rejected because of the frightening content, not science.

D. Downing and S. Davies discuss the repression of knowledge in medicine in their insightful article in the *Journal of Nutritional Medicine*.[15] They quote a statement of medical ethics made in the Declaration of Helsinki:

In the treatment of a sick person, the physician must be free to use a new diagnostic or therapeutic measure, if in his or her judgment it offers hope of saving life, re-establishing health, or alleviating suffering.

In spite of all that is written, the safe restoration of a patient's health must be given priority, at all times, over considerations of whether a procedure is "proven."[16]

■ REBUTTALS TO INSURANCE COMPANY REJECTIONS

In their denials of medical coverage on the basis of a lack of "science," various insurance companies have labeled environmental medicine as "not customary, unreasonable, experimental, investigational, unproven, anecdotal, or controversial." They tend to ignore the patients' previous poor response to traditional treatments, as well as factors of prevention, safety, and cost containment. They also fail to consider that fewer than half of current medical treatments are "proven" to the satisfaction of medical scientists and that at least a third of all Americans are presently seeking and using alternative medical therapies.

Let us critically examine, in turn, each of the eight labels that insurance companies apply to environmental medicine.

1. IS ENVIRONMENTAL MEDICINE "NOT CUSTOMARY"?

Environmental medicine specialists are certainly guilty of practicing noncustomary medicine. Contrary to customary practices, they often spend hours taking a patient's medical history, doing a physical examination, and studying his or her past medical records. How often does a conventional doctor spend one or two hours with one patient? One study showed that only two percent of hospitalized patient histories contained information about their toxic exposures, their former occupations, or even the duration of their employment.[17] Undoubtedly this aspect of patients' histories needs more serious consideration. It is both customary and routine for EM physicians to ask for such information and at times spend hours on one patient.

Nor is it customary, unfortunately, for physicians to check nutritional factors. One publication indicates that 90 percent of physicians fail to check for a magnesium deficiency in hospitalized patients,[18] even though it is estimated that about 50 percent have this problem.[19] EM physicians know about magnesium; they also recognize that zinc helps tissues heal and that C and B vitamins help restore and preserve health. They would routinely order these for patients *in advance of surgery*. Again, this is not customary medicine.

It is customary for most physicians to treat patients with appropriate drugs. They customarily do not emphasize finding and eliminating the causes of recurrent ear infections, migraine, arthritis, asthma, nose allergies, tics, bed-wetting, epilepsy, nephrosis, colitis, and so on. EM specialists frequently help these types of problems because they routinely emphasize the detection of unrecognized causes of illness[20]—namely, allergenic substances, foods, and chemicals.

Unsuspected environmental or dietary factors may well be related to the present inordinate rise in deaths in asthmatic children. This consideration is not customary, but maybe it should be. One seven-year-old in our clinic wheezes so badly that he must be rushed to the hospital if he steps outside too soon after the lawn-care truck sprays on his street. Many customary physicians are unaware of the dangers of such herbicide exposures.

Many patients seen by EM physicians have previously received customary treatment from other specialists but have not been helped. It is perplexing that insurance companies routinely pay for treatments that fail to help patients, yet refuse to pay for treatments that relieve the patients' symptoms and need for medication.

2. IS ENVIRONMENTAL MEDICINE "UNREASONABLE"?

Is it unreasonable to emphasize that the cause of an illness should be found and eliminated? Is it unreasonable to recognize the role of foods in health, especially when this role has been reported in the medical literature for more than seventy years?[21] Is it unreasonable to individualize therapy because each person is different? These fundamental principles have been part of environmental medicine for almost fifty years.

Environmental medical allergy testing using provocation/neutralization is not a "new kid on the block." It has been used for over thirty-five years.[22] Scientifically, SET (serial end-point titration) is well-documented. The AMA has published that it is an effective, useful, and scientific method for quantifying a sensitivity.[23] This testimony removes any questions about its reasonableness. *Amazingly, insurance companies do not approve of P/N testing, even though it is very similar to SET but more specific, precise, and informative.*

Why would insurance companies be willing to pay for allergy testing of many items at once but not for more precise P/N testing with one item at a time? The answer should not be that the former is faster. P/N testing can be justifiably accused of being much too time-consuming. The time, however, is well spent, because this testing often enables a physician to pinpoint the specific cause(s) of each symptom. How can a method be considered unreasonable if it enables the doctor and the patient to recognize specific causes more clearly? Why does evaluating a patient's skin-test site, pulse, breathing, appearance, actions, and handwriting between each dilution of allergy extract make an allergy test nonreimbursable? Another distinct advantage of P/N allergy extract treatment is that it can be administered at home, saving time and money. The fact that frequent office visits for allergy extract are not necessary should make this method preferred, not "unreasonable."

Is it unreasonable to acknowledge that every cell in our bodies needs certain essential nutrients? If the body needs magnesium for about three hundred intermediate metabolic processes and zinc for sixty, is it unreasonable to check the levels of these minerals in chronically ill patients? If magnesium is needed for proper heart functioning and is deficient in at least 40 percent of heart attack patients,[24] is it unreasonable to check its level in cardiac emergencies and prescribe it if indicated? Is it unreasonable to believe that if nutrients make the immune system stronger they might help those who have weakened immune systems? Yet many insurance companies routinely deny claims for nutritional evaluations by environmental or medical physicians, and others, even though the detection and treatment of biochemical deficiencies can improve the quality of some lives and in some situations, save lives, as well as money.

If a patient has had multiple evaluations by innumerable specialists without finding relief, how can it be unreasonable for an EM physician to make the effort to determine the causes of the illness? For that matter, how can it be reasonable for an insurance company to penalize both patient and doctor by nonpayment in spite of a successful response to treatment?

It would definitely be unreasonable for any EM physician to promise patients a cure. But the vast majority certainly will not make such promises. The initial fees for EM care can be high, but that is not unreasonable in view of the time required to properly evaluate the history, do a thorough physical examination and then test, teach, and treat each patient.

The outcome of many illnesses often depends upon the following:

- If the cause of an illness is found and eliminated,
- If biochemical nutrient deficiencies are corrected, and
- If therapy is individualized,

If this is done, it is possible to improve the patient's health and reduce or eliminate the need for drug therapy.

ISN'T THIS WHAT MEDICINE SHOULD BE ABOUT?

---

3. IS ENVIRONMENTAL MEDICINE "EXPERIMENTAL AND INVESTIGATIONAL"?

An experiment is a test, a trial, or a tentative procedure. The label "experimental" is hardly applicable to environmental medicine, when so many studies have long since verified its efficacy, and when it has been in use for over fifty years (see the section on allergy testing in For Further Reading). Ironically, insurance companies even deny payment for inexpensive diagnostic diets, which are often helpful in a few days.[25]

To make it even more perplexing insurance companies do make payment for procedures that are patently experimental. They pay for the treatment of symptom-free HIV infection with zidovudine, for example, even though this drug has shown no statistically significant or clinically documented benefits. Asthma treatment with methacholine inhalation was ineffective but covered.[26] Insurance companies routinely pay for drugs that are known to be ineffective, as well as for many whose mechanism of action is unknown. EM specialists, by contrast, pride themselves on needing few or no drugs to treat EI patients. On what basis do insurance companies make their exceptions?

As we have seen, EM specialists use basically the same allergy extract for testing as do traditional allergists. Yet very careful testing with one item at a time in 1:5 dilutions is called experimental, while less precise testing with innumerable allergens at one time in 1:10 dilutions is not. Monitoring each patient's skin-test site, pulse, breathing, appearance, symptoms, and handwriting should be described not as "experimental" but as "desirable, more precise, beneficial, and worthy of emulation."

The potentially sensitizing chemical phenol is commonly used as a preservative in the diluting fluid used to prepare patients' allergy extract solutions. Many EM specialists no longer use it. This is not experimental; it is a precaution to prevent the development of a sensitivity to this ubiquitous chemical[27] (see the phenol table in the Appendix).

4. IS ENVIRONMENTAL MEDICINE "UNPROVEN AND ANECDOTAL"?

What proof is required to give a medical specialty the label of legitimate? How many scientific studies in humans and animals are needed? The environmental medical literature is so extensive that it is ludicrous to state that EM is unproven. Since the 1920s articles and books have been published on the physical and behavioral effects of foods and allergenic substances.[28] Similarly, the diverse effects of chemicals on human health have been noted and written since the 1940s.[29] To date, innumerable diet, controlled and single- or double-blinded sublingual treatment, and subcutaneous treatment studies have shown that P/N allergy treatment is helpful.[30] One study has even substantiated the efficacy of EM allergy treatment on asthmatic horses.[31] How many more studies are needed before its efficacy is considered proven? Articles that refute these methods are often flawed methodologically[32] or biased in other ways.

Excellent texts for physicians have been written by Drs. Theron Randolph, Herbert Rinkel, Joseph Miller, William Rea, and Jonathan Brostoff.[33] The four encyclopedic volumes of *Chemical Sensitivity* by William Rea,

M.D., provide a wealth of essential information and a plethora of references. This entire issue is also frankly discussed for the public in Nicholas Ashford and Claudia Miller's *Chemical Exposures: Low Levels and High Stakes* and Bonnye L. Matthews's *Chemical Sensitivity*.[34]

5. IS ENVIRONMENTAL MEDICINE "CONTROVERSIAL"?

Differences of opinion should be possible in medicine without the newer approaches being labeled "controversial," implying that they are wrong. Admittedly, it can be difficult at first to distinguish a genuine medical advance from a new idea that has no merit. Environmental medicine is certainly not a panacea. But if it succeeds where traditional medicine has failed, maybe there should be rejoicing, emulation, and reflection rather than resistance and disbelief. Perhaps we should adopt the Chinese system and pay physicians only when a patient gets well. Which therapy will enable sick children to return to school and learn? What treatment will make it possible for ill teachers to resume teaching?

Many illnesses are diagnosed and treated without the basic mechanisms of the disease or the treatment being fully understood. Patients who have chemical, food, and environmental sensitivities should not be sacrificed in a debate that has so many financial implications. Quite simply, insurance and government benefits should be based on defined functional disabilities. What can the patient no longer do as a result of his or her illness?

While traditional allergy medicine is unquestionably helpful, it is more limited and less precise then environmental medicine. The restrictive present-day definition of what constitutes an allergy can miss the true scope of allergies and their causes. If traditional allergists don't accept that it is possible to diagnose and successfully treat allergies by testing one item at a time with different dilutions of allergy extracts, they have probably never personally observed, properly learned, or adequately tried it. That is their choice, but insurance companies should not be influenced by medical controversy to exclude payment for methods that are proven to be helpful and safe, especially if those who disagree are caring and competing for the same type of patients. Admittedly, the complex neuro-immuno-endocrine-physiological implications of environmental illness are not fully under-

Payment by insurance companies should be dependent not on opinion-based "position papers" written by competing medical specialists but on whether the patient is ill and the physician is qualified to treat the illness.

stood. However, the successful, safe responses of patients treated with an environmental medical approach are abundant. Unequivocal documentation shows that physiological and immune abnormalities in many chemically sensitive individuals can significantly improve after EM treatment.[35]

If the right dose of an allergy extract prevents, improves, or stops a patient's symptoms, in spite of continued exposure, is he or she not better? If a patient suddenly requires little or no drug therapy, is that not an improvement? Isn't such healing what medicine is all about? The fact that we can't explain why the human body is smarter than physicians is really not the issue.

The existence of environmental illness is presently gaining greater acceptance in the United States and abroad. The fact that this more precise method takes more time should not be a consideration for insurance reimbursement. Yet insurance companies still do not realize how much they have to gain by making it totally reimbursable. It is most perplexing that they reject a method that reduces medical costs while improving the health of their clients. Is it possible that insurers somehow gain more when patients use more drugs or are hospitalized?

When decisions regarding insurance reimbursement are investigated, examples of major inconsistencies, misinformation, and poor judgment are plentiful. Some decisions appear to be arbitrary, grossly contradictory, and illogical. Some companies claim that their decisions follow a standard national policy rather than an isolated local one. Yet the same major insurance companies will pay well in some parts of the country and poorly in others for the same environmental medical care. On what basis do they discriminate? Parents have reported that some insurance companies will pay for the medical care of a child for months, then suddenly stop the payments, and then after some time, resume reimbursement again for no apparent reason. At times, payments are made for one child and not for another—even when the children are from the same family and underwent the same allergy tests on the same day. When parents point out such obvious inconsistencies and inequities, they have been told that the previous payments were made in error. If the family seeks payment for the second child, they are intimidated and told that they will have to reimburse the previous payments for the first child. (Check with your lawyer if this happens.)

6. IS ENVIRONMENTAL MEDICINE PREVENTATIVE?

Most people will agree that the prevention of illness is a reasonable, highly desirable goal of medicine. Even insurance companies obviously believe in it, since they pay for coronary bypass surgery. They pay for stress tests before a heart attack, appendix surgery before a rupture, Pap smears before cervical cancer, and drugs to prevent strokes from increased blood pressure and cholesterol. A basic tenet of EM is prevention. Why is it not covered?

Moreover, insurance companies refuse to pay for nutrients that appear to help relieve many major illnesses caused by the oxidation of free radicals (see Chapter 15). If only 100 I.U. of vitamin E can decrease the risk of a stroke or vascular accident by 50 percent, why isn't it covered?[36]

Why do insurance companies arbitrarily refuse to pay for the time physicians spend teaching a patient how to eliminate or better tolerate an offending exposure? Why would patient education not be a priority concept in insurance coverage? If patients are educated about the cause of their illness, they can avoid future exposure and illness. They can learn to recognize impending flare-ups earlier, which can avoid hospitalization. Although it is faster to write a prescription for a drug, prevention is really the best form of medicine and is unquestionably both cost-and health-effective on a short- and long-term basis.

7. IS ENVIRONMENTAL MEDICINE SAFE?

Proven fatalities due to environmental medical care are rare, but they have occurred. Despite this record of safety, payment for environmental medicine claims is denied. In the past thirty years there have been at least thirty deaths associated with *traditional* allergy injection therapy in the United States. Other deaths are mentioned in the foreign literature.[37] According to Dr. Jean Monro, in the British Isles, the routine use of traditional allergy injection therapy is not allowed unless cardio-resuscitation equipment is available, and each patient must wait one to two hours after the injection.[38] If the safety of P/N allergy treatment is not in question in the United States, why is there discrimination against a safer form of therapy?

Although safety is said to be a key issue, insurance companies routinely cover certain unequivocally risky, unproven techniques. Costly transplants and high-dose chemotherapy for cancer are paid for, even though they are admittedly fraught with more than an element of danger. Such inconsistencies are difficult to explain.

8. IS ENVIRONMENTAL MEDICINE COST-EFFECTIVE?

An analysis in England by Jonathan Brostoff, M.D., an eminent immunologist and author, indicates that environmental medicine can markedly decrease or eliminate the need for drugs, office visits, and hospitalizations. He presents data showing that England could save millions of pounds by using it.[39] Why are American insurance companies not interested? Why are the politicians not listening?

Let us consider one common illness, cancer of the prostate. An insurance company will willingly pay $100,000 for treatment that involves surgery, chemotherapy, radiation, and hormones. With this therapy the patient has a median survival rate of six years. According to studies by J.P. Carter and colleagues, treatment using a macrobiotic diet entails minuscule costs, and the patient has a median survival rate of nineteen years.[40] Why isn't the latter treatment covered by insurance?

> **A** most perplexing question: It appears that insurance companies, at times, choose to pay for medical care that perpetuates illness and the use of drugs in preference to care that prevents and/or diminishes illness and the need for drugs. We must respectfully ask *why?*

■ WHAT SHOULD INSURANCE COMPANIES DO?

Insurance carriers can help change the system by training their staff in insurance loss control. They can contain medical costs and illness by denying coverage to companies that cannot provide truly safe products. They can force companies to create clear and specific literature regarding their products' uses and dangers. They can demand nontoxic packaging. Similarly, they can insist on safe, clean air and water in homes, workplaces, and schools. They can flag those patients who have seen fifteen or more well-trained physicians without improvement and request an evaluation for chemical sensitization or neurotoxic damage. This is actually what our federal government should be doing, but insurance companies also have the power to effectively force changes to restore the health and vitality of the American public.

NOTES

1. Cindy Duering, "Medical and Legal Briefs, a Referenced Compendium of Chemical Injury," available from Environmental Access Research Network (see Resources).

2. Earon S. Davis, "Insurance Reimbursement Challenges and Environmental Medicine," *Environmental Physician* (Spring 1992) pp. 21–22; available from The American Academy of Environmental Medicine (see Resources). See also D. Downing and S. Davies, "Allergy: Conventional and Alternative Concepts," A Critique of The Royal College of Physicians of London's Report, *Journal of Nutritional Medicine*, vol. 3 (1992), pp. 331–39.

3. Ann L. Davidoff and Linda Fogarty, "Psychogenic Origins of Multiple Chemical Sensitivities Syndrome: A Critical Review of the Research Literature," *Archives of Environmental Health*, vol. 49, no. 5 (Sept./Oct. 1994), pp. 316–24. See also G. Ziem, "Multiple Chemical Sensitivity: Treatment and Follow-up with Avoidance and Control of Chemical Exposures," *Toxicology and Industrial Health*, vol. 8, no. 4 (1992), pp. 73–86; and the numerous reference articles on MCS are available from the Environmental Access Research Network (see Resources).

4. Ziem, "Multiple Chemical Sensitivity," and Environmental Access Research Network papers.

5. Davidoff and Fogarty, "Psychogenic Origins"; and AMA Council on Scientific Affairs, "Clinical Ecology," *Journal of the American Medical Association*, vol. 2687, no. 24 (Dec. 23–30, 1992), pp. 3465–67.

6. Davidoff and Fogarty, "Psychogenic Origins."

7. MCS Referral and Resources, *Recognition of Multiple Chemical Sensitivity* (Mar. 13, 1995); see Resources for address.

8. Nicholas A. Ashford and Claudia S. Miller, *Chemical Exposures: Low Levels and High Stakes* (New York: Van Nostrand Reinhold, 1991).

9. Ziem, "Multiple Chemical Sensitivity."

10. Sherry A. Rogers, *The Scientific Basis for Selected Environmental Medicine Techniques* (Sarasota, FL: SK Publishing, 1995), pp. 69–93.

11. *Toxic Law Reporter* (June 23, 1993), p. 72. See also the National Organization of Legal Advocates for the Environmentally Injured (see Resources).

12. Glenn Beebe, *Toxic Carpet III* (Cincinnati, OH: Glenn Beebe, 1991).

13. For more information, write to Alternative Health Plan, Box 6279, Thousand Oaks, CA 91359-6279, or call (800) 966–8467.

14. Iris R. Bell, *Clinical Ecology: A New Medical Approach to Environmental Illness* (Bolinas, CA: Common Knowledge Press, 1982).

15. Downing and Davies, "Allergy."

16. Downing and Davies, "Truth."

17. Rogers, *Scientific Basis*, p. 41.

18. R. Whang, *Journal of the American Medical Association*, vol. 2364 (June 13, 1990), pp. 3063–64.

19. Rogers, *Scientific Basis*, pp. 124–25.

20. Albert H. Rowe et al., "Food Allergy, Its Manifestation and Control and the Elimination Diets: A Compendium with Important Consideration of Inhalants (Especially Pollen)," *Drug and Infectant Allergy* (Springfield, IL: Charles C. Thomas, 1972); Joseph Miller, *Relief at Last!* (Springfield, IL: Charles C. Thomas, 1987); Jonathan Brostoff and J.J. Challacombe, *Food Allergy Intolerance* (London: Bailliere Tindall, 1987); Doris J. Rapp, *Is This Your Child?* (New York: William Morrow & Co., 1991); Doris J. Rapp, *The Impossible Child* (Buffalo, NY: Practical Allergy Research Foundation, 1989); Theron G. Randolph and R. Moss, *An Alternative Approach to Allergies* (New York: Harper & Row, 1989); Theron G. Randolph, *Human Ecology and Susceptibility to the Chemical Environment* (Springfield, IL: Charles C. Thomas, 1962); K. A. Ogle and J.D. Bullock, "Children with Allergic Rhinitis and/or Bronchial Asthma Treated with Elimination Diet: A Five-Year Follow Up," *Annals of Allergy*, vol. 44 (1980), p. 273; R.S. Panush et al., "Diet Therapy for Rheumatoid Arthritis," *Arthritis and Rheumatism*, vol. 26, no. 4 (1983), pp. 462–70; and Rogers, *Scientific Basis*.

21. Rowe, "Food Allergy."

22. W.P. King et al. "Provocation/Neutralization: A Two-Part Study. Part I: The Intracutaneous Provocative Food Test: A Multi-Center Comparison Study," *Otolaryngology: Head and Neck Surgery*, vol. 99, no. 3 (Sept. 1988), pp. 263–72; W. P. King et al., "Provocation/Neutralization: A Two-Part Study. Part II: Subcutaneous Neutralization Therapy: A Multi-Center Study," *Otolaryngology: Head and Neck Surgery*, vol. 99, no. 3 (Sept. 1988), pp. 272–78.

23. AMA Council on Scientific Affairs, "In Vivo Diagnostic Testing and Immunotherapy for Allergy. Report I, Part I; Part II, Report II of the Allergy Panel," *Journal of the American Medical Association*, vol. 358, no. 10 (Sept. 11, 1987), p. 1363; see also Rogers, *Scientific Basis*, p. 116.

24. C.B. Seelig, C.E. Montano, and J.E. Ranney, "Physician Recommendation of Magnesium Status in Patients with Coronary Artery Disease Admitted to a Regional Medical Center," *American Journal of Cardiology*, vol. 72 (July 15, 1993), pp. 226–27.

25. Rogers, *Scientific Basis*, p. 115.

26. Ibid.

27. C. Skea, D. McAvoy, and L. Broder, "Phenol Amplifies Complement-Fixing Activity and Induces IgG Precipitating Activity in Grain-Dust Extract," *Journal of Allergy and Clinical Immunology*,

vol. 81 (1988), pp. 557–63; and M.F. LaVia and D.S. LaVia, "Phenol Derivatives Are Immunosuppressive in Mice," *Drug and Chemical Toxicology*, vol. 2, nos. 1 and 2 (1979), pp. 167–77.

28. Rowe, "Food Allergy."

29. Randolph, *Human Ecology*.

30. David L.J. Freed, "Part I: The Provocation-Neutralization Technique. Part II: Can We Diagnose Allergies, Do We Know What We Are Doing, Does It Matter?" in *Food Intolerance*, ed. John Dobbing (London: Bailliere Tindall, 1987), pp. 151–84. See also the sources under "Allergy Testing" in For Further Reading.

31. S.A. Rogers, "Provocation-Neutralization of Cough and Wheezing in a Horse," *Clinical Ecology*, vol. 5, no. 4 (1987/1988), pp. 185–87.

32. Kendall A. Gerdes, "Provocation/Neutralization Testing: A Look at the Controversy," *Clinical Ecology*, vol. 6, no. 1 (1989), pp. 21–29; and D. L. Jewett et al., "A Double-Blind Study of Symptom Provocation to Determine Food Sensitivity," *New England Journal of Medicine*, vol. 323 (1990), pp. 429–33. See also Davidoff and Fogarty, "Psychogenic Origins."

33. Rea, *Chemical Sensitivity*; Brostoff and Challacombe, *Food Allergy Intolerance*; Randolph and Moss, *Alternative Approach*, Herbert J. Rinkel et al., *Food Allergy* (Springfield, IL: Charles C. Thomas, 1951); and J.B. Miller, *Relief at Last!* (Springfield, IL: Charles C. Thomas, 1987).

34. Bonnye L. Matthews, *Chemical Sensitivity* (Jefferson, NC: McFarland & Co., 1992); and Ashford and Miller, *Chemical Exposures*.

35. Ziem, "Multiple Chemical Sensitivity"; Rea, *Chemical Sensitivity*.

36. Rogers, *Scientific Basis*, p. 118.

37. R.W. Weber, T.R. Vaughn, and W.K. Dolen, "A Ten-Year Review of Adverse Reactions to Immunotherapy," *Journal of Allergy and Clinical Immunology*, abs. no. 510 (Jan. 1988), p. 295.

38. Personal communications with Jean Monro, M.B., B.S., Breakspear Hospital, Hertsfordshire, England; and with Dr. M.J. Radcliffe, Hythe Medical Centre, Southampton, England.

39. Jonathan Brostoff, "Application of Financial Cost Assessment as a Measure of Clinical Outcome in Allergy and Environmental Medicine," *Cost Benefit Analysis Studies* and "Cost Benefit Analysis Studies as a Measure of Clinical Outcome," proceedings of American Academy of Environmental Medicine, Jacksonville, FL, 1991.

40. J.P. Carter et al., "Dietary Management May Improve Survival from Nutritionally-Linked Cancers Based on Analysis of Representative Cases," *JACN*, vol. 12, no. 3 (1993), pp. 209–26.

P · A · R · T

VI

SOME FINAL
CONSIDERATIONS

18 The Possibility of Chronic Illness

There are many reasons why environmentally ill youngsters go untreated. Sometimes the reason is not a lack of knowledge of environmental illness but rather denial on the part of a parent, teacher, or older child that impedes recognition of the specific cause and interferes with proper care. Informed adults sometimes know exactly what is wrong and what to do, but their health insurance supplier limits the type of medical care that they can receive by denying payment for certain forms of effective, safe treatment. Too often, despite a parents' knowledge of what is helpful and a desire to find appropriate care, they realize they are unable to pay for it. Others are reluctant or simply can't make the necessary changes in their child's physical surroundings, diet, habits, and lifestyle. Single mothers, often already pushed to the limit as they try to meet their daily family obligations, and justifiably feel they can't do more. The medicine-cabinet quick-fix orientation is pervasive in our present-day society. Too many are content to use medicines that provide only temporary relief. Some parents and teachers know and understand why a child is ill, but they don't really have the time or want to make the effort to remove the underlying cause of the illness. Their main concern is to make the child stop misbehaving or not feeling well so that learning and everyday living is less of a challenge.

Several serious consequences can occur if an environmental illness is not treated early. They include academic, physical, and emotional effects, as well as possible long-range hormonal or sex-related changes.

ACADEMIC EFFECTS

Some innately bright children may never excel in school because molds, dust, chemicals and/or foods are affecting their scholastic ability. As mentioned in Chapter 12, some youngsters learn better, attend school more regularly, earn higher grades, and concentrate better in class when they feel well. After they are treated for environmental illness, some students improve so much, they no longer need to attend special classes. The IQ scores of some youngsters increase by 20 to 30 points, and occasionally considerably higher. The exceptional Marsha demonstrated an IQ increase of 68 points (see Chapter 8). Unless environmental factors are recognized, a growing number of young children will not only be unable to learn as well as they should, but they will continuously disrupt classrooms, or need to be subdued with daily doses of quieting drugs.

Many youngsters on home teaching desperately want to go to school. At first being home may be a joy, but reality soon sets in. Many children dislike being alone, but find they are unable to play and interact normally with their friends at school. For older children, two hours a day of home schooling in a three-year period is the equivalent of only one year of school education. They become justifiably concerned about their future because they know that as each day passes, they fall further and further behind.

■ PHYSICAL EFFECTS

Many environmentally ill children cannot remember ever feeling well. Some adults have the same experience, wrongly attributing their symptoms to "growing older." Some have never been free of nose allergies, earaches, asthma, headaches, muscle aches, abdominal discomfort, or recurrent infections, and the restrictions that these illnesses cause. Some have been on medication most of their lives. Many have gone from doctor to doctor and specialist to specialist, searching for an effective treatment. After they finally do find appropriate environmental allergy treatment, some older students and adults say they had forgotten how wonderful it is to feel well. (For a checklist for possible environmental illness or allergy, see Table 3.1.)

The long-term effects of untreated illness can be disastrous. Our bodies usually give us subtle clues that something is wrong. If we ignore these warnings, more serious illness can result. For example, recurrent, relatively minor intestinal complaints, such as belching, bloating, bad breath, excessive gas, or diarrhea can surely cause uneasiness and difficulty in concentrating. If the cause is not found, these complaints can progress years later to colitis, Crohn's disease, diverticulitis, and cancer. Lung problems can lead from a simple cough to chronic bronchitis, emphysema, or possibly cancer. We have no long-term follow-up studies in children, but some pulse irregularities in certain youngsters may mean that they will eventually be prone to cardiac or vascular disease. Such diseases are prevalent in adults who live in "advanced" civilizations but are rare in remote, "uncivilized" tribes.

Although some of these long-term chronic illnesses might be reversible, no studies exist to tell us how often or to what degree this happens. Studies do confirm, however, that the incidence of leukemia is higher if parents use pesticides in their home or garden.[1] Now that we know this, why should pesticides ever be used in or around schools again? We must all start asking why 33 percent of the U.S. population will die of cancer and why the rate of birth defects has doubled in the past twenty-five years. *It is time that we as individuals begin to make the changes in our lives that can help prevent these problems.* We must also insist that our government stop procrastinating and take action to stop the continued contamination of our environment.

■ BEHAVIORAL AND LEARNING CONSEQUENCES

Some environmentally ill children have little hope for the future because they simply don't feel right or behave appropriately. Whether occasionally or on a daily basis, some can't seem to concentrate or learn. Others seem unable to control their actions. Mothers are crushed because their little ones are sent home, because of unacceptable behavior before the end of the first day in kindergarten. Many children try a number of schools, only to be told in a few days or weeks that they cannot return. Many of these children genuinely want to learn but are unable to stay awake or sit still in class. After months (or years) of ridicule and reprimands, their self-image is squashed. They feel that they have no redeeming qualities. Many children and their parents have seen counselors, psychologists, or psychiatrists, for years, as well as tried various forms of behavior modification. The children have received one quieting drug after another. Some have been threatened with prolonged separation from their loved ones by placement in residential or psychiatric institutions.

If environmental issues are not met, there may be more youngsters like Sidney described below. We cannot allow their young lives to be needlessly lost when environmental factors are the primary cause.

A SUICIDAL CHILD THREATENED WITH INSTITUTIONALIZATION

Sidney

Eight-year-old Sidney seriously considered suicide. We have no idea how many others may have succeeded in taking their own lives, with no one having a glimmer of understanding why. No, environmental illness is certainly not the cause of all suicidal children's problems, but how often is it a critical factor that was missed by one professional after another?

When we first saw Sidney, he was truly an "angry" child. His mother described him as desperate, saying she didn't "need a miracle, only a more normal child." He was irritable, wiggly, and argumentative. His parents were separated, in part because of the stress Sidney had caused in their marriage. His mother knew that she must find out what was wrong. The doctors told her that placement in a psychiatric institution for violent children might be the only solution. Her relatives agreed. Sidney's teacher thought he was schizophrenic.

It was clearly no longer safe for Sidney to remain at home. There was no doubt that he acted strangely at times. He had periods of extreme hostility and sudden outbursts when he would hurt other children, as well as his parents and himself. When upset, he would climb to the top of a high piece of furniture, flip his mattress from the bed onto the floor, or totally tear a room apart. On one occasion, he threw his tiny sister, complete with her walker, across the room. When she was three years old, Sidney tried to shove her out of a moving car. One Christmas, in spite of his young age, he became so enraged that he heaved the trimmed Christmas tree against the wall. He once tossed a chair through a school window. His mother's arms were constantly covered with his fresh and residual bite marks. At times, he felt so angry that he even bit himself if no one else was around. Each violent episode could last more than an hour.

Sidney repeatedly said he was unhappy, and from the age of six he kept repeating, "Let me die." One time he tried to hang himself with a shoelace. He grabbed knives and threatened to cut his wrists. He repeatedly ran into the street, hoping for cars to run him down. The school officials told his mother they did not want him to return. His mother was pushed beyond her limit of tolerance when he jumped from a first-story window only to be returned by a sheriff when he attempted to run away. Before this episode Sidney told his mother: "Kill me, or I will have to kill myself."

Clues to Sidney's Problems

Similar to many environmentally ill children, Sidney developed brilliant red earlobes, wiggly legs, and a spacey look, just before and during the periods when his behavior became intolerable. At other times he was the nicest, cutest, calmest, brightest little boy imaginable. On one occasion he took off his coat and gave it to a little boy who needed warmer clothes. Sidney was a caring child whose intermittent most inappropriate actions were actually screams for help.

Why did he have such frightening violent episodes? His own history and that of his family revealed typical allergies. One grandmother was repeatedly suicidal during the month of September. (Perhaps her depression was related to undetected seasonal ragweed or mold sensitivity. See Chapter 5.)

Clues of EI from Sidney's Early Life

Sidney's fetal and infant periods suggested that he had food allergies. Before his birth, he kicked so hard in the uterus that his father could not sleep next to his pregnant wife. His mother was eating excessive amounts of dairy foods at that time, so the most logical possible cause was milk and cheese. As an infant he cried constantly and had prolonged colic until his formula was changed to a soy preparation. Years later, dairy products continued to profoundly affect him though, the effect was much different. He walked at nine months, which is very early and suggests hyperactivity. He could not be cuddled, and even today, he does not like to be held. He had typical nose allergies, along with recurrent ear infections, before he was one year old.

By the time Sidney was two, intense uncontrollable temper tantrums were a daily occurrence. Sleep was always a challenge, and bedtime was known as "helltime." His mother realized that sugar set him off at an early age, but no one believed her. As time passed, he developed typical headaches and classical hay fever. (As you have read the histories of environmentally ill children in this and other books, you've probably found that they sound remarkably similar despite each child's highly individual characteristics. The major differences are related mainly to the location, intensity, and severity of specific symptoms.)[2]

Getting Appropriate Medical Care

Sidney's mother is grateful that the *Donahue* television talkshow in 1988 provided the insight that she so desperately needed. There she saw and heard about the role that diet can play in some children's behavioral problems. A year before she finally came to our clinic, she had tried to have him follow the Multiple Food Elimination Diet (Chapter 3). Sidney refused to cooperate, however. After the sheriff's visit, she knew she had no choice; she had to find the cause of his problems. She tried the diet again, and this time Sidney was cooperative. Within four days, his Conner's hyperactivity score decreased from a highly abnormal 28 to a normal 8. During the second week of the diet, she found that sugar, wheat, milk, and preservatives were the major offenders. When he adhered to an allergy diet and received allergy extract treatment, his violent moods, aggression, and irritability markedly decreased at home, although he continued to have difficulty in school. Once his hypoglycemia was also recognized, the reason for this discrepancy was obvious. At home, he ate whenever he wanted; at school, he could not.

At our medical center, we videotaped his responses to molds, sugar, orange juice, and plums during P/N allergy testing. Only one drop of specific allergy extracts caused him to revert to the behavior that had made his school suggest placement in an institution. In response to some allergy tests, he showed little or no change, but with others, his response was astounding and incredible. When one drop of a major offender was injected under his skin, he became totally uncontrollable in less than seven minutes. He would scream, bite, hit, kick, race about, crawl under furniture, refuse to be touched, and break anything within reach. Before and after each test, however, he was calm, pleasant, and playful. (The video *Environmentally Sick Schools* shows one of his reactions.)

After only one day of testing, Sidney's parents were delighted. He smiled for the first time in years and actually laughed and joked on the way home. He became more affectionate. In time, his parents became aware that the odor of auto fumes and correction fluid could cause drastic changes in his activity. After nine days of environmental medical treatment, his episodes were still evident but noticeably less severe and frequent. His mother said he was 50 percent better. After four weeks, he was 75 percent better and after one year 90 percent better.

Presently his mother no longer lives in fear that her son will need to be institutionalized. There is no doubt that the course of his life, and all the rest of his family's lives, improved immensely after environmental medical treatment.

Prior to his diagnosis of allergy, Sidney's astute, capable mother was repeatedly told that she was not raising him correctly, or that she had to be firmer and discipline him better. Others said he was "just being a boy" and was "spoiled." Ritalin, Mellaril, Clonidine, and Desipramine had all been tried unsuccessfully. They all helped initially, but his aggression, anger, temper, and suicidal statements quickly returned when they were found to provide only a temporary fix.

It is too soon to know the long-term effect of comprehensive environmental medical treatment on Sidney's future, but we do know that food and mold allergies, chemical sensitivities, and hypoglycemia were major causes of his intolerable behavior. Once he improved, his family life changed, his father returned to the family, and his mother was able to complete her education in a professional school. Almost five years later, Sidney continues to behave and learn in a manner that would make any parent proud.

Once the causes of EI are recognized and eliminated or allergy treatment begins, youngsters such as Sidney are immensely relieved. Many older youngsters have commented that they had truly feared they were "crazy." They desperately want to feel well, have energy, play sports, be accepted, and learn. As one depressed, gifted boy so aptly and succinctly put it, "I want a future."

■ POSSIBLE HORMONAL EFFECTS

Can chemical exposures in schools cause hormonal and fertility problems?

This possibility may seem far-fetched at first, but anecdotal as well as sound scientific data, in both animals and humans, indicates that further study is urgently needed.[3]

There is evidence to strongly suggest that chemicals can affect the health and sexual functioning of offspring if either parent has been exposed to toxic chemicals.[4] The families who lived in the Love Canal area of Niagara Falls, in homes that were erected on heavily chemically contaminated soil, had an increase in hormonal problems, congenital disorders, severe psychological problems, and allergies. Were their many health and emotional symptoms due in part to the chemicals buried beneath their homes? What about schools that are built near or on top of toxic dump sites?

Entire medical texts and reports are devoted to the effects of chemicals on reproduction.[5] There is no doubt that chemicals can cause mutation or DNA-genetic coding problems that can result in infertility or congenitally malformed babies. No one can deny that many poorly investigated toxic chemicals are used within and around many schools, homes, and workplaces every day.

The estrogenic effect of an immense number of chemicals has been reported in particular by Danish researchers.[6] These chemicals can act as if an individual had taken female sex hormones. As with differing concentrations of allergens, varying doses of estrogens may have totally different effects in humans.

In addition, the time of exposure can vary the response. Even babies in the uterus can have sex and hormone disruptions if they are exposed near the time of birth. The effects depend upon the sex of the infant and the time and amount of exposure. Even in the tiniest amounts estrogen can be potent and alter developing young. In animals such chemical pollution appears to cause anomalies, birth defects, abnormal sex organs, cancer, "gay" gulls and animals that have not clearly differentiated into males or females, and other effects on the brain. For example, pregnant women who ate Great Lakes fish that were contaminated with PCBs (polychlorinated biphenyls) two or three times per month had infants who weighed less, and these babies had smaller heads than did pregnant women who did not eat such fish. The chemicals were found in the umbilical cord blood. The higher this level, the greater the lag in development and short-term memory.[7]

These estrogens include alkylphenols in detergents, paints, herbicides, and cosmetics; nonylphenols found in spermicides, hair dyes, and other toiletries; phthalate esters in plastics; and herbicides or pesticides, such as endosulfan, used on vegetables.[8] Low levels of industrial chemicals in plastics, plastic water jugs, the plastic lacquer inner coating of food cans, and food wrapping materials, are all surprisingly possible sources of human hormonal medical problems.[9] Some foods contain plant estrogens, but unlike synthetic estrogenlike chemicals that remain in the body for prolonged periods of time, these are excreted quickly. The effects of estrogens were generally detected by accident, not by a scientific systematic method intended to assure the safety of chemicals.[10]

THE ROLE OF PESTICIDES

There is no doubt that most pesticides can pass through the placenta and damage an unborn infant.[11] More than half the pesticides in this country are chlorinated, even though chlorine is known to affect the reproductive and hormonal systems of animals and humans.[12] Although the use of

The EPA has the power to require certain rat or rabbit studies to determine if pesticides cause birth defects, stillbirths, infertility, or genetic changes. If this is not being done, we must ask why not? When there is a warning, why does it pertain only to acute and not to long-term effects in children and female, as well as in men?

PCBs, or polychlorinated byphenols, is no longer allowed in the United States, these chemicals are commonly found in our food, water, human fat, and breast milk. Suggestive evidence is accumulating that relates them to breast, testicular, and prostate cancer.[13] (Dioxin has been found to cause cancer in animals, and an accidental spill of this chemical in Seveso, Italy, in 1976 has been associated with an increased incidence of liver and blood cancer in humans.)[14]

SCHOOL EXPOSURES

Although they are not well-publicized, miscarriages, stillbirths, and congenital birth defects appear to be inordinately common among the offspring of some teachers in some schools. Not all pregnant women exposed to chemicals develop these serious problems, but some certainly seem to be genetically, nutritionally, and/or immunologically susceptible.[15] For example, in one middle school in Virginia, seven miscarriages were reported within a year's time; five of them occurred when the women were in the first three months of pregnancy. In most such situations, the cause is rarely found.[16] Without mandatory documentation and reporting, we have no way of knowing how many other individuals or schools may be affected.

Workplace exposures can also temporarily or permanently affect male reproductive functioning. More than fifty therapeutic, occupational, and environmental agents are believed to either irreversibly affect the genetic material or temporarily affect the quality and quantity of sperm. In studies in both animals and humans, some substances (like pesticides, benzene, tobacco, and lead) have been associated with specific types of cancer, premature infants, small infant size, and illness in male offspring.[17]

THE ESTROGENIC EFFECTS OF PESTICIDES

The following observations, as well as the evidence presented in Chapter 10, suggest that the effects of pesticides on reproductive functioning deserves intensive study. It is not unusual for Americans to come into contact with these chemicals, either directly or from air contaminated by nearby incinerators.[18]

The estrogenic or feminizing effects of pesticide exposures on the reproductive system have been observed in various ways. These observations need more scientific verification in humans and animals, but even if only a few of the following observations turn out to be valid, the implications are frightening.

In Human Males

■ Worldwide, the average male sperm count decreased from about 120 million per milliliter (M/ml) in 1938 to 20 to 80 M/ml in 1991. In many industrialized countries the sperm count has dropped by 50 percent, in quantity and quality, in the past fifty years. If this trend were to continue, the sperm count will be zero in seventy to eighty years or within two generations. Think about this dire prediction for a little while. Some of this drop is attributed to marijuana, cocaine, alcohol, and sexually transmitted diseases, but why does our wildlife manifest similar problems? They don't drink alcohol or smoke.[19]

■ Prostatic cancer has doubled in the past fifty years.

■ Testicular cancer has risen 66 percent, or tripled, in the past fifty years.[20]

■ Cases of undescended testicles and malformed or tiny penises are increasing in various countries.[21]

■ Sterility had risen from 0.5 percent to 25 percent in one cross-section study of college males.[22]

■ Exposure of adult men to pesticides may alter not only their own fertility but the health of their newborn infants.[23]

■ A study of 1,500 children of Vietnam war veterans has shown evidence of impaired immune systems, severe and chronic infections, allergies, multiple chemical syndrome, asthma, learning and attention disorders, unusual mood swings, food reactions, cysts, and cancer.[24] Another study has shown that children of veterans exposed to Agent Orange have twice the normal rate of birth defects. Twenty-some years after the war, some of these soldiers continue to have dioxin (TCDD, tetrachlorodibenzo-p-dioxin) from Agent Orange in their semen.[25]

■ Vietnam veterans showed a 2.5 percent increase in testicular cancer, compared with men who were not in Vietnam. These veterans are 70 percent more likely to father children with major birth defects.[26] A number of chemical exposures, including malathion (which is known to cause testicular damage in rats), dioxin, 2,4 D, and inert substances could also be at fault.[27]

■ One study showed that the sperm of farmers exposed to 2,4 D were less motile, more deformed, and fewer in number than those of nonexposed farmers.[28]

■ Many Gulf War veterans were exposed to a plethora of harmful chemicals. The Gulf War Syndrome is complex, but many soldiers have the classical symptoms of Multiple Chemical Sensitivities (MCS) and definite evidence of impaired neurological, musculoskeletal, respiratory, reproductive, and immune function.[29] Common complaints include nausea, chronic fatigue, joint pain, and body aches. Preliminary information certainly indicates that some of these individuals have been helped by environmental medical care. Some veterans' wives complain of vaginal burning after intercourse and difficulties conceiving babies. Is it possible that the soldiers' contaminated semen has chemically sensitized their wives? Maybe a damaged male-mediated genetic factor is also related to the congenital anomalies evident in some of their infants. Their offspring appear to be inordinately sick, with multiple complaints, that suggest possible food sensitivites and/or environmental illness. Some of these children appear to be classically allergic, but since the army does not test for allergies until a child is five years old, no official data are yet forthcoming.[30] The government has the capability to do spect brain images. If veterans have altered brain function, are they being given this test? Major Richard Haines, a U.S. Army Reserve officer, an independent researcher, has commendably collected data of this type so that everyone's awareness about these issues can be raised.[31]

■ The pesticide DBCP (dibromochloropropane) is conclusively proven to cause reproductive problems, in particular, sterility in males.[32]

In Human Females

■ In 1988, 600,000 women experienced a miscarriage or fetal death, but the cause was not always clear.[33]

■ Breast cancer has doubled in the past fifty years, and nobody knows why. It has increased by 1 percent each year since World War II.[34]

■ Breast milk, as well as semen, appears to store toxic substances.[35] Some females have more pesticides in their breast milk than is allowed in cow's milk.

■ Women who have DDE (a breakdown product of DDT) in their breast fat have a four times greater risk of developing breast cancer than women whose fat is free of chemicals.[36]

■ The incidence of breast cancer on Long Island is 27 percent higher than in the rest of the country. One suspected factor could be the pesticides used to grow potatoes there.

■ In 1934, only twenty-one cases of endometriosis existed in the entire world.[37] Now this illness, which causes sterility, has an estimated incidence of five million in the United States alone.[38] High levels of PCBs have been found in the blood of German women who have endometriosis. Female monkeys exposed to high doses of dioxin also suffer from increased endometriosis.[39] How do low dose short-term high doses of chemicals in monkeys compare with long-term exposures in humans? We don't know.

- A female needs only one exposure to a pesticide at a critical stage during her pregnancy for her offspring to be severely affected.[40] (Male sperm can be genetically altered for ninety days from one pesticide exposure.)[41]
- Industrial chemicals have been connected to the increased incidence of breast cancer in both females and males.[42]
- Some women who have elevated levels of a pentachlorophenol (from wood preservatives, leather upholstery, and carpets) or lindane (from lice treatment preparations) in their blood have habitual abortion, unexplained infertility, menstrual disorders, and premature menopausal symptoms.[43]

In Children

- In 1988, 250,000 American children had birth defects.[44]
- According to the former chairman of the International Joint Commission overseeing the water quality of the Great Lakes, ". . . Toxic chemicals are very likely harming the children in North America. . . . a threat to the health of our children emanates from our exposure to persistent toxic substances, even at very low ambient levels. . . . The scientific evidence confirming problems with human reproduction, learning, behavior, and the ability to ward off disease is now becoming broadly accepted."[45]
- Compelling evidence from industry, government, and the public shows that chemical exposures are very likely damaging North American children in many ways, reducing their ability to pay attention in school; diminishing their IQs; making them hyperactive, aggressive, hostile, and unruly or too tired; some have damaged immune systems, decreasing their ability to fight off common infections and serious diseases such as cancer; *perhaps even predetermining their sexual preferences and behavior before they are born.*[46]
- Sons of Michigan women whose breast milk contained the industrial flame-retardant chemical either Tris or (PBB, or polybrominated byphenyls) had a higher incidence of testicular abnormalities and smaller penises than normal.[47]
- Some women who, between 1948 and 1971, took DES (diethylstilbestrol) to prevent spontaneous abortions gave birth to girls who had genital abnormalities and boys who had abnormally small penises. Dioxin has had a similar estrogenlike effect on pregnant rats.[48]
- A group of boys in Taiwan who had been exposed in utero to an analogue of dioxin were found to have smaller penises than normal.[49]
- If women are exposed to PCBs, their sons can have a diminished penis size, and children of both sexes can have an array of other genital, hormonal, and immune system abnormalities and cancer.[50]

- Due to the lag time between exposure and illness, the effects of pesticides and other chemicals on today's children will not be known for another generation or two.[51]
- Researchers believe the male urogenital system is vulnerable to damage in the womb or shortly after birth. Weak estrogens have a far more potent effect on the unborn, than upon adults in both animals and humans.[52]

In Animals

- After the alligators in Lake Apopka, Florida, were exposed to a spill of DDT, the males' testicles atrophied. Sterility and a 75 percent decrease in the size of their penises were also noted.[53] When they do reproduce, the offspring are mainly females.
- If alligator eggs are painted with estrogen, many won't hatch. Those that do are mainly females.[54] Are males changed before they are born?
- Dogs who served as scouts and sentries in Vietnam were approximately twice as likely to develop cancer of the testicles.[55] The noncancerous sentry dogs had a significant increase in testicular degeneration, atrophy, and decreased sperm production. Were the many pesticides at fault?
- Pet dogs exposed to a 2,4 D lawn pesticide spray have an increased incidence of cancer (lymphomas).[56]
- Malathion and tetracyclines have been found to cause testicular atrophy and decreased sperm quality in dogs and humans.[57]
- If mice are given synthetic estrogen, they develop testicular cysts, undescended testes, and abnormal sperm.[58]
- In Florida, female panthers exposed to pesticides cannot reproduce. The males are sterile; they have low sperm counts and very high estrogen levels.[59]
- Studies show that monkeys exposed to dioxin have developed immune system defects and endometriosis.[60]
- The Great Lakes region contains fish with high PCB and DDT levels due to contamination of the water.[61] Some of the terns and gulls that eat these fish are hermaphrodites, with both male and female sex organs.[62] Their male offspring are feminized.[63] (The Great Lakes, a vast and badly polluted ecosystem, contain 20 percent of all the fresh water on earth.)
- If turtle eggs are painted with PCBs, the male hatchlings are sex reversed. They become females, complete with ovaries.[64]
- Many animals eat plants that make or contain estrogens. Moldy, estrogen-rich corn causes uterine overgrowth in pigs; estrogen-rich clover causes increased miscarriages in sheep. We need to evaluate the effects of plant estrogens more fully, even though they are readily excreted from the body in one day, in contrast to synthetic estrogens, which tend to be stored for years.[65]

Miscellaneous

■ Somewhere between 10 and 15 percent of all American couples are infertile.[66]

■ Estrogen or feminizing effects appear to be related to exposures to a number of pesticides, including DDT, DDE, PCB, and PBB.[67]

■ An estrogenic component in plastic appears to cause infertility and feminizing effects in some male animals; up to 80 percent of plastic liners in food cans may be affected. Polycarbonate plastics are found in baby bottles and water jugs. Even chemicals released from plastic test tubes appear to interfere with some animal research because of the hormonal effects. Consider for a moment the increasing number of foods and beverages sold in plastic containers, the plasticizers found in disposable diapers, and the plastic bags routinely used in hospitals to store and administer intravenous fluids and medicines.[68] Are the chemicals on plastic infant mattresses and crib guards safe?

■ Known hormonal disruption chemicals include 209 PCBs, 75 dioxins, and 135 furans.

■ Some mothers have the "impression" that their son's genitals seem to shrink when they use disposable diapers, in contrast to their more normal appearance when cotton diapers are used. (This "impression" proves nothing until it is documented scientifically, but maybe these children should be studied after they become adults—daily wet diaper exposure continues for about two years in most American children.)

■ Some forms or doses of estrogen appear to protect against cancer, while others seem to cause it. Obviously we need more research.[69]

> If pesticides can cause a feminizing effect in male animals, as well as infertility, significantly smaller male sex organs, hormone changes, and testicular or breast cancer, why are these chemicals being used in and around schools, or anywhere else?

■ SUGGESTIONS FOR FUTURE RESEARCH

As alarming as the previous information in this chapter is, it could be met with some meaningful responses. For example:

■ A governmental agency should be made responsible for compiling data about the incidence of miscarriages and congenitally abnormal births among teachers, students, and other school employees.

■ Long-term follow-up studies of students and teachers should be conducted whenever a serious environmentally triggered illness occurs in a school.

- A study should be conducted to compare the sexuality of men who were in disposable, modern, plastic diapers for two years versus those who used only pure cotton in infancy.
- Data concerning the offspring of Vietnam and Gulf War soldiers, who were exposed to many chemicals, must be contrasted with children of those stationed elsewhere. Preliminary evidence suggests that Gulf War soldiers, like those who served in Vietnam, have an inordinate number of symptoms typical of Multiple Chemical Sensitivities (MCS), allergies, and cancer.[70] Such data are necessary to provide meaningful insight about the inherent dangers in pesticides.[71]
- Research is necessary to determine whether our foods, beverages, and medications can be safely stored in plastic. Dr. J. L. Laseter has shown that if a woman receives intravenous fluids through plastic tubing immediately before delivering a baby, the newborn will have evidence of plasticizers in its blood.[72] Should hospital fluids and medications be stored for prolonged periods (months to years) in plastic bags in hot warehouses, merely because they are more convenient, less fragile, and less bulky than glass bottles? Should we knowingly give sick people intravenous plastic along with their medications and hydrating fluids because it is less expensive and more convenient than glass containers?
- We must teach students, as well as their teachers and parents, about environmentally related health concerns as part of our required academic curriculum.

The information in this chapter strongly suggests that chemicals are one possible cause of the present increase in human infertility. Businesses with heavily vested financial interests in products that have an estrogenlike effect certainly do not want an informed public that is aware of the inherent dangers of routine chemical exposures. If we continue to ignore what is happening with the future inhabitants of this planet, however, we will pay an even greater price unless we immediately begin to do everything possible to diminish the ever-increasing pollution of our air, food, water, and soil.

It took forty years and fifty studies before the surgeon general issued

---

We need much more research and strictly enforced governmental regulations concerning chemical exposures in our schools, homes, and workplaces, as well as in our food, air, water, soil, and clothing. We must decide which is more important: corporate businesses that pollute but help the economy, or everyone's children and grandchildren.

his report about cigarettes in 1964. We can't wait that long to get information about the harmful effects of chemicals on children. Protection of the youngsters who will become the parents of tomorrow's generation represents only a small facet of a much larger challenge. If the rate of increase in male infertility continues, we must be seriously concerned about the ability of our great-grandchildren to reproduce. We simply must end the thoughtless pollution of our planet.

NOTES

1. Marion Moses, *Designer Poisons* (San Francisco: Pesticide Education Center, 1995).
2. Doris Rapp, *Is This Your Child?* (New York: William Morrow, 1991).
3. Moses, *Designer Poisons*; Joan Dine, "Toxic Reduction," in Naomi Friedman, ed., *Greening Synagogues and Community Centers* (Takoma Park, MD: Shomrei Adamah, 1995); Dianne Dumanski, John Peterson Myers, and Theo Colborn, *Our Stolen Future* (New York: Dutton, 1996), and Lawrence Wright, "Silent Sperm," *New Yorker* (Jan. 15, 1996), pp. 47, 48, 53.
4. *Rachel's Environmental and Health Weekly*, no. 438 (Apr. 20, 1995); and Moses, *Designer Poisons*.
5. C. Clement and T. Colborn, "Herbicides and Fungicides: A Perspective on Potential Human Exposure"; T. Colborn and C. Clement, eds., *Chemically Induced Alterations in Sexual and Functional Development: The Wildlife/Human Connection*. Vol. 21 of *Advances in Modern Environmental Toxicology* (Princeton, NJ: Princeton Scientific Publishing Co., 1992); Ellen Grant, *Sexual Chemistry* (London: Reed Books, 1995); Council on Scientific Affairs, "Effects of Toxic Chemicals on the Reproductive System," *Journal of the American Medical Association*, vol. 253, no. 23 (June 21, 1985), pp. 3431–37.
6. *Rachel's*, no. 438 (Apr. 20, 1995).
7. See Wright, "Silent Sperm."
8. Moses, *Designer Poisons*; "Estrogen in the Environment," *Washington Post* (Jan. 25, 1994).
9. *Rachel's*, no. 438; J.A. Brotons et al., "Xenoestrogens Released from Lacquer Coatings in Food Cans," *Environmental Health Perspectives*, vol. 103, no. 6 (1995), pp. 608, 612.
10. Ibid.
11. Ibid.
12. Dine, "Toxic Reduction."
13. Dioxin/Organochlorine Center, Eugene, OR; Society for the Advancement of Women's Health Research, Washington, DC; "Estrogen in the Environment." "Assault on the Male," BBC-TV broadcast (Sept., 1994).
14. "Dioxin Indictment," *Scientific American* (Jan. 1994), p. 25.
15. Moses, *Designer Poisons*.
16. *Indoor Air Review* (Sept. 1993).
17. Devra Lee Davis, "Fathers and Fetuses," *The New York Times* (Mar. 1, 1991).
18. *Rachel's*, no. 456 (Aug. 24, 1995).
19. *Rachel's*, no. 432 (Mar. 9, 1995).
20. Lynn Lawson, *Staying Well in a Toxic World* (Chicago: Noble Press, 1993); *Rachel's*, no. 250 (Sept. 11, 1991); *Rachel's*, no. 436 (Apr. 6, 1995); Rinkel, Randolph, and Zeller, *Food Allergy*.
21. *Rachel's*, no. 438 (Apr. 20, 1995); "Estrogen in the Environment."
22. *Rachel's*, no. 438 (Apr. 20, 1995).
23. Dine, "Toxic Reduction."
24. See Lewis G. Regenstein, *Cleaning Up America the Poisoned* (Washington, DC: Acropolis Books, 1993).
25. Ibid.; R.W. Clapp et al., "Human Health Effects Associated with Exposure to Herbicides and/

or Their Associated Contaminants—Chlorinated Dioxins," *Agent Orange and the Vietnam Veteran: A Review of the Scientific Literature* (April 1990).

26. *Rachel's,* no. 250 (Sept. 11, 1991).

27. *Rachel's,* no. 463 (Oct. 12, 1995).

28. *Rachel's,* no. 250 (Sept. 11, 1991).

29. G. Ziem, "Multiple Chemical Sensitivity: Treatment and Follow-up with Avoidance and Control of Chemical Exposures," *Toxicology and Industrial Health,* vol. 8, no. 4 (1992), pp. 73–86.

30. Ibid.; Statement of Myra Shayevitz, M.D., FACP, Veterans Affairs Medical Center, Northampton, MA, presented to the Committee on Veterans' Affairs, Subcommittee on Oversight and Investigations, Nov. 16, 1993. (The statement includes a proposed treatment plan entitled "A Biopsychosocial Therapeutic Approach for the Treatment of Multiple Chemical Sensitivity Syndrome in Veterans of Desert Storm," comments from successfully treated veterans, and Dr. Shayevitz's response to questions submitted by the Honorable Lane Evans, chairman of the subcommittee.)

31. For an information packet and survey findings, please send a donation of a book of stamps to Major Richard Haines, 4247 Valley Terrace, New Albany, IN 47150.

32. Moses, *Designer Poisons.*

33. Gordon Durnil, *The Making of a Conservative Environmentalist* (Bloomington, IN: Indiana University Press, 1995).

34. Faim, *Innovation,* no. 1 (1995).

35. *Rachel's,* no. 438 (Apr. 20, 1995).

36. Lawson, *Staying Well;* "Estrogen in the Environment."

37. Lawson, *Staying Well.*

38. Sherry Reir et al., "Endometriosis in Rhesus Monkeys (Macaca mulatta) Following Chronic Exposure to 2,3,7,8-Tetrachlorodibenzo-p-dioxin," *Fundamental and Applied Toxicology,* vol. 21 (1993), pp. 433–41.

39. "Estrogen in the Environment."

40. Moses, *Designer Poisons.*

41. Colborn and Colborn, "Chemically Induced Alterations."

42. *Rachel's,* no. 438 (Apr. 20, 1995).

43. Ingrid Gerhard, "Prolonged Exposure to Wood Preservatives Induces Endocrine and Immunologic Disorders in Women," *American Journal of Obstetrics and Gynecology,* vol. 165, no. 2 (Aug. 1991), pp. 487–88.

44. Durnil, *Conservative Environmentalist.*

45. Fifth biennial report of the International Joint Commission (IJC) to study the water quality and pollution in the Great Lakes (1990).

46. Ibid.

47. Regenstein, *Cleaning Up America;* Durnil, *Conservative Environmentalist;* "Estrogen in the Environment."

48. *Rachel's,* no. 432 (Mar. 9, 1995); and no. 463 (Oct. 12, 1995).

49. Davis, "Fathers and Fetuses"; "Estrogen in the Environment."

50. Dine, "Toxic Reduction"; "Dioxin Indictment"; and Colborn, Dumanski, and Myers, *Our Stolen Future.*

51. *Rachel's,* no. 438 (Apr. 20, 1995).

52. Colborn, Dumanski, and Myers, *Our Stolen Future.*

53. Lawson, *Staying Well; Rachel's,* no. 438 (Apr. 20, 1995); CBS, *Eye to Eye With Connie Chung* (July 28, 1994); *Chemical and Environmental Health News* (Jan. 13, 1994).

54. "Estrogen in the Environment."

55. *Rachel's,* no. 436 (Apr. 6, 1995).

56. *Rachel's,* no. 250 (Sept. 11, 1991); no. 436 (Apr. 6, 1995).

57. *Rachel's,* no. 436 (Apr. 6, 1995).

58. Lawson, *Staying Well.*

59. Ibid.; *Rachel's,* no. 438 (Apr. 20, 1995).

60. Reir et al., "Endometriosis"; "Dioxin Indictment."

61. Durnil, *Conservative Environmentalist.*

62. Lawson, *Staying Well.*
63. *Rachel's,* no. 438 (Apr. 20, 1995).
64. Ibid.; "Estrogen in the Environment."
65. Colborn, Dumanski, and Myers, *Our Stolen Future.*
66. Durnil, *Conservative Environmentalist.*
67. Lawson, *Staying Well.*
68. *Rachel's,* no. 438 (Apr. 20, 1995).
69. "Estrogen in the Environment."
70. Ziem, "Multiple Chemical Sensitivity"; statement of Myra Shayevitz.
71. Moses, *Designer Poisons.*
72. J.L. Laseter et al., "Chlorinated Hydrocarbon Pesticides in Environmentally Sensitive Patients," *Clinical Ecology,* vol. 4, no. 1 (1983), pp. 3–12.

19 Fast, Easy, Practical Tips for Parents, Teachers, and School Administrators

■ FOR PARENTS

This section is directed mainly to parents of schoolchildren. However, it is as applicable to homes and workplaces as it is to schools.

1. Observe your child carefully before and after school. If you see a change in how your child feels, behaves, or learns, ask yourself what was eaten, touched, or smelled that could have caused it. Was the change related to an indoor or outdoor exposure, a food, or a chemical? Teach your older youngsters to help you figure out why they aren't feeling up to par. No one knows a child as well as an older child, the parents, and sometimes the teacher. Document your observations. Present your information and conclusions to school officials and to your physician. If you encounter skepticism, videotape your child's responses, for example, to being in a particular classroom. Videotape your child before, during, and after an offending exposure in school; demonstrate any changes in behavior, handwriting, walking, speaking, appearance, or breathing.

2. Read all the articles and books you can about environmental illness (see For Further Reading). Educate others by presenting your information to your local PTA. Be sure your school and the public libraries and bookstores carry the major books and videotapes on environmental medicine. Use self-help methods to find answers and eliminate problems. Some mothers have held bake sales or rummage sales to raise funds to purchase books and videos to donate to public and school libraries, school health offices, and specific teachers, principals, and school superintendents.

3. Keep your detailed records in a bound notebook, not on bits of paper.

Record the pertinent facts in detail, including the time, place, and your child's symptoms. For older children, teach them to record their own symptoms. Try to correlate the onset of symptoms with exposures. Don't exaggerate or understate. Just document the facts fairly.[1] Urge other parents to keep similar records if a change at school seems to affect their children.

4. If your youngster is not well, consult a physician to document that something is wrong. Be explicit, and be sure the doctor's records are complete. Take photographs if your child has a rash or other visible symptoms. If his handwriting changes, record the date and time on the samples you take. Make "before, during, and after" videos to document changes in how your child feels and looks, record the gait, speech, attitude, and ability to learn.

5. Try to work with, not against, school officials, teachers, physicians, and psychologists. They want to help.

6. Be concerned if someone adamantly refuses to listen, pats you on the back, and says self-righteously, "If you want to believe that some food or exposure causes this problem in your child, it's all right," or "You'll simply have to learn to live with it."

7. If no one seems to know what's wrong or believes your suspicions about an environmental concern, find a doctor who has expertise in environmental medicine and chemical sensitivities (see Resources).

8. If certain physicians, principals, or teachers are skeptical about environmental illness, give or loan them a video or book that discusses the subject, or refer them to appropriate scientific material. Many informative books are listed in For Further Reading. They describe why many individuals are chronically ill and show how elusive the causes can be unless one is aware of environmental factors.

9. The more environmentally safe and allergy-free you can make your home, the better your child will be able to tolerate unavoidable allergenic or chemical exposures outside your home. (For books on less toxic living, see For Further Reading.)

10. Eat organically grown foods, and drink filtered or glass-bottled water. Choose "natural" substances whenever you can, like cotton clothing and safer cleaning agents. Use a less toxic flea control for your pet. These and other measures will decrease your family's total exposure to chemicals (see Resources).

11. Ask for the MSD sheet for any chemical used on the school grounds or in renovations if you are the least bit concerned about it. Ask school officials pointed questions: Why are synthetic carpets or potentially toxic disinfectants being used, for example, if some can possibly damage the nervous system?

12. Check on the lawn sprays and other pest-control measures that are being used in your child's school. Insist on written information about which ones are being used and when. If harmful pesticides are being sprayed on lawns where children play, ask why. Urge that your school use safer, natural biocides to effectively control pests, such as an integrated pest management program (see Chapter 10).

13. If your school plans to install a synthetic carpet, ask for a piece of it in advance. Have your child sniff it and sleep on it by placing it between her pillow and the pillowcase. Watch for symptoms the next day: Does your child feel, write, breathe, think, behave differently? If the pulse increases or your youngster becomes ill, send a square foot of the carpet to Anderson Laboratories for testing (see Resources). If the carpet appears to be the cause of her illness, but you can't persuade the school to change the plan to install it, go directly to the school board. Ask why a financially pressed school is buying carpets anyway, if tile costs much less and lasts longer.[2]

14. If you see that something is wrong, follow through. Research the problem thoroughly, and organize your information. Stand up and make yourself heard. Go to PTA meetings and educate other parents. Increase the awareness of school nurses, principals, superintendents, school board members, and state education commissioners. Share your knowledge, books, and videos. Encourage teachers and school psychologists, in particular, to become interested in environmental issues as they relate to learning and behavior.

15. If school bus engines idle and pollute the air outside the school, be assertive about having them moved. The fumes can have an adverse effect on chemically sensitive children. Present articles about the harmful effects of auto exhaust to the school board.[3] If the buses idle near ventilation intake ducts, take pictures of the scene. Take them to the school principal, superintendent, or school board. You have a right to urge that your child's school have quality indoor air. If a ventilation inspection is conducted, ask about the results. What levels of carbon monoxide and other problem gases and chemicals were found in the air? Always be certain that a thorough evaluation was made for chemicals. Sometimes reports state all is fine but this aspect of the evaluation was not done or done incompletely. A school might purposely not request this type of evaluation or hire evaluators who have vested interests in writing reports which indicate little is wrong with a particular school. Ask why a ventilation system is dusty or moldy. Take photographs or videos of polluted areas.

16. Get involved in the pollution issues in your city. If the trees near your child's school, your house, or in a park where he plays are about to be

sprayed, find out about the spray and ask if a safer yet equally effective chemical is available.

17. If you are told that it is impossible to transfer your child to a different school, have an environmental medical specialist evaluate the circumstances so that an informed decision can be made. Get everything in writing or ask to tape record comments.

18. Work with the environmental agencies in your area. On Earth Day organize an exhibit stressing the effects of environmental problems on schoolchildren and teachers. Urge older children to select school projects related to environmental issues. Do not allow today's children to become the rain forest of tomorrow.

19. If a new school is to be built in your area, endeavor to have some input in the planning. Read the many books on this topic.[4] Work to make your area the first in our country to have a completely environmentally sound school. If this isn't possible, encourage your school officials to emulate the practical, progressive, and economical clean-classroom approach used in Canada (see Chapter 12).

20. Urge your school to bring in the two-hour workshop, "How Environmentally Safe Are Our Schools?" produced by Safe Schools (see Resources) or discuss "Environmentally Sick Schools" at a PTA meeting. (See For Further Reading)

21. Seek cost-effective ways to aid your school administrators and teachers in helping your child and themselves.

22. Spoil the teachers who listen to you and help. Give them books, flowers, and candy, and be lavish with your praise. Write to the school superintendent and the principal, telling them that a particular teacher is exceptional. Teachers are truly special and deserve appreciation and understanding. They already had more than enough to do before they also had to "watch" your child for health or learning problems. Any "above and beyond" cooperation should be valued very highly. Similarly, write the commissioner of education in your state, when a principal, superintendent, or other school official is exceptionally understanding or negligent about an environmental health issue.

23. If your child's school remains a concern, write detailed letters to your local and state legislators. They are elected to represent you.

24. Check with your state education department in your capital on the rights of children to receive an education.[5]

25. If you are threatened, be it in person, by phone, or in writing, contact a lawyer. If someone acts this way, something may be **terribly** wrong with the school building. Seek the cause of an anonymous caller's worry or fear. It's possible that you have asked exactly the right probing questions.

26. Enlist the help of any local specialists in environmental medicine. Obtain a consultation, and judge for yourself before you make decisions.

    Once you have seen an environmental specialist, is it possible that skeptical physicians will sometimes refuse to see your child in the future. If your child's previous treatments have failed, maybe it is time to consider other options. Ask your doctor if your child could be a "test" patient to see if an environmental medical approach really helps. With this attitude it is possible for a doctor to personally evaluate the outcome.

27. If your insurance company will not pay for environmental medical care, make a list of all the office visits, medical and drug bills, symptoms, hospitalizations, and surgeries; include school attendance records, your personal observations, and your child's grades for the previous few years. Add up these costs and compare the total with the cost of several months of environmental care. Let the records speak for you. Provide this comparison to your insurance company. Seeing those figures, third-party payers should listen. For details, see Chapter 17, and if you have doubts, have your lawyer read over the letter before you send it.

28. Organize a group of interested parents to spread the message that what we breathe, eat, and touch can indeed make us ill. Start a newsletter. Figure out better ways to educate children about environmental issues. Children can sometimes communicate the message to other children better than adults.

29. If no one listens to you, and your child's problems are truly serious, go to your local newspaper and ask to speak to the editor. Tell a reporter how environmental illness has affected your child and/or yourself. Write a "letter to the editor." You are probably not alone, but you may be the only one willing to stand up and speak out. By speaking out you might prevent illness in many others in your child's school.

30. Write to television talk-show hosts about your concerns and the persistent injustices you encounter. You will find you are not the only person who has this problem. Talk shows help millions of people quickly, easily, and effectively by bringing critically important issues before the public. Two talk-show hosts who would like to hear from you are:

Sally Jessy Raphael
CBS TV
51 West 52nd Street
New York, NY 10019

Jerry Springer
NBC Tower
454 North Columbus Drive
Chicago, IL 60611

31. Consider going on your local public access television to discuss the problem. There is no fee. Remember, tell the straight, honest facts—no exaggeration.

32. If you are overwhelmed by all of these suggestions, slow down. Begin with what is sensible, practical, and pertinent to your personal situation. Remember, no one else is going to do it for you; many who state they would like to help are simply too busy. Few people care as much as you do about your child. And only the rare soul will care equally about all the other children, teachers, and staff at your child's school.

■ FOR TEACHERS

1. Read as much as you can about environmental medicine. Study the video *Environmentally Sick Schools* (see video listings in For Further Reading). Have you seen children react similarly to exposures and foods? Some youngsters may have perplexed you with their erratic changes in health, handwriting, behavior, and learning ability. Observe your students more carefully, and you will be amazed at how easily you can spot why some children can't learn and behave appropriately.

2. Similarly, study the stressful experiences of the teachers and youngsters who react to environmental factors in this book and others. Learning about school-related environmental illness will help you prevent similar health problems from developing in yourself and others. You will find comfort in seeing that other teachers have had problems similar to yours. You may have never understood why you did feel unwell, why your doctors seemed equally perplexed, or why no one believed you.

3. Note what particular students breathed, ate, drank, or smelled just prior to a change in behavior. The physical clues will usually be evident. Watch for the sudden onset of red earlobes, dark eye circles, nose rubbing, throat clearing, wiggly legs, and/or voice or handwriting changes, followed by some major outburst, loss of attention, or physical complaints. Respect the need of these children for special diets, particularly with regard to food rewards and school parties. Learn what emergency procedures to use to treat their reactions to foods, chemical vapors, and stinging insects.

4. Study your students' response patterns to environmental or food exposures. Many children have a consistent sequential pattern. Just with this knowledge you can anticipate and abort some outbursts. The problem with a spirited difficult youngster might not be the fault

of a child but a brain-related reaction to some allergen, food, or chemical.

5. Gather evidence of handwriting, drawing, and learning changes that occur before and after meals, snacks, parties, certain classes, and unusual exposures to dust, mold, pollen, chemicals, pets, and plants. Share your evidence with older students, the child's parents, other teachers, and school administrators.

6. Carefully note the circumstances before, during, and after problem periods in children classified as having Attention Deficit Hyperactivity Disorder. ADHD is not a Ritalin deficiency! Possibly as many as two-thirds of these youngsters actually suffer from an environmental illness that has been overlooked. You can help turn a child's life around by increasing the parent's knowledge about environmental medicine. This can ultimately relieve health and learning problems, and decrease the need for drugs in some children. Be aware that you might be the best or even only person in a position to help.[6]

7. Listen carefully to observations made by the parents of challenging students. They sometimes provide amazingly shrewd insight. Also, listen to the students. Sometimes their insight is equally beneficial but no one has asked them the obvious questions or listened to them before.

8. You *should not* recommend specific physicians or specific types of medical care to parents, but you can urge the school and the public library to carry books, literature, and videos about environmental medicine. Encourage students, other teachers, health assistants, school nurses, and parents to look over or critique such self-help materials. There must be communication and teamwork between you, the parents, and other school staff members.

9. Diplomatically, but assertively, urge school administrators to recognize the many advantages of making environmental changes in your school. Such changes can improve the attendance and academic performance of some students, decrease the need for special classes and home teaching, and sometimes provide an economic boon to the school (see Chapter 12). Every teacher's and student's health should be enhanced by a cleaner classroom.

10. Talk to your school administration and union about how you can obtain employee insurance that will cover environmental medicine. Some of the more progressive insurance companies now realize they can save money on a short- and long-term basis if they cover environmental medical care and other less drug-oriented treatments. (See Chapter 17 regarding the new insurance available for alternative health care.)

11. If a number of teachers are greatly concerned but there has been little administrative response, go directly to your union and enlist its help. Send letters with your concerns to your school administrators, school board, school supervisor, or state education commissioner. Notify the health department. Call a specialist in environmental medicine for more information and guidance. (see Resources).

12. If you are threatened, directly or indirectly, keep a detailed record in a spiral notebook. There is safety and strength in numbers, so enlist the help of others who are similarly concerned. Check on the health and well-being of other teachers who have previously used your classroom. (See Chapter 3 for sample history forms.)

13. Avoid personally using scented body products or tobacco. Do not wear clothing that smells of a fabric softener, dry-cleaning fluid, or mothballs. Similarly, discourage your students from wearing perfumed body and hair products. Some children are so sensitive that the slightest whiff of an aroma can quickly cause them to feel unwell and impair their ability to learn and/or behave. Even fingernail polish or remover can cause symptoms. In some sensitive children, even the scent from chewing gum or a chemical imprint on a sweatshirt can cause a dramatic physical change or emotional outburst.

14. Be equally aware that minute odors from many commonly used items—like chalk, freshly printed paper, marking pens, ordinary crayons—can cause symptoms. Be careful to select nonodorous substances for use in your classroom.

15. Do not use candy as a reward. Some children will act in an inappropriate manner within 15 minutes to an hour of eating sugar. Notice which children routinely become the "life of the party" at junk-food school celebrations. Which ones become noisy, undisciplined, hyperactive, withdrawn, untouchable, or unable to write? Organize a vegetable party—do the same students react in that way? A comparison will show it is not always excitement that causes misbehavior at party time.

16. Remember that it is *how sensitive* a child is, not *how much* of a chemical he is exposed to, that determines whether he will react. A child who is exquisitely allergic to peanuts or eggs may become desperately ill from merely smelling these items in someone else's lunch. Exposures have the potential to cause many different symptoms. Everyone is special, and an individualized approach is imperative.

17. Note exactly when changes occur in your students or yourself. *When,* not *how often,* can provide important clues. If a child is exposed to the wrong thing every day, the problem will occur daily. If the contact is intermittent, the problem will occur intermittently. Always compare the good days versus the bad. For example, a child may have behav-

ioral problems only on the "pizza day." Ask why. To help parents pinpoint the cause when an item contains several foods, see Chapter 5. If possible, remind the affected child to avoid known offending exposures at least during school hours. A child who thinks unclearly or becomes uncontrollable because of sugar or food coloring should not eat a dyed sugary cereal for breakfast, drink a sweet red beverage just before an exam, or eat colored candy before playing sports.

18. Children are sensitive souls with delicate, easily crushed natures. If red earlobes or wiggly legs routinely precede a child's tantrum, discreetly advise that youngster to see the school nurse as soon as you spot these clues, *before* an outburst erupts. You may have to give a child such advice shortly after arrival at school, if the spacey-eyed look, dark eye circles, the expression, or walk indicates a "ticking behavioral time bomb."

19. Some children must urinate frequently, or have accidents in their pants, because of their sensitivities. Those children should be seated near the door so they can come and go discreetly with a minimum of distraction. If a child must eat special lunch or party foods, allow them to be eaten surreptitiously, so that hardly anyone will notice. If you handle it casually, without fanfare, others may do likewise. Never belittle, embarrass, or mock a child, especially in front of other students.

20. If a child has hypoglycemia, seat this youngster on the far-right or left-front corner of the classroom, so a non-sweet snack can be eaten without drawing attention to the child.

21. Enlist the help of other teachers who may have environmental illness. Together you can look for patterns. Do problems consistently recur only in certain rooms or at specific times? Find out why. Think of molds on damp, rainy days, or pollen when the count is high. Did you initially note a problem during or immediately after building renovations? Check the health records with the school nurse or health assistant for individualized characteristic patterns of illness.

22. Remember that environmental illness can affect any child, including the gifted and the learning disabled. Whether youngsters are bright, normal, or slow, many cannot begin to realize their full potential because of an unrecognized environmental illness. Although only part of a bright child's academic performance might be adversely affected by certain exposures; much is to be gained from appropriate therapy. For a seriously disabled child, a small improvement can provide a giant step welcomed by all concerned. Occasionally you may see a miracle, as in an exceptional autistic child, who becomes perfectly normal after a week or two on a dairy or grain free diet.

23. If you have an opportunity to suggest a speaker for a teachers' conference, suggest an environmental medical specialist. Facts and figures,

as well as videos, can be presented to raise awareness of environmental illness. For speakers, contact the American Academy of Environmental Medicine (see Resources).

24. No, you were not hired as a nursemaid or a doctor, but twentieth-century education demands much more of teachers than ever before. You can't teach well and your students can't learn well if one child is repeatedly disrupting the class. If your school's ventilation system is poor or if the carpet is a problem, finding and eliminating the cause can help everyone. Your own stress load can be significantly diminished by identifying and eliminating the cause of one student's outbursts.

25. It is not always easy to distinguish an exuberant youngster from one who is reacting to an adverse exposure. If a child has the characteristic physical appearance of an environmental illness, and suddenly and inexplicably can't behave or learn normally, at least consider the possibility of some adverse environmental factors. You may be the *only* knowledgeable person to understand a child's puzzling problems.

26. Remember: Many parents, especially single working mothers, are forced to spend fewer waking hours with their children than their teachers. Sometimes a family's entire future may depend solely upon your expertise and analytical ability, as well as on your caring, sharing nature. More than one family has been on the verge of breakup because a child's unrecognized environmental illness has caused so much upheaval. Your personal satisfaction can be immense when the opportunity for greatness is thrust upon you. There are times when you alone may make the crucial difference in a child's or family's life. Willingly accept this opportunity.

■ FOR SCHOOL ADMINISTRATORS

1. All schools' boards should have an advisory board with knowledge of environmental illness. The EPA offers educational material on the subject, as do the states of New York and Maryland, as well as several Canadian school districts (see Chapter 13). Making informed decisions will save your district money and raise the academic performance in your school.

2. Find consultants who have the expertise to properly and thoroughly assess air quality and building maintenance. They can suggest safer cleaning and maintenance materials. If certain students and teachers routinely become ill shortly after entering a school building in spite of various changes, something has been overlooked.

3. If problems arise, consult an environmental medical specialist immedi-

ately for advice about possible missed factors. Early recognition can prevent distressing expensive sequelae.

4. Be sure your health personnel are knowledgeable so that they can properly assist each environmentally ill child and teacher.

5. An environmental health questionnaire should be completed for all children prior to the beginning of school (see Chapter 3). This form might provide clues to help predict which children are most apt to become the school problems of tomorrow. Toxic environmental factors should be eliminated as soon as possible.

6. When the health needs of challenging students are reviewed at regular intervals, always consider elusive environmental factors as a source of their difficulty. The health personnel should look for patterns of illness that correspond to days of the week, times of the month, or certain classroom exposures.

7. Each PTA should have a health and safety committee to help monitor the children's health records and recurrent health problems. Are the records up to date?

8. Many children's parents have special expertise in environmental issues. At times their input can be most beneficial and cost-effective.

9. Make every effort to communicate openly and honestly with parents and students when health issues arise. A coverup can backfire causing stress for everyone.

10. Help teachers accommodate their own special needs as well as those of their students by:
    - providing an environmentally safer classroom within the school building (avoid portable classrooms—they "outgas" formaldehyde)
    - insisting upon carpet-free classrooms
    - using slightly aged or sealed furniture that no longer "outgasses" chemicals
    - cleaning with safer, better tolerated, less odorous products
    - upgrading dusting and cleaning routines

11. To ensure a safer school environment:
    - Closely monitor the maintenance of the heating and ventilation systems, especially the filters. Are dusty or moldy ventilation systems cleaned as often as necessary. If a ventilation inspection is conducted, critically evaluate the results. What levels of carbon monoxide and other problem gases and chemicals were found in the air? Why are levels elevated in certain areas.
    - Eliminate the routine use of herbicides and pesticides on school grounds. Use only integrated pest management or safer biocide measures.
    - Build schools with classrooms which contain windows that can be opened. Provide sufficient full-spectrum lighting.

- Schedule painting and renovation projects at the *beginning* of school vacation so no "fresh remodelling" odors remain when school is resumed.
- Be sure that office copiers, printers, and laminating equipment are located in adequately vented rooms. Allow no school district printing presses within a school building.
- Establish procedures to ensure that substitute teachers are adequately aware of the special needs of environmentally sensitive students.

12. Involve the school nurse, as well as all students and staff, in an in-depth program to increase everyone's awareness about environmental illness.

13. Exhaust fumes from school buses can have an adverse effect on many children and teachers. Provide less polluted nondiesel transportation with nonsmoking drivers, especially for very allergic children. Do not allow buses to idle near the school's ventilation intake ducts.

14. Enforce a **total** absence of smoking in teachers' lounges as well as in student lavatories. If this can't be done, provide smoke-free lavatories for the youngsters who are sensitive to tobacco smoke.

NOTES

1. For more details on record-keeping, see Doris J. Rapp, *Is This Your Child?* (New York: William Morrow & Co., 1991), chap. 9.

2. Mary Oetzel, *The Comparative Cost of School Floorcoverings* (Austin, TX: Environmental Education and Health Services, 1992, 1994).

3. National Education Association, *Healthy School Handbook* (Washington, DC: NEA Professional Library, 1995).

4. Ibid.; Lynn Marie Bower, *The Healthy Household* (Bloomington, IN; Healthy House Institute, 1995); David Rousseau, W.J. Rea, and Jean Enwright, *Your Home, Your Health, and Well-Being* (Vancouver, BC: Hartley & Marks, 1988); and John Bower, *Healthy House Building* (Bloomington, IN: Healthy House Institute, 1993).

5. The New York booklet on this subject is entitled "A Parent's Guide to Special Education for Children Ages 5–21—Your Child's Right to an Education in New York State." This free publication must be requested in writing, from New York State Education Department, Publication Sales Office, R 309 EB, 89 Washington, Albany, NY 12234.

6. M. Boris, and F.S. Mandel, "Foods and Additives Are Common Causes of the Attention Deficit Hyperactive Disorder in Children," *Annals of Allergy*, vol. 72 (May 1994), pp. 462–68; J. Egger et al., "Controlled Trial of Oligoantigenic Treatment in the Hyperkinetic Syndrome," *Lancet 1* (1985), pp. 540–45; D.J. Rapp, "Does Diet Affect Hyperactivity?" *Journal of Learning Disabilities*, vol. 11 (1978), pp. 56–62; and J.A. O'Shea and S.F. Porter, "Double-Blind Study of Children with Hyperkinetic Syndrome Treated with Multi-Allergen Extract Sublingually," *Journal of Learning Disabilities*, vol. 14 (1981), p. 1899.

Afterword: What Is a Utopian School?

In a utopian world, *every* school and *every* classroom would be environmentally safe, free of allergens and offending chemicals. The food and water would not contain chemicals such as pesticides and dangerous toxic metals. All personnel would be aware that environmental factors can cause impaired learning, physical illness, and activity and behavioral problems. They would consider the possibility that these types of symptoms could be caused by dust, mold, or chemicals in classrooms, as well as by foods or beverages ingested in school and at home.

It is disappointing that such a visionary, caring, and enterprising country such as the United States has no such school. There are only a handful of environmentally safe classrooms in all of North America, and most of those are located in Canada. As more school systems become aware of the multiple advantages of environmentally cleaner and safer schools, they may well adopt the ECO classroom approach so ably modeled by some of the more progressive school districts in Canada. Gary Oberg, M.D., is helping to create an entirely environmentally sound school in Chicago at the present time.

Perhaps community-minded philanthropists will consider the creation of model environmental schools for their cities. These schools could become beacons of light for education, worthy of universal emulation. Most ordinary, caring individuals can create only tiny ripples of goodness, but the wealthy are capable of generating gigantic waves of magnificence. What better way is there to have a truly successful fulfilling life than to be the 1 person who improved the health, learning, and lives of many by providing a nontoxic, safe model school worthy of universal evaluation. We must all work together to consider practical ways to help others and preserve our well-being as well as that of our precious planet universe.

Let us hope that, for the sake of present and future generations, a universal change in attitude will take place. An expanding number of children are destined never to reason, think, act, feel well, or reproduce at a level that is considered to be normal or comparable to their innate ability. They will never reach their maximum academic potential because of adverse environmental exposures that persist because of denial, deception, ignorance, and a desire for short-term economic rewards.

In time, we shall have schools that provide clean air, pure water, nonharmful chemical- and pesticide-free foods and beverages in a totally safe environment. We can no longer tolerate the casual, indiscriminate use of chemicals that endanger the health, in particular the brains and nervous systems, of our present and future generations.

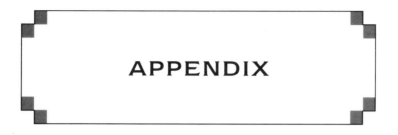

APPENDIX

Chemicals Found Frequently in Schools and Homes

As informed parents and teachers, you need to know the following information about chemicals commonly found in schools, as well as in homes and workplaces:

- the common or trade names
- the areas in schools and homes where they are found
- the sources of these substances
- the possible health effects of exposure to them

This information will enable you to better understand the reasons why certain products should not be used in your child's school or your home.

TABLE A.1

Formaldehyde, Hydrocarbons, and Phenol

Common or Trade Name	Where Found	Sources (Many of these items contain multiple chemicals; check the Material Safety Data sheets for more information)	Health Effects & Precautions
Formaldehyde	Art Class Auditorium Cafeteria Cooking class Gym Industrial arts Laboratories Library Locker room Miscellaneous Music room Shower room Swimming pool Welding class	Adhesives, aerated waste, air fresheners, air pollution, alcoholic beverages, animal feed, antifreeze, antihistamines, antiperspirants, antiseptics, antislip agents, antistatic agents, automotive exhaust, bactericide, binding (paper bag seams), brake drums, building material, butcher paper, buttons, carpets/pads, catalytic heaters, cellophane, chalk, chemical stabilizers, chewing gum, chickens (to whiten skin), chip board, cleaning compounds, coated papers (cartons/labels), coatings (appliances), coffee, combustion (diesel/ fossil fuel/gas/kerosene/oil/wood),	Allergies. Cause of cancer. Toxic to the immune system. Asthma, eye, respiratory tract, & skin irritation; dizziness, nose congestion, nausea.

Common or Trade Name	Where Found	Sources (Many of these items contain multiple chemicals; check the Material Safety Data sheets for more information)	Health Effects & Precautions
		concrete, cosmetics, cotton fabric (sanforized), dental fillings, deodorants, deodorizers, detergents (some), dialysis units, disinfectants, dry-cleaning compounds/disinfectant solutions, dust sterilizing solutions, dyes (some), eggs (to increase shelf life), elastic, embalming fluids, enamels, explosives, fabrics (polyester/artificial silk), fabric finishes (permanent press, water-repellent, dye-fast, flame- & water-resistant, shrink-, moth- & mildew-proof), fertilizers (nitrogen), fiber preservative (jute/hemp), fiberboard, fibers (acrylic/wool/nylon), filters (air/furnace), fish (preservative rinse), flame retardants, floor coverings, flour (preservative), flower arrangements (some), foam insulation, foundries, fur, furnishings, furniture, gas appliances, gelatin capsules, germicides, glass manufacturing, glue, hair products, hardeners, hardware or hardware stores, hospital bed sheets, incinerators, ink, insecticides, insulation (urea formaldehyde/foam/fiberglass/wool), laboratories, lacquers, laminates, laundry starch, lawn/garden equipment, leather & tanning agents, lubricants (synthetic), maple syrup (some), mascara, meat smokehouses, medicines (some), melamine tableware, mildew prevention, milk, mimeo paper, mineral wool production, mobile homes, molding compounds, mothproofing, mouthwash, mushroom farms, nail polish/hardener/undercoat/remover, napkins, napping agents, newsprint, orthopedic casts & bandages, paint (all), paint stripper/remover, paneling, paper products, particle board, perfume, pesticides, pharmaceuticals, phenol formaldehyde & thermosetting resin, photochemical smog, photographic chemicals/film, plaster, plastic, plastic cleaners, plywood furniture, polishes, preservatives, razor blades, refrigerator hardware, roden-	

Common or Trade Name	Where Found	Sources (Many of these items contain multiple chemicals; check the Material Safety Data sheets for more information)		Health Effects & Precautions
		ticides, roofing, rubber hose production, sanitary products (disposable), seeds, shampoo, smoke (cigarette/wood), soap, softeners, sporting goods, spray starch, sterilizing solutions, stucco, textiles, tires, tissues (facial), toilet paper, toilet seats, toothpaste, urea formaldehyde foam insulation (UFFI), urethane coatings & resins, utensil handles, vaccine preparations, varnish, vinyl resins, vitamin A & E preparations, wallpaper, water filters, water-softening chemicals, wax (floor/household), waxed paper, wines, wood-burning stoves, wood preservative/stain/veneer.		
Hydrocarbons (chemical compounds containing only hydrogen & carbon bonds)	Art class Auditorium Cafeteria Cooking class Gym Industrial arts Laboratories Library Locker room Miscellaneous Music room Shower room Swimming pool Welding class	Air fresheners, alcoholic beverages, anesthetics, art & decorating supplies, automotive exhaust, baked goods, bath oils, beverages, bubble bath, butane, candy, catalytic heaters, cigarette smoke, cleaning agents containing naphtha, coal heat, coal & petroleum products including:		Cause of cancer. Toxic to immune system. Loss of appetite, anemia, blurred vision, bone marrow & central nervous system depression, disorientation, drowsiness, drunken behavior, eye, nose, throat & lung irritation, silly feeling, fatigue, gastrointestinal irritation, headache, kidney, liver & lung damage, leukemia, lightheadedness, loss of appetite, low white blood cell count, multiple myeloma, nerve problems, brain damage, paralysis, rashes, reproductive problems.
		solids:	plastics, synthetic fabrics, roof tar, asphalt, wax coatings (used to coat some fruit & vegetables);	
		liquids:	gasoline, diesel & oil (industry uses a huge number of related petrochemicals);	
		gases:	fumes from engines that burn petrochemicals (gasoline, diesel), cars, buses, lawn mowers, outboard motors, trucks, natural & bottled gas appliances, ranges, water heaters, refrigerators, dryers, oil or gas furnaces & space heaters, gas appliance pilot light, evaporating oil from electric motors (mixers, sewing machines), hydrocarbon solids or liquids, cleaning compounds, polishes, paints, insecticides,	*Aromatic hydrocarbons,* such as xylene, toluene, styrene, benzene, naphthalene, are most apt to be toxic to the nervous system, causing irritability, headaches, & fatigue.

Common or Trade Name	Where Found	Sources (Many of these items contain multiple chemicals; check the Material Safety Data sheets for more information)	Health Effects & Precautions
		newspapers, plastics, colognes, copying/duplicating machines, cosmetics, deodorants, detergents, diesel oil, disinfectant cleaning solutions, dried fruits, dyes derived from coal tar, automotive exhaust, explosives, face cream, facial tissue, fireplaces, flavoring agents, frozen pizza crust, fruits (all sprayed, even if scrubbed & peeled), gelatin desserts, glycerol, hair care products, hand lotions, ice cream, ink, insecticides, kerosene, lighter fluid, lip balm, lipstick, liquors, lotions, machine oil, meat (stored in the animal's fat cells), metal polish, mineral oil, mineral spirits, motor oil, nail polish/hardener/undercoat/remover, newsprint, oil products, paints/stains, paraffin, perfume, petroleum jelly, photographic film, pine scent, pine wood & turpentine (affects those sensitive to hydrocarbons: coal, oil & gas all developed from organic material such as pine trees), plastics, polyester, preparation of essences, extracts & tinctures, rubbing alcohol, sauces, soaps, space heaters, spray propellants, stationery, sterilization of medical instruments, synthetic fibers, tires, toilet tissue, treated papers & adhesives, varnish, vegetables (all sprayed, especially the cabbage family), wax-coated fruits/vegetables, wax-coated paper cups, waxes, wood-burning by-products.	*Halogenated hydrocarbons* contain chlorine as in tri- or tetrachlorethylene or ethane dichlorobenzene or chloroform. Some of these can cause cancer.

Common or Trade Name	Where Found	Sources (Many of these items contain multiple chemicals; check the Material Safety Data sheets for more information)	Health Effects & Precautions
Phenol	Art class Laboratories Library Miscellaneous	Acne medications, adhesive, aerosol disinfectants, aftershave, traditional allergy extract as a preservative, aluminum foil (plastic on dull side "outgasses" phenol when heated), antiseptics, baking powders, bronchial mists, calamine lotion, canned foods (can liner), caulking agents, cleaning compounds, cosmetics, deodorants, detergents, disinfectants (pine), dyes, epoxy/glue, explosives, fiberglass, fiber preservative (jute/hemp), flame-retardant finishes, food additives, gasoline additives, hair products (dyes, hair sprays, setting lotions, shampoos), hand lotion, herbicides, inks, insulation, laminated boards, laundry starches, lozenges, matches, metal polishes, mildew, mildew-proofing, molded plastic (telephones, toys), mouthwashes, nasal sprays, nylon, odors (soaps, perfumes, scented stationery, polishes, cleaning compounds, paints, insecticides), ointments (first aid cream), over-the-counter drugs (antihistamines, aspirin, cold capsules, cough syrups, decongestants, eye drops), paints (all), perfumes (all), pesticides, pharmaceuticals, phenolic thermo-setting resins (hard plastics "outgas" phenol vapors when warmed: sauce-pan handles, TV sets, computers, radios), photographic chemicals, plastic coatings on electric wires, plastic dishes & wraps (when heated in microwave), plastics, plywood, polishes, polyurethane, preservatives, refrigerator storage dishes, resorcinol, shaving preparations, smoke (tobacco), solvents, spandex (girdles, support hose), sugar substitute, sunscreens & lotions, transparent tape, trinitrophenol (picric acid), vaccines, wallpaper (vinyl-coated), waterbeds, wood preservatives & sealants.	Possibly fatal. Extremely caustic, burns. Absorbed by lungs & skin, central nervous damage, heart-rate irregularities, numbness, pneumonia, respiratory tract & skin irritation & burning, vomiting, kidney & liver damage. Can cause cancer and damage genes, causing birth defects.

TABLE A.2

Other Chemicals Frequently Found in Schools

Common or Trade Name	Where Found	Sources	Health Effects & Precautions
Acetone	Auditorium Cafeteria Cooking class Industrial arts Library Locker room Music room Shower room Swimming pool Welding class	Caulking, cologne, concrete, dishwashing liquid & detergent, glue, laminated plastic, nail polish/hardener/undercoat/remover, paint, paneling, particle board, phenolic thermosetting resins, plywood, roofing, polyurethane wood finish stain/sealants, tires, wall coverings, water.	Toxic. Absorbed by breathing & skin penetration, dizziness, eye, nose, & throat irritation, liver & skin damage, skin burns. Can cause gene changes & birth defects.
Alkylphenol Novolac Resin	Miscellaneous	Carbonless paper, hydrocarbons.	Extremely toxic. Central nervous system damage, lung & mucous membrane irritation.
Ammonia	Art class Miscellaneous	Cleaning compounds, deodorants, disinfectants, duplicating machines.	Possibly fatal. Conjunctivitis, irritation of eye, nose, throat, & lungs, laryngitis, pneumonitis, lung fluid, chemical burns.
Benzene (benzol)	Art class Cafeteria Cooking class Gym Miscellaneous Swimming pool	Adhesives, aerosol propellants, air fresheners, anthraquinone colors, automotive exhaust, carpets, cigarette smoke, cleaning solutions, dyes, degreasers, deodorizers, eggs, floor tile, fossil fuel, fungicide, furniture polish & stripper, gasoline, glue, metal polish, mothballs/crystals, paint, plastics, polyurethane wood finish stain/sealants, refrigerants, solvents, spot removers, synthetic fibers, tobacco smoke, VOCs, water, wood finish.	Cause of leukemia. Toxic to immune system. Anemia, blurred vision, bone marrow & central nervous system depression, birth defects, disorientation, drowsiness, drunken behavior, silly feeling, eye, gastrointestinal, nose, throat, & lung irritation, fatigue, headache, lightheadedness, loss of appetite, low white blood cell count, multiple myeloma, nerve problems, paralysis, rashes, reproductive problems.
Benzyl alcohol	Lavatories Classrooms Cafeteria	Acne medications, aftershave preparations, anesthetic (local/topical), antiseptics, artificial flavorings, baked goods, beverages, candy, chewing	Allergies. Intestinal damage.

Common or Trade Name	Where Found	Sources	Health Effects & Precautions
		gum, cleaning compounds, cologne, cosmetics, cough drops, deodorants, dusting powder, ear drops, gelatin desserts, hair spray, heat-sealing polyethylene film, ice cream, ink, lip balm, lipstick, nylon dyes, ointments, perfume, photographic chemicals, polyethylene film, preservatives in medications, raspberries, solvents, synthetic flavoring & scents (blueberry, cherry, floral, fruit, grape, honey, liquor, loganberry, muscatel, nut, orange, raspberry, root beer, rose, vanilla, violet, walnut), tea (some).	
Cadmium	Miscellaneous	Cigarette smoke, water.	Cause of cancer. Possibly fatal. Anemia, eye, nose, throat, lung, & skin irritation, cyanosis, emphysema, headache, kidney & lung damage, reproductive problems. On exposure to heat or acid, releases hydrogen sulfide gas.
Caprolactam	Miscellaneous	Adhesives, carpets, caulk, laser printers, latex-based wall covering (some), paint (some), plastics, polyethylene, polyurethane, rubber products & clothing, sealants, tires, styrofoam, water.	Suspected cause of cancer. Narcotic. Blood, central nervous system, eye, & liver damage, headache, loss of appetite, menstrual irregularities, mucous membrane irritation, nausea, nose, throat, lung, & skin irritation.
Carbon monoxide	Miscellaneous	Incomplete combustion of gasoline (automotive exhaust), natural gas, oil, wood, kerosene, etc., sidestream smoke (passive or secondhand smoke).	Odorless gas. Displaces oxygen in the blood, can trigger flulike symptoms, headache, decreased hearing, dizziness, disorientation, fatigue, loss of appetite, intestinal upsets, muscle weakness, eye irritation, diminished sight, personality changes, heart irregularities, seizures, psychosis, heart

Common or Trade Name	Where Found	Sources	Health Effects & Precautions
			palpitations, coma, suffocation, death.
			Slight exposure (3–5%): Fatigue, flu, headaches, nausea, shortness of breath, weakness.
			Moderate exposure (15%): Dim vision, fainting.
			Extreme exposure (40%): Brain damage, coma, convulsions, blood problems, possibly fatal.
Chlorine	Industrial arts Miscellaneous Swimming pool	Aging & oxidizing agents, anesthetics, antiseptics, bleach (including: laundry, cleansers, textiles, wood pulp, foods [flour]), cleaning agents, de-tinning & de-zincing iron, disinfectants, fire extinguishers, food processing (fish, flour, meat, fruit, vegetables), industrial preparations of various compounds (dyes, plastics, & synthetic rubber), metallurgy, oil refining, oven cleaners, pool chemicals, production of organic & inorganic chemicals, showers, shrinkproofing of wool, sugar refining, water sources (bathtubs, hot tubs, municipal water systems), sewage systems.	Allergies. Cause of cancer. Anemia, bronchitis, circulatory collapse, coma, confusion, delirium, diabetes, dizziness, eye, mouth, nose, throat, lung, skin, & stomach irritation, fainting, heart disease, high blood pressure, nausea, lung fluid.
Cresol	Miscellaneous	Air deodorizers & fresheners, dandruff shampoos, disinfectants, mouthwash, toothpaste, typewriter correction fluid, permanent-ink pens & markers.	Absorbed by breathing and skin penetration, blood, kidney, liver, & spleen damage, eye, mucous membrane, and skin irritation, depression, irritability, and hyperactivity.
Dichlorobenzene	Miscellaneous	Air deodorizers & fresheners, carpets, disinfection of drinking water, fumigants (building, grain, soil), mothballs & crystals, paint remover/ stripper.	Possible cause of cancer. Neurotoxic.

Common or Trade Name	Where Found	Sources	Health Effects & Precautions
Diethylene glycol (cellosolve)	Miscellaneous	Antifreeze, carpets, cosmetics, furniture polish, lubricants, plastics, propylene glycol, softening agents, triethylene.	Absorbed by breathing and skin penetration, blood, kidney, & liver damage, eye, mucous membrane, & skin irritation, reproductive problems.
Diisocyanates	Miscellaneous	Adhesives, carpets, paint, paint stripper, phenolic thermosetting resins, photocopiers, plastics, plastic coatings.	Allergies. Toxic to immune system. Asthma, lung damage, nose, throat, & lung irritation.
Ethanol (ethyl alcohol)	Auditorium Cafeteria Cooking class Industrial arts Library Locker room Miscellaneous Music room Shower room Swimming pool Welding class	Adhesives, aftershave, alcoholic beverages, automotive exhaust, bath oil, cleaning compounds, cologne, deodorants, deodorizers, dishwashing liquid & detergent, disinfectants, duplicating fluids, dusting powder, fabric softener, gas appliances, gasoline, glue, hair spray, lavatory deodorizers, metal cleaners & polishes, oil furnaces, oven cleaner, paint & varnish remover, paneling, perfume, polyurethane wood finish, propane gas, soap, shampoo, smoke (cigarette/wood), varnish, vinyl floor tiles.	Intoxication if ingested, hoarseness, liver damage, reproductive problems. Highly flammable.
Ethylene glycol	Miscellaneous	Antifreeze, hydraulic fluid, solvents.	Extremely toxic. Brain, kidney, & liver damage.
Fiberglass	Miscellaneous	Insulation.	Nose, throat, lung, & skin irritation.
Fluoride	Cooking class Industrial arts Library Locker room Miscellaneous Music room Shower room Swimming pool Welding class	Aerosol propellants, aluminum refining, cutting steel, fire extinguishers, hair spray, insecticides, insulation, isotope separation, lubricants, mouthwashes, paneling, plastics, pills, refrigerants, rocket fuel, rodenticide, roofing, soil-release agents, solvents, steel cutting, textile treatment, toothpastes, water.	Cause of cancer. Anemia, bone hardening, fluorosis, gastric, respiratory, & nervous system damage, ligament calcification, skin rashes, tooth discoloration.
Fluorocarbons	Cooking class Industrial arts Library Locker room Music room Shower room Swimming pool Welding class	Aerosol propellants, hair spray, insecticide, insulation, lubricants, paint, plastics, refrigerants, rocket fuel, rodenticide, roofing, Teflon, textile treatments.	Anesthetic. Dizziness, kidney & liver damage. On exposure to heat, release chlorine, hydrogen chloride, hydrogen fluoride, phosgene, & sulfur dioxide gases.

Common or Trade Name	Where Found	Sources	Health Effects & Precautions
Glycerine	Cafeteria Cooking class Industrial arts Library Locker room Miscellaneous Music room Shower room Swimming pool Welding class	Adhesives, allergy extracts, animal fat (beef, chicken, lamb, pork), anti-freezes, astringents, capsules (soft gelatin), cements, coconut, cleaning compounds, cosmetics (especially cake or compact form), cough drops, disinfectants, dry-cleaning agents, emollients, eye drops, fabric soften-ers, face masks, fire retardant for tex-tiles, flavorings, food additives, freckle-removal lotions, glues, hand lotion, ink, insulation, latex paints, lavatory deodorizers, leather, marga-rine, modeling clay, mouthwashes, oven cleaners, paint, paneling, paper, perfume, pharmaceuticals, plastics, polishes, polyurethane foam, regen-erated cellulose, roofing, shaving creams/lotions, shortenings, soaps, solvents, styptic pencils, suntan prep-arations, textile finishes, tobacco, toothpaste, window cleaners.	Allergies in different body areas.
Hexane	Art class Miscellaneous	Adhesives, agricultural seeds, carpets, gasoline, ink, paint thinner, rubber cement, solvents, urea formaldehyde glue, varnish.	Toxic to immune sys-tem. Brain damage.
Lead	Art class Miscellaneous	Cans (food), paint (old), water foun-tains, pipes, polyurethane wood fin-ish, solder.	Possibly fatal. Brain & nervous system dam-age, colic, convulsions, coma, fatigue, head-aches, high blood pres-sure, hyperactivity, mental retardation, muscle aches, repro-ductive problems.
Methanol (wood alcohol)	Library Miscellaneous	Adhesives, duplicating machines, epoxy/glue, phenolic thermosetting resins, polyurethane wood finish, stain, & sealants.	Possibly fatal. Ab-sorbed by lungs & skin, blindness, central ner-vous system damage, delirium, headache, liver damage, nausea & vomiting, skin irrita-tion. Highly flam-mable.
Methyl ethyl ketone	Auditorium Cafeteria Cooking class Gym	Insulation, paint, paneling, roofing, furniture strippers, latex paint, sol-vents, varnish, wall coverings.	Central nervous sys-tem & liver damage.

Common or Trade Name	Where Found	Sources	Health Effects & Precautions
	Industrial arts Library Locker room Music room Printing class Shower room Swimming pool Welding class		
Methylene chloride	Art class Auditorium Cafeteria Cooking class Gym Industrial arts Library Locker room Music room Printing class Shower room Swimming pool Welding class	Adhesives, coffee, cologne, epoxy/glue, insulation, paint, paneling, roofing, furniture strippers, latex paint, lubricants, paint remover/stripper, pesticides, pharmaceuticals, phenolic thermosetting resins, shampoo, wall coverings.	Converts to carbon monoxide in the blood. Bronchitis, central nervous system, & heart damage, eye, lung, & skin irritation, lung fluid. Can damage genes, causing birth defects or cancer.
Nitropyrenes	Miscellaneous	Diesel exhaust, photocopier toners (may be a by-product of carbon-black production, the substance that is the ink of photocopies).	Can cause cancer.
Ozone	Miscellaneous	Computer terminals, laser printers, disinfectant, photocopiers & dry-process copiers, lightning, electric-arc welding.	Possibly fatal. Blood damage, eye, nose, & throat irritation, burning and swelling of the lungs, chronic obstructive lung disease, possible cause of cancer.
Paradichlorobenzene	Some students' clothing	Mothballs	Nose, throat, & lung irritation, liver & kidney damage, depression.
Perchloroethylene: for sources & health effects, see Tetrachloroethylene	Miscellaneous		
Phenylcyclohexene (4-PC)	Miscellaneous	Adhesives, carpet & pad (causes odor), fiber preservative (jute or hemp; carpet backing, burlap, area rugs, rope, twine).	Anesthetic. Central nervous system damage.

Common or Trade Name	Where Found	Sources	Health Effects & Precautions
Bis (2-ethylhexyl) Phthalate (phthalates, phthalic acid esters)	Miscellaneous	Adhesives, carpets, paint, paint stripper, phenolic thermosetting resins, photocopiers, to soften plastic, and in polyvinyl chloride to make medical devices. For injections and intravenous tubing and plastic containers. It is a widely used solvent for pesticides, a fixative in perfumes, found in cosmetics & nail polish. Foods or beverages stored in plastic. Some types are priority toxic pollutants & in hazardous wastes.	Toxic birth defects, liver & testes disease, respiratory illness, asthma, some forms are possibly carcinogenic.
PCBs (polychlorinated biphenyls)	Miscellaneous	Adhesives, carbonless carbon paper, insulating coolants in electrical transformers, lubricants, paints, plastics, stain retardants, varnishes.	Possible irritation of nose, throat, & lungs, central nervous system depression, headaches, & skin rashes. Some cause animal cancer & reproductive problems, i.e., in rats, testicular atrophy.
Styrene, butadiene (ethylbenzene)	Miscellaneous	Adhesives, carpets, caulk, laser printers, latex-based wall covering (some), paint (some), plastics, polyethylene, polyurethane, rubber products & clothing, sealants, tires, Styrofoam, water.	Suspected cause of cancer. Narcotic. Blood, central nervous system, eye, & liver damage, headache, loss of appetite, menstrual irregularities, mucous membrane irritation, nausea, nose, throat, lung, & skin irritation.
Tetrachloroethylene (perc, perchloroethylene)	Art class Miscellaneous	Degreaser/solvent, dry-cleaning, fumigant (building, grain, soil), paint, paint thinner, typewriter correction fluid.	Cause of cancer. Toxic to immune system. Central nervous system, kidney, & liver damage, memory and personality changes.
Toluene (methyl benzene)	Auditorium Cafeteria Cooking class Industrial arts Library Locker room Music room Shower room	Adhesives, carpets, cleaning fluids, composite wood products, degreasers, deodorizers, fossil fuel, gasoline refining, glue, insulation, latex paint, lipstick, typewriter correction fluid, paint, paint stripper, paneling, petroleum products, plastic, polyethylene, polyurethane wood finish, printing	Cause of cancer. Narcotic. Central nervous system damage, depression, disorientation, eye, lung, nose, & skin irritation, fatigue, hoarseness, irritability, kidney, liver, & spleen

Common or Trade Name	Where Found	Sources	Health Effects & Precautions
	Swimming pool Welding class	materials, roofing, rubber cement, solvents, styrene, tobacco smoke, vinyl floor tile, wall coverings, water.	damage, loss of coordination, bone marrow damage, reproductive problems.
Trichloroethane (methyl chloroform, TCA)	Art class Miscellaneous	Degreasers, dry-cleaning, duplicating fluid, fumigants (building, grain, soil), insecticides, insulators, paint, paint thinner, solvents, vinyl floor tile, VOCs, water.	Cause of cancer. Dizziness, headaches, possible liver damage.
Trichlorethylene (TCE, acetylene trichloride)	Art class Miscellaneous	Adhesives, coffee, copy machines, dry-cleaning fluids, fire retardant (textile), floor polish, food additives, fumigant, glue, ink, lacquers, machine & oil solvent/degreaser, paint, paint thinner, rug shampoos, stencil machines, typewriter cleaners, typewriter correction fluid, varnish, wax (coating, household).	Narcotic. Central nervous system damage & depression, dizziness, fatigue, headache, heart, intestinal, & liver damage, loss of coordination, nausea, paralysis, psychosis. On exposure to heat, releases hydrochloric acid & phosgene.
Trinitrofluorenone (TNF)	Miscellaneous	Dry-process copiers.	Can damage genes, causing birth defects or cancer.
Vinyl chloride	Miscellaneous	Electrical wires, furniture upholstery, laminates, lighting fixtures, pipes, plastics, polyethylene, synthetic carpeting, wall coverings, water, weatherstripping.	Can damage genes, causing birth defects or cancer. Bronchitis, eye, nose, throat, lung, skin, & stomach irritation, numbness, cold, blue hands & feet.
Xylene (xylol)	Art class Auditorium Biology Cafeteria Cooking class Industrial arts Library Locker room Miscellaneous Music room Shower room Swimming pool Welding class	Adhesives, carpets, cleaning compounds, degreasers, disinfectants, epoxy/glue, fossil fuel, furniture strippers, gasoline, gums, inks, insecticides, microscope lens cleaners, paint, paint thinner/stripper, paneling, pesticides, phenolic thermosetting resins, photocopiers & photographic solutions, plastics, resins, roofing, solvents, synthetic fibers, varnish, wall coverings.	Narcotic. Possibly fatal. Central nervous system damage, coma, confusion, dizziness, fatigue, headache, heart problems, hoarseness, kidney & liver damage, lung irritation, bone marrow suppression, nausea, rashes, reproductive problems, short-term memory loss. Highly flammable.

TABLE A.3

Chemicals Found in Scented Products

Common or Trade Name	Where Found	Health Effects & Precautions
Acetone	Cologne, dishwashing liquid & detergent, nail polish/hardener/undercoat/remover.	If inhaled, causes dry mouth & throat, dizziness, nausea, incoordination, slurred speech, drowsiness, & in severe exposures, coma. Dulls the central nervous system (CNS).* Considered hazardous waste by the EPA, RCRA, and CERCLA.
Benzaldehyde	Perfume, cologne, hair spray, laundry bleach, deodorants, detergent, hand lotion, shaving cream, shampoo, bar soap, dishwasher detergent.	Irritation to the mouth, throat, eyes, skin, lungs, & GI tract causing nausea and abdominal pain; may cause kidney damage. Acts as a narcotic, local anesthetic, dulls the nervous system.
Benzyl acetate**	Perfume, cologne, shampoo, fabric softener, stick-up air freshener, dishwashing liquid & detergent, soap, hair spray, bleach, aftershave, deodorants.	Can cause cancer, especially of the pancreas, vapors irritate eyes & lungs, cough. Can be absorbed through the skin.
Benzyl alcohol**	Perfume, cologne, soap, shampoo, nail enamel remover, air freshener, laundry bleach & detergent, hand lotion, deodorants, fabric softener.	Irritates nose, throat, lungs, headache, nausea, vomiting, dizziness, drop in blood pressure, dulls the nervous system, death in severe cases due to respiratory failure.
Camphor	Perfume, shaving cream, nail enamel, fabric softener, dishwasher detergent, stick-up air freshener.	Irritates eyes, nose, & throat, dizziness, confusion, nausea, twitchy muscles & convulsions. Stimulates nervous system. Do not inhale.
Ethanol	Perfume, hair spray, shampoo, fabric softener, dishwashing liquid & detergent, laundry detergent, shaving cream, soap, hand lotion, air fresheners, nail polish/hardener/undercoat/remover, paint & varnish remover.	Fatigue, irritates eyes & nose, throat and lungs, in low concentrations. If inhaled or ingested, drowsiness, impaired vision, loss of coordination, stupor. Hazardous waste, according to the EPA.
Ethyl acetate	Aftershave, cologne, perfume, shampoo, nail polish/hardener/undercoat/remover, fabric softener, dishwashing liquid & detergent.	Irritates eyes & nose, throat & lungs, headache, stupor, dries skin, may cause anemia & liver & kidney damage. Acts as a narcotic & is a hazardous waste, according to the EPA.
Limonene**	Perfume, cologne, disinfectant spray, bar soap, shaving cream, deodorants, nail polish/hardener/undercoat/remover, fabric softener, dishwashing liquid & detergent, air	Causes cancer. Prevent contact with skin, as it irritates and sensitizes. Do not inhale. Wash hands thoroughly after using this material & before eating, drinking, & applying cosmetics.

Common or Trade Name	Where Found	Health Effects & Precautions
	fresheners, aftershave, bleach, paint & varnish remover.	
Linalool**	Perfume, cologne, bar soap, shampoo, hand lotion, nail enamel remover, hair spray, laundry detergent, dishwashing liquid & detergent, hand lotion, air fresheners, bleach powder, fabric softener, shaving cream, aftershave, solid deodorant.	Breathing problems, attracts bees, in animal testing it has been shown to produce a peculiar walk, affects muscles, depression. Acts as a narcotic, drowsiness.
Methylene chloride	Shampoo, cologne, paint, & varnish remover.	Headache, giddiness, stupor, irritability, fatigue, tingling in limbs. Can cause cancer. When absorbed, is stored in body fat. Reduces the oxygen in the blood. Considered hazardous waste by EPA, RCRA, and CERCLA.
a-pinene	Bar and liquid soap, cologne, perfume, shaving cream, deodorants, dishwashing liquid & detergent, air freshener.	Damages the immune system. Makes sensitive to other substances.
g-terpinene	Cologne, perfume, soap, shaving cream, deodorant, air freshener.	Causes asthma & nervous disorders.
a-terpineol**	Perfume, cologne, laundry detergent, bleach powder, laundry bleach, fabric softener, stick-up air freshener, hand lotion, cologne, soap, hair spray, aftershave, roll-on deodorant.	Highly irritating to mouth, nose, & eyes. Causes excitement, headache, loss of muscular coordination, hypothermia, CNS depression, difficulty breathing. Can cause pneumonia or fatal edema. Prevent prolonged or repeated skin contact.

*CNS (central nervous system) disorders include multiple sclerosis, Parkinson's disease, Alzheimer's disease, and sudden infant death syndrome.

**An FDA analysis (1968–1972) of 138 compounds used in cosmetics that most frequently involved adverse reactions identified five commonly used in fragrance products: a-terpineol, benzyl acetate, benzyl alcohol, limonene, and linalool.

Source: The information in this table was taken from a 1991 EPA study entitled ''Twenty Most Common Chemicals Found in Thirty-One Fragrance Products.''

TABLE A.4

Gas and Vapor Exposures

Common or Trade Name	Sources	Health Effects
Acetaldehyde	Breakdown of alcohol, carpet, and fabric fumes, plastic fumes, formaldehyde-coated paper, sidestream smoke (passive or second-hand smoke), smog, vehicle exhaust.	Upper respiratory tract irritation, coughing, wheezing, central nervous system depression and disruption.
Acetonitrile (methyl cyanide)	Sidestream smoke (passive or secondhand smoke).	Liver and blood damage, eye and skin irritation, shock.
Acetylene	Industrial arts class.	Flammable, asphyxiating (reduces necessary volume of oxygen in air).
Ammonia	Cleaning compounds, deodorants, disinfectants, duplicating machines, industrial use, sidestream smoke (passive or secondhand smoke).	Conjunctivitis, irritation of eye, nose, throat, & lungs, laryngitis, pneumonitis, lung fluid, chemical burns, blindness. Possibly fatal.
Argon	Industrial arts class.	Inert noninflammable gas, asphyxiating (reduces necessary volume of oxygen in air).
Bromine	In some pools; industrial use.	Coughing, nosebleed, feeling of oppression, dizziness, headache, stomach pains, diarrhea, rash, burns, ulcers, thyroid abnormalities, chronic sore throat, heart disease, low blood pressure.
Butane	Industrial arts class, chemistry class	Flammable, asphyxiating (reduces necessary volume of oxygen in air).
CO_2 (carbon dioxide)	Ordinary breathing, industrial use, sidestream smoke (passive or secondhand smoke).	Asphyxiating (reduces necessary volume of oxygen in air).
CO (carbon monoxide)	Idling school buses or automobiles, incomplete combustion of gasoline, natural gas, oil, wood, kerosene, etc., sidestream smoke (passive or secondhand smoke). 1% is 1,000 ppm, 2% is 2,000 ppm, etc.	<5% drowsiness, fatigue, flu, nausea, shortness of breath, weakness; <15% eye, intestinal complaints, headaches evident, fainting; <40% brain damage, coma, convulsions, blood problems, death.
Chlorine	Tap water, showers, & pools, aging & oxidizing agents, anesthetics, antiseptics, bleach (including: laundry, cleaners, textiles, wood pulp, foods [flour]), cleaning agents, de-tinning & de-zincing iron, disinfectants, fire extinguishers, food processing (fish, flour, meat,	Asthma, hay fever, anemia, bronchitis, circulatory collapse, coma, confusion, delirium, diabetes, dizziness, eye, mouth, nose, throat, lung, skin, & stomach irritation, fainting, heart disease, high blood

Common or Trade Name	Sources	Health Effects
	fruit, vegetables), industrial preparations of various compounds (dyes, plastics, & synthetic rubber), metallurgy, oil refining, oven cleaners, production of organic & inorganic chemicals, shrinkproofing of wool, sugar refining, water sources (bathtubs, hot tubs, municipal water systems), sewage systems.	pressure, nausea, lung fluid. Possible cause of cancer.
Ethane	Industrial arts class.	Flammable, asphyxiating (reduces necessary volume of oxygen in air).
Ethylene	Antifreeze, solvents, industrial use.	Flammable, asphyxiating (reduces necessary volume of oxygen in air).
Fluorine	Industrial arts class.	Skin, eye, mouth, throat, & respiratory tract irritation, lung swelling, thermal burns.
Helium	Industrial arts class, physics class.	Asphyxiating (reduces necessary volume of oxygen in air).
Hydrogen	Industrial arts class.	Flammable, asphyxiating (reduces necessary volume of oxygen in air).
Hydrogen cyanide	Blast furnaces, gas works, coke ovens, fumigation, sidestream smoke (passive or secondhand smoke).	Headache, mental confusion, nausea & vomiting, unconsciousness, cessation of breathing, death.
HS (hydrogen sulfide)	Industrial arts class, manufacture of chemicals, dyes, & pigments, petroleum refining.	Eye & upper respiratory tract irritation, suffocation, chronic lung disease.
Iodine vapor	Industrial arts class.	Lung irritation & swelling, eye irritation, inflammation of respiratory tract, runny nose, mouth & throat sores, nervousness, thyroid damage, weight loss.
Methane	Industrial arts, home economics, & chemistry classes; heating units.	Flammable, asphyxiating (reduces necessary volume of oxygen in air).
Neon	Industrial arts class.	Asphyxiating (reduces necessary volume of oxygen in air).
Nitrogen	Industrial arts class.	Asphyxiating (reduces necessary volume of oxygen in air).
NO_2 (nitrogen dioxide)	Faulty combustion, sidestream smoke (passive or secondhand smoke).	Respiratory & eye problems, particularly in asthma-prone children.
Nitrogen oxide	Dyes, lacquers, celluloid, incomplete combustion.	Eye & upper respiratory tract irritation, coughing & chest pain, lung swelling, cold sweat, nausea, severe

Common or Trade Name	Sources	Health Effects
		shortness of breath, air hunger, anxiety, death.
Nitrous oxide	Industrial arts class, incomplete combustion.	Asphyxiating (reduces necessary volume of oxygen in air).
Ozone	Can be produced in oxygen in the air by lightning, shop (electric-arc welding), computer terminals, photocopiers, dry-process copiers, laser printers.	Burning & swelling of the lungs, chronic obstructive lung disease, possible cause of cancer.
Propane	Industrial arts class.	Flammable, asphyxiating (reduces necessary volume of oxygen in air).
Radon	Produced in soil.	Colorless, odorless. Lung damage, cause of cancer, death.
SO_2 (sulfur dioxide)	Industrial arts class incomplete combustion causes odor of rotten eggs. When fluorocarbons (from aerosol propellants, hair spray, insecticide, insulation, lubricants, paint, plastics, refrigerants, rocket fuel, rodenticide, roofing, textile treatment) are heated, this gas is released.	Upper respiratory tract irritation, lung swelling, changes in the senses of taste & smell, fatigue.
Volatile organic compounds (VOCs)	Solvent VOCs: lacquers, cleaners, adhesive, paints, strippers, degreasers, cosmetics containing benzene, toluene, methyl & ethyl compounds, mineral spirits & ethers, freshly dry-cleaned clothes. Organochloride VOCs: pesticides, cleaning agents, and preservatives such as 1,1,1-trichloroethane, trichloroethylene, carbon tetrachloride, chlorobenzene, heptachlor & chlordane, pentachlorophenol, & hexachlorophene. PCBs & vinyl chloride are also in this category. Phenol VOCs: coal tar & petroleum compounds, disinfectants, antiseptics, plastics, cleaners, perfumes, air fresheners, mouthwashes, polishes, waxes, & glues.	Toxic to immune system. Anemia, blurred vision, bone marrow & central nervous system depression, birth defects, disorientation, drowsiness, drunken behavior, silly feeling, eye, gastrointestinal, nose, throat, & lung irritation, fatigue, headache, leukemia, lightheadedness, loss of appetite, low white blood cell count, multiple myeloma, nerve problems, paralysis, rashes, reproductive problems. Particularly significant during painting & cleaning activities. In poorly ventilated indoor settings, levels can reach 100 ppm or more. Also can be absorbed by building materials & fabrics, which can pose potential long-term exposure risks. A potential cause of leukemia.

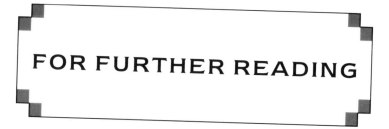

FOR FURTHER READING

Books for the General Reader

ALLERGY

Krohn, Jacqueline, F. A. Taylor, and E. M. Larson. *The Whole Way to Allergy Relief and Prevention* (Port Roberts, WA: Hartley and Marks, 1991).

Mandell, Marshall. *Dr. Mandell's Five Day Allergy Relief System* (New York: Thomas Y. Crowell, 1979).

Miller, Joseph B. *Relief at Last!* (Springfield, IL: Charles C. Thomas, 1987).

Randolph, Theron G. "Human Ecology and Susceptibility to the Chemical Environment" (questionnaire), *Annals of Allergy*, vol. 19 (May 1961), pp. 533–38.

———. "Allergic-Type Reactions to Industrial Solvents and Liquid Fuels; Mosquito Abatement Fogs and Mists; Motor Exhausts; Indoor Utility Gas and Oil Fumes; Chemical Additives of Foods and Drugs; Synthetic Drugs and Cosmetics," *Journal of Laboratory and Clinical Medicine*, vol. 44 (1954), pp. 910–14.

———, and R. W. Moss. *An Alternative Approach to Allergies* (New York: Harper and Row, 1989).

Rapp, Doris J. *Allergies and Your Family* (Buffalo, NY: Practical Allergy Research Foundation, 1989).

———. *The Impossible Child at School and at Home* (Buffalo, NY: Practical Allergy Research Foundation).

———. *Is This Your Child?* (Buffalo, NY: Practical Allergy Research Foundation).

Rinkel, Herbert J., et al. *Food Allergy* (Springfield, IL: Charles C. Thomas, 1951).

Rowe, Albert, and Albert Rowe, Jr. *Food Allergy* (Springfield, IL: Charles C. Thomas, 1972).

ALLERGY DIETS

Golos, Natalie, and F. Golos Golbitz, *If This Is Chicken, It Must Be Tuesday* (New Canaan, CT: Keats Publishing Co., 1983).

Powell, Donna. *Why 5?* (Waterdown, Ont.: Cobra Limited, 1989). The publisher's address is Box 25, Waterdown, Ontario, Canada L0R 2H0.

Rockwell, Sally. *The Rotation Game* (Seattle: Sally Rockwell Publishing, 1981).

CARPETS

Beebe, Glenn. *Toxic Carpet III* (Cincinnati, OH: Glenn Beebe, 1991). The publisher's address is P.O. Box 53344, Cincinnati, OH 45253.

Carpet and Rug Institute. *Floorcovering Products for Schools* (Dalton, GA: Carpet and Rug Institute, 1995). A report by carpet industry representatives. The publisher's address is P.O. Box 204B, Dalton, GA 30722.

Oetzel, Mary. *The Comparative Cost of School Floorcoverings* (Austin, TX: Environmental Education and Health Services, 1992, 1994). The publisher's address is P.O. Box 92004, Austin, TX 78709.

CHEMICAL SENSITIVITY

Board on Environmental Studies and Toxicology Commission on Life Sciences. *Multiple Chemical Sensitivities; Addendum to Biologic Markers in Immunotoxicology* (Washington, DC: National Academy Press, 1992).

Calabrese, E. J. *Genetic Variation in Susceptibility to Environmental Agents* (New York: Wiley Interscience, 1984).

———. *Pollutants and High Risk Groups: The Biological Basis of Increased Human Susceptibility to Environmental and Occupational Pollutants* (New York: Wiley Interscience, 1977).

Hilman, B. *Multiple Chemical Sensitivity* (Washington, DC: American Chemical Society, 1991).

Matthews, Bonnye L. *Chemical Sensitivity* (Jefferson, NC: McFarland & Co., 1992).

Rea, William. *Chemical Sensitivity*, 4 vols. (Chelsea, MI: Lewis Publishers, 1991–1996). The publisher's address is 121 South Main, Chelsea, MI 48118.

Small, B. M. *The Susceptibility Report: Chemical Susceptibility and Urea Formaldehyde Foam Insulation* (Goodwood, Ont.: Small and Associates, 1982). The publisher's address is R.R. #1, Goodwood, Ont., L0C 1A0 Canada.

Wilson, Cynthia. *Chemical Exposures and Human Health* (Jefferson, NC: McFarland and Co., 1993).

ENVIRONMENTAL ILLNESS

Ali, Majid. *The Canary and Chronic Fatigue* (Denville, NJ: Life Span Press, 1995). The publisher's address is 95 East Main Street, Denville, NJ 07834.

———. *RDA: Rats, Drugs and Assumptions* (Denville, NJ: Life Span Press, 1995). The publisher's address is 95 East Main Street, Denville, NJ 07834.

American Association of School Administrators. *Schoolhouse in the Red* (Arlington, VA: AASA, 1992). The publisher's address is 1801 North Moore Street, Arlington, VA 22209.

Ashford, Nicholas, and Claudia Miller. *Chemical Exposures: Low Levels and High Stakes* (New York: Van Nostrand Reinhold, 1991).

Colborn, Theo, Dianne Dumanski, and John Peterson Myers. *Our Stolen Future: Are We Threatening Our Fertility, Intelligence, and Survival?—A Scientific Detective Story* (New York: Dutton, 1996).

Durnil, Gordon. *The Making of a Conservative Environmentalist* (Bloomington, IN: Indiana University Press, 1995).

Freydberg, N., and W. A. Gortner. *The Food Additives Book* (New York: Bantam, 1982).

Green, Nancy S. *Poisoning Our Children: Surviving in a Toxic World* (Chicago: Noble Press, 1991).

Makower, J. *Office Hazards* (Washington, DC: Tilden Press, 1981).

Moses, Marion. *Designer Poisons* (San Francisco: Pesticide Education Center, 1995).

National Research Council. *Indoor Pollutants* (Washington, DC: National Academy Press, 1981).

Rapp, Doris J. *Is This Your Child?* (New York: William Morrow & Co, 1991).

——. *The Impossible Child, at School and at Home* (Buffalo, NY: Practical Allergy Research Foundation, 1989).

Regenstein, Lewis G. *Cleaning Up America the Poisoned* (Washington, DC: Acropolis Books, 1993). The publisher's address is 2311 Calvert Street, N.W., Washington, DC 20008.

Rogers, Sherry. *Tired or Toxic?* (Syracuse, NY: Prestige Publishing, 1990).

Sahley, Billie. *The Anxiety Epidemic*, 2d ed. (San Antonio, TX: Pain and Stress Center, 1995).

Tate, Nicholas. *The Sick Building Syndrome* (Far Hills, NJ: New Horizon Press, 1994).

Taylor, Joyal. *The Complete Guide to Mercury Toxicity* (San Diego, CA: Scripps, 1988).

Thrasher, Jack, and Alan Broughton. *The Poisoning of Our Homes and Workplaces* (Santa Ana, CA: Seadora, 1989).

Winter, Carl K., J. N. Seiber, and C. F. Nuckton. *Chemicals in the Human Food Chain* (New York: Van Nostrand Reinhold, 1990).

HEALTHY LIVING

Ali, Majid. *The Butterfly and Life Span Nutrition* (Denville, NJ: Life Span Press, 1992). The publisher's address is 95 East Main Street, Denville, NJ 07834.

Berthold-Bond, Annie. *Clean and Green* (Woodstock, NY: Ceres Press, 1990).

Bower, John. *Healthy House Building: A Design and Construction Guide* (Bloomington, IN: Healthy House Institute, 1993).

——. *The Healthy House* (Bloomington, IN: Healthy House Institute, 1989).

Bower, Lynn Marie. *The Healthy Household* (Bloomington, IN: Healthy House Institute, 1995).

Dadd, Debra Lynn. *The Nontoxic Home and Office* (New York: Jeremy P. Tarcher, 1992).

——. *Nontoxic, Natural, and Earthwise* (Los Angeles: Jeremy P. Tarcher, 1990).

Dine, Joan. "Toxic Reduction," in *Greening Synagogues and Community Centers*, ed. Naomi Friedman (Wyncote, PA: Shomrei Adamah, 1995).

Gorman, Carolyn P. *Less Toxic Living* (Texarkana, TX: Optima Graphics, 1993).

Inlander, Charles B., and Eugene I. Pavalon. *Your Medical Rights* (Boston: Little, Brown, 1990).

Krohn, Jacqueline. *The Whole Way to Natural Detoxification* (Port Roberts, WA: Hartley and Marks, 1996).

Lawson, Lynn. *Staying Well in a Toxic World* (Chicago: Noble Press, 1993).

Marinelli, Janet, and Paul Bierman-Lytle. *Your Natural Home* (Boston: Little, Brown, 1995).

McGowen, Jeannie. *Your Home and Your Health*, 3rd ed. (Dallas, TX: Bruce Miller, 1994). The publisher's address is Bruce Miller Enterprises, P.O. Box 743244, Dallas, TX 75374.

Murray, Frank. *The Big Family Guide to All Minerals* (New Canaan, CT: Keats Publishing, 1995). The publisher's address is Keats Publishing, 27 Pine Street, Box 876, New Canaan, CT 06840.

National Education Association, *The Healthy School Handbook* (Washington, DC: NEA Professional Library, 1995).

Rogers, Sherry. *Wellness Against All Odds* (Syracuse, NY: Prestige, 1995).

——. *The Scientific Basis for Selected Environmental Medicine Techniques* (Sarasota, FL: SK Publishing, 1995). The publisher's address is P.O. Box 40101, Sarasota, FL 34242.

Ross, James W. *Social Security Benefits: How to Get Them! How to Keep Them!* (Slippery Rock, PA: Ross Publishing Co., 1984).

Rousseau, David, William J. Rea, and Jean Enwright. *Your Home, Your Health and Well-Being* (Vancouver, BC: Hartley and Marks, 1989).

Sahley, Billie. *The Natural Way to Control Hyperactivity with Amino Acids and Nutrient Therapy*, 2d ed. (San Antonio, TX: Pain and Stress Center, 1994).

———, and Katherine Birkner. *Breaking Your Addiction Habit* (San Antonio, TX: Pain and Stress Center, 1990).

Small, B. M. *Recommendations for Action on Pollution and Education in Toronto* (Ont.: Small and Associates, 1985). The publisher's address is R.R. #1, Goodwood, Ont., L0C 1A0 Canada.

Smith, Lendon H. *Feed Your Body Right* (New York: M. Evans and Co., 1995).

Steinman, David, and Samuel Epstein. *The Safe Shopper's Bible* (New York: Macmillan, 1995).

Steinman, David, and R. Michael Wisner. *Living Healthy in a Toxic World* (New York: Putnam, 1996).

Wright, Jonathan. *Dr. Wright's Guide to Healing with Nutrition* (New Canaan, CT: Keats Publishing, 1991). The publisher's address is 27 Pine Street, Box 876, New Canaan, CT 06840.

INDOOR AIR QUALITY

Maryland Department of Education. *Air Cleaning Devices for HVAC Supply Systems in Schools.* For address, see Resources.

National Air Duct Cleaners Association. *The Mechanical Cleaning of Nonporous Air Conveyance System Components* (Oct. 23, 1982). For address, see Resources.

U.S. Environmental Protection Agency. *Building Air Quality: A Guide for Building Owners and Facility Managers*, no. 055-000-00390-4 (Washington, DC: U.S. Government Printing Office, 1991).

U.S. Environmental Protection Agency. *Indoor Air Quality Tools for Schools.* (Washington, DC: U.S. Government Printing Office).

U.S. Environmental Protection Agency. *Indoor Air Pollution*, no. 523-217-81322 (Washington, DC: U.S. Government Printing Office, 1994).

U.S. Environmental Protection Agency. *Indoor Allergens*, no. IAQ-0057 (Washington, DC: U.S. Government Printing Office).

U.S. Environmental Protection Agency. *Inside Story: A Guide to Indoor Air Quality*, no. 055-000-00441-2. (Washington, DC: U.S. Government Printing Office, 1995).

U.S. Environmental Protection Agency. *Residential Air Cleaning Devices*, no. IAQ-0010 (Washington, DC: U.S. Government Printing Office).

U.S. Environmental Protection Agency and National Institute for Occupational Safety and Health. *Building Air Quality* (Washington, DC: U.S. Government Printing Office).

U.S. Occupational Safety and Health Administration. *Indoor Air Quality Investigation*, no. 1910-1033 (Washington, DC: U.S. Government Printing Office).

U.S. Occupational Safety and Health Administration. *Indoor Air Quality and Workplace Smoking Rules* (Washington, DC: U.S. Government Printing Office).

PESTICIDES AND SAFER PEST MANAGEMENT

Abrams, R., et al. *Pesticides in Schools: Reducing the Risks* (New York State, 1993). Available from New York State: Department of Law, Environmental Protection Bureau, 120 Broadway, New York, NY 10271.

Lieberman, A., P. Hardman, and P. Preston. *Academic, Behavioral, and Perceptual Reactions in Dyslexic Children When Exposed to Environmental Factors: Malathion and Petrochemical Ethanol* (Tallahassee, FL: Dyslexia Research Institute, 1981). The publisher's address is 4745 Centerville Road, Tallahassee, FL 32308.

Mott, L., and K. Snyder. *Pesticide Alert: A Guide to Pesticides in Fruits and Vegetables* (San Francisco: Sierra Club Books, 1987).

Olkowski, W., S. Daar, and H. Olkowski. *Common-Sense Pest Control* (Albany: New York Coalition for Alternatives to Pesticides, 1991, 1994). The publisher's address is 353 Hamilton Street, Albany, NY 12210-1709.

Snell, P., and K. Nichol. *Pesticide Residues and Food: The Case for Real Control* (London Food Commission, 1986).

U.S. Environmental Protection Agency. *Information on Wood Preservatives in Playground Equipment* (Washington, DC: U.S. Government Printing Office).

U.S. Environmental Protection Agency. *Information on Lawn Care Alternatives* (Washington, DC: U.S. Government Printing Office).

U.S. Environmental Protection Agency. *Parents, Teachers and Administrators Make the Difference Around the Country* (Washington, DC: U.S. Government Printing Office).

U.S. Environmental Protection Agency. *Pest Control in Schools: Adopting Integrated Pest Management* (Washington, DC: U.S. Government Printing Office).

U.S. Environmental Protection Agency. *The Recognition and Management of Pesticide Poisonings*, 4th ed., no. EPA-540-9-88-001 (Washington, DC: U.S. Government Printing Office, 1989).

U.S. Environmental Protection Agency. *Sample Indoor IPM Contracts* (Washington, DC: U.S. Government Printing Office).

RADON

U.S. Environmental Protection Agency. *Radon Measurement in Schools* (1993), no. 402-R-92-014 (Washington, DC: U.S. Government Printing Office, 1993).

U.S. Environmental Protection Agency. *Radon Reduction Techniques in Detached Houses*, no. 625/5/86-0/9 (Washington, DC: U.S. Government Printing Office, 1988).

Periodicals

Human Ecologist
Human Ecology Action League
P.O. Box 49126
Atlanta, GA 30359-1126
(404) 248–1898

Mastering Food Allergies
2615 North Fourth Street, Suite 616
Coeur d'Alene, ID 83814-3781
(208) 772-8213

Rachel's Environment and Health Weekly
Environmental Research Foundation
P.O. Box 5036
Annapolis, MD 21403-7036
(410) 463-1584
fax (410) 263-4894

Toxic Law Reporter
1231 Twenty-fifth Street, N.W.
Washington, DC 20037
(800) 372-1033

Toxic Times
Chemical Injury Information Network
P.O. Box 301
White Sulphur Springs, MT 59645
(406) 547-2255

Studies of Allergy Testing

(You may submit references or copies of these articles to your insurance company to document your claim for environmental medical care.)

STUDIES OF FOOD ALLERGIES

Crook, W. G., et al. "Systemic Manifestations Due to Allergy." *Pediatrics*, vol. 27 (1961), p. 790.

Finn, R., and H. N. Cohen. "Food Allergy: Fact or Fiction." *Lancet 1* (1978), pp. 426–28.

Green, M. "Sublingual Provocative Testing for Foods and F, D, and C Dyes." *Annals of Allergy*, vol. 33 (1974), pp. 274–81.

O'Banion, D. B., B. Armstrong, and R. H. Cummings. "Disruptive Behavior: A Dietary Approach." *Journal of Autism and Childhood Schizophrenia*, vol. 8 (1978), p. 325.

Randolph, T. G., and J. P. Rollins. "Beet Sensitivity: Allergic Reactions from Ingesting Beet Sugar (Sucrose) and Monosodium Glutamate of Beet Origin." *Journal of Laboratory and Clinical Medicine*, vol. 366 (1950), pp. 407–14.

———. "Allergic Reactions from Ingestion or Intravenous Injection of Cane Sugar (Sucrose)." *Journal of Laboratory and Clinical Medicine*, vol. 36 (1950), pp. 242–48.

———, and C.K. Walter. "Allergic Reactions Following Intravenous Injection of Corn Sugar (Dextrose)." *Archives of Surgery*, vol. 61 (1950), pp. 554–64.

STUDIES SUPPORTING THE CONNECTION BETWEEN FOOD ALLERGIES AND ILLNESS

Bernstein, M. "Double-Blind Food Challenge in the Diagnosis of Food Sensitivity in the Adult." *Journal of Allergy and Clinical Immunology*, vol. 70 (1982), pp. 205–10.

Finn, R., and T. M. Battcock, "A Critical Study of Clinical Ecology." *Practitioner*, vol. 229 (1985), pp. 883–85.

Gerrard, J. "Just Food Intolerance." *Lancet 2* (1984), p. 413.

Goldman, J. A., et al. "Behavioral Effects of Sucrose on Preschool Children." *Journal of Abnormal Psychology*, vol. 14, no. 4 (1986), pp. 585–87.

Radcliffe, M.J. "Food Allergy in Polysymptomatic Patients." *Practitioner*, vol. 225 (1981), pp. 1652–54.

Rapp, D. J. "A Prototype for Food Sensitivity Studies in Children (Abstract No. 25)." *Annals of Allergy*, vol. 47 (1981), pp. 123–24.

———. "Weeping Eyes in Wheat Allergy." *Trans American Society of Ophthalmology and Otolaryngology*, vol. 18 (1978), p. 149.

Rowe, Katherine S., and Kenneth J. Rowe, "Synthetic Food Coloring and Behavior: A Dose Response Effect in a Double-Blind, Placebo-Controlled, Repeated-Measures Study." *Journal of Pediatrics*, vol. 125, no. 5, part 1 (Nov. 1994), pp. 691–98.

Colitis

Soothill, J. F., et al. "Food Allergy: The Major Cause of Infantile Colitis." *Archives of Disease in Childhood*, vol. 59 (1983), pp. 326–29.

Eczema

Atherton, D. J., et al. "A Double-Blind Controlled Crossover Trial of an Antigen Avoidance Diet in Atopic Eczema." *Lancet 1* (1978), pp. 401–03.

Epilepsy

Crayton, J. W. "Epilepsy Precipitated by Food Sensitivity: Report of a Case with Double-Blind Placebo-Controlled Assessment." *Clinical Electroencephalography*, vol. 12 (1981), p. 192.

Egger, J., et al. "Oligoantigenic Diet Treatment of Children with Epilepsy and Migraine." *Journal of Pediatrics*, vol. 114, no. 1 (1989), pp. 51–58.

Hyperactivity

Boris, Marvin, and Francine S. Mandel. "Foods and Additives Are Common Causes of the Attention Deficit Hyperactive Disorder in Children." *Annals of Allergy*, vol. 72 (1994), pp. 462–68.

Carter, C. M., et al. "Effects of a Few Food Diets in Attention Deficit Disorder." *Archives of Diseases of Childhood*, vol. 69 (1993), pp. 564–68.

Egger, J., et al. "Controlled Trial of Oligoantigenic Treatment in the Hyperkinetic Syndrome." *Lancet 1* (1985), pp. 540–45.

Kaplan, B. J., et al. "Dietary Replacement in Preschool-Aged Hyperactive Boys." *Pediatrics*, vol. 83 (1989), pp. 7–17.

Levy, F., et al. "Hyperkinesis and Diet: A Double-Blind Crossover Trial with a Tartrazene Challenge." *Medical Journal of Australia*, vol. 1 (1978), pp. 61–64.

Prinz, R. J., W.A. Roberts, and E. Hantman. "Dietary Correlates of Hyperactive Behavior in Children." *Journal of Consulting and Clinical Psychology*, vol. 48 (1980), pp. 760–69.

Rapp, D. J. "Does Diet Affect Hyperactivity?" *Journal of Learning Disabilities*, vol. 11 (1978), pp. 56–62.

———. "Food Allergy Treatment for Hyperkinesis." *Journal of Learning Disabilities*, vol. 12 (1979), pp. 42–50.

———. "Double-Blind Confirmation and Treatment of Milk Sensitivity." *Medical Journal of Australia*, vol. 1 (1978), pp. 571–72.

Shaywitz, B. A., J. R. Goldenring, and R.S. Wool. "Effects of Chronic Administration of Food Colorings on Activity Levels and Cognitive Performance in Normal and Hyperactive Developing Rat Pups." *Annals of Neurology*, vol. 4 (1978), p. 196.

Swanson, J. "Food Dyes Impair Performance of Hyperactive Children on a Laboratory Learning Test." *Science*, vol. 207 (1980), pp. 1485–87.

Trites, R. W., H. Tryphonas, and B. Ferguson. *Case Studies in Treatment of Hyperactivity in a Child with Allergies to Food* (Springfield, IL: Charles C. Thomas, 1978).

Tryphonas, H., and R. Trites. "Food Allergy in Children with Hyperactivity, Learning Disabilities, and/or Minimal Brain Dysfunction." *Annals of Allergy*, vol. 42 (1979), pp. 22–27.

Weiss, B. "Behavioral Responses to Artificial Food Colors." *Science*, vol. 207 (1980), pp. 1487–89.

Williams, J. I., et al. "Relative Effects of Drugs and Diet on Hyperactive Behaviors: An Experimental Study." *Pediatrics*, vol. 61 (1978), pp. 811–17.

Kidney Disease

Lagrue, G., et al. "Food Sensitivity and Idiopathic Nephrotic Syndrome." *Lancet 2*, issue 8458 (Oct. 5, 1985), p. 777.

Sandberg, D. H., et al. "Severe Steroid-Responsive Nephrosis Associated with Hyperactivity." *Lancet* (1977), 1:388.

Learning Difficulties

Colgan, M., and L. Colgan. "Do Nutrient Supplements and Dietary Changes Affect Learning and Emotional Reactions of Children with Learning Difficulties? A Controlled Series of 16 Cases." *Nutrition and Health*, vol. 3 (1984), pp. 69–77.

Lung Disease

Gerdes, K. A., and J. C. Selner. "Bronchospasm Following IV Dextrose (Abstract No. 25)." *Annals of Allergy*, vol. 48 (1980), p. 4.

Migraine

Egger, J., et al. "Is Migraine Food Allergy? A Double-Blind Controlled Trial of Oligoantigenic Diet Treatment." *Lancet*, vol. 11 (1983), pp. 865–69.

Egger, J., et al. "Oligoantigenic Diet Treatment of Children with Epilepsy and Migraine." *Journal of Pediatrics*, vol. 114, no. 1 (1989), pp. 51–58.

Monro, J. "Food Allergy and Migraine." *Clinical Immunology and Allergy*, vol. 42 (1983), pp. 241–46.

P/N ALLERGY TESTING: OVERVIEWS

Davidoff, Ann L., and Linda Fogarty. "Psychogenic Origins of Multiple Chemical Sensitivities Syndrome: A Critical Review of the Research Literature." *Archives of Environmental Health*, vol. 49, no. 5 (1994), pp. 316–24.

Freed, David L. J. "Part I. The Provocation-Neutralization Technique. Part II. Can We Diagnose Allergies, Do We Know What We Are Doing, Does It Matter?" in *Food Intolerance,* ed. John Dobbing (London: Bailliere Tindall, 1987), pp. 151–84.

Gerdes, Kendall A. "Provocation/Neutralization Testing: A Look at the Controversy." *Clinical Ecology,* vol. 6, no. 1 (1991), pp. 21–29.

Podell, Richard N. "Intracutaneous and Sublingual Provocation and Neutralization." *Clinical Ecology,* vol. 2, no. 1 (1993), pp. 13–20.

Rapp, Doris J. "Environmental Medicine: An Expanded Approach to Allergy." *Buffalo Physician* (1986), pp. 16–24.

STUDIES SUPPORTING THE EFFICACY OF SUBCUTANEOUS P/N TREATMENT

Single-Blinded Studies

Bentley, S. J., D. J. Pearson, and K. B. Rix. "Food Hypersensitivity in Irritable Bowel Syndrome." *Lancet 2,* issue 8345 (Aug. 8, 1983), pp. 295–97.

Draper, W. L. "Food Testing in Allergy." *Archives of Otolaryngology,* vol. 95 (1972), pp. 169–71.

Finn, R., and T. M. Battcock. "A Critical Study of Clinical Ecology." *Practitioner,* vol. 229 (1985), pp. 883–85.

Lee, C. H., R. I. Williams, and E. I. Binkley, Jr. "Provocative Inhalant Testing and Treatment." *Archives of Otolaryngology,* vol. 190 (1960), p. 81.

Lee, C. H., et al. "Provocative Testing and Treatment for Foods." *Archives of Otolaryngology,* vol. 90 (1969), pp. 113–20.

Lee, L. K., W. T. Kniker, and T. Campos. "Aggressive Coseasonal Immunotherapy in Mountain Cedar Pollen Allergy," *Archives of Otolaryngology,* vol. 108 (1982), p. 782.

Miller, J. B. "The Optimal-Dose Methods of Food Allergy Management." In *Otolaryngologic Allergy,* ed. H. C. King (Symposia Specialists, 1981), pp. 253–83.

———. "Management of Migraine Headaches." In *Current Therapy of Allergy,* ed. C.A. Frazier. (New York: Medical Examination Publishing Co., 1978), pp. 93–98.

Double-Blinded Studies

Boris, M., et al. "Antigen-Induced Asthma Attenuated by Neutralization Therapy." *Clinical Ecology,* vol. 3 (1985), pp. 59–62.

———. "Bronchoprovocation Blocked by Neutralization Therapy." *Journal of Allergy and Immunology,* vol. 71, no. 1, part 2 (1983 abstract), p. 92.

Boris, M. N., M. Schiff, and S. Weindorf. "Injection of Low-Dose Antigen Attenuates the Response to Subsequent Broncho-Provocative Challenge." *Otolaryngology: Head and Neck Surgery,* vol. 98 (1988), pp. 539–45.

King, W. P., et al. "Provocation-Neutralization: A Two-Part Study. Part I. The Intracutaneous Provocative Food Test: A Multi-Center Comparison Study." *Otolaryngology: Head and Neck Surgery,* vol. 99 (1988), pp. 263–77.

———. "Provocation-Neutralization: A Two-Part Study. Part II. The Intracutaneous Provocative Food Test: A Multi-Center Comparison Study." *Otolaryngology: Head and Neck Surgery,* vol. 99, no. 3 (1988), pp. 272–78.

Miller, J. B. "A Double-Blind Study of Food Extract Injection Therapy: A Preliminary Report." *Annals of Allergy,* vol. 38 (1977), pp. 185–91.

Rapp, D. J. "Food Allergy Treatment for Hyperkinesis." *Journal of Learning Disabilities*, vol. 12 (1979), pp. 42–50.

———. "Possible New Way to Treat Herpes Progenitalis." Letter to the Editor (Abstract No. 61), *New York State Journal of Medicine*, vol. 78 (1978), p. 693.

Rea, W. J., et al. "Elimination of Oral Food Challenge Reaction by Injection of Food Extracts." *Archives of Otolaryngology*, vol. 110 (1984).

Rogers, S. A. "Provocation-Neutralization of Cough and Wheezing in a Horse." *Clinical Ecology*, vol. 5, no. 4 (1987–88), pp. 185–87.

STUDIES SUPPORTING THE EFFICACY OF SUBLINGUAL P/N TREATMENT

Single-Blinded Studies

Monro, J. "Food Allergy and Migraine." *Clinical Immunology and Allergy*, vol. 42 (1983), pp. 241–46.

Morris, David L. "Use of Sublingual Antigen in Diagnosis and Treatment of Food Allergy." *Annals of Allergy*, vol. 27 (1969), pp. 287–94.

Rapp, D. J. "A Prototype for Food Sensitivity Studies in Children." Abstract No. 25. *Annals of Allergy*, vol. 47 (1981), pp. 123–24.

———. "Food Allergy Treatment for Hyperkinesis." *Journal of Learning Disabilities*, vol. 12, no. 9 (1979), pp. 42–50.

———. "Hyperactivity and Food Allergy: Are They Related?" *Annals of Allergy*, vol. 40 (1978), p. 297.

———. "Does Diet Affect Hyperactivity?" *Journal of Learning Disabilities*, vol. 11 (1978), pp. 56–61.

Double-Blinded Studies

Bjorksten, B., and Janet Dewdney. "Oral Immunotherapy in Allergy: Is It Effective?" *Clinical Allergy*, vol. 17 (1987), pp. 91–94.

Brostoff, J., and G. Scadding. *Study: Double-Blind Sublingual Treatment and Immunological Studies* (London: Department of Immunology, Middlesex Hospital, 1988).

Fellziani, V., et al. "Rush Immunotherapy with Sublingual Administration of Grass Allergen Extract." *Allergology et Immunopathology*, vol. 21, no. 5 (1993), pp. 173–78.

Giovane, A. L., et al. "A Three-Year Double-Blind Placebo-Controlled Study with Specific Oral Immunotherapy to Dermatophagoides: Evidence of Safety and Efficacy in Pediatric Patients." *Clinical and Experimental Allergy*, vol. 24 (1994), pp. 53–59.

Holt, P. G., et al. "Sublingual Allergen Administration I. Selective Suppression of IgE Production in Rats by High Allergen Doses." *Clinical Allergy*, vol. 18 (1988), pp. 229–34.

King, D. S. "Can Allergic Exposure Provoke Psychological Symptoms? A Double-Blind Test." *Biological Psychiatry*, vol. 16 (1981), pp. 3–19.

Leng, Xiao, et al. "A Double-Blind Trial of Oral Immunotherapy for Artemisia Pollen Asthma with Evaluation of Bronchial Response to the Pollen Allergen and Serum-Specific IgE Antibody." *Annals of Allergy*, vol. 64 (1990), pp. 27–31.

Mandell, M., et al. "The Role of Allergy in Arthritis, Rheumatism, and Polysymptomatic Cerebral, Visceral, and Somatic Disorders: A Double-Blind Study." *Journal of International Academy of Preventive Medicine*, vol. 7, no. 2 (1982), pp. 5–16.

Moller, C., et al. "Oral Immunotherapy of Children with Rhinoconjunctivitis Due to Birch Pollen Allergy." *Allergy*, vol. 41 (1986), pp. 271–79.

Morris, David L. "Treatment of Respiratory Disease with Ultra-Small Doses of Antigens." *Annals of Allergy*, vol. 28 (1970), pp. 494–500.

O'Shea, J. A., and S. F. Porter. "Double-Blind Study of Children with Hyperkinetic Syndrome Treated with Multi-Allergen Extract Sublingually." *Journal of Learning Disabilities*, vol. 14 (1981), p. 189.

Rapp, D. J. "Chronic Headache Due to Foods and Air Pollution." *Annals of Allergy*, vol. 40 (1978), p. 289.

———. "Herpes Progenitalis Responding to Influenza Vaccine." *Annals of Allergy*, vol. 40 (1978), p. 302.

———. "Weeping Eyes in Wheat Allergy." *Trans American Society of Ophthalmology and Otolaryngology*, vol. 18 (1978), p. 149.

———. "Double-Blind Confirmation and Treatment of Milk Sensitivity." *Medical Journal of Australia*, vol. 1 (1978), pp. 571–72.

———. "Water as Cause of Angio-Edema and Urticaria." Letter to the Editor. *Journal of the American Medical Association*, vol. 221, no. 3 (1972), p. 305.

Sabbah, A., et al. "A Double-Blind Placebo-Controlled Trial by the Sublingual Route of Immunotherapy with a Standardized Grass Pollen Extract." *Allergy*, vol. 49 (1994), pp. 309–13.

Scadding, Glenis K., and J. Brostoff. "Low Dose Sublingual Therapy in Patients with Allergic Rhinitis Due to House Dust Mite." *Clinical Allergy*, vol. 16 (1986), pp. 483–91.

Tari, M. G., et al. "Efficacy of Sublingual Immunotherapy in Patients with Rhinitis and Asthma Due to House Dust Mite: A Double-Blind Study." *Allergology et Immunopathology*, vol. 18, no. 5 (1990), pp. 277–84.

Taudorf, Ebbe, et al. "Oral Immunotherapy in Birch Pollen Hay Fever." *Journal of Allergy and Clinical Immunology*, vol. 80, no. 2 (1987), pp. 153–61.

———. "Specific IgE, IgC, and IgA Antibody Response to Oral Immunotherapy in Birch Pollinosis." *Journal of Allergy and Clinical Immunology*, vol. 83, no. 3 (1989), pp. 589–94.

Troise, C., et al. "Sublingual Immunotherapy in Parietaria Pollen-Induced Rhinitis: A Double-Blind Study." *Journal of Investigational Allergology and Clinical Immunology*, vol. 5, no. 1 (1995), pp. 25–30.

Van Nierkerk, C. H., and J. I. DeWet. "Efficacy of Grass-maize Pollen Oral Immunotherapy in Patients with Seasonal Hay Fever; a Double-Blind Study." *Clinical Allergy*, vol. 17 (1987), pp. 507–13.

Wortman, F. "Oral Hyposensitization of Children with Pollinosis or House-Dust Asthma." *Allergology et Immunopathology*, vol. 5, no. 15 (1977), pp. 15–26.

Other Media

VIDEOTAPES

Available from Practical Allergy Research Foundation (PARF) (P.O. Box 60, Buffalo, NY 14223, (800) 78-78-78-0):

Environmentally Sick Schools, an 85-minute videotape.

Allergies Do Alter Activities and Behavior, a 3-part 40-minute videotape shows why some children can't learn or behave. It shows how to recognize EI from how a child looks and acts, what causes such reactions, and includes many children's reactions from infancy to adolescence, including a Tourette's syndrome patient. The first part is also available in Spanish.

Why a Clean Classroom, is a 60-minute videotape.

Specific individual videotapes that demonstrate tics, depression, arthritis, fatigue, hyperactivity, headaches, withdrawal, walking, speech, vision, and multiple behavior disorders are also available.

Impossible or Allergic Child—Five Allergic Children, and *How to Prepare an Indoor Air Allergy Extract* are short videos.

Video 1-2-3
A basic overview of environmental illness. *Video 1:* How to recognize children who have allergies. *Video 2:* How to detect the cause of allergies and environmental illness. *Video 3:* Shows a hyperactive toddler, a child with Tourette's Syndrome, and a retarded child.

PARF also offers videotapes on hyperactivity, learning problems, aggression, withdrawal, fatigue, intestinal symptoms, headaches, and arthritis, as well as videotapes showing patient reactions to P/N allergy testing.

AUDIOTAPES

Allergy Diets, a 70-minute audiotape that discusses various simple and more complex allergy diets.

Environmental Aspects of Allergy, a 66-minute audiotape that discusses making homes more allergy-free and environmentally safe.

Infant Food Allergies, a 50-minute audiotape that discusses common challenges of allergic infants.

Allergy Songs by Steven Lemberg and Doris Rapp.

Also Available from Practical Allergy Research Foundation:

Allergy Diets

Environmental Aspects of Allergy

Infant Food Allergies

Many books written about environmental illness

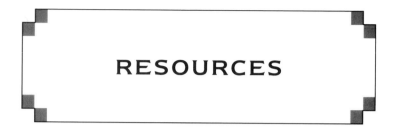

RESOURCES

Advocacy and Various Organizations

American Academy of Environmental Medicine (AAEM)
4510 West 89th Street
Prairie Village, KS 66207
(913) 642-6062
fax (913) 341-3625

They can provide the name of the nearest EI specialist and suggest speakers for conferences and other events.

American Conference of Governmental Industrial Hygienists (ACGIH)
6500 Glenway Avenue, Building D7
Cincinnati, OH 45211
(513) 742-2020

They publish a yearly list of threshold limit values related to potential health hazards in the workplace.

American Society of Heating, Refrigeration and Air Conditioning Engineers (ASHRAE)
1791 Tullie Circle, N.E.
Atlanta, GA 30329
(404) 636-8400
(800) 527-4723

They have recommended indoor air limits for six contaminants: sulfur dioxide, particulate matter, carbon monoxide, ozone, nitrogen dioxide, and lead. ASHRAE 62-1989 appears to be the most quoted and accepted standard.

Citizens Clearinghouse for Hazardous Waste (CCHW)
P.O. Box 6806
Falls Church, VA 22040
(703) 237-2249

CCHW trains and assists local people fighting to protect their communities from toxics in our environment.

Enviro–Health
2605 Meridian Parkway, Suite 115
Durham, NC 27713
(800) 643-4794
fax (919) 361-9408

This clearinghouse provides free information on environmental health issues. They can refer you to an appropriate governmental or private agency.

Environmental Access Research Network (EARN)
P.O. Box 426
Williston, ND 58802-0426
(701) 859-6363

They publish the newsletter Medical and Legal Briefs: A Reference Compendium of Chemical Injury. *They do computer searches on lawsuits and provide information on expert witnesses; they can also provide copies of court decisions.*

Environmental Education and Health Services
Mary Oetzel, President
P.O. Box 92004
Austin, TX 78709
(512) 288-2369

This company provides technical information on indoor air quality issues for architects, home-owners, schools, and businesses.

Environmental Health Network
Great Bridge Station
P.O. Box 16267
Chesapeake, VA 23328
(804) 424-1162
fax (804) 424-1517

This national nonprofit organization provides technical information, counseling, referrals, organizing, and networking to injured workers, individuals, and communities with environmental health problems so they can better their quality of life.

Environmental Research Foundation
P.O. Box 5036
Annapolis, MD 21403
(410) 463-1584
Internet: erf@igc.apc.org

They publish Rachel's Environment and Health Weekly.

Green Seal
1730 Rhode Island Avenue, N.W., Suite 1050
Washington, DC 20036
(202) 331-7337

This organization sets standards to protect air, water, and energy. It reviews public standards, packaging, and quality of "environmental" products.

HealthComm International
5800 Southview Drive
Gig Harbor, WA 98335
(206) 851-3943

They offer a video series on nutrition for physicians; they refer patients with nutritional concerns to knowledgeable physicians.

Human Ecology Action League (HEAL)
P.O. Box 49126
Atlanta, GA 30359-1126
(404) 248-1898

They publish Human Ecologist, *which contains a wealth of information for those with environmental illness.*

International Health Foundation
Billy Crook, M.D.
P.O. Box 3494
Jackson, TN 38303
(901) 427-8100

They provide information on yeast-related illness.

Job Accommodation Network
P.O. Box 6122
Morgantown, WV 26506
(800) 526-7234

This international toll-free consulting service provides information about job accommodations and the employability of people with functional limitations, including those with environmental illness. Consultants also provide information concerning employment rights in relation to the Americans with Disabilities Act and other pieces of similar legislation.

MCS Referral and Resources
2326 Pickwick Road
Baltimore, MD 21207
(410) 448-3319
fax (410) 448-3317

They provide detailed information and advice regarding the diagnosis and rights of those with chemical sensitivities.

National Air Duct Cleaners Association
1518 K Street, N.W., Suite 503
Washington, DC 20005
(202) 737-2926
fax (202) 638-4833

They will recommend an air duct cleaner in your area.

National Center for Environmental Health Strategies
Mary Lamielle
1100 Rural Avenue
Voorhees, NJ 08043
(609) 429-5358

They provide a wealth of information about environmental illness.

National Education Association
1201 Sixteenth Street, N.W.
Washington, DC 20036
(202) 833-4000

They publish educational material for teachers.

National Environmental Health Association
720 Colorado Boulevard, no. 970, South Tower
Denver, CO 80222
(303) 756-9090

An environmental/health/consumer organization for educators.

National Institute of Environmental Health Sciences
P.O. Box 12233
Research Triangle Park, NC 27709
(919) 541-3212

This center for toxicological and environmental health science research has as its mission to reduce environmental illness. They publish Environmental Health Perspectives.

National Institutes of Health
9000 Rockville Pike
Bethesda, MD 20892
(301) 496-4000

This organization does research into health-related medical issues.

National Organization of Legal Advocates for the Environmentally Injured
P.O. Box 29507
Atlanta, GA 30329
(404) 264-4445
fax (404) 325-2569

National Parent-Teacher Association
330 North Wabash Avenue, Suite 2100
Chicago, IL 60611-3690
(312) 670-6782

They provide information to parents and teachers.

Natural Resources Defense Council
40 West 20th Street
New York, NY 10011
(212) 727-2700

They publish The Amicus Journal.

New York Coalition for Alternatives to Pesticides
353 Hamilton Street
Albany, NY 12210-1709
(518) 426-8246

They publish a booklet on pesticides.

Nontoxic Environments
P.O. Box 384
Newmarket, NH 03857
(800) 789-4348

They provide books and videotapes related to environmental illness.

OMB Watch
1742 Connecticut Avenue, N.W.
Washington, DC 20009
(202) 234-8494

This nonprofit watchdog group focuses on advocacy, government accountability, and the budget-
   ary process. Their databases—the Right to Know Net and the Toxic Release Inventory—
   provide access to environmental issues.

Practical Allergy Research Foundation (PARF)
P.O. Box 60
Buffalo, NY 14223
(800) 787-8780

Dr. Rapp's foundation provides many of the materials mentioned throughout this book, includ-
   ing many EI books, audiotapes, and videotapes of patients discussed in this book and others
   reacting to common environmental and food exposures. They provide helpful information to
   physicians and parents, and provide nontoxic products, including air purifiers, air extract
   machines, Peak Flow Meters for asthma, mold absorbers, charcoal masks, water purifiers,
   and water filters.

Safe Schools
205 Paddington Drive
Lafayette, LA 70508
(318) 984-2766
fax (318) 904-3342

They offer a two-hour workshop, "How Environmentally Safe Are Our Schools?" and a video.
   Send a SASE for more information.

Well Mind Association of Greater Washington, D.C.
3205 Wake Drive
Kensington, MD 20895-0201
(301) 949-8282
fax (301) 946-1402

They offer educational materials and an environmentally aware newsletter about alternative ways to treat mental disorders.

State and Federal Government Agencies

Advocates for the Disabled

Contact information may be found in the state government section of your telephone book.

Architectural and Transportation Barriers Compliance Board (Access Board)
1331 F Street, N.W., Suite 1000
Washington, DC 20004
(800) USA-ABLE

Consumer Product Safety Commission (CPSC)
5401 Westbard Avenue
Bethesda, MD 20207
(301) 492-6580
Hotline: (800) 638-2772

Reviews complaints about the safety of consumer products and takes action to ensure product safety.

Environmental Protection Agency (EPA)
401 M Street, S.W.
Washington, DC 20460
(202) 382-2090
Public Information Center: (202) 829-3535
Indoor Air Division: (202) 233-9030
Indoor Air Quality Information Clearinghouse: (800) 438-4318

EPA provides information, literature, and referrals.

Equal Employment Opportunity Commission (EEOC)
1801 L Street, N.W., Room 9024
Washington, DC 20507
(800) 669-4000

They provide information about employment rights and inequities.

Food and Drug Administration (FDA)
5600 Fishers Lane
Rockville, MD 20857
(301) 443-1544

They provide information about food and drug standards in the United States.

Maryland Department of Education
200 West Baltimore Street
Baltimore, MD 21201
(410) 333-2508

They provide information about school environmental issues.

National Council on Disability
800 Independence Avenue, S.W., Suite 814
Washington, DC 20591
(202) 272-2004

They provide disability information.

National Institute for Occupational Safety and Health (NIOSH)
Hazard Evaluation and Technical Assistance Branch (R-9)
4676 Columbia Parkway
Cincinnati, OH 45226
(800) 356-4674

They offer publications, including the Pocket Guide to Chemical Hazards, *as well as databases and information on indoor air quality; they do on-site evaluations of potential health hazards; they provide training programs, materials, and videos.*

Occupational Safety and Health Administration (OSHA)
U.S. Department of Labor
200 Constitution Avenue, N.W.
Washington, DC 20210
(202) 523-8017
Information and Consumer Affairs: (202) 219-8151

This government agency works to ensure a healthy and safe workplace environment.

Environmental Medicine

SOURCES OF REFERRALS TO ENVIRONMENTAL MEDICAL SPECIALISTS

American Academy of Environmental Medicine (AAEM)
4510 West 89th Street
Prairie Village, KS 66207
(913) 642-6062

Call for nearest well-trained specialist.

American Academy of Otolaryngic Allergy
8455 Colesville Road, Suite 745
Silver Spring, MD 20910
(301) 588-1800

American College for Advancement in Medicine (ACAM)
23121 Verdugo Drive, Suite 204
Laguna Hills, CA 92653
(800) 532-3688

Pan American Allergy Society
P.O. Box 947
Fredericksburg, TX 78624
(210) 997-9853

PHYSICIANS AND CLINICS
(a listing here is not necessarily an endorsement by the author)

FOR SPECT BRAIN IMAGING TESTS

Advanced Metabolic Imaging
Theodore Simon, M.D.
12200 Preston Road
Dallas, TX 75230
(214) 490-0536

Med-Health, Ltd.
Thomas Callender, M.D.
1101 Hugh Wallis Road South, Suite 106
Lafayette, LA 70508
(313) 233-6022
fax (318) 269-0171

Ismael Mena, M.D.
Chief Division of Nuclear Medicine
Lac Harbor, UCLA Medical Center
Box #23, P.O. Box 2910
Torrance, CA 90509
(310) 222-2842
fax (310) 328-7288

SPECIALTY EI MEDICAL CENTERS IN U.S. AND ABROAD

Airedale General Hospital and Airedale Allergy Centre
D. Jonathan Maberly, M.D.
Steeton, Keighley
West Yorkshire BD20 6SB
England
053-023-3622
fax 053-022-3622

An inpatient facility to evaluate and treat environmentally ill patients.

Allergy and Environmental Health Center
Kalpana Patel, M.D.
65 Wehrle Drive
Buffalo, NY 14225
(716) 833-2213

Board certified in the practice of environmental allergy with special expertise in occupational and nutritional medicine. She has a detoxification unit.

Breakspear Hospital
Jean Monro, M.D.
Diagnostic Medicine, Allergy and Environmental Diagnostic Medicine
Belswains Lane, Hemel Hempstead
Herts. HP #9HP
England
0923-261333
fax 0922-261876

Vast EI knowledge including electromagnetic illness.

Adrienne Buffaloe, M.D.
964 Third Avenue
New York, NY 10155
(212) 355-2315

Board certified in environmental emergency medicine. She has a detoxification unit and special expertise in eating and digestive disorders.

Center for Environmental Medicine
Allan D. Lieberman, M.D.
7510 Northforest Drive
North Charleston, SC 29420
(803) 572-1600

Board certified in pediatric and environmental medicine with special expertise in infectious disease.

Environmental Health Center
William Rea, M.D., Alfred Johnson, D.O., and Gerald H. Ross, M.D.
8345 Walnut Hill Lane, Suite 220
Dallas, TX 75231-4262
(214) 368-4132
fax (214) 691-8432

They are "super"specialists in environmental medicine, internal medicine, vascular medicine, and electromagnetic illness and they have vast experience with extremely medically ill patients. They have a detox unit and hospital unit.

Environmental Health Psychologists
P.O. Box 399
Dewey, OK 74029

They conduct clinical investigations, as well as education and training concerning the psycho-logical versus environmental sensitivity aspects of a patient's complaints.

Institut für Umweltkrankheiten
Klaus Runow, M.D.
Im Kurpark 1
W34308 Bad Emstal
Germany
56 24 8061
fax 56 24 8695

This is an inpatient diagnostic and teaching evaluation center.

Charles R. Mabray, M.D.
4204 North Laurent Street
Victoria, TX 77901
(512) 578-5233

A gynecologist with expertise in female hormonal imbalances and EI.

Starcare Family and Preventive Medicine
Fran Rose, M.D.
1701 W. Walnut Hill, Suite 200
Irving, TX 75038
(214) 594-1111
fax (214) 518-1867

Integrated medicine with western, eastern, homepathy, naturopathy, nutritional, and chelation.

Drs. Robert and Marsa Trossel
Joost Banchert Plaza 24-29
3012 and 3065 BB
Rotterdam, Holland
31010-414-7633
fax 31010-414-7990

DIET, NUTRITION, AND FOOD ADVISERS

Jeffrey Bland, Ph.D. and Associates
HealthComm International
5800 Southview Drive
Gig Harbor, WA 98335
(206) 851-3943

They offer Ultraclear, Ultrasustain, and UltraKids oral detoxification products plus educational tapes on nutrition for physicians.

Susan Brown, Ph.D.
1200 East Genesee Street, Suite 310
Syracuse, NY 13210
(315) 471-0264

Knows rotation and yeast diets, plus practical information.

Susan E. Busse, M.D.
909 East Palatine Road
Palatine, IL 60067
(847) 776-2111

Board certified in family medicine. She has special expertise in nutrition and uses alternative methods of healing such as chelation.

Ilene Buchholz, R.N.
c/o Klaire Laboratories, Inc.
1573 W. Seminole Street
San Marcos, CA 92069
(619) 744-9680
(800) 533-7255

Kelly Dorfman, M.S., L.N., L.D.
10828 Tuckahoe Way
North Potomac, MD 20878

Natalie Golos
Women's Wellness Institute
9707 Medical Center Drive
Suite 210
Rockville, MD 20850
(301) 279-0488

This author has in-depth knowledge of environmental illness.

Bonnie Holtz, R.D.
2112 Norcross Road
Erie, PA 16510

An E.I. rotation diet nutrition specialist.

MAST Enterprizes
Marjorie Hurt Jones, R.N.
2615 North Fourth Street, Suite 616
Coeur d'Alene, ID 83814-3781
(208) 772-8213

She is the source of much allergy information—three cookbooks and ten years of Mastering Food Allergies *newsletters, now* The MFA Collection.

Majid Ali, M.D.
95 East Main Street
Denville, NJ 07834
(201) 586-4111

Author of several books for patients (see For Further Reading), Dr. Ali teaches courses for physicians on nutritional therapies and healing.

James A. Neubrander, M.D.
23 Barrington Road
Belle Mead, NJ 08502
(908) 874-7783

Board certified in the practice of environmental allergy. He has expertise in nutritional and environmental medicine.

Northeast Center for Environmental Medicine
Sherry A. Rogers, M.D.
2800 West Genesee Street
Box 2716
Syracuse, NY 13220
(315) 488-2856

Emphasizes self-healing, nutrition, and macrobiotic diets; has written many "how to" books.

Pain and Stress Center
Billie Sahley, Ph.D. and Katherine Birkner, Ph.D.
5282 Medical Drive, Suite 160
San Antonio, TX 78229
(210) 614-7246

They provide nutritional counseling, guidance, books, and products.

Donna Powell, BScN.
Box 25
Waterdown, Ontario
L0R 2H0 Canada

The author of an excellent rotation diet cookbook.

Sally Rockwell, C.N., Ph.D.
P.O. Box 31065
Seattle, WA 98103
(206) 547-1814

The creator of exceptional teaching videos, audiotapes, and other excellent material about rotation diets and environmental control.

Aubrey M. Worrell, Jr., M.D.
3900 Hickory Street
Pine Bluff, AR 71603
(501) 535-8200

Board certified in pediatrics, allergy, immunology, and environmental medicine, with a special interest in MCS, Chronic Fatigue Syndrome, and nutritional deficiencies.

Jonathan V. Wright, M.D.
24030 132nd Southeast
Kent, WA 98042
(206) 854-4900

A specialist in family practice, environmental medicine, nutritional biochemistry, and allergy.

DETOXIFICATION MEDICALLY SUPERVISED CENTERS

See listings under "Physicians and Clinics" for the following centers. (a listing here is not necessarily an endorsement by the author)

U.S.

Allergy and Environmental Health Center
Kalpana Patel, M.D.
65 Wehrle Drive
Buffalo, NY 14225
(716) 833-2213

Center for Environmental Medicine
Allan D. Lieberman, M.D.
7510 Northforest Drive
North Charleston, SC 29420
(803) 572-1600

Enviro-Med Clinics, Inc.
Jeffrey White, M.D.
3715 Azeele Street
Tampa, FL 33609
(813) 876-5442

Environmental Health Center—Dallas
William Rea, M.D.
8345 Walnut Hill Lane
Suite 205
Dallas, TX 75231-4262
(214) 368-4132
fax (214) 691-8432

Healthcare for the 21st Century, LLC
Adrienne Buffaloe, M.D.
964 Third Avenue
Fourth Floor
New York, NY 10155
(212) 355-2315
fax (212) 355-4496

HealthMed
David Root, M.D.
5501 Power Inn Road, Suite 140
Sacramento, CA 95820
(916) 924-8060

Jacqueline Krohn, M.D.
Los Alamos Medical Center
3917 West Road, Suite 136
Los Alamos, NM 87544
(505) 662-0960
fax (505) 662-0024

Author of new book entitled Detoxification of Chemicals.

Rittenhouse Cleanse Center
Ronald C. Maugeri, D.C.
1930 Chestnut Street, Lower Mezzanine
Philadelphia, PA 19130
(215) 665-1662
fax (215) 563-2426

FOREIGN

Airedale General Hospital and Airedale Allergy Center
D. J. Maberly, M.D.
Steeton, Keighley
West Yorkshire BD20 6SB
England (an inpatient center)
053 022 3622
fax 053 022 3622

Institut für Umweltkrankeiten
Klaus Runow, M.D.
Klaus-Dietrich Runow Center
Im Kurpark
D-34308 Bad Emstal, Germany
56 24 8061
fax 56 24 8695 (inpatient and outpatient center)

Wasserschlob Klinik Betriebs-GmbH
Dr. Thomas Meyn
26427 Nordseebad
Neuharlingersiel, Germany
04974/160
fax 04974/1673

Chemical detoxification center for children in Germany.

NUTRITIONAL AND OTHER SUPPLEMENTS

Allergy Research Group
400 Preda Street
P.O. Box 489
San Leandro, CA 94577-0489
(800) 545-9960

A source of many helpful nutrients.

American Biologics
1180 Walnut Avenue
Chula Vista, CA 91911
(800) 227-4473

*They carry the InFla-zyme Forte digestive adjunct, as well as the Bio-Bifidus Complex lactoba-
cillus blend, and other nutritional supplements.*

Amino Acid and Botanical Supply Company/Tyson and Associates
P.O. Box 356
Cedar Knolls, NJ 07927
(800) 952-7921

*They supply Tyson brand amino acids, as well as Aminotate capsules (helpful for hypoglycemia),
and other nutritional supplements.*

Carlson Laboratories
15 College Drive
Arlington Heights, IL 60004
(800) 323-4141

They offer L-glutamine capsules by Vital Life, and other nutritional supplements.

Klaire Laboratories
1573 West Seminole Street
San Marcos, CA 92069
(619) 744-9680
(800) 533-7255

*They provide Vital Life food supplements, including amino acid supplements, the Vitalplex lacto-
bacillus, L-glutamine capsules, and other nutritional aids.*

L&H Vitamins
32-33 47th Avenue
Long Island City, NY 11101
(800) 221-1152

They offer the Vitalplex lactobacillus and discounted quality nutrients.

Nutritional Enzyme Support System (NESS)
2903 Northwest Platte Road
Riverside, MO 64150
(800) 637-7893

They offer vegetable-derived digestive enzymes.

Pain and Stress Center
5282 Medical Drive, Suite 160
San Antonio, TX 78229
(210) 614-7246

They offer advice and booklets as well as many nutritional products, especially for hyperactivity.

Practical Allergy Research Foundation
(see "General Suppliers")

They offer alka aid and a number of nutrient preparations.

Tyler Encapsulations
2204-8 Northwest Birdsdale
Gresham, OR 97030
(800) 869-9705

They carry the Similase digestive adjunct and many other nutrients.

Vitaline Formulas
385 Williamson Way
Ashland, OR 97520
(800) 648-4755

Manufacturer of Vitaline brand food supplements and other nutritional products.

For preparations that appear to help in detoxification:

Cell Tech
22719 North 92nd Street
Scottsdale, AZ 85255
(602) 502-5022

They distribute Lake Klamath Blue-Green Algae.

HOMEOPATHY AND NATUROPATHY CENTERS AND RESOURCES

American Association of Naturopath Physicians
2366 Eastlake Avenue East, Suite 322
Seattle, WA 98102
(206) 323-7610

They can refer you to your nearest naturopath.

BioActive Nutritional
1803 North Wickham Road, Suite 6
Melbourne, FL 32935
(407) 254-9525
(800) 288-9525

They distribute homeopathic/naturopathic preparations such as Chemtox and Environtox that appear to lessen symptoms of chemical sensitivity.

Bioenergetics
P.O. Box 127
Sandy, OR 97055
(800) 334-4043

Provides homeopathic remedies for allergies and detoxification.

MarcoPharma International
15810 West Sixth Avenue
Golden, CO 80401
(800) 999-3001

They distribute nutritional supplements, including Hepatica for natural detoxification.

Mountain States Health Care Products
P.O. Box 1129
Lyons, CO 80540
(800) 647-0074

They offer Liver Liquescence by PHP for natural detoxification.

National Center for Homeopathy
801 North Fairfax, Suite 306
Alexandria, VA 22314
(703) 548-7790

They provide books and kits on homeopathic treatments and can direct you to your nearest homeopath.

Southwest College of Naturopathic Medicine and Health Sciences
2140 E. Broadway Road
Tempe, AZ 85282
(602) 990-7424

NEWER CHIROPRACTIC AND OTHER HEALING APPROACHES

Wolfgang Gerz, M.D.
Sonnenlang Strasse 2
81369 Munchen, Germany
089-7809331
fax 089-7809824

Robert R. Moore, D.C.
15227 N. 10th Street
Phoenix, AZ 85022
(602) 789-6774

He specializes in balancing body energies to promote natural healing.

Neuro-Emotional Training (NET) seminars
Scott Walker, D.C.
524 Second Street
Encinitas, CA 92024
(800) 888-4638

Offers seminars for doctors and Ph.D.s.

Steel Alternative Health Care Clinic
Harvey Steel, D.C.
390 Wellington Street, West
Chatham, Ontario N7M 1K4
(519) 354p36560

A chiropractor who uses newer techniques and nutrition to heal.

Total Body Modification (TBM) seminars
Victor Frank, D.C.
1907 East Foxmoor Circle
Sandy, UT 84092
(800) 243-4826

Offers seminars for doctors and the public.

UNPROVEN METHODS

American Biologics
1180 Walnut Avenue
Chula Vista, CA 91911
(800) 227-4473

They interpret blood samples and provide nutritional products.

For Edgar Cayce approaches:

Association of Research and Enlightenment (ARE)
P.O. Box 595
Virginia Beach, VA 23451
(804) 428-3588

They provide books and other educational materials.

Logos Center
Herbert Puryear, Ph.D.
P.O. Box 12880
Scottsdale, AZ 85267-2880

They provide books and other educational materials.

Diagnostic Laboratories

AccuChem Laboratories
990 North Bowser, Suite 800
Richardson, TX 75081
(214) 234-5412

They provide blood, urine, and water testing, after chemical exposures.

American Environmental Health Foundation
(see ''General Suppliers'')

They provide testing of carpets, air samples, and foods; they also do ''on-the-spot'' immediate gas chromatography and mass spectrometry tests for chemicals and gases.

Anderson Laboratories
773 Main Street
West Hartford, VT 05084-0323
(802) 295-7344
fax (802) 295-7648

They provide bioassay testing on carpets and other common household items, by exposing and monitoring mice.

Antibody Assay Laboratory
1715 East Wilshire, Suite 715
Santa Ana, CA 92705
(800) 522-2611

They do various blood antibody, autoantibody, immune system, and chemical detection testing after toxic or chemical exposures.

Bionostics
Lincoln Center, Suite 104
4513 Lincoln Avenue, Route 53
Lisle, IL 60532
(708) 960-5146

They provide amino acid testing, as well as mineral and element testing.

Citizens Environmental Laboratory
160 Second Street
Cambridge, MA 02142
(617) 876-6505

They test carpets for chemicals.

Doctor's Data
170 West Roosevelt Road
West Chicago, IL 60185
(800) 323-2784

They do nutrient testing, amino acid testing, and hair analysis tests for toxic metals.

Great Smokies Diagnostic Laboratory
18A Regent Park Boulevard
Asheville, NC 28806
(800) 522-4762

They test for intestinal parasites, yeast, and digestive problems, including stool examinations.

Immunosciences Laboratory
8730 Wilshire Boulevard, Suite 305
Beverly Hills, CA 90211
(800) 950-4686

They do immunology, autoantibody, and chemical detection, and immunotoxicology testing.

MetaMetrix Medical Laboratory
5000 Peachtree Industrial Boulevard, Suite 110
Norcross, GA 30071
(404) 446-5483
(800) 221-4640

They do amino acid analysis, hair analysis for toxic metals, and many other nutritional and metabolic tests for patients referred by physicians.

National Medical Services
2300 Stratford Avenue
Willow Grove, PA 19090
(215) 657-4900

They provide poison testing.

SmithKline Beecham
Clinical Laboratories
1201 S. Collegeville Lab
Collegeville, PA 19426
(610) 454-6000

They provide blood nutrient testing.

SpectraCell Laboratories
515 Post Oak Boulevard, Suite 830
Houston, TX 77027
(800) 227-5227

They provide nutrient testing.

Vitamin Diagnostics
2 Industrial Drive, Suite A
Cliffwood Beach, NJ 07735
(908) 583-7773

They provide nutrient, EFA, and amino acid testing.

General Suppliers of Nontoxic Products

AFM Enterprises
350 West Ash Street, Suite 700
San Diego, CA 92101-3404
(619) 239-0321

Supplies many nontoxic products, including a variety of safer paints, sealers, carpet cleaners, radon testing kits, etc.

Allerx (formerly Allergy Asthma Shopper)
P.O. Box 239
Fate, TX 75132
(800) 447-1100

They supply many nontoxic products, including safer carpet cleaners, safer sealers, bacteria and mold tests, computer-screen shields, lead testing kits, radon testing kits, gaussmeters, formaldehyde test and analysis kits, Neolife Rugged Red, and carbon monoxide detectors needed by the environmentally ill.

American Environmental Health Foundation
8345 Walnut Hill Lane, Suite 225
Dallas, TX 75231-4262
(800) 428-2343
(214) 361-9515
fax (214) 361-2534

They supply many nontoxic products and are distributors for home saunas and water purifiers. They also test indoor and outdoor air, foods, and carpets. This foundation has a store that funds research and education. A separate office or clinic cares for patients.

Environmental Medicine and Engineering
5133 North Central Avenue, Suite 102
Phoenix, AZ 85012
(602) 274-6563
(800) 953-2678

Living Source
7005 Woodway Drive, Suite 214
Waco, TX 76712
(817) 776-4878

They supply Nature Clean products; Purisol.

National Ecological and Environmental Delivery System (NEEDS)
527 Charles Avenue, Suite 12A
Syracuse, NY 13209
(800) 634-1380

They supply an immense range of discounted EI products.

Practical Allergy Research Foundation (PARF)
P.O. Box 60
Buffalo, NY 14223
(716) 875-0398
(800) 787-8780

They supply many of the books, videos, and audiotapes about EI, air and water purifiers, and other nontoxic products mentioned throughout this book.

Suppliers for Specific Hazards

AIR QUALITY CONSULTANTS

Environmental medical evaluation consultants:

Electro-Analytical Laboratories
7118 Industrial Park Boulevard
Mentor, OH 44060
(216) 951-3514

They do environmental testing for asbestos, radon, lead, formaldehyde, PCBs, pesticides, and herbicides.

Engineers:

Green Eclipse
Bruce Small
R.R. #1
Goodwood, Ontario
L0C 1A0 Canada
(905) 649-1356

An expert on construction for EI.

Marc Cree Jackson, M.S.E.
1703 John Smith Drive
Irving, TX 75061
(214) 259-1522

An advocate for indoor air quality

HVAC consultants:

Alternative Building Consultants
444 Brickell Avenue Plaza 51-273
Miami, FL 33131
(305) 674-9716

American Environmental Health Foundation
(see "General Suppliers")

Ameritec
8732 North 66th Place
Paradise Valley, AZ 85253
(602) 274-6563

Enviro Health
77 West Coolidge, Suite 132
Phoenix, AZ 85013
(602) 274-6624

Environmental Medicine and Engineering
5133 North Central Avenue, Suite 102
Phoenix, AZ 85012
(602) 274-6563
(800) 953-2678

They provide in-depth building evaluations with a well-qualified team of experts and provide products for environmentally safer buildings.

Environmental Testing and Technology
P.O. Box 369
Encinitas, CA 92024
(619) 436-5990
fax (619) 436-9448

They conduct indoor environmental building surveys, are very familiar with environmental illness and tests for indoor air quality, mold problems, and electromagnetic fields.

J. May Home Inspections
1522 Cambridge Street
Cambridge, MA 02139
(617) 354-0152

They do indoor environmental evaluations mainly on real estate, but also on homes.

RH of Texas
c/o Chris Rea
10050 Monro Street
Dallas, TX 75229
(214) 351-6681

Provides thorough environmental evaluations of all types of buildings.

Tennessee Valley Authority
Occupational Hygiene Department
3328 Multipurpose Building
Muscle Shoals, AL 35660
(205) 386-2314

Provides building surveys and assessments.

Texas Power Vac
1721 Franklin Avenue
Waco, TX 76701
(817) 754-7606
(800) 525-9005

Services and consultation for environmentally safe HVAC cleaning and decontamination.

For control of pet dander:

Dr. Goodpet
P.O. Box 4728
Inglewood, CA 90309
(800) 222-9932

They supply homeopathic products for animals.

AIR QUALITY PRODUCTS

Air purifiers:

Environmental Medicine and Engineering
(see "Air Quality Consultants")

Practical Allergy Research Foundation (PARF)
(see "General Suppliers")

Also supplied by other general distributors.

Air quality badges:

Occupational Health and Environmental Safety Division
3M Corporation
3M Center
St. Paul, MN 55144
(800) 243-4630

Mold treatments and tests:

Allerx
(see "General Suppliers")

American Environmental Health Foundation
(see "General Suppliers")

They provide mold identification plates and reports.

National Ecological and Environmental Delivery System (NEEDS)
527 Charles Avenue, Suite 12A
Syracuse, NY 13209
(800) 634-1380

This distributor of nontoxic products offers the Odor Trap bag.

Northeast Center for Environmental Medicine
Sherry Rogers
P.O. Box 2716
2800 West Genesee Street
Syracuse, NY 13220
(315) 488-2856

They provide mold identification plates and reports.

Practical Allergy Research Foundation (PARF)
(see ''General Suppliers'')

They provide mold adsorbers.

Carbon monoxide detectors:

American Environmental Health Foundation
(see ''General Suppliers'')

They will make on-site inspections using a portable Gas Chromatograph Mass Spect Apparatus for the immediate detection of innumerable gases and chemicals in air and water (the cost is $500 or more).

RCI Environmental, Inc.
17772 Preston Road, Suite 202
Dallas, TX 75252
(214) 250-6608
fax (214) 250-6706

For inexpensive single dosimeter tubes to detect gases and chemicals and a water soluble pesticide test kit.

Dehumidification units:

(also available from a number of ''General Suppliers'')

Crispaire Corporation
3285 Saturn Court
Norcross, GA 30092
(770) 734-9696
fax (770) 453-9323

They carry MarVent units.

Semco
907 Forest Pond Drive
Marietta, GA 30068
(404) 643-1664

They carry a central dehumidification unit.

General Household cleaning products (including Purisol and Neolife Rugged Red):

Allerx
(see "General Suppliers")

AFM Enterprises
(see "General Suppliers")

They carry Safechoice carpet-cleaning products.

American Environmental Health Foundation
(see "General Suppliers")

International Health Foundation
1099 Southwest Columbia, Suite 300
Portland, OR 97201
(503) 221-1779

Living Source
(see "General Suppliers")

PARF
(see "General Suppliers")

Ozone treatments, including the Tri-O System:

Global Pollution Control
323 Industrial
McKinney, TX 75069
(214) 542-5333

National Ecological and Environmental
Delivery System (NEEDS)
527 Charles Avenue, Suite 12A
Syracuse, NY 13209
(800) 634-1380

They rent ozone machines.

Yezbak Enterprises
108 North Beeson
Uniontown, PA 15401

They rent ozone machines.

Safe moisture barrier:

AFM Enterprises
(see "General Suppliers")

Allerx
(see "General Suppliers")

American Environmental Health Foundation
(see "General Suppliers")

Living Source
(see "General Suppliers")

Environmental Medicine and Engineering
(see "HVAC consultants")

Texas Power Vac
(see "HVAC consultants")

ART SUPPLIES

For safer, nonodorous art supplies, including water-based markers:

Arts, Crafts and Theater Safety
181 Thompson Street, no. 23
New York, NY 10012-2586
(212) 777-0072

Center for Safety in the Arts
care of New York Foundation for the Arts
155 Avenue of the Americas, 14th floor
New York, NY 10013
(212) 366-6900, x333 (voice mail only)

They distribute arts and crafts literature on environmental and industrial hygiene; for publications list, enclose a SASE.

ASBESTOS

Asbestos and Small Business Ombudsman
Environmental Protection Agency
(800) 368-5888

They provide information about asbestos for the general public and small businesses.

COTTON AND COTTON PRODUCTS
(Request nonpesticided cotton only)

Allergy Relief Shop, Inc.
3371 Whittle Springs Road
Knoxville, TN 37917
(800) 626-2810

The Cotton Place
P.O. Box 59721
Dallas, TX 75229
(214) 243-4149

Heart of Vermont
Old Schoolhouse
Route 132, P.O. Box 183
Sharon, VT 05065
(800) 639-4123

They offer cotton futons.

KB Cotton Pillows, Inc.
P.O. Box 57
DeSoto, TX 75123
(214) 223-7193
(800) 544-3752

The Natural Bedroom
P.O. Box 2048
Sebastopol, CA 95473-2048
(800) 365-6563

Organic Cotton
9760 Owensmouth Avenue
Chatsworth, CA 91311
(818) 886-7471

Otis Bedding
367 Hamburg Street
Buffalo, NY
(716) 852-2076

The Vermont Country Store
P.O. Box 3000
Manchester Center, VT 05255-3000
(802) 824-6932

CARPETING

Diagnostic laboratories:

Anderson Laboratories
773 Main Street
West Hartford, VT 05084-0323
(802) 295-7344

They provide well-designed, extensive, and impartial evaluations of the effects on mice after exposure to air blown over carpets and carpet materials, as well as other common items.

Reed and Associates
2017 Dixie Highway, no. 117
Edgewood, KY 41017
(606) 344-8686

Determine chemicals in carpets.

For formaldehyde test and analysis kits:

Allerx
(see "General Suppliers")

Northeast Center for Environmental Medicine
(see "Mold Tests")

Carpets examined by Anderson Laboratories:

Nature's Carpet
distributed by Colin Campbell & Sons
1428 West Seventh Avenue
Vancouver, British Columbia
B6H 1C1 Canada
(604) 734-2758
fax (604) 734-1512

This carpet was one of the very best that Anderson examined.

Foreign Accents
2825 East Broadbent Parkway, N.E.
Albuquerque, NM 87107
(505) 344-4833

For safer carpet cleaners:
See "General Suppliers" for the following:

AFM Enterprises

Allerx

American Environmental Health Foundation

Environmental Medicine and Engineering

NEEDS

CONSTRUCTION MATERIALS

General:

Green Eclipse
Bruce Small
R.R., #1
Goodwood, Ontario
LOC 1AA Canada
(905) 649-1356

The Healthy House Institute
430 North Sewell Road
Bloomington, IN 47408
(812) 332-5073

Author John Bower will provide consultation by phone or on site about existing or new house designs and safer construction.

For safer sealers:

American Environmental Health Foundation
(see "General Suppliers")

They carry sealers for use on wood, concrete, grout, and carpet.

Environmental Medicine and Engineering (see "General Suppliers")

Fletco Corporation
1000 45th Street
Oakland, CA 94608
(510) 655-2470
(800) 635-3286

They carry Vara Phane-Elite Diamond Finish.

Safer, low-odor wall paint brands:

Benjamin Moore Prestige or Low Odor Paint
Glidden Spred 2000 Low VOC Paint

ELECTROMAGNETIC ENERGY

For general information:

Electrical Sensitivity Network Midwest
P.O. Box 645
Elkhorn, WI 53121

Electro Ecology Services
7122 Poverty Hill Road
Ellicottville, NY 14731
(716) 699-4128

Institute for Bau-biologie and Ecology
P.O. Box 387
Clearwater, FL 84615
(813) 461-4371

Cyril Smith, Ph.D.
Department of Electronic/Electrical Engineering
University of Salford
Salford M54WT
England

For gaussmeters:
See "General Suppliers" for the following:

AFM Enterprises

Allerx

American Environmental Health Foundation

Environmental Medicine and Engineering

NEEDS

For computer-screen shields:

Less Gauss
187 East Market Street, Suite 160
Rhinebeck, NY 12572
(914) 876-5432

They carry the Clarifier, a protective computer screen.

NoRad Corporation
1549 Eleventh Street
Santa Monica, CA 90401
(800) 262-3260

For box enclosures for electric equipment:

Safe Reading and Computer Box Company
1158 North Huron
Linwood, MI 48634
(517) 697-3989

For low-radiation monitors:

Body America
6847 Urubu Street
Carlsbad, CA 92009
(407) 781-0519

They carry the Ultra 7000 monitor, made by Safe Technologies.

Also see "General Suppliers" for the following:

AFM Enterprises

Allerx

American Environmental Health Foundation

NEEDS

LEAD

For lead testing kits:

Allerx
(see "General Suppliers")

They offer the Lead Only water test.

Frandon Enterprises
P.O. Box 300321
Seattle, WA 98103
(800) 359-9000

They offer the Frandon Lead Alert Kit.

Also see "General Suppliers" for the following:

AFM Enterprises

American Environmental Health Foundation

NEEDS

Laboratories that test water supplies for lead:

Clean Water Lead Testing
UNCA, One University Heights
Asheville, NC 28804-3299
(704) 251-6895
fax (704) 251-6913

They provide lead testing of water, dust, soil, and paint samples while conducting research on the effectiveness of various lead-based paint abatement methods.

National Testing Laboratory
6555 Wilson Mills Road
Cleveland, OH 44143
(800) 458-3330

They test water for bacteria, lead, and pesticides.

Suburban Water Testing Laboratories, Inc.
4600 Kutztown Road
Temple, PA 19560
(800) 433-6595
fax (610) 929-8321

They provide home water testing, including testing for bacteria, lead, and pesticides.

For referrals to state-certified laboratories in your area:

Environmental Protection Agency
Safe Drinking Water Hotline
(800) 426-4791

For more information:

National Lead Information Center
1019 Nineteenth Street, N.W., Suite 401
Washington, DC 20036
(800) 424-5323

This organization aims to educate the public about the cause of lead intoxication and the means to prevent it.

LIGHTING

For sources of full-spectrum light:

Cutting Edge Catalogue
Befit Enterprises
P.O. Box 5034
Southampton, NY 11969
(516) 287-3813 or (800) 497-9516

Duro-Test Corporation
9 Law Drive
Fairfield, NJ 07007
(800) 289-3876

Electro Ecology Services
7122 Poverty Hill Road
Ellicottville, NY 14731
(716) 699-4128

Network Marketing
25 West Fairview Avenue
Dover, NJ 07801
(800) 777-INFO

Ott BioLight Systems
28 Parker Way
Santa Barbara,CA 93101
(800) 234-3724

These lighting retrofit specialists offer books and a video, Light, Radiation, and You, *as well as fluorescent lighting materials that may decrease hyperactivity in some children.*

Simmons Company
P.O. Box 3193
Chattanooga, TN 37404
(800) 622-1308

PESTICIDES AND PEST CONTROL

For information on pesticides:

Bio-Integral Resource Center
P.O. Box 7414
Berkeley, CA 94707
(510) 433-2814
fax (510) 524-1758

They do research and education on specific pest problems.

National Pesticide Telecommunications Network
Ag Chem Extension
Oregon State University
333 Weniger
Corvallis, OR 97331-6502
(800) 858-7378

They provide information about specific chemicals and their toxic effects.

Pesticide Education Center
P.O. Box 420870
San Francisco, CA 94142-0870
(800) 732-3733
fax (415) 391-9159

They provide books and other information about pesticides.

To join a school IPM network:

National Coalition Against the Misuse of Pesticides
701 E Street, S.E., Suite 200
Washington, DC 20003
(202) 543-5450

For natural pest-control solutions:

Concept
213 S.W. Columbia Street
Bend, OR 97702
(800) 367-8727

Nontoxic, nonchemical pest-control products for consumer and agricultural purposes.

Earthtek Corporation
177 West Cass Street
P.O. Box 166
Greenville, MI 48838
(800) 695-9956
(616) 754-9290

The Bug Banisher is a negative-ion generator that helps to reduce ants, roaches, ticks, scorpions, moths, flies, aphids, and other pests from specific areas in 3 to 10 days. It uses no chemicals and no ultrasonic or electrical frequencies. Earthtek offers a free video on the Bug Banisher and will refer you to the dealer nearest you.

Praxis
2723 116th Street
Allegan, MI 49010-9023
Tel./fax (616) 873-2795

This advisory group on integrated pest management provides schools, municipalities, and businesses with Biotool Kits, which helps to control pests, gypsy moths, and odors from drains and septic tanks. They use no pesticides in any form.

Also see "General Suppliers" for the following:

AFM Enterprises

Allerx

American Environmental Health Foundation

NEEDS

For formal pest-management programs:

Environmental Health Coalition
1717 Kettner Boulevard
San Diego, CA 92101
(619) 235-0281

They offer the 40-page School Pesticide Use Reduction (SPUR) guide, plus an 11-minute video.

Get Set
2530 Hayes Street
Marne, MI 49435-9752
(800) 221-6188, or (616) 677-1261

Human Ecology Action League
(see "Advocacy and Other Organizations")

They provide detailed information on low-emission and pest-resistant materials.

Montgomery County Schools
16651 Crabbs Branch Way
Shady Grove Depot
Rockville, MD 20855
(301) 840-8122

New York Coalition for Alternatives to Pesticides
P.O. Box 6005
Albany, NY 12206-0005
(518) 426-8246

They offer informative, inexpensive booklets on safer pest management.

Residents for Alternative Pest Policy
1408 East Rosemonte Drive
Phoenix, AZ 85024
(602) 582-0266

They offer the Hug-a-Bug curriculum.

PLANTS

For plants that help remove specific pollutants:

Behnke's Nursery
Beltsville, MD 20705
(301) 937-4035

RADON

For radon testing kits:

National Safety Council Radon Test Kit Offer
P.O. Box 33435
Washington, DC 20033-0435
(800) SOS-RADON
(also see "General Suppliers")

SAUNAS

Distributors of home saunas:

American Environmental Health Foundation
(see "General Suppliers")

Heavenly Heat Saunas
1106 Second Street, Suite 162
Encinitas, CA 92024-5008
(800) 533-0623

Safe Reading and Computer Box Company
158 North Huron
Linwood, MI 48634
(517) 697-3989

SWIMMING POOL PRODUCTS

American Biologics
1180 Walnut Avenue
Chula Vista, CA 91911
(800) 227-4473

They offer Dioxychlor.

Bio-Prep Laboratories
P.O. Box 12770
Palm Desert, CA 92255-2770
(619) 345-9293
fax (619) 345-8766

They provide Pool Magic and Cooling Tower Magic.

Dolphin Pools
3544 Forest Lane
Dallas, TX 75234
(214) 357-0446

Environmental World
1555 West Seminole
San Marcos, CA 92069
(800) 288-0230

They carry the Boss Oxygen Purification System.

Oxygen Technologies Corporation
8229 Melrose Drive
Lenexa, KS 66214
(913) 894-2828
fax (913) 894-5455

*They sell ozonation equipment to kill bacteria, remove odors, control molds, and decrease con-
tamination in cooling towers, fountains, aquariums, etc. They can decrease chlorine odor
and the need for chlorine in pools.*

Water Savers World Wide
9450 Skillman, Suite 103
Dallas, TX 75243
(214) 503-1113
(800) 886-9283
fax (214) 503-8160

They offer copper and silver alloys.

Zeneca
P.O. Box 15438
Wilmington, DE 19897
(800) 456-3669

This chemical company carries Baquacil.

VACUUM SYSTEMS

The top six systems as rated by *Consumer Reports* (Jan. 1995) are:

Eureka Bravo! The Boss (#334DT)
Eureka Powerline Plus (#9741AT)
Hoover Power Drive Supreme (#U6323-930)
Kirby (#G4)
Sears Kenmore Whispertone (#35612)
Sharp Twin Energy (#EC-12TXT)

American Environmental Health Foundation
(see ''General Suppliers'')

Environmental Medicine and Engineering
(see ''General Suppliers'')

Texas Power Vac
(see ''HVAC consultants'')
(also see ''General Suppliers'')

Vacuum cleaners:

AFM Enterprises
(see ''General Suppliers'')

They carry the Nilfisk GS90.

WATER

Water test kits:

(see ''General Suppliers'')

Water purifiers without plastic:

American Environmental Health Foundation
(see ''General Suppliers'')

Practical Allergy Research Foundation
(see ''General Suppliers'')

All Federal Agencies

Information Center for All Federal Agencies:
(800) 688-9889

Americans with Disabilities Act (ADA)

The medical disability called MCS is considered an illness in some individuals because the ADA, the Social Security Administration, and HUD have recognized it as such. For extensive practical information contact EARN (see ''Legal Advice'') or the National Center for Environmental Health Strategies (see ''Advocacy and Other Organizations'').

DEPARTMENT OF JUSTICE (DOJ)

ADA requires the DOJ to provide technical assistance to affected entities and individuals. The department encourages voluntary compliance by providing education and technical assistance to business, industry, government, and the general public through a variety of means.

Telephone Information Line

The DOJ provides toll-free 800 service for callers in English and Spanish who wish to receive ADA information or discuss an ADA-related problem.

Nationwide:
(800) 514-0301 (voice)
(800) 514-0383 (TDD)

Washington, DC, area:
(202) 514-0301 (voice)
(202) 514-0383 (TDD)

Grants

ADA technical assistance grants are awarded primarily to target specialized information to specific audiences. To date, $6.5 million in grant funds have been awarded for such projects to thirty organizations.

Publications

The DOJ regulations for ADA Titles II and III, the ADA's Questions and Answers booklet, the ADA Handbook, and information about the DOJ's technical assistance grant program can be obtained by writing:

Public Access Section
Civil Rights Division
Department of Justice
P.O. Box 66738
Washington, DC
(202) 514-6193

They are available in several formats: standard print, large print, Braille, audiotape, and computer disk.

The DOJ's Technical Assistance Manuals for ADA Titles II and III can be obtained by subscription from the Government Printing Office in Washington. Order forms can be obtained through the ADA information line. Contact:

Department of Justice
Honorable Janet Reno
Attorney General of the USA
10th and Constitution Ave. N.W.
Room 4400
Washington, DC 20520
fax (202F) 514-4371

Copies of legal documents and settlement agreements can be obtained from:

Freedom of Information/Privacy Act Branch
Civil Rights Division, Room 7337
Department of Justice
Washington, DC 20530

Funded by the DOJ:

Disability Rights Education and Defense Fund (DREDF)
2212 Sixth Street
Berkeley, CA
Hotline on ADA Titles II and III:
(510) 544-2555
(800) 466-4232

OTHER GOVERNMENT AGENCIES RELEVANT TO ADA

Department of Education

The National Institute on Disability and Rehabilitation Research (NIDRR) of the Department of Education has funded Disability and Business Technical Assistance Centers (DBTACs) in ten regions in the United States, to provide technical assistance to the general public on ADA Titles I, II, and III.

For ADA technical assistance:
(800) 949-4232 (voice and TDD)

Department of Health and Human Services (DHHS)

The DHHS has basic regulations pertaining to schools and teachers. If changes within a school, a move to a different classroom, or a transfer to another school does not resolve an affected teacher's health problems, a disability exists.

200 Independence Avenue, S.W.
Washington, D.C.
(202) 619-0257

Civil Rights Hot Line: (202) 863-0100

Department of Housing and Urban Development (HUD)

HUD recognizes chemical sensitivities as a disability requiring reasonable protection by landlords on a case-by-case basis. (See the MCS memo dated Mar. 5, 1992, available from the assistant general counsel for fair housing enforcement.) If the federal government helps pay for a school, apartment, or housing project, those who occupy it cannot willfully pollute the premises if doing so causes another tenant to become seriously ill.

Department of Housing and Urban Development
Washington, DC 20410-0500
(202) 708-0570

Department of Labor

The Occupational Safety and Health Administration (OSHA) has a "right to know" clause (Standards 1910.20) that discusses "claimant sustained causally related disability." In simple terms, this clause means that an employer is supposed to be responsible for direct or indirect work-related exposures that cause a current disability, regardless of a prior existing health problem.

Occupational Safety and Health Administration (OSHA)
U.S. Department of Labor
200 Constitution Avenue, N.W.
Washington, DC 20210
(202) 523-8017

Also:
4676 Columbia Parkway
Cincinnati, OH 45226
(800) 356-4674

Department of Transportation (DOT)

The Department of Transportation offers technical assistance to the general public on the public transportation provisions of ADA Titles II and III.

400 7th Street, S.W.
Washington, D.C. 20590
(202) 366-4000

For ADA documents and general questions:
(202) 366-1656 (voice)
(202) 366-2979 (TDD)

For legal questions about ADA:
(202) 366-9306 (voice)
(202) 755-7687 (TDD)

For questions about the National Easter Seal Society "Project Action" grant:
(202) 347-3066 (voice)
(202) 347-7385 (TDD)

For questions about Air Carrier Act:
(202) 376-6406 (voice)

Environmental Protection Agency (EPA)

In 1989 the EPA recognized that MCS is a genuine health concern and acknowledged that such health problems can be caused by low-level nontoxic exposures. These levels can be well below those allowed by existing regulations. The EPA issues a number of publications related to environmental compliance (see For Further Reading).

Environmental Protection Agency
401 M Street, S.W.
Washington, DC 20460
(202) 382-2090
Public Information Center: (202) 829-3535

Equal Employment Opportunity Commission (EEOC)

The EEOC protects workers who instigate legal action from retaliation by their employers. If a worker is qualified for the job, the employer cannot discriminate against him or her on the basis of disability. The EEOC handles complaints under ADA Titles I, II, and III. It offers particular assistance to the general public concerning Title I.

Office of Communication and Legislative Affairs
1801 L. Street, N.W., Rm. 9405
Washington, D.C. 20507

To order documents:
(800) 669-3362 (voice)
(800) 800-3302 (TDD)

To ask questions:
(800) 669-4000 (voice)
(800) 949-4232 (TDD)

The Baltimore office of the EEOC has recognized MCS as a disability requiring workplace accommodation. (See Mary Helinski v. Bell Atlantic, charge no. 120 93 0152 [May 1994], a determination letter signed by the director of the Baltimore EEOC office.)

Federal Communications Commission (FCC)

The Federal Communications Commission offers technical assistance to the general public concerning ADA Title IV.

1919 M Street, N.W.
Washington, D.C. 20554
(202) 418-0200

For ADA documents and general questions:
(202) 632-7260 (voice)
Use relay service for TDD.

For ADA legal questions:
(202) 634-1808 (voice)
(202) 632-6999 (TDD)

For questions on the Hearing Aid Compatibility Act:
(202) 634-7150 (voice)
Use relay service for TDD.

Internal Revenue Service (IRS)

The IRS provides tax benefits for the disabled (publication number 907) and guides for employers who provide necessary accommodations. Contact HEAL for more information.

Protection and Advocacy Systems for the Rights of Individuals with Disability

This agency provides funding to various organizations that help people make ADA-related claims. Call them to learn which agency in your state or county receives funding.

c/o Office of Special Education and Rehabilitation Services
Department of Education
Washington, D.C. 20202
(202) 205-5465

Social Security Administration (SSA)

The SSA states that evaluations of MCS should be made on a case-by-case basis to determine whether the impairment substantially prevents gainful activity.

Social Security Administration
6401 Security Boulevard
Baltimore, MD 21235
(800) 772-1213 *or your local office*

Legal Advice

These organizations can provide help and information to the environmentally ill and disabled. Their staff are often caring, knowledgeable people who are available for consultations and/ or presentations on the rights of people with environmental illness.

American Academy of Environmental Medicine
4510 West 89th Street
Prairie Village, KS 66207
(913) 642-6062

They can send you informal copies of successful court cases against insurance companies.

Environmental Access Research Network (EARN)
P.O. Box 426
Williston, ND 58802-0426
(701) 859-6363

Ellie Goldberg, M.Ed.
79 Elmore Street
Newton, MA 02159

Send a SASE to this education rights specialist for more information.

Environmental Access Research Network (EARN)

They publish the newsletter Medical and Legal Briefs: A Reference Compendium of Chemical Injury. *They do computer searches on lawsuits and provide information on expert witnesses; they can also provide copies of court decisions.*

HALT
1319 F Street N.W., Suite 300
Washington, DC 20004
(202) 347-9600

This organization for legal reform can send you the citizens' legal manual Small Claims Court.

Human Ecology Action League (HEAL)
P.O. Box 41926
Atlanta, GA 30359-1126
(404) 248-1898

They publish Multiple Chemical Sensitivities and the Americans with Disabilities Act: A Guide to Accommodation. *They can also send you copies of court decisions against insurance companies.*

National Center for Environmental Health Strategies
(see ''Advocacy and Other Organizations'')

They provide copies of pertinent documents, case reports, legal cases, information packets, insurance and legal packages, and books on chemical sensitivities.

Safe Schools
(see ''Advocacy and Other Organizations'')

LEGAL AIDS AND ATTORNEYS

These organizations can provide referrals to attorneys knowledgeable about environmental illness.

Agreements Unlimited
9042 Canterbury Riding
Laurel, MD 20723
(301) 498-1193

They provide mediators.

American Arbitration Association
205 South Salina Street
Syracuse, NY 13202
(315) 472-5483

They provide mediators.

Chemical Injury Information Network
P.O. Box 301
White Sulphur Springs, MT 59645
(406) 547-2255

They publish Toxic Times.

Human Ecology Action League (HEAL)
(see ''Advocacy and Other Organizations'')

Legal Services Corporation

They provide free legal services to, among many others, individuals with handicapping conditions.

MCS Referral and Resources
2326 Pickwick Road
Baltimore, MD 21207
(410) 448-3319
fax (410) 448-3317

They provide detailed information and advice concerning the diagnosis and rights of those who have chemical sensitivities.

National Social Security Disability Advocates
2603 Main Street, Suite 820
Irvine, CA 92714
(800) 662-4633 (English)
(800) 742-9696 (Spanish)

A network of lawyers who specialize in providing inexpensive aid related to denial of Social Security Disability benefits.

Society of Professionals in Dispute Resolution
815 Fifteenth Street, N.W., Suite 530
Washington, DC 20005
(202) 783-7277

They provide mediators.

Trial Lawyers for Public Justice
1717 Massachusetts Avenue, N.W., Suite 800
Washington, DC 20036
(202) 797-8600
fax (202) 232-7203

**These attorneys are knowledgeable about EI. Inclusion here does not
constitute endorsement:**

Robert Amidon
3900 West Alameda Avenue, Suite 1700
Burbank, CA 91505-4316
(818) 972-1800
fax (818) 920-1650

Gerald Eddins
Gerald Eddins and Associates
P.O. Box 2564
Port Arthur, TX 77643
(409) 962-7800

William Eddins
900 North Palafox Street
Pensacola, FL 32501
(904) 432-4277

Michael N. Friedman
1901 Avenue of the Stars, Suite 1901
Los Angeles, CA 90067-6020
(310) 552-3336

Lewis Golinker
225 Ridgedale Road
Ithaca, NY 14850
(607) 277-7286

Jonathan Gould, Daniel Livingston, and Mary Kelly
Gould, Livingston, Adler, Pulda
557 Prospect Avenue
Hartford, CT 06105-2922
(203) 233-9821

Barry F. Greenberg
Barry F. Greenberg Associates
Front Street and Route 202
Bridgeport, PA 19405
(610) 275-5500

James Hooper
O'Brien and Hooper
400 North Ashley Street, Room 2080
Tampa, FL 33602
(813) 223-9133

Robert W. Katz
Gordon, Feinblatt, Rothman, Hoffberger, Hollander
Garrett Building
233 East Redwood Street
Baltimore, MD 21202
(410) 576-4287

Alan S. Levin, M.D.
P.O. Box 4703
Incline Village, NV 89450
(702) 831-5604
(415) 986-2625

Few have his level of expertise as an E.I. specialist, immunologist, and lawyer.

Kent Lilly
800 South Florida Avenue
Lakeland, FL 33801
(941) 683-1111

James Olson
Lawton and Cates, S.C.
P.O. Box 2965
Madison, WI 53701-2965
(608) 256-9031

Tom L. Pettiette
33229 D'Amico, Suite 200
Houston, TX 77019
(713) 650-1776

Jeffrey A. Rabin
Cook, Lake and DuPage Counties
223 West Jackson Boulevard, Suite 1110
Chicago, IL 60606

Peter K. Skivington
Jones and Skivington
31 Main Street
P.O. Box 129
Geneseo, NY 14454
(716) 243-0313

Ann Snieg
4750 North Milwaukee Avenue, Suite 18
Chicago, IL 60630
(312) 283-3388

Jeffery F. Speer
725 South Washington Street
P.O. Drawer 4303
Lafayette, LA 70502
(318) 232-0405
fax (318) 237-3415

He is most knowledgeable about carpets.

Eli I. Taub
705 Union Street
Schenectady, NY 12305
(518) 370-5515

Influencing Federal Legislation

To write your senators:

U.S. Senate
Washington, DC 20510
(202) 224-3121

To write your congressperson:

U.S. House of Representatives
Washington, DC 20515
(202) 225-3121

To obtain a copy of a particular bill:

Senate Document Room
Hart Senate Office Building, Room B-04
Washington, DC 20510
(202) 224-7701

House Document Room
Ford Building, Room B-18
Washington, DC 20515
(202) 225-3456

For information on the status of a particular bill:

Legislative Information and Status
(202) 225-1772

INDEX